MANUAL OF HIGH-RISK PREGNANCY

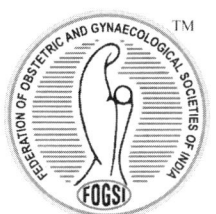

Federation of Obstetric and Gynaecological Societies of India (FOGSI)

MANUAL OF HIGH-RISK PREGNANCY

Editors

Richa Baharani
MD FICOG Dip Endoscopy
Senior Consultant
Department of Obstetrics and Gynecology
Jabalpur Hospital and Research Center
Jabalpur, Madhya Pradesh, India

Pushpa Pandey
MD
Senior Consultant
Department of Obstetrics and Gynecology
Bombay Hospital and Research Center
Jabalpur, Madhya Pradesh, India

Shashi Khare
MS FICOG
Former Dean, Professor and Head
Department of Obstetrics and Gynecology
Netaji Subhash Chandra Bose Medical College
Jabalpur, Madhya Pradesh, India

Sushma Dikhit
MS MRCOG
Senior Consultant and Head
Department of Obstetrics and Gynecology
Max Superspecialty Hospital
Ghaziabad, Uttar Pradesh, India

———— **A FOGSI Publication** ————

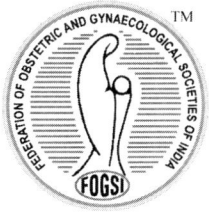

JAYPEE *The Health Sciences Publisher*

New Delhi | London | Panama

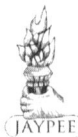

Jaypee Brothers Medical Publishers (P) Ltd.

Headquarters
Jaypee Brothers Medical Publishers (P) Ltd
4838/24, Ansari Road, Daryaganj
New Delhi 110 002, India
Phone: +91-11-43574357
Fax: +91-11-43574314
E-mail: jaypee@jaypeebrothers.com

Overseas Offices

J.P. Medical Ltd
83, Victoria Street, London
SW1H 0HW (UK)
Phone: +44 20 3170 8910
Fax: +44 (0)20 3008 6180
E-mail: info@jpmedpub.com

Jaypee-Highlights Medical Publishers Inc
City of Knowledge, Bld. 235, 2nd Floor, Clayton
Panama City, Panama
Phone: +1 507-301-0496
Fax: +1 507-301-0499
E-mail: cservice@jphmedical.com

Jaypee Brothers Medical Publishers (P) Ltd
17/1-B, Babar Road, Block-B, Shaymali
Mohammadpur, Dhaka-1207
Bangladesh
Mobile: +08801912003485
E-mail: jaypeedhaka@gmail.com

Jaypee Brothers Medical Publishers (P) Ltd
Bhotahity, Kathmandu
Nepal
Phone: +977-9741283608
E-mail: kathmandu@jaypeebrothers.com

Website: www.jaypeebrothers.com
Website: www.jaypeedigital.com

© 2018, Jaypee Brothers Medical Publishers

The views and opinions expressed in this book are solely those of the original contributor(s)/author(s) and do not necessarily represent those of editor(s) of the book.

All rights reserved. No part of this publication may be reproduced, stored or transmitted in any form or by any means, electronic, mechanical, photocopying, recording or otherwise, without the prior permission in writing of the publishers.

All brand names and product names used in this book are trade names, service marks, trademarks or registered trademarks of their respective owners. The publisher is not associated with any product or vendor mentioned in this book.

Medical knowledge and practice change constantly. This book is designed to provide accurate, authoritative information about the subject matter in question. However, readers are advised to check the most current information available on procedures included and check information from the manufacturer of each product to be administered, to verify the recommended dose, formula, method and duration of administration, adverse effects and contraindications. It is the responsibility of the practitioner to take all appropriate safety precautions. Neither the publisher nor the author(s)/editor(s) assume any liability for any injury and/or damage to persons or property arising from or related to use of material in this book.

This book is sold on the understanding that the publisher is not engaged in providing professional medical services. If such advice or services are required, the services of a competent medical professional should be sought.

Every effort has been made where necessary to contact holders of copyright to obtain permission to reproduce copyright material. If any have been inadvertently overlooked, the publisher will be pleased to make the necessary arrangements at the first opportunity. The **CD/DVD-ROM** (if any) provided in the sealed envelope with this book is complimentary and free of cost. **Not meant for sale.**

Inquiries for bulk sales may be solicited at: jaypee@jaypeebrothers.com

Manual of High-Risk Pregnancy

First Edition: **2018**

ISBN: 978-93-5270-392-0

Printed at Sanat Printers

Dedicated to
All expectant women and all members of
The Federation of Obstetric and Gynaecological Societies of India (FOGSI)

CONTRIBUTORS

Aashita Shrivastava MS
Senior Resident
Department of Obstetrics and Gynecology
Nalanda Medical College and Hospital
Patna, Bihar, India

Ajay Sinha
Assistant Professor
Department of Medicine
Nalanda Medical College and Hospital
Patna, Bihar, India

Alka Kriplani MD FRCOG FAMS FICOG FICMCH
Professor and Head
Department of Obstetrics and Gynecology
All India Institute of Medical Sciences
New Delhi, India
President, FOGSI 2016

Alka Pandey MD PhD
Professor
Department of Obstetrics and Gynecology
Nalanda Medical College and Hospital
Patna, Bihar, India
Chairperson, FOGSI

Amit Bharadiya MBBS MD (General Medicine)
DNB (Cardiology)
Resident
Department of Cardiology
Apollo Hospital
Hyderabad, Telangana, India

Anamika Dwivedi MS
Assistant Professor
Department of Obstetrics and Gynecology
Government Medical College
Rewa, Madhya Pradesh, India

Anand Baharani MD (Gen Med)
Consultant Physician
Baharani Medicine and Gynae Center
Jabalpur, Madhya Pradesh, India

Anita Singh MBBS MS DGO DNB FICOG
Diploma Endoscopy
Former Professor
Department of Obstetrics and Gynecology
Patna Medical College
Patna, Bihar, India
Chairperson
Endocrinology Committee, FOGSI

Anupama B Solanki MS (Obs & Gyn)
Assistant Professor
Department of Obstetrics and Gynecology
Sukh Sagar Medical College and Hospital
Jabalpur, Madhya Pradesh, India

Anu Pathak MS
Associate Professor
Department of Obstetrics and Gynecology
SN Medical College
Agra, Uttar Pradesh, India

Anuradha Dang MS
Consultant
Department of Obstetrics and Gynecology
Suvidha Hospital
Jabalpur, Madhya Pradesh, India

Archana Verma MD FICOG
Chairperson
Public Awareness Committee
FOGSI (2016–2018)
Ghaziabad, Uttar Pradesh, India

Asha Baxi MS FRCOG
Director and Head
Department of Infertility and
Gynecological Endoscopy
Disha Fertility and Surgical Centre
Indore, Madhya Pradesh, India
Chairperson, Infertility Committee FOGSI

Ashutosh Gupta DM (Genetics)
Consultant
Department of Obstetrics and Gynecology
Max Hospital
New Delhi, India

Beenu Kushwah MD DNB FICOG
Associate Professor
Department of Obstetrics and Gynecology
Shyam Shah Medical College
Rewa, Madhya Pradesh, India

Bharati Dhorepatil DNB DGO FICS FICOG
Dip (Endo, Germany) PGDCR
Head
Department of Obstetrics and Gynecology
Cloudnine Hospital
Pune, Maharashtra, India
Vice President, FOGSI 2016

Bharti Sahu MS
Associate Professor
Department of Obstetrics and Gynecology
Netaji Subhash Chandra Bose
Medical College
Jabalpur, Madhya Pradesh, India

Deepak Dwivedi MD (Pediatrics)
PGD (Development Neurology)
Assistant Professor
Shyam Shah Medical College
Rewa, Madhya Pradesh, India

Deepti Gupta MS
Consultant
Ankur Fertility Clinic and IVF Centre
Jabalpur, Madhya Pradesh, India

Deepti Shrivastava MBBS MD PhD
Professor and Head
Department of Obstetrics and Gynecology
Jawaharlal Nehru Medical College (JNMC)
Wardha, Maharashtra, India
Past President, DSOGS

Devanshi Mishra Vyas MD DNB
Senior Resident
Department of Obstetrics and Gynecology
Sawai Man Singh Medical College
Jaipur, Rajasthan, India

Geetha Balsarkar MS
Consultant
Department of Obstetrics and Gynecology
Nowrosjee Wadia Maternity Hospital
Seth GS Medical College
Mumbai, Maharashtra, India

Girija Wagh MD FICOG Dip Endoscopy
Professor and Head
Department of Obstetrics and Gynecology
Bharati Vidyapeeth Medical College
Pune, Maharashtra, India
Chairman
Medical Disorders Committee
FOGSI (2013-16)

Gita Guin MS LLB FICOG
Associate Professor and Incharge
Obstetric Critical Care Unit
Department of Obstetrics and Gynecology
Netaji Subhash Chandra Bose
Medical College
Jabalpur, Madhya Pradesh, India

Gorakh G Mandrupkar MBBS DGO FCPS
FICOG FICMCH MCSEP(I)
Consultant (Reproductive Medicine)
Prakash Memorial Clinic and
Research Center
Islampur, Maharashtra, India
Chairman, Medical Disorders in
Pregnancy Committee
FOGSI 2016–2019

Hema J Shobhane MD (Obs & Gyn)
Associate Professor
Department of Obstetrics and Gynecology
Maharani Laxmibai Medical College
Jhansi, Uttar Pradesh, India

Hitesh J Bhatt MD PGDMLS
Chairperson
Ethics and Medicolegal Committee, FOGSI
Mumbai, Maharashtra, India

Jagruti Murkey
Department of Obstetrics and Gynecology
Nowrosjee Wadia Maternity Hospital
Seth GS Medical College
Mumbai, Maharashtra, India

Jaideep Malhotra MD FICMCH FICOG
FIAJAGO FICMU FICS
Director
Rainbow IVF
Agra, Uttar Pradesh, India
President, FOGSI 2018

Jignesh Shah MD FICMCH Dip USG
Senior Consultant
Dr Shah Institute for Women's Health
Ahmedabad, Gujarat, India

Jigyasa Dengra MD (Obs & Gyn)
Consultant Gynecologist
Mahi IVF Centre
Jabalpur, Madhya Pradesh, India

Jyoti Bindal MS FACS FICS FICOG LLB PGDHM
Professor and Head
Department of Obstetrics and Gynecology
Government Medical College
Gwalior, Madhya Pradesh, India

Jyotsna Gupta MS Fellowship
(Feto-maternal Medicine)
Assistant Professor
Department of Obstetrics and Gynecology
Punjab Institute of Medical Sciences
Clinical Director
Promise Ultrasound and
Fetal Medicine Centre
Jalandhar, Punjab, India

Kanchan Gulbani MD
Senior Resident
Matru Sewa Sangh
Nagpur, Maharashtra, India

K Aparna Sharma MS
Associate Professor
Department of Obstetrics and Gynecology
All India Institute of Medical Sciences
New Delhi, India

Kavita Bapat MS FICOG
Director
Bapat Hospital
Indore, Madhya Pradesh, India
Chairperson, Breast Committee, FOGSI

Kavita N Singh MS PhD (Gyn Oncology) FICOG
FICMCH
Associate Professor and Head
Department of Obstetrics and Gynecology
Netaji Subhash Chandra Bose
Government Medical College
Jabalpur, Madhya Pradesh, India

Kirtan M Vyas MS (Obs & Gyn)
Assistant Professor
Department of Obstetrics and Gynecology
Pandit Deendayal Upadhyay Government
Medical College
Rajkot, Gujarat, India

Madhuri Alwani MS FICOG
Associate Professor
Department of Obstetrics and Gynecology
Sir Aurobindo Medical College
Indore, Madhya Pradesh, India

Madhuri Chandra MD DNB FICOG CMCL
FAIMER (Fellow)
Professor and Head
Department of Obstetrics and Gynecology
Mahaveer Institute of Medical Sciences
and Research
Bhopal, Madhya Pradesh, India
Chairperson
HIV-AIDS Committee, FOGSI 2014–2016
President, AMPOGS RPWS 2015-2017

Madhuri Gawande MS
Consultant
Department of Obstetrics and Gynecology
NKP Salve Institute of Medical Sciences
and Lata Mangeshkar Hospital
Nagpur, Maharashtra, India

Mahesh Gupta MD (Gyn)
Past President
Ahmedabad Obstetrics and
Gynecological Society, Ahmedabad
Director
Pushpam and Indus II Hospital
Ahmedabad, Gujarat, India

Mamta Sai MBBS
Resident Medical Officer
Pt Jawahar Lal Nehru Memorial
Medical College
Raipur, Chhattisgarh, India

Meenu Agarwal DGO DNB
Director
Morpheus Bliss Fertility Centre
Pune, Maharashtra, India
Vice-President, POGS (2012–2014)

Nafisa Husain DGO
Consultant
Department of Obstetrics and Gynecology
Global Hospital
Jabalpur, Madhya Pradesh, India

Nalini Mishra MD DGO DNB FICOG MNAMS
Professor and Head
Department of Obstetrics and Gynecology
Government Medical College
Ambikapur, Chhattisgarh, India

Contributors | ix

Neha Khatik MD
Assistant Professor
Department of Obstetrics and Gynecology
Shyam Shah Medical College
Rewa, Madhya Pradesh, India

Nidhi Jain MBBS DGO
Consultant Gynecologist
Department of Obstetrics and Gynecology
Bombay Hospital and Research Center
Jabalpur, Madhya Pradesh, India

Niraj Jadav MBBS DGO
Past President
(Rajkot Obstetrics and
Gynecological Society)
West Zone Coordinator Adolescent Health
Committee, FOGSI

Nisha Sahu DGO
Senior Consultant
Lady Elgin Hospital
Jabalpur, Madhya Pradesh, India

Padma Shukla MS
Assistant Professor
Department of Obstetrics and Gynecology
Government Medical College
Rewa, Madhya Pradesh, India

Phagun Shah MD (Obs and Gyn)
Senior Consultant
Zeal Maternity and Nursing Home
Ahmedabad, Gujarat, India

Poorva Badkur MS
Senior Resident
Department of Obstetrics and Gynecology
Netaji Subhash Chandra Bose
Medical College
Jabalpur, Madhya Pradesh, India

Prachi Dixit MS
Assistant Professor
Department of Obstetrics and Gynecology
NKP Salve Institute of Medical Sciences
and Lata Mangeshkar Hospital
Nagpur, Maharashtra, India

Pragya Dhirawani DGO FICOG
Senior Consultant (Obstetrics and
Gynecology)
Director
Jabalpur Hospital and Research Centre
Jabalpur, Madhya Pradesh, India

Priti Kumar MD (Obs and Gyn)
Associate Professor
Department of Obstetrics and Gynecology
King George's Medical University
Lucknow, Uttar Pradesh, India

Priyanka Kukrele MD (Medicine)
Assistant Professor
Government Medical College
Jabalpur, Madhya Pradesh, India

Pushpa Pandey MD
Senior Consultant
Department of Obstetrics and Gynecology
Bombay Hospital and Research Center
Jabalpur, Madhya Pradesh, India

Rana Khan Chowdhry DNB (Obs & Gyn)
DGO FCPS DFP MNAMS
Consultant
Ankoor Fertility Clinic
Mumbai, Maharashtra, India

Ranjana Gupta MS (Obs & Gyn)
Joint Director Rewa, an
develop division Health
Jabalpur, Madhya Pradesh, India

Richa Baharani MD FICOG Dip Endoscopy
Senior Consultant
Department of Obstetrics and Gynecology
Jabalpur Hospital and Research Centre
Jabalpur, Madhya Pradesh, India

Richa Dhirawani MD
Consultant (Obstetrics and Gynecology)
Director
Jabalpur Hospital and Research Centre
Jabalpur, Madhya Pradesh, India

Ritu Choubey MBBS DDV
Consultant
Department of Dermatology
Deshmukh Hospital
Pune, Maharashtra, India

Rooplekha Chauhan MS FICMCH
Former Dean, Professor and Head
Department of Obstetrics and Gynecology
Netaji Subhash Chandra Bose
Medical College
Jabalpur, Madhya Pradesh, India

Roza Olyai MBBS MS MICOG FICOG FICMCH
Director
Olyai Hospital
Gwalior, Madhya Pradesh, India

Rubina Vohra MD DM (Nephro)
Consultant Nephrologist and
Transplant Physician
Sir Aurobindo Medical College
Indore, Madhya Pradesh, India

Rujuta Fuke MD DNB
Associate Professor
Department of Obstetrics and Gynecology
Government Medical College and Hospital
Nagpur, Maharashtra, India

Sadhana Gupta MS (Obs & Gyn) MNAMS
FICOG FICMU FICMCH
Senior Consultant
(Obstetrics and Gynecology)
Jeevan Jyoti Hospital and
Medical Research Centre
Gorakhpur, Uttar Pradesh, India
Vice President, FOGSI 2016

Sangeeta Shrivastava MD FICOG
Senior Consultant
Department of Obstetrics and Gynecology
Jabalpur Hospital and Research Centre
Jabalpur, Madhya Pradesh, India

Sarita Agrawal MD FICOG
Professor and Head
Department of Obstetrics and Gynecology
All India Institute of Medical Sciences
Raipur, Chhattisgarh, India
Vice President FOGSI 2015

Saroj Singh MS MAMS FICOG FICMCH FIAJAGO
Professor and Head
Department of Obstetrics and Gynecology
SN Medical College
Agra, Uttar Pradesh, India

Shabbir H Husain MS MCh
Assistant Professor
Government Medical College
Jabalpur, Madhya Pradesh, India

Shalini Agrawal DGO DNB
Consultant
Department of Obstetrics and Gynecology
Max Superspecialty Hospital
Ghaziabad, Uttar Pradesh, India

Shally Gupta DGO DNB
Consultant
Rainbow IVF
Agra, Uttar Pradesh, India

Shashi Khare MS FICOG
Former Dean, Professor and Head
Department of Obstetrics and Gynecology
Netaji Subhash Chandra Bose
Medical College
Jabalpur, Madhya Pradesh, India

Sheetal K Gujral MS
Gynecologist
Port Trust Hospital
Mumbai, Maharashtra, India

Shirish Vaidya DMRD DNB
Assistant Professor
Department of Radiodiagnosis
Jawaharlal Nehru Medical College (JNMC)
Wardha, Maharashtra, India

Shivani Dwivedi MDS
Associate Professor
Department of Periodontics
People's Dental Medical College
Bhopal, Madhya Pradesh, India

Shreya Goenka MS DNB FMAS
Senior Resident
Department of Obstetrics and Gynecology
All India Institute of Medical Sciences
Raipur, Chhattisgarh, India

Shruti Agrawal MS
Associate Professor
Department of Obstetrics and Gynecology
Sukh Sagar Medical College and Hospital
Jabalpur, Madhya Pradesh, India

Shubhada Neel MD DGO DNB
Consultant
Neel Clinic
Mumbai, Maharashtra, India

Shweta Bhandari MS
Consultant
Department of Obstetrics and Gynecology
Sri Aurobindo Institute of Medical Sciences
Indore, Madhya Pradesh, India

Shweta Sirsikar MS
Assistant Professor
Department of Obstetrics and Gynecology
Netaji Subhash Chandra Bose
Government Medical College
Jabalpur, Madhya Pradesh, India

Sneh Chaube MD
Senior Consultant
Department of Obstetrics and Gynecology
City Hospital
Jabalpur, Madhya Pradesh, India

Sonam Baxi MS
Consultant, Obstetrician and Gynecologist
Disha Fertility and Surgical Centre
Indore, Madhya Pradesh, India

S Sampathkumari MD DGO FICOG FC (Diab)
Professor (Obstetrics and Gynecology)
Chengalpattu Medical College
Chengalpattu, Tamil Nadu, India
Chairperson
FOGSI Adolescent Health Committee

Suchitra N Pandit MD DNB FRCOG (UK) FICOGDFP MAMS
Senior Consultant and Head
Department of Obstetrics and Gynecology
Kokilaben Dhirubhai Ambani Hospital
and Research Centre
Mumbai, Maharashtra, India
President, FOGSI 2014

Sushma Dikhit MS MRCOG
Senior Consultant and Head
Department of Obstetrics and Gynecology
Max Superspecialty Hospital
Ghaziabad, Uttar Pradesh, India

Swaraj Naik MS
Senior Gynecologist
Naik Hospital
Jabalpur, Madhya Pradesh, India

Tasabieh Ali
Resident
Department of Obstetrics and Gynecology
Sultan Qaboos Hospital (SQH)
Salalah, Oman

Tripti Deb MBBS MD (General Medicine) DNB (Cardiology)
Interventional Cardiologist
Apollo Hospital
Hyderabad, Telangana, India

Tripti Nagaria MD
Professor and Head
Department of Obstetrics and Gynecology
Pt Jawahar Lal Nehru Memorial
Medical College
Raipur, Chhattisgarh, India

Vaishali A Deshpande MD
Gynecologist
Port Trust Hospital
Mumbai, Maharashtra, India

Vasumati S Upadhye MD
Chief Gynecologist
Port Trust Hospital
Mumbai, Maharashtra, India

Veena Paliwal MS FRCOG
Senior Consultant and Head
Department of Obstetrics and Gynecology
Sultan Qaboos Hospital (SQH)
Salalah, Oman

Vineeta Ghanghoriya MS
Assistant Professor
Department of Obstetrics and Gynecology
Netaji Subhash Chandra Bose
Medical College
Jabalpur, Maharashtra, India

PREFACE

Science is ever changing and steadily moving forward. Explosion of knowledge in medicine is phenomenal and fast.

The Federation of Obstetric and Gynaecological Societies of India (FOGSI) over the years has been active in bringing out more and more recent literature with a view to updating its member's knowledge with the latest developments in our field.

Pregnancy and childbearing are attended by certain challenges and risks to the mother as well as to the fetus. The aim is to improve our management of high-risk situations and optimize the outcome of pregnancy in current era. The purpose of this book is to provide information necessary for high-risk pregnancy because they have the potential for high mortality and morbidity for mother and fetus because of unique anatomic and physiological changes that influence diagnosis and management. The book covers various aspects which puts the fetus at risk, and presents update on prenatal care, management of various medical disorders, hematological disorders, and infections during pregnancy, etc. A number of new chapters have been added like missing dimensions in antenatal care. Chapters have been written in a way so that they provide contemporary information and stimulate clinical thinking. Presentation of all the chapters in a precise and systematic manner is a joint collaborative effort.

This is a multi-authored book and the views expressed herein are those of authors.

We are most grateful to all the esteemed contributors for sparing their valuable time to write these chapters.

We are especially indebted to our FOGSI, Secretary General, Dr HD Pai, FOGSI Presidents and stalwarts, Professors Suchitra N Pandit, Alka Kriplani, and Jaideep Malhotra, for providing their useful inputs and being instrumental in this assignment, at the cost of their precious time despite their multifarious academic, clinical and social activities.

On the completion of this major task, we feel more humble and ever so grateful to the governing body of FOGSI, Secretary General FOGSI, for having given us this opportunity to carry out this job for and on behalf of our parent organization.

During entire course of past two years of compiling of this book, our family members were a source of great strength and motivation. For all their support, we wish to place on record our heartfelt thanks.

In this Universe, nothing happens without the grace and blessings of God. Above all, it is the almighty God who gave us power and creative thoughts. The book is into existence because of His blessings.

Richa Baharani
Pushpa Pandey
Shashi Khare
Sushma Dikhit

ACKNOWLEDGMENTS

On the occasion of successful completion of this marathon job, it would be appropriate to acknowledge, and express our gratitude to all those who have helped in getting this job well done.

We are grateful to all the authors for giving their valuable time and contributing various chapters.

We acknowledge the vast contribution of all our seniors, mentors, teachers who always supported and inspired us.

We would like to thank Dr T Chakma, a brilliant scientist from ICMR, Jabalpur, Madhya Pradesh, India, for his endless support and guidance for this book. We appreciate his advice on planning the layout and for constant encouragement for the entirety of the project.

The final production of the book has been possible due to the hard work put in by Shri Jitendar P Vij (Group Chairman), Mr Ankit Vij (Group President), Ms Samina Khan (Executive Assistant to Director–Content Strategy); Mr Sunil Kumar Dogra (Production Executive); Mr Gurnam Singh (Sr Proofreader), Mr Chandra Dutt (Typesetter) and Mr Amit Mathur (Graphic Designer) of M/s Jaypee Brothers Medical Publishers (P) Ltd, New Delhi, India.

CONTENTS

SECTION 1: UPDATE ON ANTENATAL CARE

1. Changing Trends in Antenatal Care 1
Padma Shukla, Pushpa Pandey, Nidhi Jain

- Epidemiology *1*
- Diagnosis *1*
- Physical Examination *2*
- Other Screening Tests *2*
- Treatment *3*
- Prognosis *4*
- Prophylaxis *5*

2. Missing Dimensions in Antenatal Care 7
Pushpa Pandey, Deepak Dwivedi, Shashi Khare, Shubhada Neel

- Mental Health *7*
- Social Health *8*
- Spiritual Health *9*

3. Nutrition in Pregnancy 13
Roza Olyai, S Sampathkumari

- Energy Requirements *13*
- Protein Requirements in Pregnancy *13*
- Fat Requirements During Pregnancy *13*
- Carbohydrate Requirements During Pregnancy *14*
- Water Requirements During Pregnancy *14*
- Iron Requirements During Pregnancy *14*
- Folic Acid Requirements During Pregnancy *14*
- Calcium Requirements During Pregnancy *14*
- Vitamin D Requirements *15*
- Magnesium Requirements *15*
- Sodium Requirements *15*
- Potassium Requirements *15*
- Iodine Requirements *15*
- Zinc *15*
- Thiamine *15*
- Riboflavin *15*
- Niacin *15*
- Pyridoxine *16*
- Vitamin B_{12} *16*
- Vitamin C *16*
- Vitamin A *16*

4. **Antenatal Fetal Surveillance and Identification of High-risk Pregnancy** 18
   Gita Guin, Poorva Badkur

   - Who to Screen (Patients at Risk) *18*
   - Previous Obstetrical History *18*
   - Current Pregnancy *18*
   - Initiation and Frequency of Antenatal Testing *19*
   - Methods *19*
   - Identification of High-risk Factors *22*

SECTION 2: FETAL ADVANCES

5. **Prenatal Genetic Screening and Testing** 25
   Jyotsna Gupta

   - Screening for Prenatal Aneuploidies *25*
   - Antenatal Screening for Down Syndrome *26*
   - Current Limitations of NIPS (ACMG Statement 2016, ACOG 2015) *30*
   - SOGC Recommendations for Aneuploidy Screening *30*
   - Abnormal Maternal Serum Screening *30*
   - Recommnedations for Screening in Multiple Pregnancies *32*
   - Invasive Fetal Tests *32*
   - Common Indications for Karyotyping Analysis *32*
   - Screening for Gene Mutations that Lead to Fetal Disease *33*
   - Preimplantaion Genetic Diagnosis *33*

6. **Impact of Advances in Genetics in Prenatal Diagnosis** 36
   Shweta Bhandari, Ashutosh Gupta

   - Genetic Techniques *36*
   - Current Limitations of NIPT (ACMG Statement 2016, ACOG 2015) *39*
   - Future of NIPT *40*
   - Preimplantation Genetic Diagnosis *40*

7. **Ultrasonography-guided Interventions in Pregnancy** 42
   Jaideep Malhotra, Shally Gupta

   - Chorionic Villus Sampling *42*
   - Amniocentesis *43*
   - Cordocentesis (Percutaneous Umbilical Blood Sampling) *44*
   - Placental Biopsy *45*
   - Fetoscopy *45*

SECTION 3: HEMATOLOGICAL DISORDERS DURING PREGNANCY

8. **Anemia During Pregnancy and New Parenteral Iron** 49
   Archana Verma, Pushpa Pandey, Richa Baharani

   - Introduction and Magnitude of Problem *49*
   - Definition *49*
   - Causes and Classification of Anemia *49*
   - Iron Metabolism in Pregnancy *50*

- Effect on Anemia on Maternal and fetal Outcome *51*
- Symptoms and Signs *51*
- Laboratory Investigations *52*
- Management *52*
- Indications *54*
- Advice about Family Planning *56*
- Megaloblastic Anemia *56*

9. Non-nutritional Anemia in Pregnancy   59
Vasumati S Upadhye, Sheetal K Gujral, Vaishali A Deshpande

- Etiology of Non-Nutritional Anemia *59*
- Approach to the Patient *59*
- Clinical Examination *59*
- Laboratory Evaluation of Anemia *59*

10. Rh-incompatibility During Pregnancy   66
Pragya Dhirawani, Richa Dhirawani

- Prevalence *66*
- Pathophysiology *66*
- Prevention *67*
- Investigations *67*

11. Management of Rh-alloimmunized Pregnancy   70
Jyotsna Gupta

- Follow-up after Positive Maternal Antibody Screening Test (ICT Positive Mothers) *70*
- Clinical Management of First Affected Pregnancy *73*
- Clinical Management of Previous Fetal or Neonatal Affection *73*
- Fetal Blood Transfusion *73*
- Timing of Subsequent Transfusion *76*
- Fetal Hydrops *76*
- Severely Anemic Early Second Trimester Fetus *77*
- Timing of Delivery *77*
- Postnatal Care *78*
- Outcome *78*
- Alternative Treatment Modalities *78*
- Pre-Pregnancy Counseling *79*
- Prevention of HDFN Fetus in Future Pregnancies *79*

12. Disseminated Intravascular Coagulation in Pregnancy   81
Saroj Singh, Anu Pathak

- Epidemiology *81*
- Normal Coagulation Cascade *81*
- Physiological Changes in Pregnancy *81*
- Triggering Factors for DIC *81*
- Etiology *81*
- Pathophysiology of DIC *82*
- Mechanism of DIC in Different Obstetric Conditions *82*
- Symptoms *83*
- Diagnosis *83*
- Management *83*

SECTION 4: EARLY PREGNANCY COMPLICATIONS

13. Recurrent Pregnancy Loss   85
K Aparna Sharma, Alka Kriplani

- When to Investigate: Defining RPL *85*
- Prevalence and Etiology of RPL: Evidence-based Investigations and Treatment *85*
- Hereditary Thrombophilias *88*
- Managing Idiopathic RPL *89*
- Summary of Work-up and Diagnosis: Do's and Don'ts *89*

14. Hyperemesis Gravidarum   91
Richa Baharani, Pushpa Pandey

- Epidemiology *91*
- Signs and Symptoms *91*
- Risk Factors *91*
- Diagnosis *91*
- Differential Diagnosis *91*
- Investigations *92*
- Complications *92*
- Management *92*
- Summary of Treatment (Medication) *92*

15. Early Pregnancy Hemorrhage   94
Girija Wagh

- Miscarriage *94*
- Gestational Trophoblastic Disease (GTD) *97*
- Ectopic Gestation *99*
- Implantation Bleeding (Physiologic) *100*
- Lower Genital Tract Pathology or Other Sites Bleeding *100*
- Iatrogenic Causes—Medications and Trauma *101*
- Important Issues to be Understood in Interpretation of Early Pregnancy Hemorrhage *101*

16. Unsafe Abortions and its Consequences   103
Kavita Bapat, Vineeta Ghanghoria

- Magnitude of the Problem *103*
- Causes of Unsafe Abortion *103*
- Consequences of Unsafe Abortion *104*
- Prevention of Unsafe Abortion *106*

SECTION 5: MEDICAL DISORDERS DURING PREGNANCY

17. Gestational Diabetes   107
Jigyasa Dengra, Meenu Agarwal

- Pathophysiology of Gestational Diabetes Mellitus *107*
- Screening and Diagnosis *108*
- Management of Gestational Diabetes Mellitus *110*

- Treatment *110*
- Surveillance During Pregnancy *112*
- Complications of GDM *113*
- Postpartum Care *113*
- Preconception Care *114*
- Prevention of GDM *114*

18. Cardiac Diseases in Pregnancy   116
Niraj Jadav, Kirtan M Vyas

- Preconceptional Counseling *116*
- Hemodynamic Changes During Pregnancy *117*
- Effect of Pregnancy on Maternal Cardiac Disease *118*
- Effects of Maternal Cardiac Disease on Pregnancy *118*
- General Measures for the Care of Pregnant Patients with Heart Disease *118*
- Evaluation of Cardiac Function During Pregnancy *118*
- Complications of Cardiac Diseases in Pregnancy *119*
- Management of Women with Heart Disease *119*

19. Specific Cardiac Conditions and Complications During Pregnancy   122
Tripti Deb, Amit Bharadiya, Richa Baharani

- Physiological Changes in the Cardiovascular System During Pregnancy *122*
- Assessment of Risk in Patients with Cardiac Disease *123*
- Specific Cardiac Lesions *125*
- Cardiomyopathy *129*
- Effect of Heart Disease on Pregnancy Outcomes *130*
- Diagnostic Approach *130*
- Management Principles *131*

20. Peripartum Cardiomyopathy   135
Anita Singh, Aashita Shrivastava

- Epidemiology *135*
- Etiology *135*
- Inflammation *135*
- Myocarditis *135*
- Abnormal Immunologic and Hemodynamic Responses to Pregnancy *136*
- Prolactin *136*
- Genetic Factors *136*
- Diagnosis *136*
- Breastfeeding *139*

21. Respiratory Diseases During Pregnancy   141
Priyanka Kukrele, Shashi Khare

- Alteration in Respiratory Physiology During Pregnancy *141*
- Asthma *141*
- Pneumonia *142*
- Cystic Fibrosis *143*
- Pulmonary Edema and Acute Respiratory Distress Syndrome *143*
- Other Respiratory Diseases in Pregnancy *145*

22. Pregnancy and Chronic Kidney Disease — 147
Rubina Vohra, Shabbir H Husain, Nafisa Husain

- Anatomical and Physiological Changes in Kidney During Pregnancy *147*
- Systemic Hemodynamics *147*
- Renal Hemodynamics *148*
- Pregnancy in Patient with Kidney Disease *148*
- Renal Biopsy During Pregnancy *150*
- Dialysis in Pregnancy *150*
- Diagnosis of Pregnancy *150*
- Maternal Complications *151*

23. Thyroid Disorders During Pregnancy — 154
Shreya Goenka, Sarita Agrawal

- Definition of Thyroid Dysfunction *155*
- Causes of Hypothyroidism in Pregnancy *155*
- Complications of Hypothyroidism in Pregnancy *155*
- Treatment *156*
- Hyperthyroidism *157*
- Caveats and Goals of Antithyroid Drug Treatment *158*
- Autoimmune Thyroiditis and Postpartum Thyroiditis *158*

24. Jaundice in Pregnancy — 162
Sangeeta Shrivastava, Richa Dhirawani

- Obstetric Cholestasis (*Synonyms:* Intrahepatic Cholestasis, Icterus Gravidarum, Recurrent Jaundice of Pregnancy) *162*
- Acute Fatty Liver of Pregnancy *163*
- Viral Hepatitis in Pregnancy *164*

SECTION 6: OBSTETRIC COMPLICATIONS

25. Prediction and Prevention of Pre-eclampsia — 169
Beenu Kushwaha, Neha Khatik, Swaraj Naik

- Etiopathogenesis of Pre-eclampsia *169*
- The Rationale for Prediction *170*
- Which Should be a Good Predictive Test? *170*
- Maternal Characteristics and Obstetric History *171*
- Biophysical Markers *172*
- Biochemical Markers *173*
- What is the Most Effective Method? *173*
- Recent Advances *174*
- Prevention of Pre-eclampsia *174*
- WHO Recommendations for Prevention of Pre-eclampsia *175*

26. Management of Pregnancy-induced Hypertension — 178
Richa Baharani, Bharti Sahu

- Physiological Changes in Blood Pressure During Pregnancy *178*
- Classification of Hypertensive Disorders During Pregnancy *178*
- When to Treat Hypertension During Pregnancy? *178*
- Timing of Delivery of Women with Pre-eclampsia/Eclampsia *180*

27. Maternal Assessment in Hypertensive Disease of Pregnancy 182
Suchitra N Pandit, Gorakh G Mandrupkar, Rana Khan Chowdhry

- Classification *182*
- Measurement of Blood Pressure *183*
- Recommendations for Measurement of BP *184*
- Recommendations for Diagnosis of Hypertension *184*
- Recommendations for Measurement of Proteinuria *185*
- Recommendations for Diagnosis of Clinically Significant Proteinuria *185*
- Recommendations for Classification of HDP *185*
- Recommendations for Investigations to Classify HDP *185*
- Recommendations for Prognosis (Maternal and Fetal) in Pre-eclampsia *185*

28. Eclampsia and HELLP Syndrome 187
Gorakh G Mandrupkar

- Incidence *187*
- Pathophysiology *187*
- Events *187*
- Management *187*
- Investigations and Treatment *187*
- Magnesium Sulfate *188*
- Pritchard Regimen *188*
- Zuspan IV Regimen *188*
- Other Regimens *189*
- Which Regimen to Use? *189*
- Antihypertensive Medicines *189*
- IV Fluids *189*
- HELLP Syndrome *189*
- Delivery Decision and Conduct *191*

29. Eye in Pregnancy 192
Anamika Dwivedi, Richa Baharani

- Ocular Adnexal Changes *192*
- Corneal Changes *192*
- Intraocular Pressure *192*
- Pregnancy Specific Eye Diseases *192*
- Pre-existing Eye Diseases *193*

30. Placenta Previa: An Obstetrical Resurgence 195
Shashi Khare, Anupama B Solanki

- Epidemiology *195*
- Etiopathogenesis *195*
- Clinical Features *195*
- Classification *196*
- Diagnosis *196*
- Differential Diagnosis *197*
- Complications of Placenta Previa *197*
- Management *197*
- Conduct of Expectant Management (McAfee and Johnson Regimen) *197*
- Cesarean Section in Placenta Previa *198*

31. Placenta Accreta — 200
Rooplekha Chauhan

- Development of Human Placenta *200*
- Placenta Accreta *200*
- Diagnosis *201*
- Management *201*

32. Placental Abruption — 204
Sadhana Gupta, Hema J Shobhane

- General Consideration *204*
- Clinical Features *204*
- Examination *204*
- Etiology *205*
- Investigations *205*
- Prevention *205*
- Management *205*
- Recurrence *207*
- Long-term Maternal Cardiovascular Mortality *207*
- Counseling *207*

33. Preterm Labor: Diagnosis and Treatment — 209
Anuradha Dang, Pushpa Pandey, Sneh Chaube

- Definition *209*
- Pathophysiology of Preterm Labor *209*
- Risk Factors *209*
- Interventions *211*

34. Premature Rupture of Membranes — 216
Jyoti Bindal

- Definition *216*
- Incidence *216*
- Pathophysiology *216*
- Etiology *216*
- Diagnosis *217*
- Management *219*

35. Management of Multiple Pregnancy: The Recent Evidence — 226
Sushma Dikhit, Shalini Agrawal

Classification of Twin Pregnancies *226*

36. Teenage Pregnancy: A Global Issue — 234
Shruti Agrawal, Nisha Sahu

- A Rising Issue *234*
- Factors Influencing Adolescent Pregnancy and Childbirth *234*
- Complications *235*
- Care of the Adolescents During Pregnancy, Childbirth and the Postnatal Period *236*
- Prevention *237*
- Initiatives by FOGSI *237*

37. Obesity and Pregnancy   238
Bharati Dhorepatil

- Definition of Obesity *238*
- Effects of Obesity on Fertility and Early Pregnancy *238*
- Antepartum Complications *239*
- Intrapartum Complications *240*
- Fetal Complications *241*
- Postpartum Complications *243*

38. Cesarean Scar Pregnancy   248
Mahesh Gupta, Richa Baharani

- Epidemiology *248*
- Diagnosis *248*
- Magnetic Resonance Imaging *249*
- Management *249*
- Differential Diagnosis *250*
- Complications *250*

SECTION 7: INFECTIONS DURING PREGNANCY

39. Malaria During Pregnancy   252
Richa Baharani, Pushpa Pandey, Anand Baharani

- Introduction and Magnitude of Problem *252*
- Epidemiology *252*
- Pathophysiology *252*
- Clinical Manifestations of Malaria *252*
- Malaria in Pregnancy *252*

40. Management of Influenza, Swine Flu and Dengue During Pregnancy   257
Priti Kumar, Phagun Shah

- Influenza and Swine Flu in Pregnancy *257*
- Pregnancy and Dengue Fever *259*
- Word of Caution *262*

41. Tuberculosis in Pregnancy: Update on an Archenemy   264
Alka Pandey, Ajay Sinha

- Diagnosis of Tuberculosis in Pregnant Women *264*
- Treatment *265*
- Breastfeeding *265*
- Multidrug Resistant Tuberculosis in Pregnancy *265*
- HIV Coinfection and Pregnant Women with Tuberculosis *265*

42. Viral Infections in Pregnancy and Labor   267
Madhuri Chandra

- Rubella (German Measles) *267*
- Cytomegalovirus *268*
- Herpes Simplex *269*

- Varicella Zoster (Chickenpox) *271*
- Hepatitis B *272*
- HIV-AIDS *273*

43. Toxoplasmosis During Pregnancy — 278
Alka Pandey, Richa Baharani

- Epidemiology *278*
- Toxoplasmosis in Pregnancy *278*
- Mode of Transmission *278*
- Routes of Transmission *279*
- Diagnosis *279*
- Preventive Measures *280*
- Prevention *280*
- Management *280*
- Dose *281*
- Intrapartum Care *281*

44. Zika Fever and Parvovirus Infection During Pregnancy — 282
Shruti Agrawal, Pushpa Pandey

***Zika Virus Disease** 282*
- Virology *282*
- Epidemiology *282*
- Pathogenesis *282*
- Diagnosis *283*
- Screening in Pregnancy *284*
- Precautions and Prevention *284*
- Treatment *284*
- Vaccines *285*

***Parvovirus B19 (PB19)** 285*
- Epidemiology *285*
- Clinical Presentation *285*
- Diagnosis *286*
- Management *286*

SECTION 8: FETAL DYSMATURITY AND DYSMORPHOLOGY

45. Fetal Growth Restriction: Monitoring and Management — 289
Geetha Balsarkar, Jagruti Murkey

- Rules of Fetal Growth *289*
- History *289*
- Examination *289*
- Monitoring the Growth Restricted Fetus *289*
- Early-onset Fetal Growth Restriction *290*
- Late-onset Fetal Growth Restriction *290*
- Monitoring in Fetal Growth Restriction *291*
- Stage-based Classification and Management of FGR *294*

46. Fetal Dysmorphology 296
Prachi Dixit, Madhuri Gawande, Shirish Vaidya
- Fetal Craniospinal Abnormalities *296*
- Open Neural Tube Defects *296*
- Hydrocephalus *297*
- Holoprosencephaly *298*
- Dandy-Walker Malformation *298*
- Hydranencephaly *299*
- Agenesis of Corpus Callosum *299*
- Abnormality of Neck-Cystic Hygroma *299*
- Fetal Cardiovascular Abnormalities *300*
- Structural Cardiac Disease *300*
- Hypoplastic Left Heart Syndrome *301*
- Outflow Tract Obstruction *301*
- Cardiac Arrhythmias *302*
- Irregular Heart Rate *302*
- Tachycardia *302*
- Bradycardia *302*
- Fetal Gastrointestinal Abnormalities *303*
- Body Stalk Anomaly *304*
- Bladder and Cloacal Exstrophies *305*
- Esophageal Atresia *305*
- Duodenal Atresia *305*
- Jejunal and Ileal Atresia *306*
- Anal Atresia, Imperforate Anus *306*
- Hyperechogenic Bowel *306*
- Fetal Genitourinary Abnormalities *306*
- Fetal Uropathies *306*
- Kidney Abnormalities *308*
- Fetal Skeletal Abnormalities *309*
- Conditions Associated with Early Onset Severe Symmetrical Shortening of Long Bones *309*
- Conditions Associated with Bowed or Fractured Limbs *310*
- Conditions Associated with Mild-to-moderate Symmetrical Shortening of Long Bones *310*
- Achondroplasia *310*
- Joint Deformities *311*
- Abnormalities of Amniotic Fluid *311*
- Postnatal Examination of a Stillborn or Anomalous Neonate *314*

SECTION 9: AUTOIMMUNE DISEASES AND OTHER DISORDERS DURING PREGNANCY

47. Systemic Lupus Erythematosus in Pregnancy 317
Anupama B Solanki, Shashi Khare
- Incidence and Prevalence *317*
- Clinical Manifestations of SLE *317*
- Diagnosis of Systemic Lupus Erythematosus *317*

48. Antiphospholipid Antibody Syndrome — 323
Deepti Shrivastava

- Epidemiology *323*
- Obstetric Implications *324*
- Etiopathogenesis *324*
- Diagnosis *324*
- Differential Diagnosis *326*
- Treatment *326*

49. Dermatological Disorders in Pregnancy — 331
Ritu Choubey, Pushpa Pandey

- Physiological Skin Changes *331*
- Pigmentary Changes *331*
- Hair and Nail Changes *331*
- Vascular Changes *332*
- Connective Tissue Changes *332*
- Glandular Changes *332*
- Mucosal Changes *332*
- Skin Infections and Pre-existing Skin Disorders in Pregnancy *333*
- Pregnancy-specific Dermatoses *334*
- Atopic Eruption of Pregnancy *335*
- Polymorphic Eruption of Pregnancy (PEP) *336*
- Intrahepatic Cholestasis of Pregnancy *337*
- Pemphigoid Gestationis *337*
- Impetigo Herpetiformis *338*
- Dermatological Drug Safety in Pregnancy *340*

50. Pregnancy and Oral Health — 341
Shivani Dwivedi, Pushpa Pandey, Richa Baharani

- Oral Conditions Effecting Pregnancy *341*
- Biological Hypotheses Linking Preterm Birth and Periodontal Diseases *341*

51. Epilepsy in Pregnancy — 349
Deepti Gupta

- Etiopathogenesis *349*
- Investigations *349*
- Differential Diagnosis *349*
- Preconception Counseling *349*
- Pregnancy and Disease Progression *350*
- Management of Pregnancy and Delivery *350*

SECTION 10: COMPLICATIONS DURING DELIVERY

52. Rupture Uterus — 352
Tripti Nagaria

- Classification of Rupture Uterus *352*
- Management of Rupture Uterus *354*
- Cautions while Doing Repair *356*

- Rupture Uterus if Detected after Delivery 357
- Future Pregnancy 357

53. Medical Management of Postpartum Hemorrhage 360
Madhuri Alwani

- Definition 360
- Etiology and Risk Factors Associated with PPH 360
- Management 361
- Treatment 361
- What is New in the Management of Postpartum Hemorrhage? 365

54. Balloon Tamponade in Postpartum Hemorrhage 368
Nalini Mishra, Devanshi Mishra Vyas, Kanchan Gulbani, Mamta Sai

- Tamponade Test 368
- Types of Balloon Tamponade 368
- Varieties of Condom Balloon Tamponade Prepared on the Spot 369
- Contraindications to use of CBT 371

55. Surgical Management of Postpartum Hemorrhage: A Review 374
Kavita N Singh, Shweta Sirsikar

- Uterine Compression Sutures 374
- Uterine and Ovarian Artery Ligation (Stepwise Devascularization of the Uterus) 375
- Uterine Artery Ligation 376
- Ovarian Artery Ligation 376
- Vaginal Uterine Artery Ligation 377
- Internal Iliac (Hypogastric) Artery Ligation and Aortic Compression 377
- Hysterectomy 377
- Logothetopulos Pack 377
- Arterial Embolization 377
- Special Situations 378

SECTION 11: MISCELLANEOUS

56. Intrauterine Fetal Death (Its Impact on Maternal Morbidity and Mortality and Preventive Strategies) 379
Rujuta Fuke

- Epidemiology 379
- Recent Nomenclature 379
- Risk Factors 379
- Causes 380
- Diagnosis 380
- Complications of IUFD 381
- Recommended Evaluation of a Stillborn 382
- Counseling and Prevention 382

57. Cerebrovascular Accidents in Pregnancy 384
Jignesh Shah

- Possibility and Risk Factors 384
- Etiology 385

- Diagnostic Work-up *386*
- Signs and Symptoms of Stroke *388*
- Causes of CVA *388*
- Prevention of CVA *390*

58. ART Pregnancies: Are They Different? 394
Asha Baxi, Sonam Baxi

- Risk of Multifetal Gestation *394*
- Management of ART Pregnancies: Practical Tips *395*

59. Adnexal Masses in Pregnancy 398
Veena Paliwal, Sushma Dikhit, Tasabieh Ali

- Patient Presentation *398*
- Other Clinical Presentations *398*
- Types of Adnexal Masses *398*
- Surgical Management *401*
- Oncologic Prognosis *404*
- Pregnancy Outcomes *404*

60. Medicolegal Aspects of High-risk Pregnancy 407
Hitesh J Bhatt

- Legal Implications *407*
- What are the Litigant Situations? *408*
- What Prevents Litigation or Saves a Doctor in Court? *408*
- Role of Consent *408*
- Documents *408*
- High-Risk Pregnancy *408*

61. Destination Far Ahead: Strategies to Reduce MMR 409
Bharti Sahu, Padma Shukla, Ranjana Gupta

- Maternal Health Services *409*
- Sustainable Developmental Goal *409*
- But why are we Unable to Save these Mothers *409*
- First Delay *410*
- Second Delay *410*
- Causes of Maternal Mortality in India *410*
- Causes of Maternal Mortality Worldwide *410*
- Road Blocks!!! *411*
- Strategies to Reduce MMR *411*
- In a Nutshell: To Reduce MMR *412*
- Myth *412*
- Lessons and Future Directions *412*
- Key to Success *412*

Index *415*

Plate 1

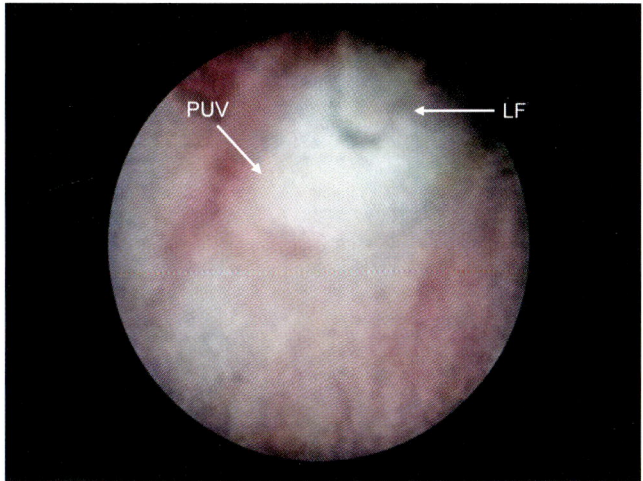

Fig. 7.5B: Cystoscopic view of a dilated posterior urethra

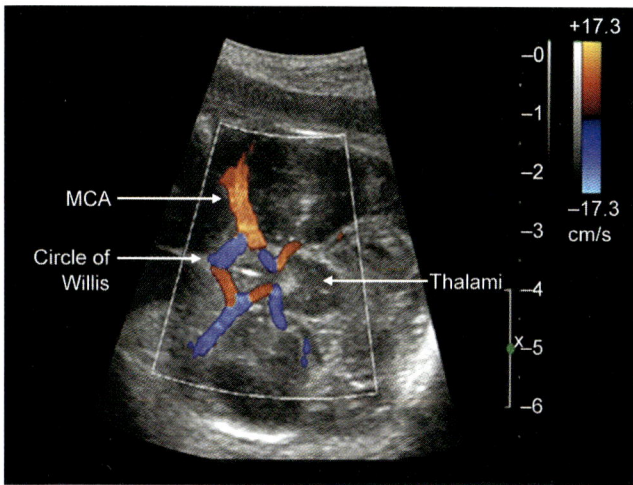

Fig. 11.1A: Middle cerebral artery

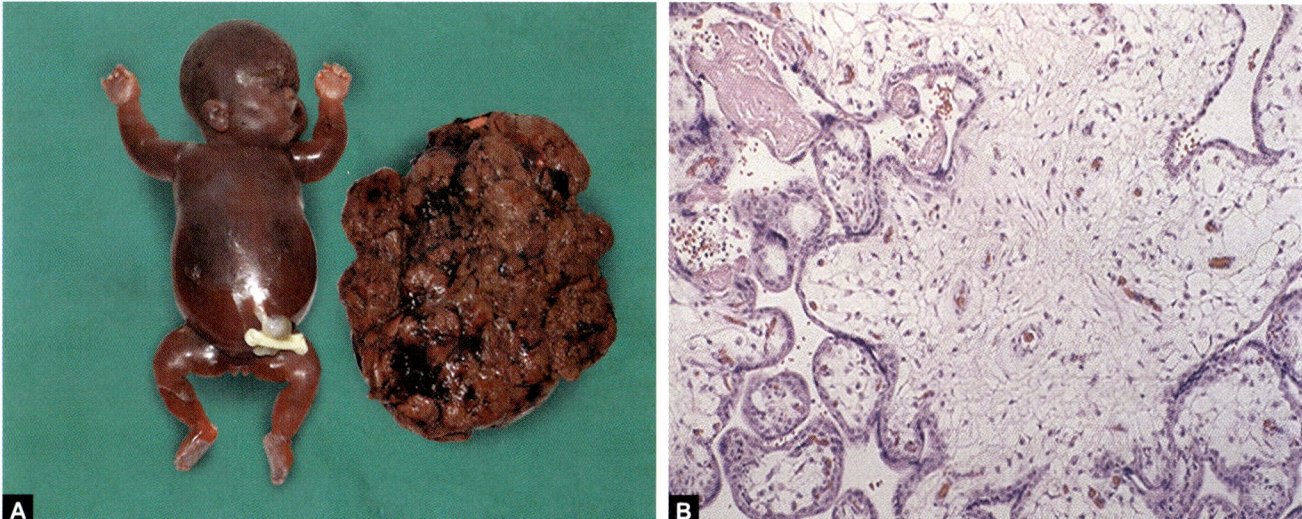

Figs 11.6A and B: (A) Hydropic fetus with large placenta seen in cases of severe Fetal affection due to Rh-alloimmunization (http://accessmedicine.mhmedical.com/content.aspx?bookid=1057&sectionid=59789153); (B) Histopathology of hydropic placenta showing chorionic villi edema and accumulation of fluid and abundant stroma with intact vessels and no trophoblast proliferation (http://library.med.utah.edu/WebPath/PLACHTML/PLAC030.html)

Plate 2

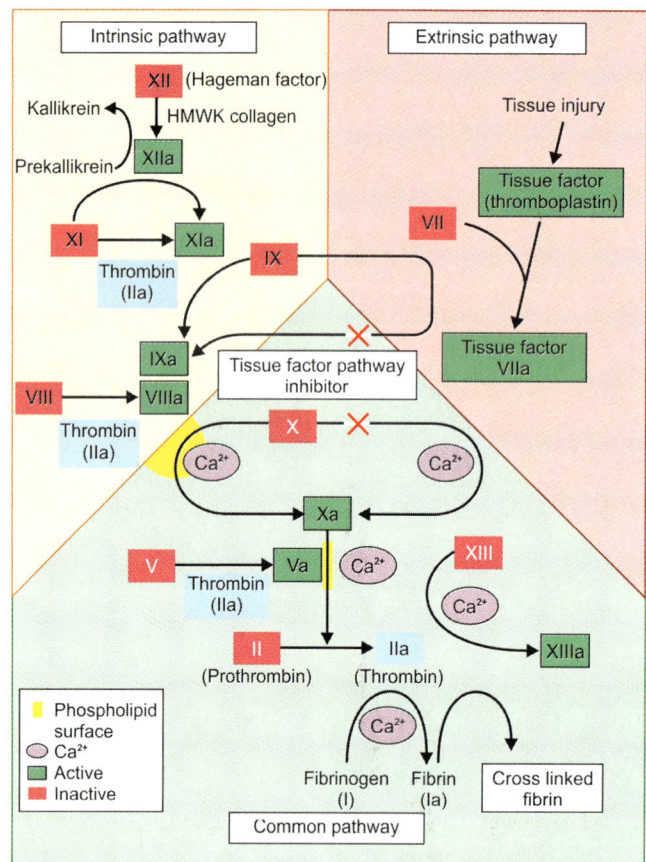

Fig. 12.1: The coagulation cascade. Factor IX can be activated by either factor XIa or factor VIIa. In laboratory tests, activation is predominantly dependent on factor XIa, whereas *in vivo*, factor VIIa appears to be the predominant activator of factor IX. Factors in red boxes represent inactive molecules; activated factors, indicated with a lowercase a, are in green boxes. Note that thrombin (factor IIa) (in light blue boxes) contributes to coagulation through multiple positive feedback loops. The red X's denote points at which tissue factor pathway inhibitor (TFPI) inhibits activation of factor X and factor IX by factor VIIa

Abbreviations: HMWK, high-molecular-weight kininogen; PL, phospholipid[4]

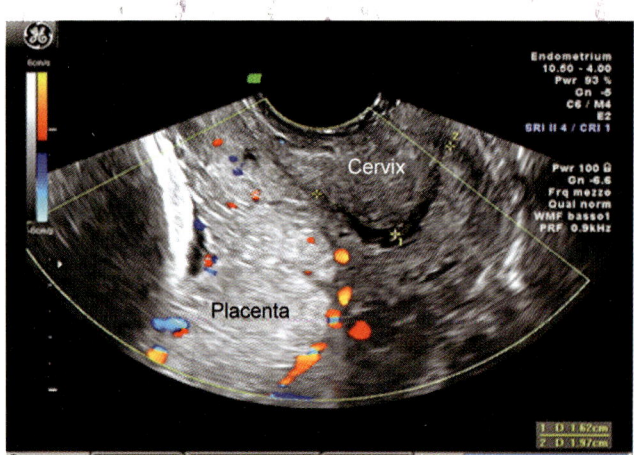

Fig. 30.1: Transvaginal sonography showing complete placenta previa

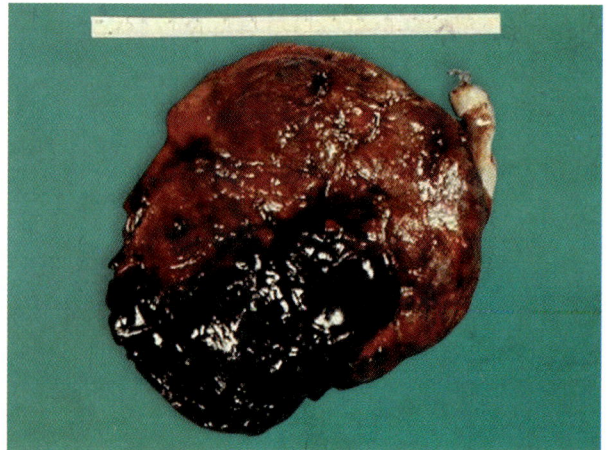

Fig. 32.1: Placenta with retroplacental hemorrhage

Plate 3

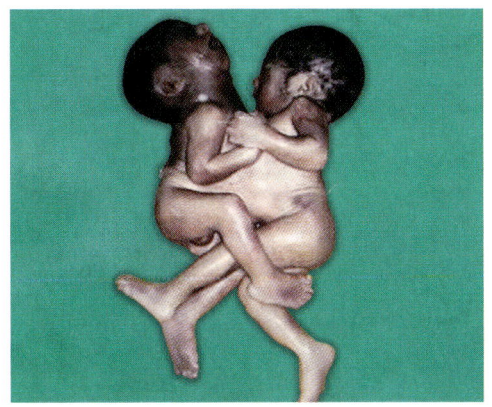

Fig. 35.4: Conjoined twins (monozygotic)

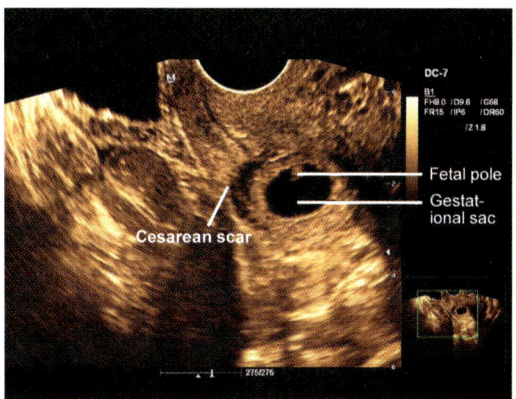

Fig. 38.1: Transvaginal sonography showing cesarian scar pregnancy

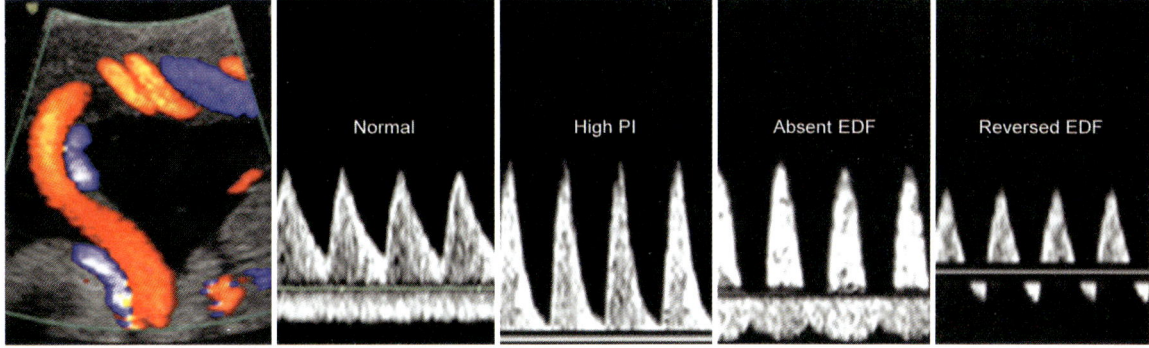

Fig. 45.3: Umbilical artery Doppler

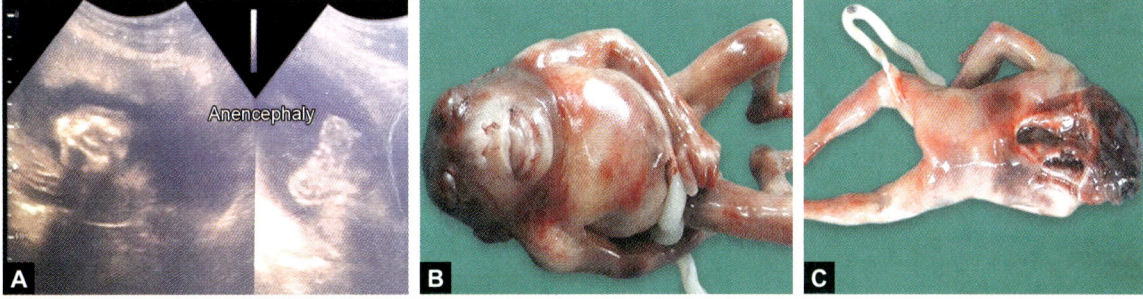

Figs 46.1A to C: Anencephaly

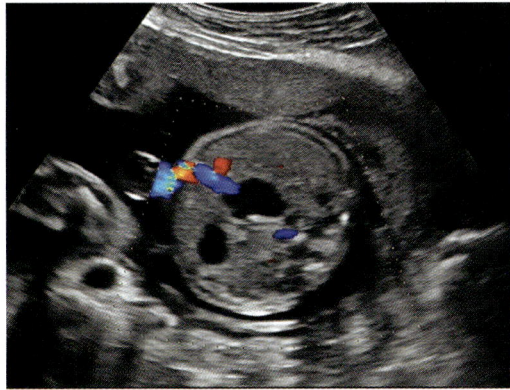

Fig. 46.7: Duodenal atresia (double bubble sign)

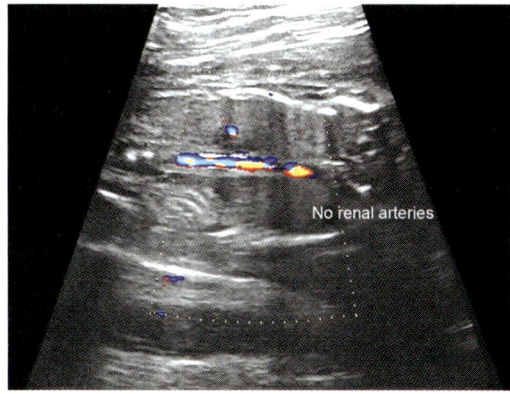

Fig. 46.10: Bilateral renal agenesis—no renal arteries

Plate 4

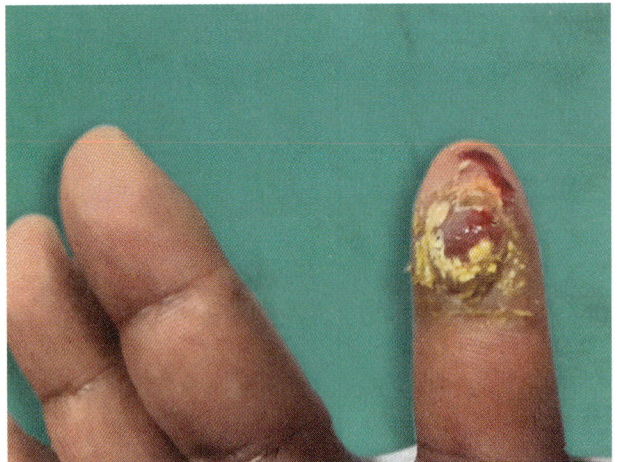

Fig. 49.1: Depicting granuloma gravidarum (pyogenic granuloma on the index finger)

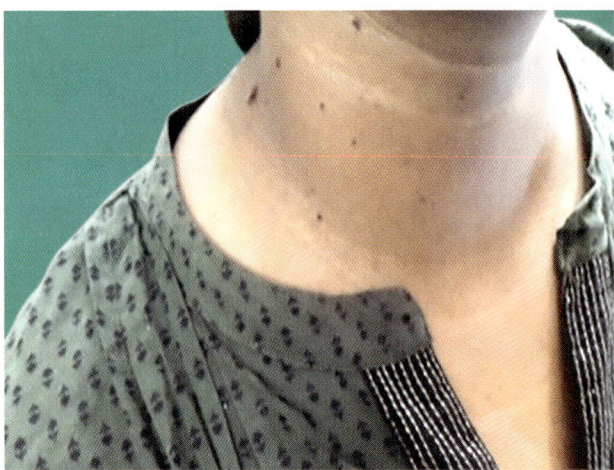

Fig. 49.2: Pseudoacanthotic changes on the neck with skin tags

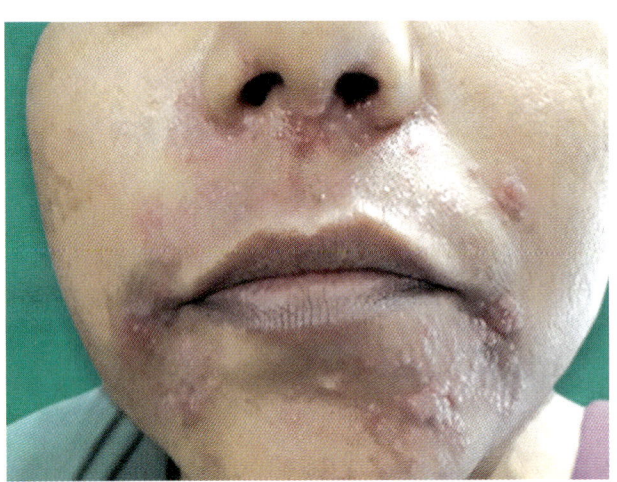

Fig. 49.3: Perioral dermatitis

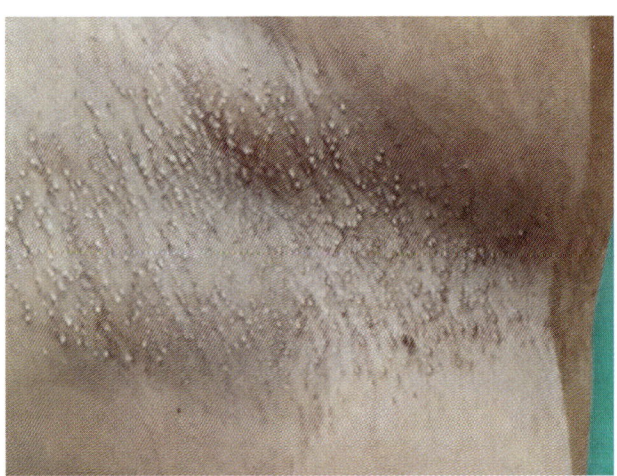

Fig. 49.4: Fox Fordyce's disease (axilla)

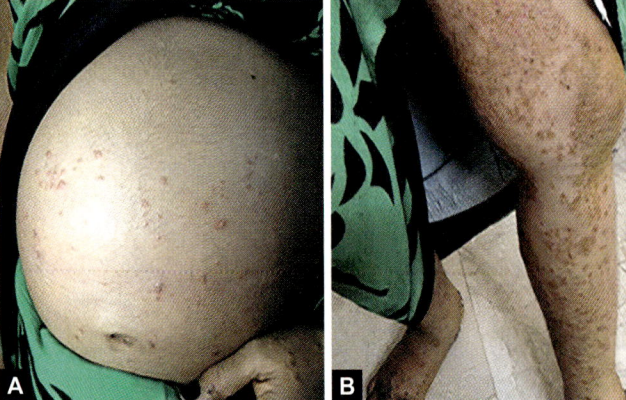

Figs 49.5A and B: (A) Pruritic papular lesions (periumbilical) of PEP; (B) Erythematous papules and plaques with targetoid lesions on the lower extremity of PEP

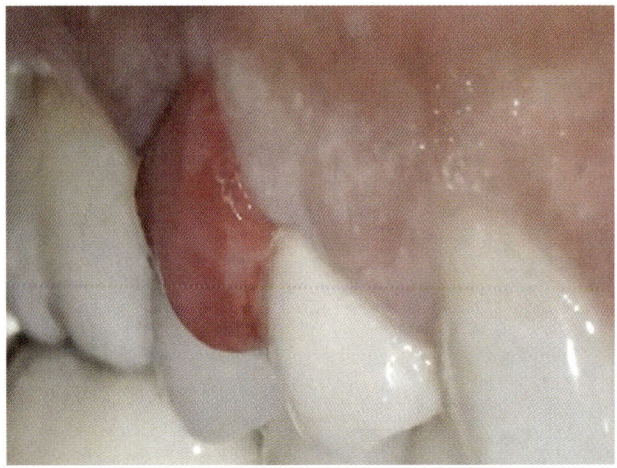

Fig. 50.1: Pyogenic granuloma

SECTION 1: UPDATE ON ANTENATAL CARE

Chapter 1

Changing Trends in Antenatal Care

Padma Shukla, Pushpa Pandey, Nidhi Jain

INTRODUCTION

Pregnancy is a normal physiological process; however, complications that increase the mortality or morbidity to the mother and fetus occur in 5-20% of pregnancies. Our system of prenatal care should be focused on prevention. Ideally, a woman planning for pregnancy should have a medical evaluation before conception; this allows the physician to determine the presence of risk factors to complicate a pregnancy. The purpose of prenatal care is to ensure a successful pregnancy outcome with the delivery of a live-healthy fetus and a healthy mother.

The standard schedule for antenatal visits in uncomplicated patients is every 4 weeks from 0 to 32 weeks gestation, every 2 weeks from 32 weeks to 36 weeks gestation and weekly visit after 36 weeks gestation. As our knowledge and information about fetal development and pregnancy is increasing, initial antenatal contacts are crucial even in normal pregnancy. WHO 2016 ANC model replaces the previous four visits focused model ANC (FANC). New guideline increases the number of contacts of a pregnant for antenatal care from four to eight. First contact at 12 weeks gestation, subsequent visit should be at 20, 26, 30, 34, 36, 38 and 40 weeks gestation. Within this model, the word 'contact' has been used instead of 'visit', as it implies an active connection between a pregnant women and a healthcare provider that is not implicit with the word 'visit'.[1]

Antenatal care should be initiated as soon as the pregnancy is confirmed. Major goals are to define health status of the mother and fetus, estimate the gestational age, identify the high-risk factors and initiate a plan for continuing obstetrical care. Concept of turning the pyramid prenatal care was introduced by Kypros Nicolaides.[2] This review presents evidence that many pregnancy complications can now be predicted at an integrated first hospital visit at 11-13 weeks.

Pregnancy is usually identified, when a woman misses her menses and presents with symptoms. Some of the woman presents with a positive home urine pregnancy test result. Common symptoms which bother woman are amenorrhea, nausea, vomiting, breast, skin and reproductive changes. Step-by-step evaluation of woman should be done by taking history, physical examination, laboratory tests, genetic screening and by ultrasonography.

Early estimation of patient specific risks for pregnancy complications would improve pregnancy outcome by shifting antenatal care to a more individualized and disease specific approach in trend of schedule and purpose of each visit.

EPIDEMIOLOGY

According to WHO, trends of maternal mortality annually estimate that 45,000 women die due to preventable pregnancy related causes in India. But with improving antenatal care the maternal mortality ratio reduced from 212 in 2007 to 178 in 2012. Individualized care of all pregnant women can further reduce maternal and fetal mortality and morbidity.

DIAGNOSIS

History: Obstetrics history should include a discussion of current symptoms, outcome of all previous pregnancies. Information about duration of gestation, birth weight, length of labor, type of delivery, fetal/neonatal outcome, anesthesia and any complications occurring in previous pregnancies.

Medical history should be taken regarding, anemia, hemoglobinopathy, epilepsy, cardiovascular, respiratory, gastrointestinal, renal, endocrine disorders and psychological disorders. Autoimmune disease and dental problems require careful evaluation. A history of previous gynecological, abdominal, uterine surgery or cervical surgery must be obtained. History of consanguineous marriage, family history of diabetes or familial disorder needs further evaluation. Documentation of tobacco and alcohol use, blood transfusion, any contact with intravenous drugs or other drug use is must. Detailed history of vaccination, fever with rashes, genital ulcers, food habit should be taken.

PHYSICAL EXAMINATION

A complete physical examination should be performed at the first obstetric visit including maternal weight, pelvic/cervical examination.

At the first prenatal visit, pregnant women should be offered information about antenatal care services, life-style modification, diet and screening tests. Screening tests include complete blood count, blood group and Rh-typing (ABO/Rh), VDRL or RPR for syphilis, hepatitis B surface antigen and serology to detect antibodies against HIV and rubella IgG. Complete urine analysis is integral part of prenatal testing midstream urine culture is recommended method for diagnosing asymptomatic bacteriuria in pregnancy.[1] Women should be screened for Rh-antibodies at first visit, and again at 28 weeks in cases of Rh-negative pregnancy.

OTHER SCREENING TESTS

Gestational diabetes: According to WHO criteria (2013)[1] hyperglycemia first detected at any time during pregnancy should be classified as either gestational diabetes mellitus (GDM) or diabetes mellitus in pregnancy. Universal screening at first contact should be done if negative, repeat using single step 2 hour value during 24–28 week.[3] Dipsi has endorsed the WHO 1999 criteria and adopted a non-fasting OGTT as a single step screening and diagnostic test for GDM in India. This guideline recommends 75 g glucose, which can be given in non-fasting or a fasting state. One blood sample to be withdrawn 2 hours after glucose load, and acute point of 140 mg/dL is diagnostic for GDM **(Table 1.1)**.[4,5]

'Maternal Health Division of Ministry of Health and Family Welfare', Government of India, released the National Guidelines for the Diagnosis and Management of GDM in December 2014. These guidelines also recommend the single step test twice during pregnancy.

Thyroid screening: ACOG does not recommend universal screening for thyroid disorder in pregnancy. As it is endemic in many areas across India, especially in northern region, thyroid screening should preferably be done at least once, especially in all pregnant women hailing from these areas.[5] Upper limit of TSH is 2.5 mU/L in first trimester and 3 mU/L in second and third trimester.[5]

Table 1.1: OGTT with 75 gm glucose (WHO Criteria)[5]

Plasma glucose	In pregnancy	Outside pregnancy
2 hours > 200 mg/dL	Diabetes	Diabetes
2 hours >140 < 199 mg/dL	GDM	IGT
2 hours >120 mg/dL < 139 mg/dL	GGI	–
2 hours < 120 mg/dL	Normal	Normal

Abbreviations: GDM, gestational diabetes mellitus; GGI, graded glucose infusion; IGT, impaired glucose tolerance.

Non-nutritional anemia: As beta-thalassemia is most common single gene disorder in India with prevalence of carrier, universal screening is required to detect more carrier. Sickle cell should be screened in all antenatal clinic.[6]

Screening tests for fetal aneuploidies (11–13 weeks): As per the understanding regarding fetal development and the screening tests to be performed to rule out pregnancy complications frequent initial visits of the woman is required. Ultrasonography should be utilized to monitor growth and development of embryo/fetus. Fetal nuchal translucency measurement and appearance of nasal bone should be seen to rule out trisomy. Fetal nuchal translucency measurement and maternal serum analysis of PAPP-A and free β-hCG is used to screen trisomy in 1st trimester. Combining the maternal age, biochemical test and nuchal translucency, the detection rate of trisomy 21 is up to 90% with false positive rate of 5%. It can be done in two visits or as one stop clinic for assessment of risk (OSCAR).[7-15]

Improvement in the performance of first trimester screening can be achieved by carrying out the biochemical test and ultrasound scan at 11–13 weeks and inclusion in the ultrasound examination assessment of nasal bone and flow in the ductus venosus, hepatic artery and across the tricuspid valve.[16-18]

For patients who did not receive 1st trimester maternal serum, quadruple screening is offered at 16–18 weeks to screen for neural tube defects and aneuploidy. Analysis include serum β-hCG, unconjugated estriol, alpha-fetoprotein and inhibin.

Invasive genetic testing is offered to all women of 35 years of age or older or who have a history of an abnormal fetus/baby. Chorionic villus sampling is performed between 10 to 13 weeks gestation and amniocentesis is performed between 15 and 20 weeks gestation. Detection rate of aneuploidy is greater than 99% with these procedures.[16]

Noninvasive Prenatal Testing (NIPT)

Cell-free DNA of fetus (cf DNA) from mother's blood can be done in high-risk patients as early as 10 weeks. It has 99.5% specificity, and 99% sensitivity. It is still an expensive screening modality.[19]

Anomalies which are always detectable at 11 to 13 weeks, include body stalk anomaly, anencephaly, alobar holoprosencephaly, exomphalos, gastroschisis and megacystitis.

Major Cardiac Defects

Abnormalities of the heart and great arteries are the most common congenital defects leading to 20% of all stillbirths and 30% of neonatal deaths due to congenital defects. The traditional method of screening for cardiac defects, which relies on family history of cardiac defects, maternal history of diabetes mellitus and maternal exposure to teratogens, identify only about 10% of the affected fetus. Specialist fetal echocardiography for cases with nuchal translucency above the 99th centile and those with reversed a wave in the ductus venosus or tricuspid regurgitation irrespective of NT, would require cardiac scanning in 4% of the population and would detect about 50% of major cardiac defect.[20-22]

Screening for spina bifida, miscarriage and stillbirth: In open spina bifida, caudal displacement of the brain is apparent at 11-13 weeks.[23-24] The rate of miscarriages and stillbirths after demonstration of live fetus at 11-13 weeks are about one and 0.4% respectively.[24] Risk is increased with increasing maternal age and maternal weight, previous miscarriages or stillbirth. Miscarriages and stillbirths are also associated with abnormal results of first trimester screening for aneuploidies such as increased fetal nuchal translucency thickness, reversed a-wave in the fetal ductus venosus and low maternal serum pregnancy-associated plasma protein-A (PAPP-A).[25]

Screening for Pre-eclampsia

Maternal characteristics, biophysical and biochemical tests at first trimester (11-13 weeks) could potentially identify about 90, 80 and 60% of pregnancies that subsequently develop early (before 34 weeks) intermediate (34-37 weeks) and late (after 37 weeks) pre-eclampsia, with a false positive rate of 57%.[26] Maternal characteristics include higher weight, African or South Asian racial origin, conception after ovulation induction, personal or family history of pre-eclampsia and in those with pre-existing chronic hypertension or diabetes mellitus. Biochemical tests include PAPP-A, placental growth factor, endoglin, activin-A and inhibin-A. Biophysical tests are increased uterine artery pulsatility index and mean arterial pressure. Increased uterine artery pulsatility index reflects the underlying mechanism for development of pre-eclampsia.[26]

Small for Gestation Age

Risk factor for small for gestational age (SGA) are maternal age, cigarette smokers, those with a medical history of chronic hypertension, women with a previous SGA neonate, assisted conception and women of African or Asian Origin. In pregnancies with SGA in the absence of pre-eclampsia, there is evidence of impaired placental perfusion and function from the first trimester of pregnancy. Uterine artery pulsatility index and mean arterial pressure are increased and placental volume and serum PAPP-A, free β-hCG, PLGF, PP13 and ADAM 12 are decreased.[27, 28]

Preterm birth: Routine vaginal examination is not done for predicting preterm birth. Although cervical shortening identified by transvaginal ultrasound and increased levels of fetal fibronectin from 13-14 weeks are associated with increased risk of preterm birth.[5]

Placenta previa: Most low lying placentas detected at 20 weeks anomaly scan will resolve by them, another scan at third trimester should be offered.[5] One ultrasound scan before 24 weeks is recommended by WHO.[29] Three ultrasounds are usually done in routine antenatal cases first at 11-13, second at 18-20 weeks (Target Scan), and third at 32-34 weeks for fetal growth.[30] Routine Doppler ultrasound is not recommended.[29] Routine cardiotocography is not recommended for pregnant women to improve maternal and perinatal outcomes.[29]

TREATMENT

Most of the women who are in first trimester of pregnancy visit to the clinician for nausea and vomiting and this provides opportunity to evaluate them in early pregnancy. Folic acid 5 mg daily, ginger, chamomile, vitamin B_6 and/or acupuncture are recommended for the relief of nausea in early pregnancy, based on a woman's preferences and availability.[31]

Other common complaints are urinary frequency, breast soreness, joint pain and backache, leg cramps, pica and discomfort in hands. Treatment of these common complaints and counseling of the women regarding regular antenatal visit is a must. Daily elemental 30-60 mg iron and 400 µg (4 mg) folic acid is recommended for pregnant women from second trimester to prevent maternal anemia, puerperal sepsis, low birth weight and preterm birth.[32]

Intermittent oral iron and folic acid supplementation with 120 mg of elemental iron and 2800 µg (2.8 mg) of folic acid, once weekly is recommended for pregnant women to improve maternal and neonatal outcomes, if daily iron is not acceptable due to side-effects, and in populations with an anemia prevalence among pregnant women of less than 20%.

In population with low calcium intake daily calcium supplementation (1.5-2 g oral elemental calcium) is recommended to reduce the incidence of pre-eclampsia. Tetanus toxoid vaccination is recommended for all pregnant women, depending on previous tetanus vaccination exposure, to prevent neonatal mortality from tetanus.[33] In endemic areas, preventive anthelminthic treatment is recommended for pregnant women after the first trimester as part of worm infection reduction programs.[34]

The pregnant women should be encouraged to eat a balanced diet and should be made aware of special needs for iron folic acid, calcium, vitamin A and zinc. Lowering caffeine intake is recommended to reduce risk of pregnancy loss and low birth weight. Healthy life style and physical activity is recommended for pregnant women to stay healthy and to prevent excessive weight gain during pregnancy.[35-37] The average woman weighing 58 kg has a normal dietary intake of 2300 kcal/day. An additional 300 kcal/day is needed during pregnancy. Antenatal prophylaxis with anti-D immunoglobulin in nonsensitized Rh-negative pregnant women at 28 and 34 weeks of gestation to prevent RhD-alloimmunization is only recommended in the context of rigorous research.

Context-specific Recommendation (Research) (Table 1.2) [29,38]

Termination of pregnancy can be advised to women with major anatomical defect. In high-risk cases of pre-eclampsia aspirin beginning in the first trimester can improve placentation and reduce the prevalence of the disease. [39] Other high-risk woman should be managed according to the individual needs.

PROGNOSIS

Women in developing countries are dying from simple preventable conditions. The importance of antenatal care for maternal health lies in its capacity for detection of preclinical or early morbid states in expectant mothers and the opportunity for health promotion. Antenatal care services

Table 1.2: Summary of prenatal care [40,41]

First trimester or first visit	Detailed history, general systemic examination, blood pressure, weight, pelvic examination, investigations • Complete hemogram • Blood sugar 2 hours after 75 g glucose • Double marker test • USG 11–13 weeks NT, NB, cervical length, DV, TR, uterine artery (PI), color Doppler, if indicated • Blood group, ABO and Rh-typing • Urine-R, M, urine culture • VDRL, HIV test • HbsAg • TSH • Indirect Coombs' test (Rh-negative) • Hb electrophoresis • HbA$_{1c}$ (if B sugar high) • Rubella IgG (preconceptionally or first visit) • Pap smear	• *Folic acid 5 mg daily:* Ginger, chamomile, vitamin B$_6$ and/or acupuncture are recommended for the relief of nausea in early pregnancy, based on a woman's preferences and available
Second trimester	Blood pressure, height, weight, fundal height, fetal heart rate *Investigations:* • Hemoglobin, urine routine and microscopic, • USG 18–20 weeks target scan • Fetal echo • Blood sugar 2 hour after 75 g glucose (24–28 weeks), if negative in first trimester • Quadruple marker (16–20 weeks) if double marker not done	• Inj T Toxoid (5 mL) IM 2 doses 4–6 weeks apart second dose at least two week before delivery • Anthelmintic A single dose of albendazole (400 mg) or mebendazole (500 mg) endemic area • Iron, calcium
Third trimester	Blood pressure, height, weight, fundal height, fetal heart rate, breast examination at term Investigation: • Hemoglobin, urine • Indirect Coombs' test (28 weeks) • USG 32–34 weeks (growth scan) • NST, if indicated • Pelvic assessment at 36 weeks	• Antenatal prophylaxis with anti-D immunoglobulin in non-sensitized Rh-negative pregnant women at 28 and 34 weeks of gestation to prevent RhD-alloimmunization is only recommended in the context of rigorous research • Continue iron, calcium

Abbreviations: NT, nuchal translucency; NB, nasal bone; VDRL, veneral disease research laboratory; Urine-R, M, urine-routine microscopically; TSH, thyroid-stimulating hormone; HBsAg, hepatitis B surface antigen; DV, ductus venous; TR, tricuspid regurgitation.

also contribute immensely to newborn survival, it is for this reason that they must be strengthened.

PROPHYLAXIS

Although even by effective antenatal care certain conditions like postpartum hemorrhage, abruptio placentae, amniotic fluid embolism cannot be predicted but effective antenatal care can prevent anemia and other high-risk conditions. Early detection of pre-eclampsia, GDM and IUGR cases can improve maternal and fetal morbidity and mortality.

CONCLUSION

Antenatal period provides clinician, windows of opportunity to predict, and prevent the worse outcome in pregnancy. Early antenatal visit of women should be utilized to screen high-risk and low-risk groups. The high-risk groups need frequent visits for effective management and for desirable outcome. Woman of low-risk groups also needs cluster of visits in initial pregnancy to be differentiated as low-risk woman and their further visits can be reduced as per requirement. That is how we can say that trend of antenatal visits is changing due to better understanding of obstetrics and newer developments in biophysical, biochemical and genetic tests.

IMPORTANT POINTS

- Early diagnosis of fetal abnormalities can be done at 11–13 weeks by detail examination of fetal anatomy.
- Specialist fetal echocardiography should be done in whom presence of reversed a wave in the ductus venosus or tricuspid regurgitation at 11–13 weeks is demonstrated.
- The rate of miscarriage an stillbirth after demonstration of live fetus at 11–13 weeks are about 1 and 0.4% respectively.
- Increased uterine artery pulsatility index reflects the underlying mechanism for development of pre-eclampsia.
- Universal screening for gestational diabetes should be offered to every antenatal patient at first antenatal visit.
- Early estimation of patient specific risk for pregnancy complications would improve pregnancy outcome by shifting antenatal care to a more individualized and disease-specific approach.

REFERENCES

1. Implementation of ANC guideline and recommendations: introducing the 2016 WHO-ANC new model pg 2015. WHO recommendations on antenatal care for appositive pregnancy experience, 2016 [Internet] [cited on 28 nov 2016] Available from *www.Who.int/reproductivehealth/publications/maternal_ perinatal_health/anc-positive-pregnancy-experience/ en.*
2. Nicolaides KH. A model for a new pyramid of prenatal care based on 11–13 weeks assesement. Prenatal Diag. 2011;31(1): 3-6. doi: 10.1002/pd.2685
3. M Hod, et al. FIGO initiative on gestational diabetes mellitus: apragmatic guide for diagnosis, management and care. International Journal of Gynecology and Obst. 2015;131(3): 173-211.
4. Seshiah V, Das AK, Balaji V, Joshi SR, Parikh MN, Gupta S, Diabetes in Pregnancy study group. Gestational diabetes, Guidelines. J Association Physicians India. 2006;54:622-8.
5. Sujata Mishra. Effect of endocrine disorders on neonate. In: Thanawala U, Wani R (Eds). FOGSI Focus, the Healthy Generation X, 2015.
6. Shrivastava M, Malay SB, Saxena R, Shrivastava A. Screening guidelines for haemoglobinopathy in antenatal care. In: Gupta S (Ed). FOGSI Focus, Update in Antenatal Care, 2016.
7. Nicolaides KH, Azar G, Byrne D, Mansur C, Mark K. Fetal nuchal translucency: ultrasound screening for chromosomal defects in first trimester of pregnancy. BMJ. 1992;304:867-89.
8. Snijiders RJ, Noble P, Sebire N, Souka A, Nicolaides KH. UK multicentre project on assessment of risk of trisomy 21 by maternal age and fetal nuchal—translucency thickness at 10–14 weeks of gestation. Fetal Medicine Foundation First Trimester Screening Group. Lancet. 1998;352:343-6.
9. Brizot ML, Snijders RJM, Bersinger NA, Kuln P, Nicolaides KH. Maternal serum pregnancy associated placental protein A and fetal nuchal translucency thickness for the prediction of fetal trisomies in early pregnancy. Obstet Gynecol. 1994;84:918-22.
10. Bindra R, Heath V, Liao A, Spencer K, Nicolaides KH. One stop clinic for assessment of risk for trisomy 21 at 11–14 weeks: a prospective study of 15,030 pregnancies. Ultrasound Obstet Gynecol. 2002;20:219-25.
11. Spencer K, Spencer CE, Power M, Dawson C, Nicolaides KH. Screening for chromosomal abnormalities in the first trimester using ultrasound and maternal serum biochemistry in a one stop clinic: a review of three years prospective experience. Br J Obstet Gynaecol. 2003;110:281-6.
12. Wald NJ, Rodeck C, Hackshaw AK, Walters J, Chitty L, Mackinson AM. SURUSS Research Group: First and Second trimester antenatal screening for Down's syndrome: the result of the serum, urine and ultrasound screening Study (SURUSS). Health technol Assess. 2003;7:1-77.
13. Kagan KO, Wright D, Baker A, Sahota D, Nicolaides KH. Screening for trisomy 21 by maternal age, fetal nuchal translucency thickness, free beta-human chorionic gonadotropins and pregnancy-associated plasma protein A. Ultrasound Obstet Gynecol. 2008;31:618-24.
14. Wright D, Spencer K, Kagan KO, Torring N, Petersen OB, Christou A, Kallikas J, Nacolaids KH. First trimester combined screening for trisomy 21 at 7–14 weeks' gestation. Ultrasound Obstet Gynecol. 2010;36:404-11.
15. Nicolaides KH, Spencer K, Avgidou K, Faiola S, Falcon O. Multicenter study of first trimester screening for trisomy 21 in 75, 821 pregnancies: result and estimation of the potential impact of individual risk-oriented two stage first trimester screening. Ultrasound Obstet Gynaecol. 2005;35:221-6.
16. American College of Obstetrician and Gynaecologist, screening for fetal chromosomal abnormalities. ACOG practice Bulletin No. 77. Obstet Gynaecol. 2007;109:217-27. PMID17197615.

17. Kagan KO, Cicero S, Staboulidou I, Wright D, Nicolaides KH. Fetal nasal bone in screening for trisomies 21, 18 and 13 and turner syndrome at 11–13 weeks of gestation. Ultrasound Obstet Gynaecol. 2009;33:259-64.
18. Maiz N, Valenlcia C, Kagan KO, Wright D, Nicolaides KH. Ductus venosus Doppler in screening for trisomies 21, 18 and 13 and Turner syndrome at 11–13 weeks of gestation. Ultrasound Obstet Gynaecol. 2009;33:512-7.
19. How accurate is the new blood test for Down Syndrome. Mark Leach. 2013;30 downsyndromeparenting.com.
20. Allan LD. Echocardiographic detection of congenital heart disease in the fetus: present and future. Br heart J. 1995;74:103-6.
21. Hyett J, Perdu M, Sharland G, Snijders R, Nicolaides KH. Using fetal nuchal translucency to screen for major congenital cardiac defects at 10–14 weeks of gestation population based cohort study. BMJ. 1999;318:81-5.
22. Matias A, Huggon I, Areias JC, Montengro N, Nicolaids KH. Cardiac defects in chromosomally normal fetuses with abnormal ductus venosus blood flow at 10–14 weeks. Ultrasound Obstet and Gynecol. 1999;14:307-10.
23. Chaoui R, Benoit B, Mitkowska Wozniak H, Heling KS, Nicolaides KH. Assessment of intracranial translucency (IT) in the detection of spinal bifida at the 11 to 13 weeks scan. Utrasound Obstet Gynecol. 2009;34:249-52.
24. Lachman R, Chaoui R, Moratolaa J, Piciarelli G, Nicolaides KH. Posterior brain in fetuses with spina bifida at 11–13 weeks. Prenat Diagn. 2011:31:103-6.
25. Akolekar R, Bower S, Flack N, Bilardo CM, Nicolaides KH. Prediction of miscarriage and stillbirth at 11–13 weeks and the contribution of chorionic villus sampling. Prenatal diagn. 2011;31:38-45.
26. Akolekar R, Syngelaki A, Sarquis R, Wright D, Nicolaides KH. Prediction of preeclampsia from biophysical and biochemical markes at 11–13 weeks. Prenatal Diagnosis. 2011;31;66-74.
27. Poon LC, Karagiannis G, Staboulidou I, Shefici A, Nicolaides KH. Reference range of birth weight with gestation and first trimester prediction of small for gestation neonates. Prenat Diagn. 2011;31:58-65.
28. Karagiannis G, Akolekar R, Sarquis R, Wright D, Nicolaides KH. Prediction of small for gestation neonates from biophysical and biochemical markers at 11–13 weeks. Fetal Diagn Ther 2010, E- Pub Ahead of print. DOI: 10, 1159/000321694.
29. Evidence and recommendations, WHO recommendations on antenatal care for appositive pregnancy experience 2016. [Internet][cited on28nov2016] Available from *www.Who.int/reproductivehealth/publications/maternal_perinatal_health/anc-positive-pregnancy-experience en/37.*
30. Sharma A, Gupta N. Optimum use of ultrasound in antenatal care. In: Sadhna Gupta (editor). FOGSI Update in Antenatal Care, FOGSI Focus; 2016.
31. Intervention for common physiological symptom, WHO recommendations on antenatal care for appositive pregnancy experience 2016. [Internet][cited on 28 nov 2016] Available from *www.Who.int/reproductivehealth/publications/maternal_perinatal_health/anc-positive-pregnancy-experience/en/37.*
32. Guideline: daily iron and folic acid supplementation in pregnant women. Geneva: World Health Organization; 2012 (*http://www.who.int/nutrition/publications/micronutrients/guidelines/daily_ifa_supp_pregnant_women/en/*).
33. Maternal immunization against tetanus: integrated management of pregnancy and childbirth (IMPAC). Standards for maternal and neonatal care 1.1. Geneva: Department of Making Pregnancy Safer, World Health Organization; 2006 (*http://www.who.int/reproductivehealth/publications/maternal_perinatal_health/immunization_tetanus.pdf,*).
34. Guideline: preventive chemotherapy to control soil-transmitted helminth infections in high-risk groups. Geneva: World Health Organization; 2016 (in press).
35. Healthy diet. Fact sheet No. 394. Geneva: World Health Organization; 2015 (*http://www.who.int/mediacentre/factsheets/fs394/en/*, accessed 1 November 2016).
36. Exercise in pregnancy. RCOG Statement No. 4. Royal College of Obstetricians and Gynaecologists. 2006:1-7. *(https://www.rcog.org.uk/en/guidelines-research-services/guidelines/exercise-in-pregnancy-statement-no.4/, accessed 24 October 2016).*
37. Rasmussen KM, Yaktine AL. Institute of Medicine and National Research Council. Weight gain during pregnancy: re-examining the guidelines. Washington (DC): The National Academies Press; 2009 (*http://www.nationalacademies.org/hmd.*
38. Crowther C, Middleton P. Anti-D administration after childbirth for preventing rhesus alloimmunization. Cochrane Database Syst Rev. 1997;(2):CD000021.
39. Bujold E, Riberge S, Lacasse Y, Bureau M, Giguere Y. Prevention of preeclampsia and intrauterine growth restriction with aspirin started in early pregnancy. A meta-analysis Obstet Gynaecol. 2010;116:402-14.
40. Pawar AP, Damania KR. Identification and antipartum surveillance of high risk pregnancy. Arias Practical Guide to High Risk Pregnancy and Delivery, 4th edn; 2015. pp. 116-31.
41. Lodha P. Screening guide line for fetal aneuploidies. Gupta S (editor). Update in Antenatal Care. FOGSI Focus; 2016.

Chapter 2

Missing Dimensions in Antenatal Care

Pushpa Pandey, Deepak Dwivedi, Shashi Khare, Shubhada Neel

INTRODUCTION

Antenatal care of the mother is a key component of a healthy pregnancy. Effective antenatal care translates into having a healthy mother and a healthy baby. Good antenatal care engenders a healthy behavior, and a healthy life style. WHO defines 'health as a state of physical, mental and social well-being of an individual and not merely the absence of disease'. Many more dimensions which have been cited such as, spiritual, emotional and vocational dimensions. The human being is a continuum of spiritual, mental and physical energy. Health is a dynamic process of harmony in the flow of spiritual, mental and physical energy. The current conventional approach addresses only one dimension, i.e. physical body. This might explain why despite the state-of-the-art advancements in the field of medical sciences, the epidemic of any syndrome has not been restrained.[1]

The fact that a human being (who is made up of physical body and psyche or consciousness) is not one-dimensional, now calls for a new model of health. Pregnancy is a boon to a lady. From the moment mother discovers the pregnancy, she has to take care of two human beings, herself and the baby inside the womb (*The fetus has the same energy (life) as an adult*).

Scientific Evidence of Wise Life *In Utero*

- Fetus begins to swallow amniotic fluid at 12 weeks of gestation and can learn tastes experienced only prenatally. Fetus favors its mother's meal and pick up the food taste culture in the womb. Healthy food habit of expectant mother is necessary to develop a positive taste culture of child which is the root cause of many diseases.[2]
- Fifer has found that fetal heart rate slows when the mother is speaking, suggesting that fetus not only hears and recognizes the sound, but calmed by it.[2]
- A premature baby is aware of and responds to the sound around it.
- Fetus reacts to loud voice and, prefers mother's voice.
- Newborn prefers a story read to it repeatedly in the womb.
- The nervous system develops fully from eight months onwards as they start thinking and memorizing the events.[3]
- The fetus experiences the rapid eye movement (REM) sleep of dream, just as adult do.

Due to advancement in technology, antenatal care is not only routine palpation, supplying folic acid, iron, calcium but it includes diagnostic modality of imaging, biochemical, biophysical marker, vaccination, screening for medical and obstetric disorders. WHO proposes eight clinical goals oriented and focused antenatal visits. Traditional concept of impetus on third trimester during antenatal care is changing to inversion of traditional pyramid with main emphasis on first trimester. However in the conventional antenatal care, even now no attention is being given to mental and social health or wellbeing of developing fetus.

It has been studied, that unfavorable conditions, events during early development, in womb also have a profound impact on the risk of behavioral abnormalities or future adult diseases. Researchers have also confirmed that babies exposed to nutritional and non-nutritional stress, during critical periods of development are more prone to diseases. It has been proven, that personality begins to take shape in the womb and that it is greatly influenced by mother's feeling and state of mind, during pregnancy. Likewise behavioral traits also originate in the womb. Infants, toddlers and adolescents largely suffer from many emotional and behavioral problems, the seeds of which are sown on the unborn baby due to negative hormonal secretions that are activated by mother's thoughts in response to stress.

MENTAL HEALTH

Mental health is not mere absence of mental illness. It is a state of well-being in which an individual realizes his or her own abilities to cope with normal stressors of life. Tension, anger and stress are increasing day by day. During pregnancy such mental stress, directly or indirectly, influences the health of the mother and the fetus.

Causes of Stress during Pregnancy

Stress is a reaction to change:
- *Internal*: Body, mind
- *External*: Unwanted pregnancy, family, environmental, sex of baby, job stress, economic fluctuation, etc.

Harmful Effects of Stress on Pregnant Mother

Stress causes increase in the level of stress-hormone, miscarriage,[4] PIH,[5] IUGR,[6] intrauterine infection, preterm delivery. Chronic maternal stress is a significant and independent risk factor for preterm birth. Maternal stress may act by one or both of the two physiological pathways, *neuroendocrine* pathway, where in maternal stress may ultimately result in premature activation of the maternal placental fetal endocrine system that promote parturition or *immune/inflammatory* pathway, in which maternal stress modulate systemic and local (placental-decidual) immunity to increase susceptibility to intrauterine and fetal infectious processes and thereby promote labor through proinflammatory process.[7]

Antenatal Psychological Stress

Influence on Fetal Physiology and Behavior

Maternal stress and anxiety during pregnancy is associated with a host of negative consequences for the fetus and its subsequent development. Fetal heart rate, activity, sleep pattern and movement have been shown to influenced by maternal psychological state. Dipietro et al. 2003 studied fetal response to induced maternal stress in 137 expectant mothers at 24 weeks and 36 weeks gestation, fetal activity monitored via actocardiograph as well as maternal EKG (electrocardiogram) and skin conductance latency (SCL) during a lab-induced stressor and found FHR variability significantly increased ($p<0.0001$) fetal movement significantly decreased ($p<0.001$) during lab-induced stressor.[8] Early gestational stress exposure is associated with negative outcomes at different developmental stages, slowed maturation and behavioral response patterns in fetuses, alterations in neonatal stress regulation and behavioral reactions to stress, blunted cognitive functions and emotional and behavioral problems in infants and toddlers, and reduced brain volume in areas associated with cognitive function in children.
- Prenatal maternal stress and anxiety may have negative consequences for children later in life, such as autism, the development of attention deficit hyperactivity disorder or lowered performance on aspects of executive function.
- It is hypothesized that maternal stress may affect the intrauterine environment and alter fetal development during critical periods, through either activation of the placental stress system causing the release and circulation of corticotropin releasing hormone, or through diminished blood flow and oxygen to the uterus.[9,10]

SOCIAL HEALTH

Social health has been defined as the 'quantity and quality of an individual's interpersonal ties and the extent of involvement with the community'.[11]

One of the reason of not improving anemia, in women in developing countries is, inspite of free supply of iron tablet, pregnant women do not take regular iron due to social taboos, minor side effects and not having faith on free supply, even ASHA, *Anganwadi* workers are not able to counsel the beneficiaries. Nutrition Foundation India Survey in Assam showed that only 32% of pregnant women received IFA tablets out of which only 4.9% consumed them, and corresponding figure in Madhya Pradesh were 74% and 6.3%.[12]

Social health also includes relationship at home, work and family. A bad social relationship makes the environment stressful, leads to addictions, violence, bad dietary habits and unhealthy life style which affect mother's and fetus' health due to malnutrition.

It is widely accepted that chronic diseases such as type 2 diabetes and coronary heart disease, may have been triggered by circumstances before birth *in utero* nutrition in particular. Dr David Barker first popularized the concept of 'fetal origins of adult disease' **(Flow chart 2.1)**. Barker hypothesized that associations between small size at birth or during infancy and later coronary vascular disease reflect permanent effects of under nutrition. The fetus depends on nutrients of mother, inadequate supply of nutrients due to prioritization of brain growth other tissues such as an abdominal viscera causes reduced secretion of fetal growth hormones and IGF-1 (insulin-like growth factor-1) and upregulation of hypothalamopituitary adrenal axis. Fetal origins of adult disease (FOAD) hypothesis proposes that although occurring in response to a transient phenomenon fetal undernutrition, these adaptations become permanent or programmed because they occur during critical period of times. Indian figures of undernutrition are worse than those of sub-Saharan Africa.[13]

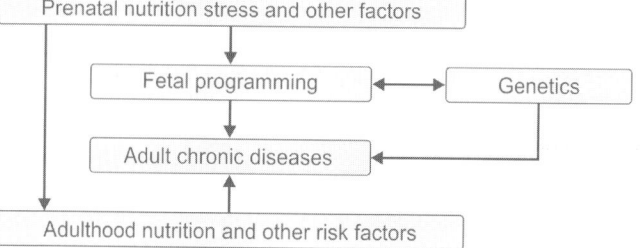

Flow chart 2.1: Fetal origins of adult disease

According to fetal origins hypothesis, effects of fetal conditions are persistent. Second, health effects can remain latent for many years. Third, effects reflect specific biological mechanism, possibly through impact of the environment on epigenome (A network of chemical compounds surrounding DNA that modify genome without altering the DNA sequences and have a role in determining which genes are active in a particular cell).[14] In Dutch Hunger-Winter 1944 series of studies, Brown and colleagues have shown that fetal development during this period is associated with a two fold increase in risk of schizophrenia, schizoid/ shizopytal personality disorder, as well as affective disorder in adulthood. There are two interpretations of the causal mechanism of these effects. First, deficiency of micro- and macronutrients such as folate or overall calorie nutrition could directly alter brain development. Second maternal stress, secondary to famine, could have neurotoxic effects on brain regions relevant to mental illness. There are extensive studies on prenatal stress in animals that support the latter interpretation.[8]

Fetus starts listening from the six months within womb.[15] Many pregnant women report a fetal jerk or kick just after a door slam. Medical advances in 3D ultrasound prove that these fetuses respond, positively or negatively, to outside voice. The negative environment (abuse or violence) affects the health of mother, may cause preterm delivery or intrauterine infection. In addition, fetal brain may get traumatized directly due to decrease in the blood supply to the brain, which may lead to many physical or behavioral disorders in children and adolescents.

The mythological story of Saint Ashtawakra depicts the traumatic effect of loud noises and abuses on the fetus. Ashtawakra is a sage mentioned in Hindu scriptures. His parents wished for an intelligent and a spiritual child. Kahod, his father, was a scholar yet arrogant. He would recite scriptures to his wife, Sujata, during her pregnancy. Consequently, the baby learned everything when inside the womb and grew up to be very intelligent. It is believed that Ashtawakra, when still in womb, interrupted his father eight times to indicate that his knowledge is pedantic and not spiritual. Kahod rebuked and cursed his own baby eight times that caused the eight curves in his body. Ashtawakra epitomizes a baby with cerebral palsy and high IQ. Cerebral palsy (CP) is a general term for a group of permanent, non-progressive movement disorders that cause physical disability. It is caused by damage to the motor control centers of the developing brain that can occur during pregnancy, during childbirth, or after birth due to some reason which is still debatable. As prenatal events are thought to be responsible for approximately 75% of all causes of cerebral palsy, although it is usually impossible to determine the nature and exact timing of event.[16]

Vice-versa is also true. If the mother listens to relaxing music, in last trimester of pregnancy, the baby responds positively to the resonant sound and after birth when it is exposed to the same music it calmed down. Feijoo paired maternal relaxation (the UCS) with music (the CS) and examined individuals as fetuses and after birth. After 24 pairings of the stimuli, when the music was played in the last weeks of pregnancy, fetuses began moving and when played to the newborn, these babies stopped crying, opened their eyes and exhibited fewer clonic movements.

In another study, researched the ability of the fetus to learn a TV theme tune. during pregnancy (and heard the theme tune) became alert stopped moving and their heart rate decreased (orienting) upon hearing the tune. In this study, the first group consisted of pregnant mothers who frequently watched "*Neighbors*", an Australian television soap opera.[3] After delivery, these mothers were asked to watch the TV show again along with their babies. It was observed that the newborn babies (2–4 days of age) became alert, stopped moving and their heart rate decreased (orienting) upon hearing the theme song. These same individuals showed no such reaction to other unfamiliar tunes. The newborns of the second group of pregnant mothers, who did not watch the same TV program during pregnancy, showed no reaction to the tune.

SPIRITUAL HEALTH

Spiritual Health refers to that part of the individual which reaches out and strives for meaning and purpose in life. However, present medical scenario is devoid of this aspect. We need to understand spirituality to comprehend and become spiritual healthy. Spirituality is to know oneself and the higher self, i.e. to explore '*swa*', the inner self (soul) and '*sth*', the consciousness. Ipso facto the Hindi word for health, '*swasth*' literally means 'the inner self-consciousness'. The inner self-consciousness encompasses aspects of the enduring and the immortal spirit. Practicing this fact will lead to stability and security, which, in-turn, would lead to peace, love and happiness. On the contrary, the outer self-consciousness encompasses aspects, role or material things that are ever-changing and mortal. Focusing merely on the of the outer leads to instability and insecurity, which, in turn, leads to anger, anxiety, depression, type-A behavior, isolation and chronic life stresses. By abstraction we can conclude that, a healthy life-style means an 'inner self-conscious life style.[1]

Traditionally, a medical personnel was a combination of priest/priestess with some medical knowledge. Gradually, the concept of spiritual principles from healing languished and in the modern medicine completely disappeared. Sadly, at present patients are being treated as machines. The word 'Holistic', as described by Jan C. Smurt, means 'whole' or 'complete'. Around 70 to 80 years ago when the dichotomy in the state of being of the human being used to be emphasized, i.e. 'spirit' the psyche and consciousness energy that drives the force 'being'. So the multidimensional health model is the need of the hour.

In holistic health model, 'consciousness (the soul), is the meta-physical and primary system of energy. At molecular and genetic level, 98% of the human body is replaced from every minute to every year; what is continuous is the 'consciousness', which recreate the body and the brain again and again including the DNA. Past birth regression therapy and cases of near death experiences, confirm the existence of meta-physical energy. It has seven innate qualities, viz. knowledge, peace, love, purity, happiness, power and bliss (spiritual energy). This metaphysical energy acts through the mind 'thoughts, judgements, feelings, emotions' and integrates with the biological energy of the body through the nervous and endocrine system, thereby nourishing every cell of body.[17] During stress internal and external pressure exceeds the inner mental strength. Inner strength can be increased by practicing spirituality.

Personality (health or behavior) is influenced by spiritual energy received at different level:
- Every one has their own innate qualities (i.e. spiritual energy)
- Spiritual energy carried forward from the past birth.
  - The spiritual energy carries forward an imprint of defects from the past birth to the next. Dr Ian Stevenson found that about 35% of children who claim to remember previous lives have birth marks and/or birth defects. These marks/defects attribute to the wounds of a person whose life the child remembers.[18] About 2700 cases of children who claim to remember previous lives have been investigated from several countries. The subjects of these cases, from a very early age, display unusual behavioral and physical features (facial appearance, gait, birth marks and birth defects, etc.) that are unusual for present circumstances but correspond with the physical features of diseased person (previous personality) whose life they claim to remember.[19] Birth defects might be result of 'memories' carried forward from the past birth that appear as abnormalities in the genes.
- Spiritual energy received from mother and father.
  - A pregnant mother has two lives within—hers and the fetuses. With spiritual energy, she can nourish both and neutralize the effect of negative energy (past *karma*), in-turn, changing physical body at molecular level (i.e.the DNA) and making both (herself and fetus) physically and mentally healthy.

Personality is colored after birth by family, company and environment.

How expectant mothers can take care of their mental, social and spiritual health?

Antenatal mothers should take care of their mental health by nourishing their minds through listening to calming music and reading positive books. This helps to create positive mental energy (thoughts, emotions, attitude and memory—a positive TEAM). Spiritual life-style and regular meditation practice (an important aspect of spirituality) helps adapt positive thinking, manage stress and improve mental, social and physical health. Spiritual energy can be increased by various methods:
- Selfless service
- Prayer
- Belief in the higher self
- Awareness of the Karmic pattern
- *Pranayama*
- *Yoga* and meditation (i.e.soul conscious life style).

Meditation

Meditation enables us to look within and make contact with our inner truth. It is to channelize the thoughts in a positive direction. It is a mental exercise and the practice of higher consciousness. Meditation and medicine has come from the greek word '*medri*' which means 'to heal. The inner peace and silence that emanate during meditation also affect our physical bodies **(Fig. 2.1)**.

Mantra meditation: Wiki describes *Mantra* as a sacred utterance, a numinous sound, a syllable, word or phonemes, or group of words in Sanskrit believed by practitioners to have psychological and spiritual powers. An alternate meaning of the sacred word is 'advice'. The *mantra* 'Om Shanti' advises us to be conscious of our essential spirituality. We should chant this *mantra* with its true understanding—'*I am, I exist, my existence is spiritual, unending, divine, eternally pure and my essence is peace*'.

Dhyan meditation: Aimed at developing concentration on a sacred object. When one focuses upon a sacred object for a long period of time, the impact of that vision can bring an internal state of sacred awareness.

Pranayama: Meditation upon breath is a favored technique, because breath is considered to be sacred life force. *Pranayama* improves our physical health **(Fig. 2.1)**.

Rajyoga meditation: '*Yoga*' means 'union'. *Rajyoga* meditation is the communion of inner self with supreme. It is the science and art of harmonizing spiritual, mental and physical energy through a connection with the ultimate source of spiritual energy called the 'Supreme soul' (Power house of spiritual energy). It is the state of soul consciousness and a positive life style. It enhances an individual's power of determination to manage and practice positive thoughts, emotions, attitudes, memories and the will to adhere to healthy diet, exercise, sleep, medication and cessation of smoking.[1]

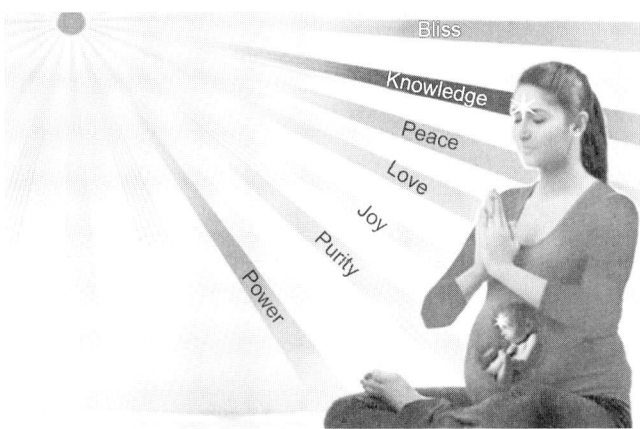

Fig. 2.1: Meditation
(*Photo courtesy:* Dr Shubhda Neel and Dr Pushpa Pandey)

How Meditation (or Spirituality) Improves Outcome of Pregnancy?

- It raises energy level and strengthens the immune system to ward of infections.
- It stimulates healthy life style changes a healthy diet, exercise, proper sleep.
- Meditation increases the spiritual energy within, neutralizes the cause and effect of *karma* and improves birth outcome.
- It nourishes the fetus with spiritual energy by creating positive thoughts as fetus gets positive chemical signals through placenta.
- It enhances positivity of a person, and reduces stress, alleviates catastrophic reaction, caused by adverse environment, unwanted pregnancy and economic problems by changing attitude and belief system.
- During the process endorphin and enkaphalin are secreted, which help to detach oneself from various kind of pain.
- It strengthens patients to tolerate various types of pains during antenatal period as well as during labor.
- It decreases metabolic rate and lowers the heart rate, which also indicate a state of deep rest. It improves sleep and decreases stress hormones, and blood lactate levels.
- In various studies, it was found that the number of preterm labor and pregnancy-induced hypertension with associated intrauterine growth restriction (IUGR), were significantly lower, in the group of mothers that practiced *Yoga*[9] and meditation[20] during their pregnancy. Also, the number of babies with birth weight of 2500 g or more was found to be significantly higher.
- It increases visualization power and subconscious mind comes to surface, visualization can be leveraged for better pregnancy outcome, a healthy happy baby and smooth progression of labor.
- It helps to give up addictions, and decrease depression anxiety, diabetes, hypertension, migraine tension headache.[21]
- It helps to instill positive *sanskars* in the fetus through mind-body-medicine approach.

Holistic health care of the expectant mother and the developing fetus is popularly known as 'Garbh Sanskar'. *Garbh Sanskar* means educating or training the mind of fetus. The famous mythological story of *Abhimanyu*, son of *Arjuna* and *Subhadra*, beautifully depicts the meaning of *garbh sanskar*. Arjuna once recounted the way to enter the 'chakravyuha' (military formation of *Kaurava* army) to *Subhadra* during her pregnancy. Abhimanyu learned it in the womb. He remembered it even in his youth and was able to apply the strategy to enter the powerful *Chakravyuha* battle. Healthy life style adopted by pregnant mother, which is taught in 'garbh sanskasr' has also great impact on their own health. The mothers are advised to consume good nutritious diet, avoid spicy food and addictive substances, practice *asanas* and sleep adequately. It is also recommended to read good books and listen to positive verses and relaxing alpha music every morning throughout the pregnancy. Reading fiction novels and watching TV serials is inadvisable. Reading out loud good stories and healthy discussions between parents improves baby's memory. These habits inculcate positive thinking in the mothers. A spiritual life style and morning meditation practice also alleviate stress.

From the mouth of a fetus:

"Dear Mom,

You are the most important person in my life. I am blessed to have divine mother like you. Please take care of your physical, mental, social and spiritual health. Healthy food and positive thinking will decide my future health and personality. Mom, I enjoy the healthy food you eat, the good stories you read to me and the good music, you listen to. I like the good vibrations when you practice meditation. The two little words "Thank You" can be never be enough to appreciate every little thing you will ever do for me.

Lots of love, Unborn little baby (Fetus)".

IMPORTANT POINTS

- Stress during pregnancy, directly or indirectly affects the mother's health and harms the fetus's growth
- In this fast-paced stressful world, calming music, good books and positive thinking are very important for improving mental and social health.
- Practice of meditation and *Yoga* during pregnancy are the important tools, to achieve spiritual health; they help alleviate stress and improve mother's health and pregnancy outcome.
- Physicians, should provide holistic health care, to expectant mothers in their antenatal clinics.

REFERENCES

1. Gupta S, et al. Regression of coronary atherosclerosis through healthy life style. Indian Heart J. 2011;63:461-9.
2. Khera N. Antenatal care beyond medicine, *Garbh Sanskar*. Sadhna Gupta (Ed). FOGSI focus, Preconception and Antenatal care, Fogsi publication. 2016. pp. 14-6.
3. Happer PG, et al. Fetal memory; does it exist? Acta Paediatri suppl. 1996;416:16-20.
4. Ishita P, Parikh RM, Sonawala S, Parikh FR. The role of stress in first trimester miscarriage. Krishna, Usha Shah D (Eds). Pregnancy at Risk, Volume 2. Jaypee Brothers Medical Publishers, 2010.
5. Parera N, et al. Psychological stress during pregnancy is a risk factor for PIH. Journal of the College of Community Physicians of Sri Lanka. 2011;16:35-9.
6. Herrichs J, et al. Maternal psychological distress and fetal growth trajectories: The generation study. Psychological Medicine. 2010;40:633-43.
7. Pathik D, Wadhwa A, et al. Stress, infection and preterm birth: A biobehavioural perspective. Paediatric and perinatal Epidemiology. 2001;15(Suppl 2):17-29.
8. Kinsella MT, Monk C. Impact of maternal stress, depression and anxiety on fetal neurobehavioral development. Clin Obstet Gynecol. 2009;52(3)425-40.
9. Curtis K, et al. Systematic Review of *Yoga* for Pregnant Women: Current Status and Future Direction. Evidence base Complementary and Alternative Medicine; 2012(internet) [cited 2016feb2]; Article ID715942. doi:10.1155/2012/715942.
10. Weinstock M. The potential influence of maternal stress hormones on development and mental health of the offspring. Brain Beha Immun. 2005;19(4):296-308.
11. K Park. Concept of Health and Disease. Preventive and social Medicine, Published by Banarilal Bhanot, Jabalpur. 23rd edn; 2015.
12. Nutrition Foundation of India. Comprehensive situational analysis on demand and supply of micronutrients supplements. Madhya Pradesh. Nutrition foundation of India; 1998.
13. Calkins K, Devaskar SU. Fetal origins of adult disease. Curr Probl Pediatr Health Care. 2011;41(6:)158.
14. "World Bank Report". Source: The World Bank (2009). Retrieved 2009-03-13. World Bank Report on Malnutrition in India.
15. Birnholz JC. The development of human fetal hearing. Science. 1983;222(4623):516-8 DOI: 10.1126/science. 6623091.
16. Reddihough DS, Jcollins K. The epidemiology and causes of cerebral palsy. Australian Journal of Physiotherapy. 2003;(49):7-12.
17. Nair N. Eternal play of physical and metaphysical energies, Mystery of Universe, published by Prajapita Brahmakumaris Ishvariya Vishwavidyalaya Mount Abu Rajasthan. 2008. pp. 10-11.
18. Stevenson I. Birth marks and birth defects corresponding to wound of diseased person. Journal of Scientific Exploration. 1993;94(7):403-10.
19. Pasricha SK. Twins who claimed to remember previous lives, Nimhans Journal, 18 (1 and 2) January and April 2000. pp. 39-51.
20. Valslan Nair. Published Glimpses of 30 years to humanity, editor by medical wing of *Rajyoga* and Research Foundation 2015; divine mother baby project 85.
21. Kiran, et al. Indian Effect of *Rajyoga* Meditation on Chronic Tension Headache. Indian J Physiol Pharmacol. 2014;58(2):157-61.

Chapter 3

Nutrition in Pregnancy

Roza Olyai, S Sampathkumari

INTRODUCTION

Nutrition in pregnancy is of vital importance as the intake of nutrients and dietary planning has to provide for the bodily requirements of both the mother and the fetus but also take care of the progressive requirement during gestation and the inadequacy will hamper the fetal development and is capable of causing delivery time problem as well as lifelong ailments for the fetus including imminent casualties. Hence, planning for nutrition for the mothers should start before conception continues through gestation and extends up to the period of lactation. An inadequate or excessive amount of some nutrients may cause malformations or medical problems in the fetus, and neurological disorders and handicaps are some of the risks run by malnourished mothers.[1] About 23.8% of babies worldwide are estimated to be born with lower than optimal weights at birth due to lack of proper nutrition.[2] Personal habits in the early stages of pregnancy such as smoking, alcohol, caffeine, use of certain medications and street drugs can negatively and irreversibly affect the developmental process of the baby.[3] Caffeine is also sometimes said to harm the unborn baby, however, there is not enough evidence to say if this is true.[2] There is also a misconception that the patient should eat for two, whereas in reality a right and balanced intake by the mother ensures the appropriate and normal fetal development. The recommended weight gain during pregnancy is based on pre-pregnancy BMI.

Pre-pregnancy BMI	BMI (kg/m^2) WHO	Total wt gain (range/kg)	Mean range kg/week
Under weight	<18.5	2.5–18.0	0.50
Normal weight	18.5–24.9	11.5–16.0	0.40
Overweight	25.0–29.9	7.0–11.5	0.27
Obese	>30.0	5.0–9.0	0.23

Source: Institute of Medicine (IOM) Resource sheet, May 2009

Nutrition is important before pregnancy, to prepare the body for the baby during pregnancy to make sure the baby is safe, after birth for lactation and post-delivery to get her body back to healthier state.

ENERGY REQUIREMENTS

Energy requirement during pregnancy comprises weight gain with protein, fat and water. The increase in BMR relative to pre-pregnancy values are 5.3, 11.4, 25.3% during first, second, third trimester.[4] Main source of energy is from carbohydrates (55–65%) from whole grain, legumes, vegetables and fruits.

PROTEIN REQUIREMENTS IN PREGNANCY

Protein is essential to meet the demand for the growth of the fetus, placenta, uterus, breasts, and blood volume. Adequate energy intake is required along with adequate protein intake to allow protein and amino acid to be used for this function. Additional protein is needed during pregnancy and lactation. Appropriate balancing of legumes with cereals advised to increase protein quality and quantity. Sources of protein include beans, pulses, fish, eggs, meat (but avoid liver), poultry and nuts.

If gestational weight gain of 10 kg additional protein required are 0.5, 6.9 and 22.7 g/day during first, second and third trimesters.[5] Protein intake should be preferably by natural and not commercial high protein supplements. Recommended safe allowance during lactation are 19 g for 1–6 months and 13 g for 6–12 months.

FAT REQUIREMENTS DURING PREGNANCY

Fat provides energy and fatty acids serve as vehicle for fat soluble vitamins and facilitate absorption. During pregnancy in earlier stage fetus uses fatty acid supplied by mother and in later stage makes its own.[6] The minimum daily energy requirement of fat should be 20%. For this, the diet of pregnant women should contain at least 30 g of visible fat and

200 mg/day of DHA for optimum adult health and fetal development. Polyunsaturated fatty acids, specifically docosahexaenoic acid (DHA) and eicosapentaenoic acid (EPA) are very beneficial. The best dietary source of omega-3 fatty acids is oily fish. Some other omega-3 fatty acids not found in fish can be found in foods such as flaxseeds, walnuts, pumpkin seeds, and enriched eggs.

CARBOHYDRATE REQUIREMENTS DURING PREGNANCY

Carbohydrate are either simple or complex and major source of energy (50-60% of total calories) simple is from fruits, vegetables, honey, milk and complex from cereals, millets, pulses and root vegetables.[7] Minimum consumption of carbohydrate is 175 g/day to accommodate fetal brain glucose utilization is recommended by IOM.[8]

WATER REQUIREMENTS DURING PREGNANCY

During pregnancy, most of added weight (6-9 L) is water because the plasma volume increases, 85% of the placenta is water and the fetus itself is 70–90% water. This means that hydration is an important aspect of nutrition throughout pregnancy. The European Food Safety Authority recommends an increase of 300 mL/day compared to the normal intake for non-pregnant women, taking the total adequate water intake (from food and fluids) to 2,300 mL, or approximately 1,850 mL/day from fluids alone.[9] Water carries nutrients to cells and waste products away, regulates body temperature and aids digestion.

Multiple micronutrient supplements taken with iron and folic acid can improve birth outcomes for women in low income countries. These supplements reduce numbers of low birth weight babies, small for gestational age babies and stillbirths in women who may not have many micronutrients in their usual diets. Undernourished women can benefit from having dietary education sessions and, balanced energy and protein supplements.

IRON REQUIREMENTS DURING PREGNANCY

Anemia is a serious health problem affecting all segments of population. About 50% of women do not have adequate iron stores for pregnancy.[10] Iron is needed for the healthy growth of the fetus and placenta, especially during the second and third trimesters. It is also essential before pregnancy for the production of hemoglobin. Iron deficiency leads to perinatal death, preterm delivery, low birth weight, fetal death and in later stage leads to disturbance in cognition, behavior and motor development.

Iron requirements are:
- *ACOG and AAP*: 27 mg of ferrous iron daily.
- *Ministry of Health and Family Welfare, India*: 100 mg of elemental iron + 500 µg of folic acid at least for 100 days in II half of pregnancy.
- *WHO*: 60 mg of iron + 500 µg folic acid.

Daily requirement of iron in pregnancy is:
- 0.8–1 mg in the 1st trimester
- 4–5 mg in the 2nd trimester
- More than 6 mg in the 3rd trimester

The total requirement during lactation is 1.27 mg/day. Pregnant women should take plant foods like green leafy vegetables, legumes, dry fruits, whole egg, meat, poultry, fish, *amla*, guava and citrus fruits. *Salads* along with meals also to be advised. So, iron rich diet and prophylactic tablets should be taken to avoid deficiency. Vitamin C will increase iron absorption.

FOLIC ACID REQUIREMENTS DURING PREGNANCY

Folate is a vitamin B that helps to prevent neural tube defects, serious abnormalities of the brain and spinal cord. The synthetic form of folate found in supplements and fortified foods is known as folic acid. Folic acid supplementation has been shown to decrease the risk of preterm delivery. Folic acid supplementation is recommended prior to conception, to prevent development of spina bifida and other neural tube defects. It should be taken as at least 0.4 mg/day throughout the first trimester of pregnancy, 0.6 mg/day throughout the pregnancy, and 0.5 mg/day while breastfeeding. Fortified cereals are great sources of folic acid. Leafy green vegetables, citrus fruits, and dried beans and peas are good sources of naturally occurring folate. Chronic and severe forms of folic acid deficiency lead to abnormal hemopoiesis and megaloblastic anemia.

CALCIUM REQUIREMENTS DURING PREGNANCY

Calcium is essential for strong bones and teeth. Calcium also helps in circulatory, muscular and nervous systems function. Normally calcium in bone plays a role in maintaining blood level even in the face of dietary calcium inadequacy. Blood Ca level is maintained within narrow limits by the interplay of vitamin D and several hormones such as parathyroid hormone (PTH), thyrocalcitonin, Cortisol and gender steroids by controlling absorption, excretion and turnover.

Pregnancy needs 1000 mg/day of calcium. Dairy products are the best absorbed sources of calcium. Non-dairy sources include broccoli and kale. Many fruit juices and breakfast cereals are fortified with calcium. Pregnant and lactating women should take 5 servings of milk and milk products.

VITAMIN D REQUIREMENTS

Vitamin D levels vary with exposure to sunlight. While it was assumed that supplementation was necessary only in areas of high latitudes, recent studies of Vitamin D levels throughout the United States and many other countries have shown a large number of women with low levels.[11] For this reason, there is a growing movement to recommend supplementation with 1000 mg of vitamin D daily throughout pregnancy. Vitamin D is necessary to prevent rickets, a disease causing weak bones.

MAGNESIUM REQUIREMENTS

Magnesium is an important cofactor of many regulatory enzymes. Magnesium is an essential mineral required for regulation of body temperature, nucleic acid and protein synthesis and in maintaining nerve and muscle cell electrical potentials. Magnesium supplementation during pregnancy may be able to reduce fetal growth restriction and pre-eclampsia, and increase birth weight.

Magnesium requirement for pregnant and lactating women is 310 mg/day.

SODIUM REQUIREMENTS

On the basis of average weight gain of 11 kg, of which 70% is water, sodium requirement is 750 mmol (sodium in ECF 145 mmol/L). Sodium need not be restricted during pregnancy, excessive use is not recommended. A diet primarily of natural foods can be safely salted "to taste." Pregnant women should avoid processed or "junk" foods that are high in sodium. Excessive intake of salt can cause high blood pressure (hypertension) and may lead to excessive weight gain. WHO recommends 5 g of salt/day. 1 g of sodium chloride contains 39% sodium. There is no place for dietary sodium restriction in the prevention or treatment of hypertension in pregnancy.

POTASSIUM REQUIREMENTS

Potassium is another very important mineral for both the pregnant and breastfeeding women. Not only does potassium help to maintain the fluid and electrolyte balance but potassium sends important nerve impulses, helps in muscle contraction, maintains blood pressure stable and normal and helps in the release of energy from protein, fat, and carbohydrates.

The current recommendation for pregnant women is 4,700 mg of potassium per day. About 5,100 mg/day when breastfeeding. Needed potassium can be received from beans, lentils, peas, milk, yogurt, bananas, tomato sauce, orange juice, broccoli, cooked green soybeans, cantaloupe, potatoes, spinach, watermelon, sweet potatoes, mushrooms, carrot juice, canned clams, prunes, etc.

IODINE REQUIREMENTS

Iodine is essential for healthy brain development in the fetus and young child. A woman's iodine requirements increase substantially during pregnancy to ensure adequate supply to the fetus. Most foods are relatively low in iodine content. To ensure that everyone has a sufficient intake of iodine, WHO and UNICEF recommend universal salt iodization as a global strategy. Intake of iodine during pregnancy has been increased from 200 to 250 µg/day.

ZINC

Zinc supplements have reduced preterm births by around 14% mainly in low income countries, and it also helps in growth and neurobehavioral development, antioxidant protection and membrane stabilization The World Health Organization does not routinely recommend zinc supplementation for pregnant women. Recommended dietary allowance (RDA) for zinc is 12 mg/day.[12] Fortified cereals and red meat are good sources of this nutrient. Oyster is a rich source of zinc but not used in pregnancy.

THIAMINE

The recommended daily allowance (RDA) for thiamine during pregnancy is 1.4 mg/day regardless of a woman's age. Thiamine, also known as vitamin B_1 enables converting carbohydrates into energy. It is essential for baby's brain development and aids the normal functioning of mothers' nervous system, muscles, and heart.

RIBOFLAVIN

Riboflavin, or vitamin B_2, is an essential vitamin that helps your body to produce energy, promotes growth, good vision, and healthy skin. It is important for baby's bone, muscle, and nerve development. National Research Council (NRC) recommends additional intake of 0.3 mg/day in pregnancy and lactation. Pregnant women: 1.4 mg per day. Milk, bread products, and fortified cereals are all good sources of riboflavin.

NIACIN

Pregnancy and breastfeeding: Niacin and niacinamide are safe for pregnant and breastfeeding women when taken in the recommended amounts. The recommended amount of niacin for pregnant or breastfeeding women is 30 mg/day for women under 18 years of age, and 35 mg for women over 18. Found in many foods including yeast, meat, fish, milk, eggs, green vegetables, beans, and cereal grains. Niacin and niacinamide are also found in many vitamin B complex supplements with other B vitamins.

PYRIDOXINE

The recommended dietary allowance (RDA) of pyridoxine (vitamin B_6) for pregnant women is 1.9 mg/day regardless of age. Pyridoxine has been reported to inhibit lactation at large doses. The RDA of pyridoxine (vitamin B_6) for lactating women is 2 mg/day, regardless of age, to ensure a vitamin B_6 concentration of milk of 130 ng/mL. Vitamin B_6 is contained in many foods including meat, poultry, fish, vegetables, and bananas. It is thought that B_6 may play a role in the prevention of pre-eclampsia, where the mother's blood pressure is high with large amounts of protein in the urine or other organ dysfunction, and in babies being born too early (preterm birth). Vitamin B_6 may be helpful for reducing nausea in pregnancy. Vitamin B_6 as oral capsules or lozenges resulted in a decreased risk of dental decay in pregnant women in one trial.

VITAMIN B_{12}

Deficiency of vitamin B_{12} leads to abnormal hemopoiesis leading to megaloblastic anemia as in the case of folic acid deficiency. Neurological manifestation can also occur.

RDA recommendation of B_{12} by ICMR for pregnant women is 1.2 µg/day and for lactating mother is 1.5/day.

VITAMIN C

Vitamin C, also known as ascorbic acid, is essential for tissue repair, wound healing, bone growth and repair, and healthy skin. Vitamin C also helps your body fight infection, and it acts as an antioxidant, protecting cells from damage. Citrus fruits are especially high in vitamin C, but leafy greens and many other fruits and vegetables are excellent sources. RDA for pregnant women is 40 mg/day and lactating women is 80 mg/day.

VITAMIN A

It is well known that vitamin A is an essential nutrient for normal cellular function, including reproduction and development. Dietary vitamin A is obtained in two forms which contain the preformed vitamin (retinol), that can be found in some animal products such as liver and fish liver oils, and as a vitamin A precursor in the form of carotene, which can be found in many fruits and vegetables. Intake of large amounts, or, conversely, a deficiency, of retinol has been linked to birth defects and abnormalities. It is noted that a 100 g serving of liver may contain a large amount of retinol, so it is best that it is not eaten daily during pregnancy

Dose: *Pregnant women:* 19 years and older: about 770 µg RAE of vitamin A (approximately 2,565 IU) per day, pregnant, 18 and younger: 750 mg (2,500 IU).

Breastfeeding women: *19 and older:* 1,300 µg RAE (4,330 IU) Breastfeeding, 18 and younger: 1,200 µg RAE (4,000 IU).

Excessive amounts of alcohol have been proven to cause fetal alcohol syndrome. The World Health Organization recommends that alcohol should be avoided entirely during pregnancy, given the relatively unknown effects of even small amounts of alcohol during pregnancy.

In spite of many nutrients, pregnant women are advised to take fruits, vegetables, greens, milk and needed tablets of folic acid, iron, B_{12} and calcium.

Proper nutrition is important after delivery to help the mother recover, and to provide enough food energy and nutrients for a woman to breastfeed her child.

IMPORTANT POINTS

- About 23.8% of babies worldwide are estimated to be born with lower than optimal weights at birth due to lack of proper nutrition.
- Recommended weight gain during pregnancy is based on prepregnancy BMI.
- Protein is essential to meet the demand for the growth of the fetus, placenta, uterus, breasts, and blood volume.
- Protein intake should be preferably by natural and not commercial high protein supplements.
- Polyunsaturated fatty acids, specifically docosahexaenoic acid (DHA) and eicosapentaenoic acid (EPA) are very beneficial.
- Iron rich diet and prophylactic tablets should be taken to prevent anemia.
- Calcium is essential for strong bones and teeth. Calcium also helps in circulatory, muscular and nervous systems function.
- Deficiency of vitamin B_{12} leads to abnormal hemopoiesis leading to megaloblastic anemia as in the case of folic acid deficiency.
- Alcohol should be avoided entirely during pregnancy, given the relatively unknown effects of even small amounts of alcohol during pregnancy.

REFERENCES

1. Barasi EM. Human Nutrition. A Health Perspective. London: Arnold. ISBN 0-340-81025-4. 2003.
2. Jahanfar S, Jaafar SH (9 June 2015). Effects of restricted caffeine intake by mother on fetal, neonatal and pregnancy outcomes. The Cochrane Database of Systematic Reviews 6: CD006965.

3. Riley L, Karpinske S. Pregnancy: The Ultimate Week-by-week pregnancy guide. Meredith Books.
4. Haider, et al. Anaemia, prenatal iron use, and risk of adverse pregnancy outcomes: systematic review and meta-analysis. BMJ, 2013.
5. Kashyap S. Maternal work and nutrition—prospective study, Delhi University.
6. Herrera E. Lipid metabolism in foetus and newborn. DM Research and Review; 2006.
7. Mann J. Scientific update on carbohydrate in human nutrition European Journal of Clinical Nutrition; 2007.
8. Food and Nutrition Board IOM National Academics 2002/2005.
9. Scientific Opinion on Dietary Reference Value of Water. EFSA Journal. 8:1459-1507.
10. Milman N. Iron and pregnancy: a delicate balance. Ann Hematol. 2006;85(9):559-65.
11. Aghajafari Fariba, et al. Association between maternal serum 25-hydroxyvitamin D level and pregnancy and neonatal outcomes: systematic review and meta-analysis of observational studies. BMJ. 2013. p. 346.
12. Zinc supplementation during pregnancy. WHO 2006 April.

Chapter 4

Antenatal Fetal Surveillance and Identification of High-risk Pregnancy

Gita Guin, Poorva Badkur

INTRODUCTION

The antenatal fetal surveillance is the method of detecting the high-risk pregnancies by using various clinical, biochemical and biophysical parameters for predicting the perinatal outcome.

The fetal surveillance during antenatal period will decrease the incidence of birth asphyxia and fetal death while maintaining the lowest possible rate of obstetrics intervention. Various adverse fetal and neonatal outcomes are associated with antepartum asphyxia, viz.

Fetal Outcome

- Stillbirth
- Metabolic acidosis at birth.

Neonatal Outcome

- Mortality
- Metabolic acidosis
- Hypoxic renal damage
- Necrotizing enterocolitis
- Intracranial hemorrhage
- Seizures
- Cerebral palsy
- Neonatal encephalopathy.

Antenatal fetal testing techniques fall into seven categories and may be used simultaneous or in hierarchical fashion. They are:
1. Fetal movements
2. Non-stress test
3. Contraction stress test
4. Biophysical profile
5. Amniotic fluid volume
6. Doppler velocimetry
7. Acoustic stimulation test.

WHO TO SCREEN (PATIENTS AT RISK)

Obstetrical history and current pregnancy conditions which are associated with increased perinatal mortality/mortality are screened in antenatal fetal surveillance and may improve perinatal outcome.

PREVIOUS OBSTETRICAL HISTORY

Maternal

- Hypertensive disorder of pregnancy
- Placental abruption
- Impaired glucose tolerance (GT) or gestational diabetes mellitus (GDM)
- Hypo- and hyperthyroidism
- Intrauterine growth restriction
- Previous surgical delivery any intrapartum complication
- Stillbirth
- Congenital malformation
- Genetic defects.

CURRENT PREGNANCY

Maternal

- Advanced maternal age
- Assisted reproductive technology
- Post-term
- Hypertensive disorders
- Pre-pregnancy diabetes
- Premature rupture of membranes
- Isoimmunization
- Abnormal maternal serum screening (hCG or AFP >2.0 MoM) in absence of confirmed fetal anomaly
- Motor vehicle accident during pregnancy
- Vaginal bleeding
- Morbid obesity.

Fetal

- Decreased fetal movement
- Intrauterine growth restriction
- Suspected oligohydramnios/polyhydramnios
- Multiple pregnancy
- Preterm labor.

INITIATION AND FREQUENCY OF ANTENATAL TESTING

The most important consideration in deciding when to begin antepartum testing is the prognosis for fetal survival. The decision to initiate and decide the frequency of antenatal fetal testing should be individualized and reflect the risk factor associated with an individual pregnancy. The severity of maternal disease is another important consideration. In general, with the majority of high-risk pregnancy, most authority recommend testing by 32–34 weeks. In pregnancy with severe complication might require testing as early as 26–28 weeks. The testing is usually performed once or twice weekly.

METHODS

Fetal Movement

Passive unstimulated fetal activity commences as early as 7 weeks, and become more sophisticated and coordinated by the end of pregnancy.

There are four fetal behavioral states:
1. *State 1F:* Quiet sleep
2. *State 2F:* Frequent gross body movements, continuous eye movements, and widen oscillation of fetal heart rate (FHR). This is active sleep in neonate.
3. *State 3F:* Continuous eye movements in the absence of body movements and no heart rate acceleration.
4. *State 4F:* Vigorous body movements with continuous fetal movements and heart rate accelerations.

Fetus spend most of their time in states 1F and 2F.

Issues Relevant for Fetal Movement Counts[1,2]

Gestational age: Fetal movements are perceived by women regularly after 24 weeks in a constant fashion.[3] Most studies initiated fetal movements at 28–32 weeks.[4] In extremely early gestational age, iatrogenic preterm delivery may have grave consequences. Therefore, fetal movement counting should not be encouraged prior to viability and possibly should start at 26–32 weeks.

Optimal time for testing: Fetal movements were found to be increased at evening time.[5,6]

Position: Fetal movements are perceived best when lying down.[7]

Food: Most studies did not show an increase of movements following food or glucose.[6,8-11]

Smoking: Smoking reduces fetal movements temporarily by increasing carboxy hemoglobin levels and reducing fetal blood flow.[12]

Drug effect: Most drugs have no effect on fetal movements. Depressant drugs and narcotics may reduce fetal movements.[13] Notably, antenatal corticosteroids may have the same effect for two days.[14]

Decreased placental perfusion and fetal acidemia and acidosis are associated with decreased fetal movements.[15] This is the basis for maternal monitoring of fetal movements or the fetal movement count test.

Methods

- *Cardiff method*: Count to 10 movements in affixed time frame. The original time required is 12 hours.
- *Sadovsky method*: A count of movements in a specific time frame.[16]

Recommendations

- Daily monitoring of fetal movements starting at 26–32 weeks should be done in all pregnancies *with* risk factors for adverse perinatal outcome.
- Healthy pregnant women *without* risk factors for adverse perinatal outcomes should be made aware of the significance of fetal movements in the third trimester and asked to perform a fetal movement count, if they perceive decreased movements **(Flow chart 4.1)**.

Nonstress Test (Table 4.1)

Nonstress test (NST) is primarily a test of fetal condition. Also incorporated in biophysical profile. Fetal heart rate normally is increased or decreased by autonomic influences mediated by sympathetic or parasympathetic impulses from brainstem center. Beat-to-beat variability is also under its control.

Recommendations

- Antepartum non-stress testing may be considered when risk factors for adverse perinatal outcome are present.
- In the presence of a normal non-stress test, usual fetal movement patterns, and absence of suspected oligohydramnios, it is not necessary to conduct a biophysical profile or contraction stress test.
- A normal non-stress test should be classified and documented by an appropriately trained and designated individual as soon as possible (ideally within 24 hours).

Frequency of Testing

This can be done weekly. But more frequently in post-term, diabetes mellitus, hypertension in pregnancy, multifetal gestation intrauterine growth restriction (IUGR).

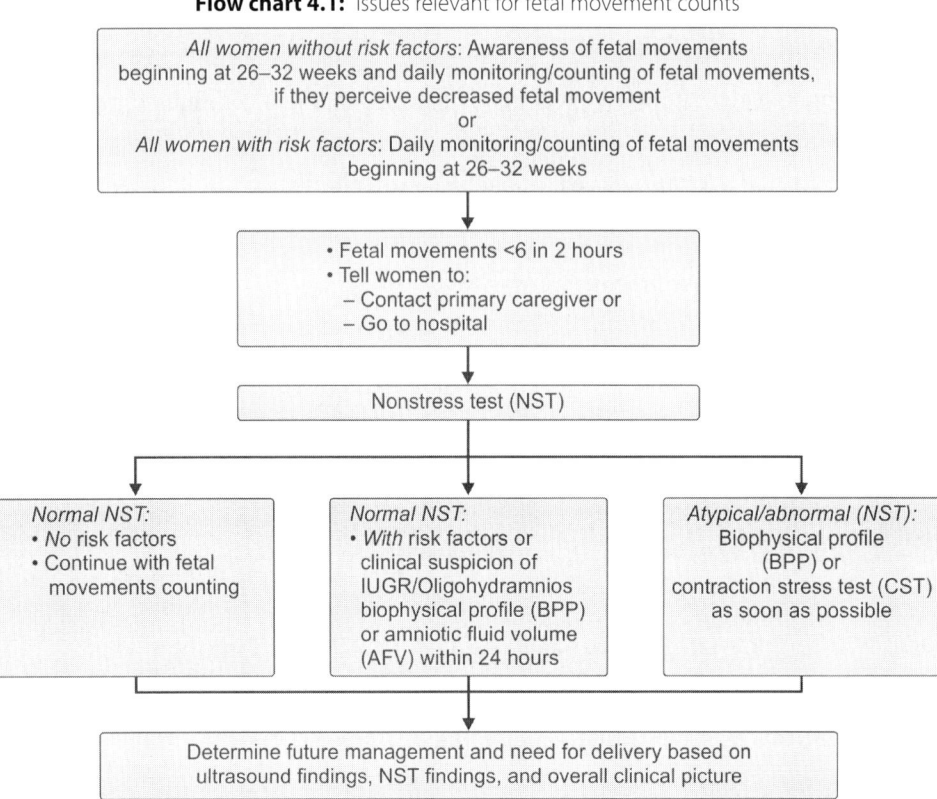

Flow chart 4.1: Issues relevant for fetal movement counts

Table 4.1: Antepartum classification: Nonstress test			
Parameter	Normal NST	Atypical NST	Abnormal NST
Baseline	110–160 bpm	100–110 bpm >160 bpm <30 min Rising baseline	Bradycardia <100 bpm Tachycardia >160 for > 30 min Erratic baseline
Variability	6–25 bpm ≥ 5 for 40 min	≤ 5 for 40–80 min	5 for >80 min 25 bpm >10 min Sinusoidal
Decelerations	None or occasional Variable <30 sec	Variable decelerations 30–60 sec. duration	Variable decelerations > 60 sec. duration Late deceleration(s)
Accelerations Term Fetus	>2 accelerations with acme of >15 bpm, lasting 15 sec <40 min of testing	<2 accelerations with acme of >15 bpm, lasting 15 sec in 40–80 min	<2 accelerations with acme of >15 bpm, lasing 15 sec in >80 min
	Action further assessment optional	Further assessment required	Urgent action required

Contraction Stress Test

Contraction stress test (CST) is primarily test for detecting uteroplacental function.

Mechanism: **Flow chart 4.2.**

Methods: **Flow chart 4.3.**

Interpretation

Negative: No late or significant variable deceleration.

Positive: Late deceleration following 50% or more of contraction.

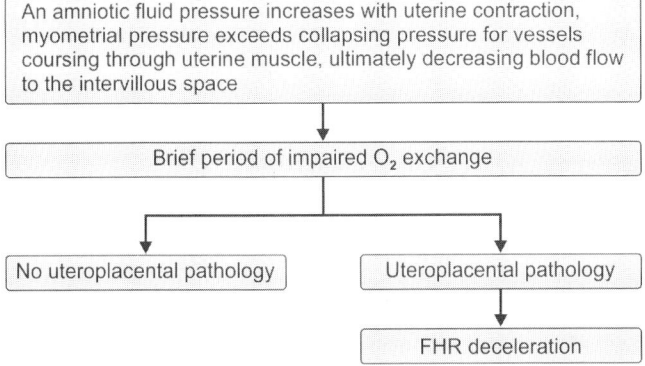

Flow chart 4.2: Mechanism of contraction stress test

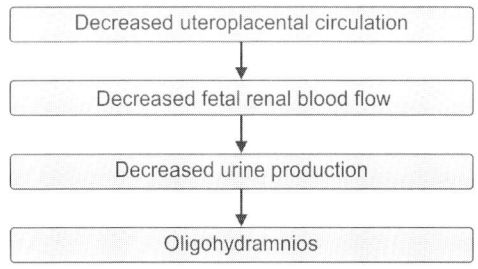

Flow chart 4.4: Mechanism of oligohydramnios development

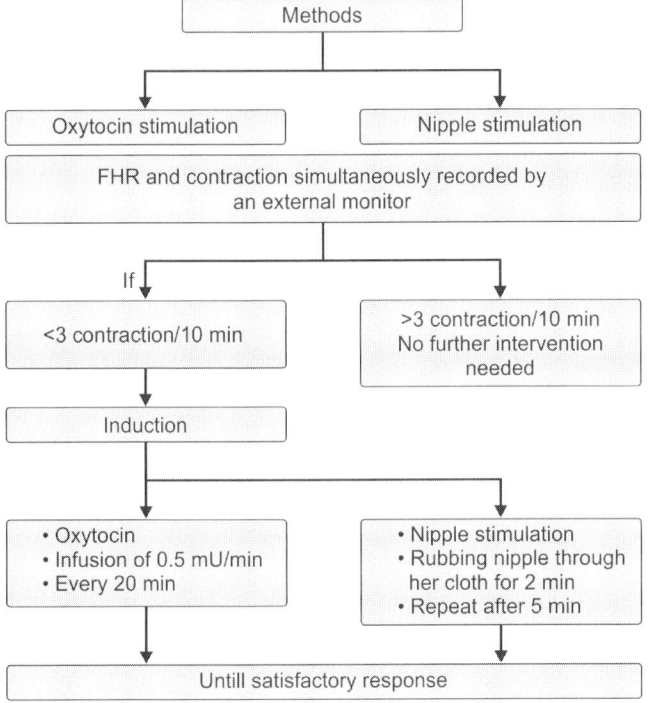

Flow chart 4.3: Method of contraction stress test

Equivocal suspicious: Intermittent late deceleration or significant variable deceleration.

Equivocal hyperstimulation: Fetal heart rate deceleration that occur in presence of contractions more frequent that every 2 min or lasting >90 sec.

Unsatisfactory: ≤ 3 contraction/10 min.

Recommendations

- The contraction stress test should be considered in the presence of an atypical non-stress test as a proxy for the adequacy of intrapartum uteroplacental function and, together with the clinical circumstances, will aid in decision making about timing and mode of delivery.
- The contraction stress test should *not* be performed when vaginal delivery is contraindicated.
- The contraction stress test should be performed in a setting where emergency cesarean section is available.

Amniotic Fluid Volume

Integral component in the assessment of pregnancies at risk of fetal death. Also included in BPP **(Flow chart 4.4)**.

An index of ≤5 cm significantly increase the risk of cesarean delivery for fetal death or a low 5 min Apgar score.

Biophysical Profile (Table 4.2)

The biophysical profile (BPP) is an evaluation of current fetal well-being. It is performed over 30 minutes and assesses fetal behavior by observing fetal breathing movement,

Table 4.2: Components and their scores for the biophysical profile

Component	Score 2	Score 0
NST	>=2 acceleration of >=15 bpm for >=15 sec within 20-40 min	0-1 acceleration within 20–40 min
Fetal breathing	>=1 episode of rhythmic breathing lasting >=30 sec within 30 min	<30 sec breathing within 30 min
Fetal movement	>=3 discrete body or limb movements within 30 min	<3 discrete movements
Fetal tone	>=1 episode of extremity extension and subsequent return of flexion	0 extension/flexion events
Amniotic fluid volume	A pocket of amniotic fluid that measures at least 2 cm in 2 planes perpendicular to each other	Largest vertical pocket <=2 cm

body movement, tone, and amniotic fluid volume.[17] In the presence of intact membranes, functioning fetal kidneys, and unobstructed urinary tract, decreased amniotic fluid reflects decreased renal filtration due to redistribution of cardiac output away from the fetal kidneys in response to chronic hypoxia.[18]

BPP score of 0 was invariably associated with significant fetal academia, whereas normal score of 8 or 10 was associated with normal pH.

An equivocal test result—a score of 6—was a poor predictor of abnormal outcome. A decrease from an abnormal result—a score of 2 or 4—to a very abnormal score was a progressively more accurate predictor of abnormal outcome.

Modified BBP: "Modified" BPP as the primary screen of antenatal surveillance. The modified BPP consists of a non-stress test and an AFI (> 5 cm is considered adequate). If either assessment measure is of concern, then the complete BPP is performed. There is less level II evidence supporting this approach.[8,19]

Recommendations of BPP

- In pregnancies at increased risk for adverse perinatal outcome and where facilities and expertise exist, biophysical profile is recommended for evaluation of fetal well-being.
- When an abnormal biophysical profile is obtained, the responsible physician or delegate should be informed immediately. Further management will be determined by the overall clinical situation.

Doppler Velocimetry

It is a noninvasive technique to assess blood flow by characterizing downstream impedance. Four fetal vascular circuits, which include the uterine artery, umbilical artery, middle cerebral artery, and ductus venosus, current used to determine fetal health and intrauterine growth restriction.

Uterine Artery Doppler

In normal pregnancy, the developing placenta implants on maternal decidua, and the trophoblast invades the maternal spiral arteries, destroying the elastic lamina and transforming these vessels into low resistance shunts in order to improve blood supply to the fetoplacental unit. Impaired trophoblastic invasion is associated with pre-existing hypertension and subsequent development of hypertensive disorders of pregnancy, IUGR, placental abruption, and intrauterine fetal demise. Doppler ultrasound of the uterine arteries is a noninvasive method of assessing the resistance of vessels supplying the placenta. In normal pregnancies, there is an increase in blood flow velocity and a decrease in resistance to flow, reflecting the transformation of the spiral arteries.

In pregnancies complicated by hypertensive disorders, Doppler ultrasound of the uterine artery shows increased resistance to flow, early diastolic notching, and decreased diastolic flow.

Recommendations

- Where facilities and expertise exist, uterine artery Doppler may be performed at the time of the 17 to 22 weeks' gestation detailed anatomical ultrasound scan in women with the following factors for adverse perinatal outcome.
- Women with a positive uterine artery Doppler screen should have the following:
  - A double marker screen (for alpha feto-protein and beta-hCG), if at or before 18 weeks' gestation.
  - A second uterine artery Doppler at 24 to 26 weeks. If the uterine artery Doppler is positive at the second scan, the woman should be referred to a maternal fetal medicine specialist for management.

Umbilical Artery

In normal pregnancy, the fetal umbilical circulation is characterized by continuous forward flow, i.e. low resistance, to the placenta, which improves with gestational age as primary, secondary, and tertiary branching of the villus vascular architecture continue to develop. Resistance to forward flow, therefore continues to decrease in normal pregnancy all the way to term. Increased resistance to forward flow in the umbilical circulation is characterized by abnormal systolic to diastolic ratio, pulsatility index (PI) or resistance index (RI) greater than the 95th centile and implies decreased functioning vascular units within the placenta.[20]

Recommendations

- Umbilical artery Doppler should not be used as a screening tool in healthy pregnancies, as it has not been shown to be of value in this group.
- Umbilical artery Doppler should be available for assessment of the fetal placental circulation in pregnant women with suspected placental insufficiency. Fetal umbilical artery Doppler assessment should be considered (1) at time of referral for suspected growth restriction, or (2) during follow-up for suspected placental pathology.
- Depending on other clinical factors, reduced, absent, or reversed umbilical artery end-diastolic flow is an indication for enhanced fetal surveillance or delivery. If delivery is delayed to improve fetal lung maturity with maternal administration of glucocorticoids, intensive fetal surveillance until delivery is suggested for those fetuses with reversed end-diastolic flow.

IDENTIFICATION OF HIGH-RISK FACTORS

A high-risk pregnancy is one in which the mother or fetus has a significantly increased chance of death or disability

(Hobel, 1979). In order to achieve optimal perinatal outcome, all factors contributing to mortality and morbidity in a particular pregnancy must be identified and acted upon early. The factors may be divided into the categories of socioeconomic, demographic, and medical.

Socioeconomic Factors

- Inadequate finances
- Poor housing
- Severe social problems
- Unwed, especially adolescent
- Minority status
- Nutritional deprivation

Demographic Factors

- Maternal age under 16 or over 35 years
- Overweight or underweight prior to pregnancy
- Height
- Less than 5 feet
- Maternal education less than 11 years
- Family history of severe inherited disorders.

Medial Factors

Obstetric History

- History of infertility
- Previous ectopic pregnancy or spontaneous abortion
- Grandmultiparity
- Previous stillborn or neonatal death
- Uterine/cervical abnormality
- Previous multiple gestation
- Previous premature labor delivery
- Previous prolonged labor
- Previous cesarean section
- Previous low-birth-weight infant
- Previous macrosomic infant
- Previous midforceps delivery
- Previous baby with neurologic deficit, birth injury, or malformation
- Previous hydatidiform mole or choriocarcinoma.

Maternal Medical History/Status

- Maternal cardiac disease
- Maternal pulmonary disease
- Maternal metabolic disease, particularly diabetes mellitus, thyroid disease
- Chronic renal disease, repeated urinary tract infections, repeated bacteriuria
- Maternal gastrointestinal disease
- Maternal endocrine disorders (pituitary, adrenal)
- Chronic hypertension
- Maternal hemoglobinopathies
- Seizure disorder
- Venereal and other infectious diseases
- Weight loss greater than 5 pounds
- Malignancy
- Surgery during pregnancy
- Major congenital anomalies of the reproductive tract
- Maternal mental retardation, major emotional disorders.

Current Obstetric Status

- Late or no prenatal care
- Rh-sensitization
- Fetus inappropriately large or small for gestation
- Premature labor
- Pregnancy-induced hypertension
- Multiple gestation
- Polyhydramnios
- Premature rupture of the membranes
- Antepartum bleeding
  - Placenta previa
  - Abruptio placenta
- Abnormal presentation
- Postdatism
- Abnormality in tests for fetal well-being
- Maternal anemia.

Habits/Habituation

- Smoking during pregnancy
- Regular alcohol intake
- Drug use.

REFERENCES

1. Baskett TF, Liston RM. Fetal movement monitoring: clinical application. Clin Perinatol. 1989;16(3):613-25.
2. Velazquez MD, Rayburn WF. Antenatal evaluation of the fetus using fetal movement monitoring. Clin Obstet Gynecol. 2002;45(4):993-1004.
3. Connors G, Natale R, Nasello-Paterson C. Maternally perceived fetal activity from twenty-four weeks' gestation to term in normal and at risk pregnancies. Am J Obstet Gynecol. 1988;158(2):294-9.
4. Froen JF. A kick from within—fetal movement counting and the cancelled progress in antenatal care. J Perinat Med. 2004;32(1):13-24.
5. Roberts AB, Little D, Cooper D, Campbell S. Normal patterns of fetal activity in the third trimester. Br J Obstet Gynaecol. 1979;86(1):4-9.
6. Patrick J, Campbell K, Carmichael L, Natale R, Richardson B. Patterns of gross fetal body movements over 24-hour observation intervals during the last 10 weeks of pregnancy. Am J Obstet Gynecol. 1982;142(4):363-71.

7. Hertz RH, Timor-Tritsch I, Dierker LJ Jr, Chik L, Rosen MG. Continuous ultrasound and fetal movement. Am J Obstet Gynecol. 1979;135(1):152-4.
8. Miller FC, Skiba H, Klapholz H. The effect of maternal blood sugar levels on fetal activity. Obstet Gynecol. 1978;52(6):662-5.
9. Birkenfeld A, Laufer N, Sadovsky E. Diurnal variation of fetal activity. Obstet Gynecol. 1980;55(4):417-9.
10. Ritchie JW. Fetal breathing and generalized fetal movements in normal antenatal patients. Br J Obstet Gynaecol. 1979;86(8):612-4.
11. Mirghani HM, Weerasinghe DS, Ezimokhai M, Smith JR. The effect of maternal fasting on the fetal biophysical profile. Int J Gynaecol Obstet. 2003;81(1):17-21.
12. Goodman JD, Visser FG, Dawes GS. Effects of maternal cigarette smoking on fetal trunk movements, fetal breathing movements and the fetal heart rate. Br J Obstet Gynaecol. 1984;91(7):657-61.
13. Jansson LM, Dipietro J, Elko A. Fetal response to maternal methadone administration. Am J Obstet Gynecol. 2005;193 (3 Pt 1):611-7.
14. Mulder EJ, Koenen SV, Blom I, Visser GH. The effects of antenatal betamethasone administration on fetal heart rate and behaviour depend on gestational age. Early Hum Dev. 2004;76(1):65-77.
15. Bocking AD. Assessment of fetal heart rate and fetal movements in detecting oxygen deprivation *in utero*. Eur J Obstet Gynecol Reprod Biol. 2003;110(Suppl 1):S108-12.
16. Sadovsky E, Weinstein D, Even Y. Antepartum fetal evaluation by assessment of fetal heart rate and fetal movements. Int J Gynaecol Obstet. 1981;19(1):21-6.
17. Manning FA. Dynamic ultrasound-based fetal assessment: the fetal biophysical profile score. Clin Obstet Gynecol. 1995;38(1):26-44.
18. Cohn HE, Sacks EJ, Heymann MA, Rudolph AM. Cardiovascular responses to hypoxemia and acidemia in fetal lambs. Am J Obstet Gynecol. 1974;120(6):817-24.
19. Nageotte MP, Towers CV, Asrat T, Freeman RK. Perinatal outcome with the modified biophysical profile. Am J Obstet Gynecol. 1994;170(6):1672-6.
20. James DK, Steer PJ, Weiner CP, Gonik B. High risk pregnancy: management options, 3rd edn. Philadelphia: Elsevier Saunders; 2006.

SECTION 2: FETAL ADVANCES

Chapter 5

Prenatal Genetic Screening and Testing

Jyotsna Gupta

INTRODUCTION

Every pregnant woman is at risk of giving birth to congenitally malformed baby. Prenatal congenital malformations occur in a frequency of 2.03–3% **(Table 5.1)**. The most common malformations in Indian population are neural tube defects and musculo-skeletal disorders.[1] The most common cause of mental retardation worldwide is Down syndrome and its incidence is approximately 1 per 1000 live births and increases with advancing maternal age. Most common structural heart defect is ventricular septal defect (VSD) and most VSD resolve spontaneously. Incidence of moderate and severe forms of congenital heart diseases is about 6/1,000 live births.[2]

Prenatal congenital disorders although low in frequency have a huge impact on the affected families and therefore screening ongoing pregnancies for genetic and structural disorders should be performed. Prenatal screening involves *family history* and pedigree analysis, population screening, fetal risk assessment, genetic counseling and fetal diagnostic tests. The genetic disorders can be divided into chromosomal aberrations, single gene mutation, polygenetic or multifactorial diseases.

Screening for genetic disorders comprises two broad categories including carrier screening and prenatal screening for aneuploidies. Carrier screening includes screening the couple or prospective parents whether they carry the affected gene for the inherited familial condition (Carrier status). Carrier screening is of two types: population prevalent genetic screening (e.g. cystic fibrosis) or specific inherited familial disorders (muscular dystrophies). After the carrier status of parents are determined, fetal risk of inheriting the disease is determined, and if present invasive fetal test for determining fetal gene aberration are done.

SCREENING FOR PRENATAL ANEUPLOIDIES

Screening tests are used to identify the possible presence of an undiagnosed genetic disorder in asymptomatic individual. Screening tests are aimed to identify individuals at risk for a particular disorder, for which a diagnostic test is required to confirm the findings. The screening tests should be positive early enough in gestation to permit safe and legal options for termination of pregnancy, if required. Screening for prenatal genetic disorders focus on detecting structural and functional problems with the fetus as early as possible, either at embryonic stage (as in preimplantation genetic diagnosis) or as early in gestation as practically possible. Blood tests and ultrasonography along with other tests are used to detect problems such as neural tube defects, chromosome abnormalities, and gene mutations.

Screening tests available include maternal serum biomarkers, ultrasonography, noninvasive cell free fetal DNA and test targeted at detecting specific inherited genetic problems. Diagnostic tests available to confirm the findings of screening test are amniocentesis, chorionic villus sampling, fetal blood sampling, fetal skin biopsy, fetal muscle biopsy or renal biopsy depending on the genetic condition.

Likelihood Ratios

Likelihood ratio is an individual's risk for a specific condition based on statistical analysis of the population. Every pregnant women has some risk for genetic disorder which is her background risk or *a priori risk*. Multiple factors such as age, serum screening markers, ultrasonography, diabetic status, IVF pregnancy, etc. may contribute to the risk so, they are

Table 5.1: Burden of genetic disorders in India (2000)

Disorder	Incidence	Births per year
Congenital malformations	1:50	678,000
Down syndrome	1:800	34,000
Metabolic disorders	1:1200	22500
Beta-thalassemia and sickle cell anemia	1:1700	16700
Congenital hypothyroidism	1:2500	10900
Duchenne muscular dystrophy	1:10000	2700
Spinal muscular atrophy	1:10000	2700

Source: The Indian Journal of Pediatrics, 2000;67(12):893-8.

given specific likelihood ratios for risk of genetic disorder. These various likelihood ratios are used to modify *the priori risk* of that pregnant women to give her final likelihood ratio for the genetic disorder.

ANTENATAL SCREENING FOR DOWN SYNDROME

Down syndrome is the most common autosomal trisomy among live births. Incidence of Down syndrome is higher with advanced maternal age. Burden of disease is significant for the family in terms of emotional, physical and financial aspect. Prenatal screening and diagnosis can help detect this syndrome and lets the parents decide upon continuation or termination of an affected baby. Counseling for the screening tests is very important. The key principle when counseling patients about prenatal screening for Down syndrome is to provide clear, easily understood, and complete information that allows them to make informed, preference-based screening and diagnostic testing decisions **(Flow chart 5.1)**.

Candidates for Prenatal Screening

The American College of Obstetricians and Gynecologists and American College of Medical Genetics recommend that:
- All women should be *offered* aneuploidy screening before 20 weeks of gestation
- All women should have the option of invasive testing, regardless of maternal age.[3,4]

Candidates for Direct Diagnostic Testing

A diagnostic test rather than screening is a reasonable choice for women of any age at high risk of Down syndrome or other fetal aneuploidies, such as women with:[3,4]
- A previous pregnancy complicated by fetal trisomy
- At least one major or two minor fetal structural anomalies in the current pregnancy
- Chromosomal translocation, inversion, or aneuploidy in the pregnant woman or her partner.
- Past history of miscarriages.
- Multifetal pregnancy

Various screening tests available to screen for Trisomy 21, 18, 13, X0 and neural tube defects are maternal age, first trimester serum screening, first trimester ultrasonography, second trimester serum screening tests, second trimester ultrasonography or a combination of various tests each having its own sensitivity and specificity. A newer screening test known as noninvasive prenatal screening test (NIPS/NIPT) is also available commercially now which can screen for various aneuploidies (21,18,13, sex chr), fetal RhD status and few microdeletions syndromes also.

Maternal Age

The incidence of fetal trisomies is directly related to maternal age.[7] The risk of having a child with Down syndrome increases in a gradual, linear fashion until about age 30 and increases exponentially thereafter **(Fig. 5.1)**. Maternal age alone as screening for Down syndrome detects only 30% of affected fetuses, so not used alone but combined with other screening tests to modify the priori risk of the pregnant women.

First Trimester Screening

First trimester screening tests in addition to maternal age are either serum screening or ultrasonography or both combined. First-trimester ultrasonography for screening evaluates fetal nuchal translucency along with other optional ultrasound markers for aneuploidy. The serum markers include pregnancy-associated plasma protein A (PAPP-A) and one of various forms of human chorionic gonadotropin, including the free beta-subunit of human chorionic gonadotropin (free beta-hCG) and total or intact hCG (hCG).[6]

Benefits of first trimester screening include earlier identification of the pregnancy at risk for fetal aneuploidy and anatomic defects, and the option of earlier diagnosis by chorionic villus sampling and first trimester termination, if required.

Ultrasound

Nuchal Translucency (NT): NT is subcutaneous fluid collection behind the neck of the fetus and can be measured between 11–14 weeks (CRL 45–84 mm). Increased NT measurement (>95th centile for the gestation) has been seen to be associated with increased incidence of Down syndrome[10] **(Fig. 5.2)**. Other aneuploidies associated with increased NT measurement are trisomy 13, 18, X0, Triploidies and rare genetic syndromes. Severe congenital heart defects, diaphragmatic hernia, skeletal dysplasia are also seen associated with increased nuchal translucency.[7,9,10] Increased nuchal translucency though seen to be associated with so many above-mentioned anomalies does not call for termination of pregnancy. It needs further confirmation with either an invasive test or follow-up sonography.

Other ultrasound markers: Other highly sensitive and specific first-trimester sonographic markers of trisomy 21 are absence of the nasal bone,[8] increased impedance to flow in the ductus venosus and tricuspid regurgitation, frontomaxillary facial angle, fetal growth restriction, tachycardia, megacystis, exomphalos and single umbilical artery.[11-13]

First trimester anatomical screening: Approximately, 50% major structural anomalies can be detected during the first-trimester scan such as acrania, holoprosencephaly,

CHAPTER 5: Prenatal Genetic Screening and Testing

Flow chart 5.1: Prenatal screening and diagnosis for chromosomal abnormalities and neural tube defects
(Based on ACOG Screening Recommendations, 2016; ACOG Committee opinion Recommendations, 2015)

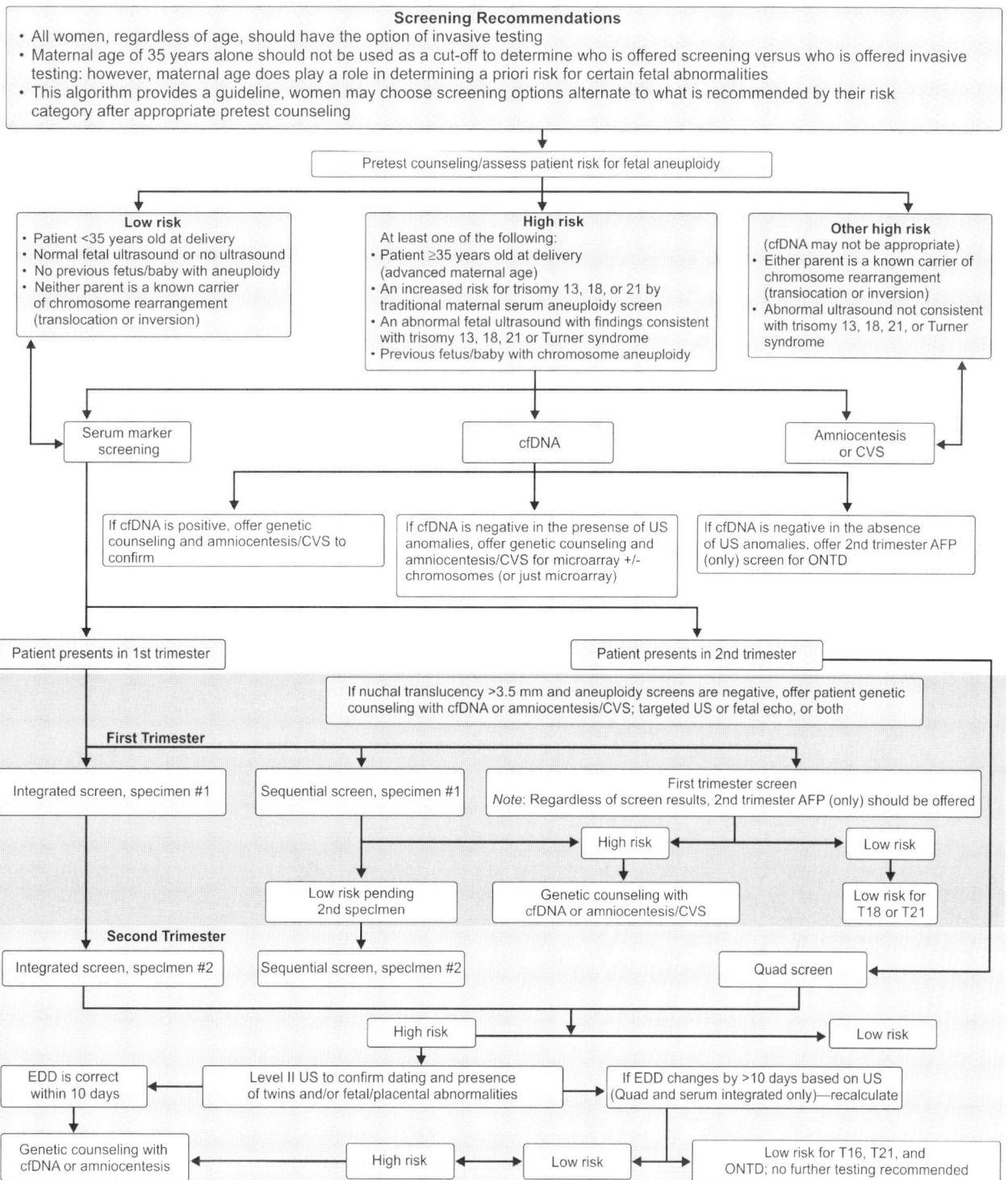

Abbreviations: AFP, alpha-fetoprotein; CRL, crown rump length; CVS, chronic villus sampling; DIA, dimeric inhibin A; DR, detection rate; EDD, estimated delivery date; hCG, human choronic gonadotropin; cfDNA-cell-free DNA; NT, nuchal transiucency; ONTD, open neural tube defect; PAPPA, pregnancy-associated placental protein A; SPR, screen positive rate; T18, trisomy 18; T21, trisomy 21 (Down syndrome); uE3, umconjugated estriol spina bifida, hypoplastic left heart syndrome, omphalocele, megacystis, missing limbs, body stalk syndrome and hydrops.[14]

First Trimester Serum Screening

Multiple markers can be used in first trimester after 9 weeks gestation for aneuploidies amongst which best are PAPP-A (Pregnancy-associated Plasma Protein-A) and Free β-hCG (human chorionic gonadotropin). Tests involving two markers in combination with maternal age, specifically PAPP-A, free β-hCG and maternal age are significantly better than those involving single markers with and without age.[5] Down syndrome detection rate using this screening protocol is close to 70% for a fixed 5% FPR[5]. Other serum biochemical markers placental growth factor (PlGF), placental protein 13 (PP13) in combination to PAPP-A and hCG can be used in first trimester serum screening in predicting pre-eclampsia, small for gestational age (SGA) and preterm delivery also.[15]

Combined Ultrasound and Serum Screening at 11–14 Weeks

Combining maternal age with sonographic measurement of fetal NT, assessment of the presence of nasal bone and maternal serum measurement of free β-hCG and PAPP-A would yield a detection rate of 95% with an invasive testing rate of about 2%.[16] Performance of various screening tests are discussed in **Table 5.2**.

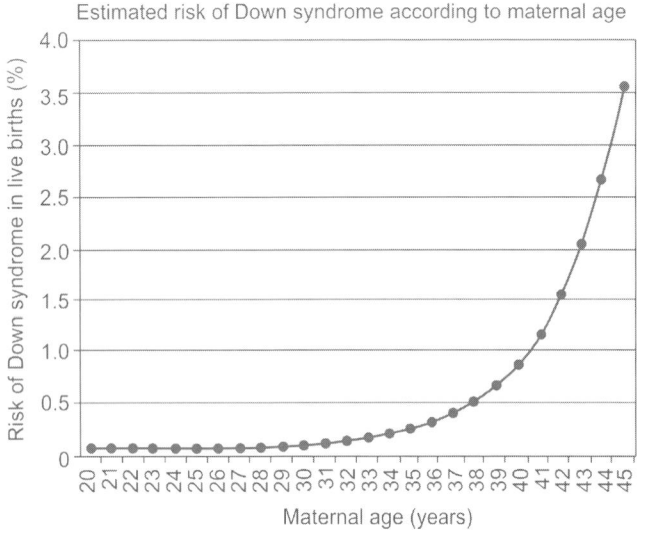

Fig. 5.1: Down syndrome risk association with maternal age

Table 5.2: Comparison of the detection rates (DR), for a false positive rate of 5%, of different methods of screening for trisomy 21

Method of screening	DR (%)
Maternal age (MA)	30
MA and maternal serum biochemistry at 15–18 weeks	50–70
MA and fetal nuchal translucency (NT) at 11–13+6 weeks	80
MA and fetal NT and maternal serum free β-hCG and PAPP-A at 11–13+6 weeks	85–90
MA and fetal NT and fetal nasal bone (NB) at 11–13+6 weeks	90
MA and fetal NT and NB and maternal serum free β-hCG and PAPP-A at 11–13+6 weeks	95

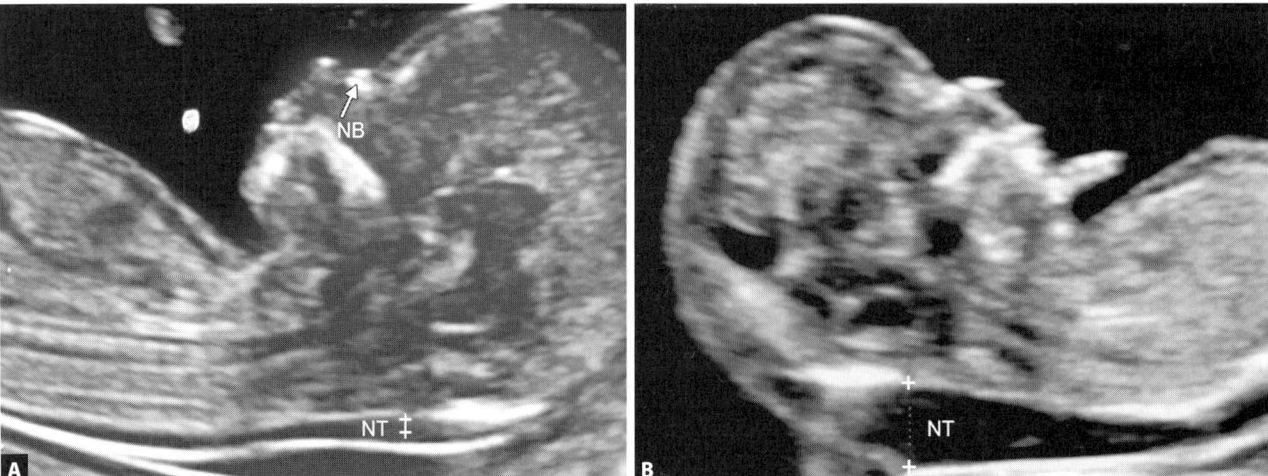

Fig. 5.2: Nuchal translucency in first trimester; Left image (A) shows a normal NT and image on the right (B) shows an increased NT

Second Trimester Serum Screening

Second trimester screening tests can be offered to women between 15–20 weeks of pregnancy. Two serum screening tests are available in the second trimester Triple test and the Quad test. Accurate pregnancy dating should be available at the time of second trimester screening test. Second trimester tests screen for trisomy 21, trisomy 18 and neural tube defects.

Triple test includes three maternal pregnancy specific hormones: AFP (Maternal serum alfa-feto-protein), hCG (human chorionic gonadotropin) and unconjugated estriol. Triple test combined with maternal age has aneuploidy detection rate, approximately 60% for a 5% screen positive rate **(Fig. 5.3)**.[17]

Quad test is a second trimester maternal blood screening test that looks for four specific hormones: AFP, hCG, estriol, and inhibin-A. Quad test combined with maternal age has down syndrome detection rate of 80% for a 5% false positive rate **(Fig. 5.3)**.[18]

Combining first and second trimester screening tests increase the detection rates of aneuploidies.[4] Various protocols are integrated screening, sequential screening and stepwise sequential screening.

Sequential Screening

This is a two-stage screening program in which first trimester combined test using both ultrasound and serum screening are done, and then second trimester serum screening is done for final risk assessment to increase the aneuploidy detection rate. The sequential screening is of two types: Stepwise sequential and contingent screening.

Stepwise sequential screening: In this the first trimester screening results are divided into:
Low risk: Continue second trimester screening
High risk: Genetic counseling and invasive testing

Contingent screening: in this protocol, based on the first trimester screening result patients are divided into three groups:
1. *High risk:* Invasive testing and genetic counseling
2. *Intermediate risk:* Proceed to second trimester screening
3. *Low risk:* No further screening required.

Integrated Screening

In this screening protocol, both the first and second trimester markers are used to adjust the patient's age-related risk. Final risk is reported after both first and second trimester tests are done. Integrated screening has the highest detection rate (94–96%) and lowest false-positive rate **(Fig. 5.3)**.

Limitations: Tests results are not declared until second trimester. Patient cannot opt for first trimester invasive tests (CVS) for confirmation.

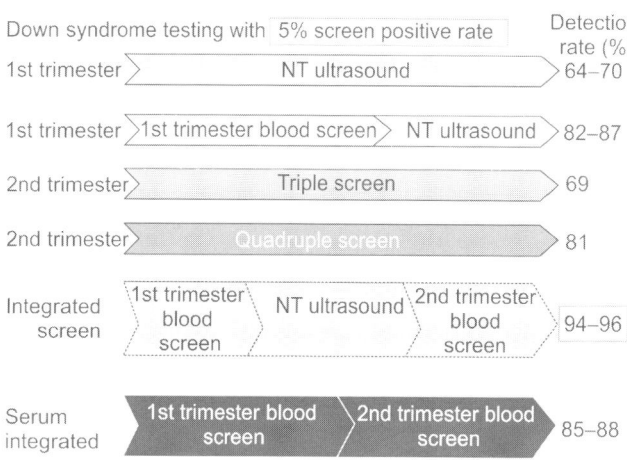

Fig. 5.3: Performance of various screening tests at 5% false positive rate. ACOG Practice Bulletin No. 7, January 2007

Second Trimester Ultrasonography

Also referred to as genetic sonogram, it can be added to the screening protocols to improve the Down syndrome detection rates. Sonographically detected major anatomical defect or soft marker are used to modify the Down syndrome risk assessment done by either first trimester combined screening or the second trimester screening tests using likelihood ratios.

Soft markers for genetic screening used to modify final risk are nuchal skin-fold, choroid plexus cyst, enlarged cisterna magna, ventriculomegaly, echogenic intracardiac focus, pericardial effusion, hydrops, echogenic bowel (with echogenicity equal to adjacent bone), liver calcification, pyelectasis, two-vessel umbilical cord, polydactyly, clinodactyly, sandal gap, and club foot. Major structural abnormality can be diaphragmatic hernia, spinal, cardiac, other thoracic, abdominal, and extremities, etc.

Genetic sonogram can be used to modify the risk, only if it is used as an adjunct to the previous screening test result to give final risk and not used alone.[19] The ultrasonography is best in gestational age window of 18–20 weeks but can be done earlier in high-risk cases. It needs to be performed by skilled personnel. No anomaly or marker detected in genetic sonogram reduces the risk by 80%.

Noninvasive Prenatal Screening (NIPS)

In 1977, it was discovered that there is cell free fetal DNA freely circulating in the maternal plasma, and it could be isolated. These DNA fragment are mostly 150–180 base pairs in length. This fetal DNA is released into the maternal circulation after apoptosis of placental trophoblasts. Cell-free fetal DNA have short half-life (4–30 min), and cleared within hours of delivery. After 10 weeks of pregnancy, they form upto

10% pool of free DNA in the maternal plasma.[21] In 2008 with the use of next generation sequencing studies proved that it can be used to detect fetal aneuploidies. Two technologies are used to study this DNA namely massive parallel sequencing (MPS) and single nucleotide polymorphism (SNP) technique. Very high sensitivity (98.6%) and specificity (99.7%) have been seen for detection of Trisomy 21.[22] Detection rates are also high for trisomy 18 (>97%) and trisomy 13 (up to 90%).[22]

Indications of NIPS

NIPS technologies have been validated in singleton pregnancies at high risk for trisomy 21 due to:
- Advanced maternal age (>35 years)
- An abnormal serum screen (either first or second trimester)
- Personal or family history of aneuploidy
- Abnormal ultrasound showing increase risk for aneuploidy
- Robertsonian translocation in parents.
- Recommending NIPS to a couple should be after thorough genetic counseling explaining the limitations and need for invasive tests, if NIPS is positive or inconclusive for aneuploidy. It should be emphasized that NIPS is a *screening* test with low false positive rate.[20]

ACOG recommends that NIPS can be offered to all pregnant patients as the most sensitive screening option for trisomies 13, 18, and 21.

CURRENT LIMITATIONS OF NIPS (ACMG STATEMENT 2016, ACOG 2015)

- Risk assessment is limited to specific fetal aneuploidies (trisomy 13, 18, and 21) now.
- Approximately 50% of cytogenetic abnormalities routinely identified by amniocentesis will not be detected.
- Chromosomal abnormalities such as unbalanced translocations, deletions, and duplications will not be detected by NIPS. Therefore, when fetal anomalies are detected, invasive diagnostic testing and cytogenomic microarray analysis are more likely to detect chromosomal imbalances than NIPS and may be a better testing option.
- NIPS is not able to distinguish specific forms of aneuploidy. For example, NIPS cannot determine if Down syndrome is due to the presence of an extra chromosome (trisomy 21), a Robertsonian translocation involving chromosome 21, or high-level mosaicism. Identification of the mechanism of aneuploidy is important for recurrence risk counseling and emphasizes the importance of diagnostic testing following NIPS.
- NIPS does not screen for single-gene mutations.
- Uninformative test results due to insufficient isolation of cell-free fetal DNA could lead to a delay in diagnosis or eliminate the availability of information for risk assessment. Biologic factors associated with reduced available cell-free fetal DNA include a high body mass index and early gestational age
- It is still not validated for use in multiple pregnancies and oocyte donors.
- If major structural anomaly is detected on ultrasound invasive fetal testing is preferred.

SOGC RECOMMENDATIONS FOR ANEUPLOIDY SCREENING[23]

- All women should be offered prenatal tests for aneuploidy screening with proper counseling regarding the same.
- Maternal age alone is a poor criterion for guiding invasive fetal testing.
- Direct invasive fetal testing should not be done without multiple marker screening tests unless: there is major ultrasound malformation, previous history of affected child with chromosomal abnormality, parents are carriers of specific genetic condition or IVF/ICSI conception.
- First trimester nuchal translucency cannot be used alone without serum biomarkers as screening test. Nasal bone and Nuchal translucency measurement are to be done only by trained sonologists.
- For women undergoing first trimester screening tests for screening, second trimester ultrasound or MSAFP is done to screen for neural tube defects.
- Ultrasound dating should always be done along with screening tests as the results are gestational age dependent.
- The presence or absence of soft markers or anomalies in the 18- to 20-week ultrasound can be used to modify the a priori risk of aneuploidy established by age or prior screening
- Information such as gestational dating, maternal weight, ethnicity, insulin-dependent diabetes mellitus, and use of assisted reproduction technologies should be provided to the laboratory to improve accuracy of testing.

ABNORMAL MATERNAL SERUM SCREENING

An unexplained level of a maternal serum marker analyte is defined as an abnormal level after confirmation of gestational age by ultrasound and exclusion of maternal, fetal, or placental causes for the abnormal level. When there are abnormally elevated or depressed values of maternal hormones with screening test; a correlation with few adverse obstetrical outcomes is discussed below.[25] Spontaneous or planned multifetal reductions may result in abnormal elevations of serum markers.

Increased alpha-fetoprotein is associated with the following conditions:

IUGR	Gestational hypertension
Antepartum hemorrhage	Oligohydramnios
Placental abruption	Spontaneous abortion
Preterm delivery	Perinatal morbidity
Fetal death < 24 weeks gestation	Gestational hypertension with proteinuria

Unexplained elevated levels of alfa-fetoprotein in cases of placenta previa should have a strong suspicion for placenta accreta, increta or percreta and an MRI should be done to rule out the same.

Low maternal serum levels of AFP < 0.25 MoM is found to be associated with the following:

Spontaneous abortion	Still birth	Increased risk of macrosomia
Preterm birth	Infant death	

Elevated hCG

About >2 MoM to >4 MoM in absences of chromosomal anomalies is seen associated with molar pregnancies, fetal demise, multifetal pregnancy, confined placental mosaicism and unexplained elevation. Adverse pregnancy outcomes are almost similar as seen with increased levels of alfa-fetoproteins.

Low levels of hCG (< 0.5 MoM) in first trimester have been associated with increased risk of spontaneous loss and also IUGR.

Unconjugated Estriol

High levels have not been associated with adverse perinatal outcomes.

The low levels of uE3 (<0.5MoM) is found to be associated with the following:

Anencephaly	Chromosomal anomalies	Hypocortisolism	Oligohydramnios
Fetal death	Sulphatase deficiency	IUGR	Pregnancy loss

Inhibin A

Its levels are elevated in triploidy and HELLP syndrome and following the loss of one twin in first trimester, gestational hypertension and proteinuria. It decreases in presence of primary antiphospholipid antibodies syndrome. Low levels of Inhibin A have not been associated with adverse obstetric outcomes in second trimester.

PAPP-A

No adverse outcomes have been reported with elevated levels of PAPP-A in the first trimester.

Low PAPP-A (< 0.4 MoM) have been found to be associated with the following:[24]

IUGR	Gest. hypertension	Gest. HT with proteinuria
Preterm delivery	Fetal death < 24 weeks	Spontaneous abortion.

SOGC Recommendations (2008) for Abnormal Maternal Serum Screening[26]

- In the first trimester, an unexplained low PAPP-A (< 0.4 MoM) and/or a low hCG (< 0.5 MoM) are associated with an increased frequency of adverse obstetrical outcomes. No specific protocol for treatment is available.
- In the second trimester, an unexplained elevation of maternal serum AFP (> 2.5 MoM), hCG (> 3.0 MoM), and/or inhibin-A (> or =2.0 MoM) or a decreased level of maternal serum AFP (< 0.25 MoM) and/or unconjugated estriol (< 0.5 MoM) are associated with an increased frequency of adverse obstetrical outcomes. No specific protocol for treatment is available.
- Pregnant woman with an unexplained elevated PAPP-A or hCG in the first trimester and an unexplained low hCG or inhibin-A and an unexplained elevated unconjugated estriol in the second trimester should receive normal antenatal care, as this pattern of analytes is not associated with adverse perinatal outcomes.
- The combination of second or third trimester placenta previa and an unexplained elevated maternal serum AFP should increase the index of suspicion for placenta accreta, increta, or percreta.
- A prenatal consultation with the medical genetics department is recommended for low unconjugated estriol levels (<0.3 MoM), as this analyte pattern can be associated with genetic conditions.
- The clinical management protocol for identification of potential adverse obstetrical outcomes should be guided by one or more abnormal maternal serum marker analyte value rather than the false positive screening results for the trisomy 21 and/or the trisomy 18 screen
- Pregnant woman who are undergoing renal dialysis or who have had a renal transplant should be offered maternal serum screening, but interpretation of the result is difficult as the level of serum hCG is not reliable.
- Abnormal maternal uterine artery Doppler in association with elevated maternal serum AFP, hCG, or inhibin-A or decreased PAPP-A identifies a group of women at greater risk of IUGR and gestational hypertension with proteinuria.

Uterine artery Doppler measurements may be used in the evaluation of an unexplained abnormal level of either of these markers.

RECOMMNEDATIONS FOR SCREENING IN MULTIPLE PREGNANCIES[27]

First trimester ultrasound should be performed for accurate dating and determining chorionicity of twin gestation. In twin pregnancies, aneuploidy screening using nuchal translucency measurements should be offered. Detailed ultrasound examination to screen for fetal anomalies should be offered, preferably between 18 and 22 weeks' gestation, in all twin pregnancies. Serum screening can be done though not very useful as it is not able to differentiate which twin is having problem. So routine serum screening in twins need further studies before introduction in the routine screening protocols. Overall aneuploidy detection rate in twins is 70% for 5% false positive rate.

INVASIVE FETAL TESTS

Prenatal invasive fetal tests are required to confirm the results of screening test or direct genetic evaluation of fetus, if required. Prenatal genetic sample for cytogenetic, molecular, biochemical studies is chorionic villi in first trimester, and amniotic fluid in early second trimester. Fetal blood is the preferred sample in late second trimester and infection studies of fetus. Tissue specific biopsy can be obtained for the relevant disease under evaluation.

There are *three primary genetic testing methods* used currently:
1. Karyotype
2. Fluorescence *in situ* hybridization (FISH)
3. Comparative genomic hybridization (CGH) (microarray).

Karyotype: It can detect whole chromosome differences, translocations and large deletions or duplications. Usually performed after culture of fetal cells and the results take 4–6 weeks to be declared.

Fluorescence in situ hybridization: It tests only specific areas of DNA so the area of interest must be known. The testing can be done on either metaphase or interphase chromosomes and it works best for identifying deletions. It is fast technique and does not require culture of fetal sample.

Comparative genomic hybridization: It can detect very small duplications or deletions and high level mosaicism. Advancement in this led to development of microarray analysis of chromosomes known as chromosomal microarray (CMA). The utility of this technology for detection of gains and losses in patients with intellectual disabilities, autism, and/or congenital anomalies has been well documented, and CMA is now recommended as a first-tier test for these indications by American College of Medical Genetics.

Advantages of CMAs

The benefits from the use of CMAs for detection of gains and losses of genomic DNA include:
- Ability to analyze DNA from nearly any tissue, including archived tissue or tissue that cannot be cultured.
- Detection of abnormalities that are cytogenetically cryptic by standard G-banded chromosome analysis.
- Better definition and characterization of abnormalities detected by a standard chromosome study.
- Interpretation of objective data, rather than a subjective visual assessment of band intensities.

COMMON INDICATIONS FOR KARYOTYPING ANALYSIS

- Advanced maternal age (more than 35 years).
- Noninvasive screening giving an abnormal report.
- USG finding which is suspicious of a chromosomal problem.
- Known inversion, translocation or insertion in one parent.
- Existing child with chromosomal abnormality.

Amniocentesis

- Typically carried out under USG guidance after 15 weeks of pregnancy.
- Approximately 15–20 mL of amniotic fluid is aspirated.
- The cultured fluid (takes about two weeks to culture) is then examined for analysis of metaphase chromosomes (numerically and structurally).
- The noncultured fluid can be used to determine the levels of alpha-fetoprotein, and if raised, then acetylcholinesterase is also measured as a marker of neural tube defects.
- The information on numerical abnormalities of chromosomes 13, 18, 21 and X and Y chromosomes can be obtained in about three days using noncultured amniotic fluid along with FISH.
- The risk specific to the procedure is 0.5 to 1%, in experienced hands.

Chorion Villus Sampling

- Performed between 11th and 13th weeks of pregnancy. Not advised to carry it out prior to 11th week due to increased risk of limb defects.
- Can be carried out transcervically or transabdominally.
- The chromosomal analysis can be carried out on non-cultured, brief cultured (1 day) or on fully cultured tissue (7 to 10 days).

- The risk specific to the procedure is about 1% in experienced hands.

Cordocentesis

- The most common indications are suspected fetal anemia associated with Rhesus disease, Parvovirus B19 infection or fetal hydrops.
- It can be used for Rapid karyotyping or molecular genetic diagnosis between 16th and 20th week of pregnancy, depending on the indication.
- The blood is collected from the umbilical vein at the site of its insertion in the placenta.
- The results of chromosomal analysis of the lymphocytes can be obtained in (3 to 5 days).

Limitations of Cytogenetic Diagnosis

- The chances of not obtaining the fetal cellular material is about (1%).
- Culture failure can happen occasionally.
- Structural chromosomal abnormalities smaller than the achievable optical resolution cannot be detected.
- Mosaicism.
- Detection of translocation or inversion often needs further investigation.

SCREENING FOR GENE MUTATIONS THAT LEAD TO FETAL DISEASE

Certain populations are at increased risk for certain inherited genetic disorders and to screen them for these specific disorders should be a part of prenatal care when dealing with such population **(Table 5.3)**. Issues concerned with these diseases work-up are patient education, counseling, inheriting pattern and individuals genetic risk along with diagnostic and therapeutic options. Family history, pedigree analysis and carrier screening are the most important points to be considered in these antenatal patients. Depending upon the type of inheritance the disease can be autosomal recessive, dominant or X-linked **(Fig. 5.4)**. Few examples are cystic fibrosis, Tay-Sachs disease(Jewish), sickle cell anemia (African-American), Thalassemia, Fragile X syndrome.

PREIMPLANTAION GENETIC DIAGNOSIS

Preimplantation genetic diagnosis (PGD) is a screening test used to determine, if genetic or chromosomal disorders are present in embryos produced through *in vitro* fertilization (IVF). Preimplantation genetic diagnosis (PGD) screens embryos before they are transferred to the uterus so couples can make informed decisions about their next steps in the IVF process. Biopsies from the embryo can be taken either at the two cell stage, 6-8 cell stage(Day 2-3) or 5-7 day blastocyst. Embryos unaffected by the genetic or chromosomal disorder can be selected for transfer to the uterus.

For couples undergoing IVF, PGD may be recommended when:

- One or both partners has a history of heritable genetic disorders
- One or both partners is a carrier of a chromosomal abnormality
- The mother is of advanced maternal age
- The mother has a history of recurrent miscarriages

PGD does not replace prenatal testing, such as chorionic villus sampling or amniocentesis. It provides diagnostic information based on the analysis of a single cell, so prenatal testing is still recommended and currently remains the standard of care.

Table 5.3: Frequency of population prevalent genetic diseases

Ethnicity	Disease(s)	Carrier frequency
Caucasian/European	Cystic fibrosis	1/25
African Americans	Sickle cell disease and other hemoglobinopathies	1/12
East/SE Asians	Thalassemia (alpha and beta)	1/20–1/50
Hispanics	Sickle cell disease and other hemoglobinopathies	Varies
Jewish ancestry	Bloom syndrome	1/100
	Canavan disease	1/40
	Cystic fibrosis	1/25
	Familial dysautonomia	1/32
	Fanconi anemia C	1/89
	Gaucher disease (type I)	1/18
	Mucolipidosis IV	1/100
	Niemann-Pick disease	1/90
	Tay-Sachs disease	1/30
French Canadians and Cajuns	Tay-Sachs disease	1/30
Middle Eastern and South Central Asia	Beta-thalassemia and other hemoglobinopathies	Varies
Mediterranean	Beta-thalassemia and other hemoglobinopathies	1/20–1/30

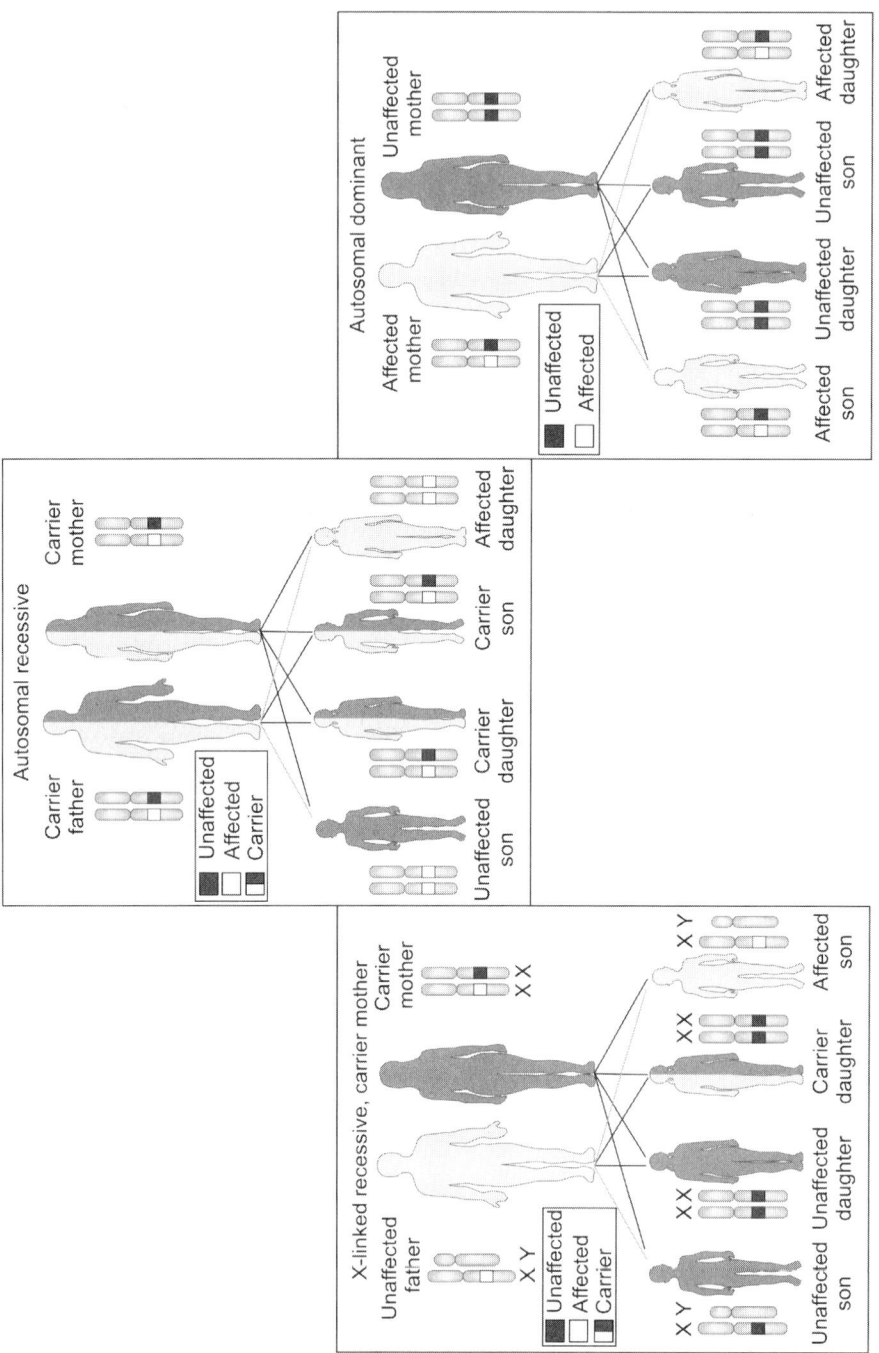

Fig. 5.4: Familial inherited disorders follow mendelian pattern of inheritance, i.e. autosomal dominant, autosomal recessive, X-linked patterns. Prenatal screening involves a positive family history, determining type of inheritance, zygosity of parents, genetic counseling regarding fetal affection, diagnostic and therapeutic options and recurrence risk

REFERENCES

1. Verma IC. Burden of genetic disorders in india. The Indian Journal of Pediatrics. 2000;67(12):893-8.
2. Hoffman JIE, Kaplan S. The incidence of congenital heart disease. J Am Coll Cardiol. 2002;39(12):1890-900.
3. American College of Obstetricians and Gynecologists. ACOG Practice Bulletin No. 88, December 2007. Invasive prenatal testing for aneuploidy. Obstet Gynecol. 2007;110:1459.
4. ACOG Committee on Practice Bulletins. ACOG Practice Bulletin No. 77: screening for fetal chromosomal abnormalities. Obstet Gynecol. 2007;109:217.
5. Alldred SK, Takwoingi Y, Guo B, Pennant M, Deeks JJ, Neilson JP, Alfirevic Z. First trimester serum tests for Down's syndrome screening. Cochrane Database Syst Rev. 2015;30(11):CD011975.
6. Glenn EP, Jo Ellen SL, Canick JA, McDowell GA, Donnenfeld AE. Technical standards and guidelines: Prenatal screening for Down syndrome that includes first-trimester biochemistry and/or ultrasound measurements. Genetics IN Medicine. 2009;11:669-81.
7. Sonek J. First trimester ultrasonography in screening and detection of fetal anomalies. Am J Med Genet C Semin Med Genet. 2007;145:45-61.
8. Cicero S, Avgidou K, Rembouskos G, Kagan KO, et al. Nasal bone in first-trimester screening for trisomy 21. Am J Obstet Gynecol. 2006;195:109-14.
9. Makrydimas G, Sotiriadis A, Huggon IC, Simpson J, et al. Nuchal translucency and fetal cardiac defects: a pooled analysis of major fetal echocardiography centers. Am J Obstet Gynecol. 2005;192(1):89-95.
10. Wapner R, Thom E, Simpson JL, Pergament E, et al. First-trimester screening for trisomies 21 and 18. N Engl J Med. 2003;349:1405-13.
11. Chelemen T, Syngelaki A, Maiz N, Allan L, Kypros H. Nicolaides. Contribution of Ductus Venosus Doppler in First-Trimester Screening for Major Cardiac Defects. Fetal Diagn Ther. 2011;29:127-34.
12. Cicero S, Curcio P, Papageorghiou A, Sonek J, Nicolaides K. Absence of nasal bone in fetuses with trisomy 21 at 11–14 weeks of gestation: an observational study. Lancet. 2001;358(9294):1665-7.
13. Nicolaides H. Screening for fetal aneuploidies at 11 to 13 weeks. Prenat Diagn. 2011;31:7-15.
14. Grande M, Arigita M, Borobio V, Jimenez JM, Fernandez S, Borrell A. First-trimester detection of structural abnormalities and the role of aneuploidy markers. Ultrasound Obstet Gynecol. 2012;39(2):157-63.
15. Zhong Y, Zhu F, Ding Y. Serum screening in first trimester to predict pre-eclampsia, small for gestational age and preterm delivery: systematic review and meta-analysis. BMC Pregnancy Childbirth. 2015;15:191.
16. Cicero S, Bindra R, Rembouskos G, Spencer K, Nicolaides KH. Integrated ultrasound and biochemical screening for trisomy 21 using fetal nuchal translucency, absent nasal bome, free β-hCG and PAPP-A at 11–14 weeks. Prenat Diagn. 2003;23:306-10.
17. Wald NJ, Cuckle HS, Densem JW, et al. Maternal serum screening for Down's syndrome in early pregnancy. BMJ. 1988;297:883-7.
18. Canick JA, MacRae AR. Second trimester serum markers. Semin Perinatol. 2005;29(4):203-8.
19. Aagaard-Tillery, Kjersti M, et al. Role of Second-Trimester Genetic Sonography After Down Syndrome Screening. Obstetrics and Gynecology. 2009;114(6):1184-96.
20. Neufeld-Kaiser WA, Cheng EY, Liu YJ. Positive predictive value of non-invasive prenatal screening for fetal chromosome disorders using cell-free DNA in maternal serum: independent clinical experience of a tertiary referral center. BMC Medicine. 2015;13:129.
21. Ashoor G, Poon L, Syngelaki A, Mosimann B, Nicolaides KH. Fetal fraction in maternal plasma cell-free DNA at 11-13 weeks' gestation: effect of maternal and fetal factors. Fetal Diagn Ther. 2012;31:237-43.
22. Nicolaides KH, Syngelaki A, Gil M, Atanasova V, Markova D. Validation of targeted sequencing of single-nucleotide polymorphisms for non-invasive prenatal detection of aneuploidy of chromosomes 13, 18, 21, X, and Y. Prenat Diagn. 2013;33:575-9.
23. Chitayat D, Langlois S, Wilson RD; Genetics Committee of the Society of Obstetricians and Gynaecologists of Canada; Prenatal Diagnosis Committee of the Canadian College of Medical Geneticists. Prenatal screening for fetal aneuploidy in singleton pregnancies. J Obstet Gynaecol Can. 2011;33(7):736-50.
24. Yuval Yaron, Sigal Heifetz, Yifat Ochshorn. Prenatal diagnosis. Decreased first trimester PAPP-A is a predictor of adverse pregnancy outcome. 2002;22(9):778-82.
25. Yaron Y, Cherry M, Kramer RL, O'Brien JE, Hallak M, Johnson MP, Evans MI. Second-trimester maternal serum marker screening: Maternal serum α-fetoprotein, β-human chorionic gonadotropin, estriol, and their various combinations as predictors of pregnancy outcome. AJOG. 1999;181(4):968-74.
26. Gagnon A, Wilson RD, Audibert F, Allen VM, Blight C, Brock JA, Désilets VA, Johnson JA, Langlois S, Summers A, Wyatt P. Obstetrical complications associated with abnormal maternal serum markers analytes. J Obstet Gynaecol Can. 2008;30(10):918-49.
27. Morin L, Lim K. Ultrasound in twin pregnancies. J Obstet Gynaecol Can. 2011;33(6):643-56.

Chapter 6

Impact of Advances in Genetics in Prenatal Diagnosis

Shweta Bhandari, Ashutosh Gupta

Prenatal congenital disorders although low in frequency have a huge impact on the affected families, and therefore screening ongoing pregnancies for genetic and structural disorders should be performed. Prenatal screening involves family history and pedigree analysis, population screening, fetal risk assessment, genetic counseling and fetal diagnostic tests. The genetic disorders can be divided into chromosomal aberrations, single gene disorders, polygenic diseases or multifactorial diseases.

Screening for genetic disorders comprises two broad categories including carrier screening and prenatal screening for aneuploidies. Carrier screening includes screening the couple or prospective parents whether they carry the affected gene for the inherited familial condition (Carrier status). Carrier screening is of two types: population prevalent genetic screening (e.g. Cystic Fibrosis) or specific inherited familial disorders (Muscular Dystrophies). After the carrier status of parents are determined, fetal risk of inheriting the disease is determined, and if present invasive fetal test for determining fetal gene aberration are done.

Prenatal screening is intended at stratifying risks as to which pregnancy is categorized as low risk or high for a genetic disorder whereas prenatal diagnosis aims at identifying genetic disorders in the fetus with an accuracy which can be best aimed at.

The traditional method of prenatal diagnosis were mainly invasive tests and the methods of analysis were principally Fluorescent *in situ* hybridization (FISH) and karyotype. However, with the advent of new technologies the diagnostic accuracy has improved.

Diagnostic methods: Prenatal detection of chromosomal abnormalities has been available for more than 40 years which was first by amniocentesis in early 1970s and later by chorionic villous sampling in 1980s. The fact there is an increasing number of aneuploid children born to women with advanced maternal age, the primary utilization of these tests was for detection of trisomy, however, now it finds its uses in diagnosis of a wide variety of chromosomal abnormalities.

- *Chorionic villous sampling*: It involves biopsy of placental cells and is usually performed between 11–13 weeks. The advantage remains in the test being performed at an early gestation. The main disadvantage lies in diagnostic ambiguity seen in 1–2% cases due to confined placental mosaicism as the sample obtained is from the trophoectoderm rather than being fetal. Also the procedure related loss rate is quoted as 1%, which is slightly higher as compared to amniocentesis (1:200 to 1:600).[1-3]
- *Amniocentesis*: It involves aspiration of the amniotic fluid and subjecting the obtained amniocytes for analysis. As the sample is derived from the fetus the chances of mosaicism do not exist and the procedure-related fetal loss is also minimized. However, the test can be performed only after 15 weeks and the yield of cells is poor, thereby the results take a longer time.
- *Fetal blood sampling*: It is usually performed after 18 weeks of gestation and the most common indications being assessment of chromosomal mosaicism after amniocentesis and hematological assessment of fetus. The main drawback is the increased risk of fetal loss nearly 1–2% as compared to other invasive procedures. The risk is mainly increased in the presence of associated structural anomalies, fetal growth restriction and when performed at a gestation earlier than 24 weeks.

The most common indications are suspected fetal anemia associated with Rhesus disease, Parvovirus B19 infection or fetal hydrops. It can be used for rapid karyotyping or molecular genetic diagnosis between 18–20 weeks of pregnancy. The blood is collected from the umbilical vein at the site of its insertion in the placenta. The results of chromosomal analysis of the lymphocytes can be obtained in (3 to 5 days).

GENETIC TECHNIQUES

- *Karyotyping:* Conventional karyotype involves culturing the fetal cells, and subsequently, isolating and treating the chromosomes to make them visible for microscopic evaluation. This enables the detection of aneuploidy, relatively larger deletions or duplications and other structural rearrangements, such as balanced and unbalanced translocations. Such classical cytogenetic G-banding (conventional karyotyping) carries the disadvantages of potential cell-culture failure and clonal selection and has a diagnostic resolution of 5–10 Mb.[4] One megabase (Mb) is a unit of length of DNA and is equivalent to 1000000 base pairs;1 kilobase (kb) is equivalent to 1000 base pairs.

- But now conventional karyotyping has largely been superseded by chromosomal microarray.[5] The conventional method for karyotype analysis is metaphase analysis of cultured amniocytes or that of placental mesenchymal cells obtained from amniocentesis or CVS, respectively. The results are available in 2 weeks. In contrast, metaphase analysis of fetal lymphocytes obtained from fetal blood sampling is available within 2–5 days. Following CVS, direct analysis of cytotrophoblastic metaphases is feasible and may be achieved within 5 days.

- Rapid testing using Fluorescent *in situ* hybridization- This is a more targeted analysis and uses chromosome specific targeted probes for diagnosis of aneuploidies and deletions. However, it cannot diagnose aneuploidies due to Robertsonian translocations and abnormalities such as inversions and translocations as it requires direct visualization of G-banded karyotype. The resolution possible with FISH is 1-2 Mb. These tests provide results in 1-2 days and are commonly employed following a screen-positive result or in fetuses with ultrasound findings or markers of common aneuploidies.

- Chromosomal microarray and array comparative genomic hybridization (CMA and Array CGH). It helps in high resolution analysis of entire genome. It is comparable to conventional karyotyping at identifying aneuploidy and unbalanced chromosomal arrangements and can also detect submicroscopic deletions that remain undiagnosed on karyotyping with a resolution of 10–400 Kb. CMA cannot identify truly balanced translocations, low level mosaicism and triploidy.[6]

  - CGH can also be used in genetic testing in miscarriage or stillbirth where cell cultures from necrotic cells is likely to fail, and therefore may not yield results with karyotype.[7-9]

  - The primary advantage of array CGH is the ability to simultaneously detect aneuploidies, deletions, duplications, and/or amplifications of any locus represented on an array. In addition, aCGH has proven to be a powerful tool for the detection of submicroscopic chromosomal abnormalities in individuals with idiopathic mental retardation and various birth defects. CMA can detect submicroscopic deletions and duplications using copy number variants (CNVs). In the first large study comparing microarrays with karyotype for prenatal diagnosis, it was found that the former could detect clinically relevant aberrations in 6.0% of fetuses with normal karyotype and structural defects and in 1.7% of those undergoing invasive testing for advanced maternal age or positive screening results.[10] Several studies have followed and pooled incremental diagnostic yields of 7.0% and 5.0% were reported with use of array CGH in fetuses with congenital heart defects or increased NT, respectively.[11,12]

  - Currently, the use of these techniques is recommended in cases of fetal structural anomalies or NT > 3.5 mm in the first trimester.[11,12] Among these groups of pregnancies, an increased rate of pathological CNV in comparison with conventional analysis is yielded by the use of microarray. But their use in an unselected population is strongly debated due to the difficult interpretation and counseling in cases of variants of unknown significance (VOUS) due to issues of counseling.[13] The American College of Obstetrics and Gynecology has recommended that prenatal CMA should be the diagnostic test of choice to investigate a prenatally identified congenital anomaly, and could also be used in structurally normal fetuses under-going invasive prenatal testing.[14]

- Next generation sequencing also called as whole genome sequencing or exome sequencing (NGS)—DNA sequencing involves determining the order of nucleotides in a DNA molecule. The classical method of DNA sequencing is Sanger technique which identifies alterations in the order of bases within a contiguous segment. Next-generation sequencing (NGS) has revolutionized genetic testing, as it enables many genes to be sequenced together in a single test. Compared with traditional Sanger sequencing methods, NGS has dramatically faster processing, and therefore a quicker turnaround of results, reducing overall cost and making the technique more feasible for use in the prenatal setting.

  Using NGS, the whole genome or exome can be sequenced; however, exome sequencing is often favored over whole-genome sequencing as it targets only exons which are the coding regions of the genome. Exons represent only 1–2% of the entire genome but contain up to 85% of mutations known to cause genetic disorders,[15] making this an efficient method of sequencing in terms of cost, time and computational resources. For exome sequencing, genomic DNA is extracted from samples (amniotic fluid, CVS or fetal blood are often used prenatally), and then fragmented into millions of small portions of DNA. A genomic library is constructed from these fragments. Finally, the DNA is sequenced and the patient DNA fragments, are typically aligned to the reference human genome, and differences between the patients DNA and reference genome are determined.

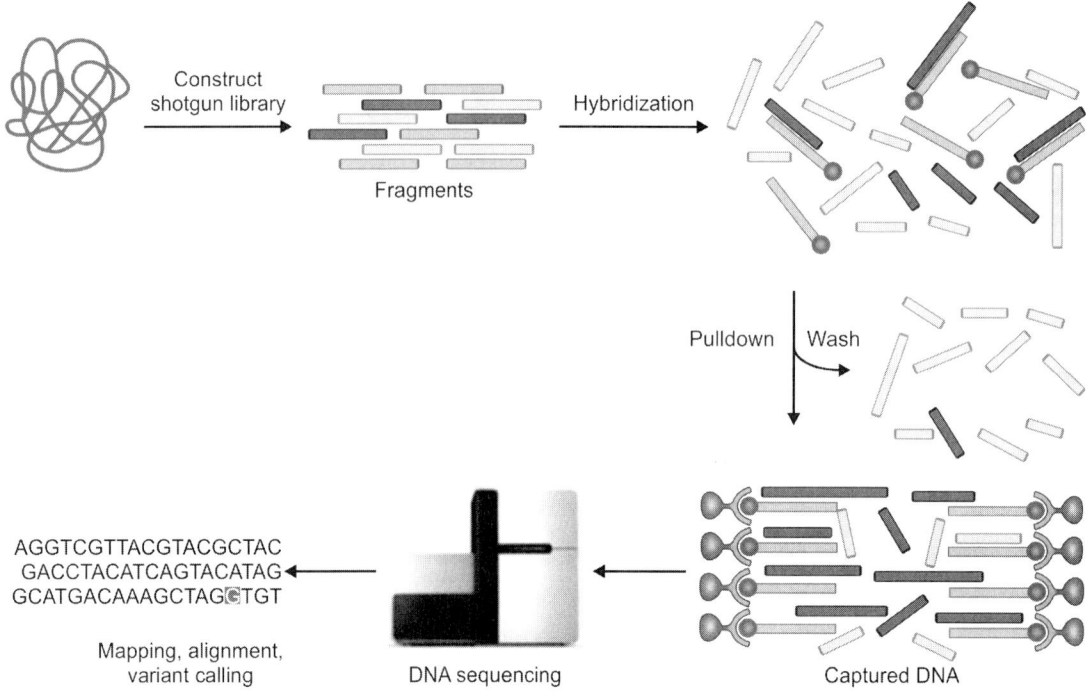

Fig. 6.1: Diagram illustrating the principle of exome sequencing. Genomic DNA is extracted from samples (e.g. amniotic fluid, chorionic villi or fetal blood) and fragmented into small sections of DNA, which are used to onstruct the genomic library. The fragments are hybridized using probes specific for exonic sequence and washed to remove unbound intronic regions. Finally, the captured exonic fragments of DNA are sequenced and compared to the reference genome. Reprinted by permission from Macmillan Publishers Ltd. Nature Rev Genet (Bamshad, et al.[27]) © 2011

NGS provides additional 10% genetic information to that provided by CMA and this is one of its drawback also as it may reveal large quantity of uninformative/unanticipated genetic information raising ethical concerns regarding disclosure **(Fig. 6.1)**.[16]

- *Noninvasive prenatal testing (NIPT):* Fetal DNA was first detected in maternal plasma by Dennis Lo in 1997 and since then it has been the aim to collect the fetal fraction from maternal plasma and utilize this as a noninvasive method for diagnosis of fetal genetic disorders. Fetal DNA is present as early as 6–7 weeks of gestation in maternal plasma and increases at the rate of 0.1% per week until 21 weeks, and then rapidly at a rate of 1% until term.[17] These DNA fragment are mostly 150–180 base pairs in length. This fetal DNA is released into the maternal circulation after apoptosis of placental trophoblasts. Cell-free fetal DNA have short half-life (4–30 min) and cleared within hours of delivery.
    - The earliest use of NIPT was for determining Rhesus status of fetus for all Rh-negative women as it avoids the need of Anti D-administration, if the fetus is identified as Rh-negative. It was also used for fetal sex determination by using real-time PCR for identification of gender in pregnancies at risk of X-linked disorders such as Duchenne muscular dystrophy (DMD), hemophilia and thereby avoid the need of invasive testing, if the fetus is not at risk but not in India due to its legal implications. NIPT is now widely used for prenatal screening of aneuploidies. In NIPT as the cell-free fetal DNA is analyzed, we cannot use traditional methods which involve counting the number of intact chromosomes. And therefore for NIPT, we need techniques which can identify the origin of DNA molecules[18] that is whether the DNA extracted is maternal or fetal and such techniques are shotgun or Sangar sequencing[19] and massive parallel sequencing (MPS).[20] Sangar technique allows analysis of sequences larger than 1000 base pairs and MPS is a form of NGS which can analyze sequences of short DNA molecules up to 100 base pairs.[21] Both the techniques facilitate digital quantification of DNA such that it may be counted and mapped to chromosome of origin. Thereafter the relative number of DNA molecules from each chromosome is found, and then it is determined whether the genome appears euploid or triploid.[19,20] The fetal fraction should atleast comprise 4% of total cell-free fetal DNA for aneuploidy detection.[22,23] The sensitivities of NIPT for detection of trisomy 21 is greater than 99%

- Released through apoptosis
  - Fetal cfDNA likely arises from cytotrophoblastic cells of placenta
- Released into bloodstream as small DNA fragments (150–200 bp)
- Maternal blood contains both fetal, maternal cfDNA
  - 2–20% of total cfDNA is fetal
- Fetal cfDNA reliable detected after 7+weeks gestation
- Fetal cfDNA undetectable within hour postpartum

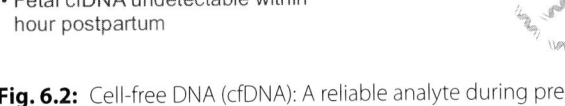

Fig. 6.2: Cell-free DNA (cfDNA): A reliable analyte during pregnancy
Source: 1. Barrett A, et al. Implementing prenatal diagnosis based on call-free fetal DNA: Accurate identification of factors affecting fetal DNA yield. PLoS One. 2011;6:e250202.
2. Nigam A, et al. Detection of fetal nucleic acid in maternal plasma: A novel noninvasive prenatal diagnostic technique. JIMSA. 2012;25:119-200.

Table 6.1: Detection rates and false positive rates of major aneuploidies using NIPT[28]

Chromosome	Detection rate (%); 95% CI	False positive rate (%); 95%CI
Trisomy 21	99.2 (98.5–99.6)	0.09 (0.05–0.14)
Trisomy 18	96.3 (94.3–97.9)	0.13 (0.07–0.20)
Trisomy 13	91.0 (85–95.6)	0.13 (0.05–0.26)
Monosomy X	90.3 (85.7–94.2)	0.23 (0.14–0.34)
Other sex chromosome aneuploidy	93.0 (85.8–97.8)	0.14 (0.06–0.24)
Multiple pregnancy trisomy 21	93.7 (83.6–99.2)	0.23 (0.00–0.92)

with a false positive rate of less than 1%.[24] In case NIPT is suggestive of abnormal or ambiguous results such as observed in confined placental mosaicism which may result in false positive results, an invasive testing is required and therefore amniocentesis remains the gold standard diagnostic prenatal test. The major limitation of NIPT is that in nearly 3% cases the results could be indeterminate or test failures.[25] Such results are known to increase in cases of high maternal BMI, presence of maternal chromosomal abnormalities, confined placental mosaicism and in pregnancies complicated by single fetal demise. Due to the small increased risk of false positive results and in those with failed results on NIPT, there is a need for undergoing confirmatory testing. NIPT is also now widely used for detection of various microdeletions and single gene disorders as well **(Fig. 6.2)**.

Indications for the use of NIPT: Currently, NIPT is indicated in women who are at increased risk of fetal aneuploidy. The American College of Obstetricians and Gynecologists (ACOG), the Society for Maternal fetal Medicine (SMFM) and The American College of Medical Genetics (ACMG) also recommend that NIPT be used for women at high-risk for aneuploidies, and they also state that invasive testing be offered to women with a fetal structural anomaly.[26,27] But the most important aspect with offering NIPT is effective pre-test and post-test counseling to discuss the implications of results **(Table 6.1)**.

NIPT in multiple gestations: Screening in NIPT is more complex than in singletons as the fetal fraction is contributed by two fetuses which may be genetically identical in monozygotic twins or non-identical in dizygotic twins discordant for aneuploidies. Dizygotic twins may contribute in different proportions to the fetal fraction. In dizygotic twins the aneuploid fetus may contribute a fetal fraction of less than 4% and therefore the results may be erroneous. To avoid this the lower fetal fraction should be used for analysis rather than the total fetal fraction[29] and therefore in twins the no results rate is higher than in singletons.[30] In twin gestation the combination of an aneuploid fetus and the euploid fetus diminishes the detection rate of aneuploidy screening. The fetal fraction contributed by a discordant twin gestation is only two-thirds of the fetal fraction as compared to a singleton pregnancy because the euploid fetus dilutes the fetal fraction of the aneuploid fetus. In about 10–15% of twin gestations, the fetal fraction per fetus may be too low to evaluate.[31] At present, there are no data for its use in triplets or higher order gestation.

The sensitivity of detection of other trisomies apart from Trisomy 21 is lower for Trisomy 18 and Trisomy 13. This is due to the lower guanine and cytosine content in chromosome 18 and 13 which makes it difficult in interpretation due to non-uniform mapping.[32] The data on individual sex chromosomal abnormalities, multiple pregnancies and egg donor pregnancies are limited. False positive results may be seen in confined placental mosaicism, vanishing twin, maternal mosaicism, maternal malignancy and in transplant recipients.

CURRENT LIMITATIONS OF NIPT (ACMG STATEMENT 2016, ACOG 2015)

- Risk assessment is limited to specific fetal aneuploidies (trisomy 13, 18, and 21) now.
- Approximately, 50% of cytogenetic abnormalities routinely identified by amniocentesis will not be detected.

- Chromosomal abnormalities such as unbalanced translocations, deletions, and duplications will not be detected by NIPS. Therefore, when fetal anomalies are detected, invasive diagnostic testing and cytogenetic microarray analysis are more likely to detect chromosomal imbalances than NIPS and may be a better testing option.
- NIPS is not able to distinguish specific forms of aneuploidy. For example, NIPS cannot determine, if Down syndrome is due to the presence of an extra chromosome (trisomy 21), a Robertsonian translocation involving chromosome 21, or high-level mosaicism. Identification of the mechanism of aneuploidy is important for recurrence risk counseling and emphasizes the importance of diagnostic testing following NIPS.
- NIPS does not screen for single-gene mutations.
- Uninformative test results due to insufficient isolation of cell-free fetal DNA could lead to a delay in diagnosis or eliminate the availability of information for risk assessment.
- It is still not validated for use in multiple pregnancies and oocyte donors.
- If major structural anomaly is detected on ultrasound invasive fetal testing is preferred.
- Maternal obesity, medical complications, early gestational age and fetal aneuploidy may lead to a lower fetal fraction, and therefore results may be affected.

FUTURE OF NIPT

In near future, widespread use of this test should result in lower cost of test. At present with some technologies it is possible to screen for other chromosomal abnormalities such as trisomy 9, 16 and 22 and a few microdeletions. Hopefully with the progress in NIPT may pave a way to diagnosis of single gene disorders, chromosomal microarray and whole genome sequencing.

NIPT with its high sensitivity is a reassuring test for those with negative results and can decrease the number of invasive procedures performed but it should not be considered a diagnostic test.

PREIMPLANTATION GENETIC DIAGNOSIS

Preimplantation genetic diagnosis (PGD) is an early for of prenatal diagnosis for couples at risk of transmitting a genetic disorder to their children. Before PGD was available the options for such couples were remaining childless, prenatal diagnosis, gamete donation or adoption.

Couples requesting PGD have to undergo *in vitro* fertilization in order to produce embryos for biopsy, even if they are fertile. Embryos that are found to be unaffected by the family's inherited condition are transferred to the uterus.

Embryo biopsy can be performed on the first and second polar body, the cleavage stage embryo or the blastocyst.

- Polar body biopsy is minimally invasive but its limitation is that it tests only the female contribution to the embryo.
- Biopsy at the cleavage stage (6–8 cell stage) allows retrieval of 1–2 cells and is the most common approach for monogenic disorders[33] however, it provides limited genetic material and time for performing analysis.[34]
- Blastocyst biopsy involves retrieval of 5–10 cells from a 5–6 day old embryo of 100–150 cells. It provides more DNA material for analysis which results in increased sensitivity and specificity of PGD. Also the implantation and live birth rates are higher as compared to the biopsy when performed at cleavage stage.[35]

REFERENCES

1. ACOG Committee on Practice Bulletins, authors. ACOG Practice Bulletin No. 77: screening for fetal chromosomal abnormalities. Obstet Gynecol. 2007;109:217-27.
2. Alfirevic Z, Sundberg K, Brigham S. Amniocentesis and chorionic villus sampling for prenatal diagnosis. Cochrane Database Syst Rev; 2003.
3. American College of Obstetricians and Gynecologists, authors. ACOG Practice Bulletin No. 88, December 2007. Invasive prenatal testing for aneuploidy. Obstet Gynecol. 2007;110:1459-67.
4. Shaffer LG, Bejjani BA. A cytogeneticist's perspective on genomic microarrays. Hum Reprod Update. 2004;10:221-6.
5. Hillman SC, Pretlove S, Coomarasamy A, et al. Additional information from array comparative genomic hybridization technology over conventional karyotyping in prenatal diagnosis: a systematic review and meta-analysis. Ultrasound Obstet Gynecol. 2011;37:6-14.
6. Caroline E Fox, Mark D Kilby. Prenatal diagnosis in the modern era. The Obstetrician and Gynecology. 2016;18:213-9.
7. Ahn JW, Bint S, Bergbaum A, et al. Array CGH as a first line diagnostic test in place of karyotyping for postnatal referrals: results from four years' clinical application for over 8,700 patients. MolCytogenet. 2013;6(1):16.
8. Ahn JW, Bint S, Irving MD, et al. A new direction for prenatal chromosome microarray testing: software-targeting for detection of clinically significant chromosome imbalance without equivocal findings. PeerJ. 2014;2:e354.
9. Evans MI, Andriole S, Evans SM. Genetics: update on prenatal screening and diagnosis. Obstet Gynecol Clin North Am. 2015;42(2):193-208.
10. Wapner RJ, Martin CL, Levy B, et al. Chromosomal microarray versus karyotyping for prenatal diagnosis. N Engl J Med. 2012;367:2175-84.
11. Jansen FA, Blumenfeld YJ, Fisher A, Cobben JM, Odibo AO, Borrell A, Haak MC. Array comparative genomic hybridization and fetal congenital heart defects: a systematic review and meta-analysis. Ultrasound Obstet Gynecol. 2015;45:27-35.
12. Grande M, Jansen FA, Blumenfeld YJ, Fisher A, Odibo AO, Haak MC, Borrell A. Genomic microarray in fetuses with increased nuchal translucency and normal karyotype: a systematic review and meta-analysis. Ultrasound Obstet Gynecol. 2015;46:650-8.
13. Ghi T, Sotiriadis A, Calda P, Da Silva Costa F, Raine-Fenning N, Alfirevic Z, McGillivray G, on behalf of the International Society of Ultrasound in Obstetrics and Gynecology. ISUOG

Practice Guidelines: invasie procedures for prenatal diagnosis in obstetrics. Ultrasound Obstet Gynecol. 2016;48:256-68.
14. American College of Obstetricians and Gynecologists Committee on Genetics. Committee Opinion No. 581: the use of chromosomal microarray analysis in prenatal diagnosis. Obstet Gynecol. 2013;122:1374-7.
15. Stenson PD, Ball EV, Howells K, Phillips AD, Mort M, Cooper DN. The Human Gene Mutation Database: providing a comprehensive central mutation database for molecular diagnostics and personalized genomics. Hum Genomics. 2009;4:69-72.
16. Reiff M, Mueller R, Mulchandani S, et al. A qualitative study of healthcare providers' perspectives on the implications of genome-wide testing in paediatric clinical practice. J Genet Couns. 2014;23:474-88.
17. Wang E, Batey A, Struble C, et al. Gestational age and maternal weight effects on fetal cell free DNA in maternal plasma. Prenat Diagn. 2013;33(7):662-6.
18. Go AT, van Vugt JM, Oudejans CB. Non-invasive aneuploidy detection using free fetal DNA and RNA in maternal plasma: recent progress and future possibilities. Hum Reprod Update. 2011;17:372-82.
19. Fan HC, Blumenfeld YJ, Chitkara U, Hudgins L, Quake SR. Noninvasive diagnosis of fetal aneuploidy by shotgun sequencing DNA from maternal blood. Proc Natl Acad Sci USA. 2008;105:16266-71.
20. Chiu RW, Chan KC, Gao Y, Lau VY, Zheng W, Leung TY, et al. Noninvasive prenatal diagnosis of fetal chromosomal aneuploidy by massively parallel genomic sequencing of DNA in maternal plasma. Proc Natl Acad Sci USA. 2008;105: 20458-63.
21. Schuster SC. Next-generation sequencing transforms today's biology. Natmethods. 2008;5:16-8.
22. Chiu RW, Akolekar R, Zheng YW, Leung TY, Sun H, Chan KC, et al. Non-invasive prenatal assessment of trisomy 21 by multiplexed maternal plasma DNA sequencing: large scale validity study. BMJ. 2011;342:c7401.
23. Palomaki GE, Deciu C, Kloza EM, Lambert-Messerlian GM, Haddow JE, Neveux LM, et al. DNA sequencing of maternal plasma reliably identifies trisomy 18 and trisomy 13 as well as Down syndrome: an International Collaborative Study. Genet Med. 2012;14:296-305.
24. Lo YM, Chiu RW. Genomic analysis of fetal nucleic acids in maternal blood. Annu Rev Genomics Hum Genet. 2012;13: 285-306.
25. Futch T, Spinosa J, Bhatt S, de Feo E, Rava RP, Sehnert AJ. Initial clinical laboratory experience in noninvasive prenatal testing for fetal aneuploidy from maternal plasma DNA samples. Prenat Diagn. 2013;33:569-74.
26. ACOG Committee on Genetics, SMFM Publications Committee. ACOG Committee opinion 545. Noninvasive prenatal testing for fetal aneuploidy. Obstet Gynecol. 2012;120(6):1532-4.
27. Gregg AR, Gross SJ, Best RG, et al. The Noninvasive Prenatal Screening Work Group of the American College of Medical Genetics and Genomics. ACMG statement on noninvasive prenatal screening for fetal aneuploidy; 2013.
28. Gil MM, Quezada MS, Revello R, et al. Analysis of cell free DNA in maternal blood in screening for fetal aneuploidies; updated meta-analysis. Ultrasound Obstet Gynecol. 2015;45(3):249-66.
29. Struble CA, Syngelaki A, Oliphant A, Song K, Nicolaides KH. Fetal fraction estimate in twin pregnancies using directed cell-free DNA analysis. Fetal DiagnTher. 2014;35:199-203.
30. Bevliacqua E, Gil MM, Nicoliades KH, et al. Performance of screening for aneuploidies by cell free DNA analysis of maternal blood in twin pregnancies. Ultrasound Obstet Gynecol. 2015;45(1):16-26.
31. Canick JA, Kloza EM, Lambert-Messerlian GM, et al. DNA sequencing of maternal plasma to identify Down syndrome and other trisomies in multiple gestations. Prenat Diagn. 2012;32(8):730-4.
32. Chez EZ, Chiu RW, Sun H, et al. Noninvasive prenatal diagnosis of fetal trisomy 18 and trisomy 13 by maternal plasma DNA sequencing. PloS One. 2011;6(7):e21791.
33. Harper JC, Wilton L, et al. The ESHRE PGD consortium: 10 years of data collection. Hum Reprod Update. 2012; 18:234-47.
34. Kokkai G, et al. Blastocyst biopsy versus cleavage stage biopsy and blastocyst transfer for preimplantation genetic diagnosis of beta thalassemia: a pilot study. Hum Reprod. 2009;24:1221-8.
35. Scott RT Jr, Upham KM, Forman EJ, Zhao T, Treff NR. Cleavage stage biopsy significantly impairs embryonic implantation potential while blastocyst biopsy does not: randomized and paired clinical trial. Fertil Steril. 2013;100:624-30.

Chapter 7

Ultrasonography-guided Interventions in Pregnancy

Jaideep Malhotra, Shally Gupta

Ultrasound is an invaluable tool in pregnancy which can be used for various prenatal diagnostic tests as well as aid in management of high-risk fetus. Starting from early pregnancy when conventional diagnostic procedures such as chorionic villus sampling (CVS) and amniocentesis help to identify the fetus at risk to more advanced interventions such as intrauterine laser therapy for twin-to-twin transfusion syndrome and other fetal diseases. Success of these procedures depends on use of high-resolution ultrasound as well as training and experience of operator. However, all invasive procedures are associated with their own risks and complications and couple should be counseled beforehand. USG-guided interventions in pregnancy can be classified as diagnostic or therapeutic.

Diagnostic interventions in pregnancy include:
- Chorionic villus sampling
- Amniocentesis
- Cordocentesis
- Placental biopsy
- Fetoscopy.

Therapeutic indications in pregnancy are:
- Amnioinfusion
- Fetal Therapy
- Fetal therapy for twin-to-twin transfusion syndrome
- Fetal reduction or selective termination
- Percutaneous procedures in the fetus
- Intrauterine shunts
- Fetal therapy for Rh-isoimmunization
- Ultrasound-guided management of ectopic pregnancy.

CHORIONIC VILLUS SAMPLING

Chorionic villus sampling (CVS) is performed for first trimester prenatal diagnosis between 11 and 13 weeks of gestation and involves aspiration or biopsy of chorionic villi. It should not be performed before 10 weeks as reports of limb defects and technical difficulty due to smaller and thinner placenta. CVS was performed for the first time by Italian biologist, Giuseppe Simoni, Scientific Director of Biocell Center, in 1983.[1] Chorionic villi are fetal in origin, and as such are also an appropriate source of tissue for the evaluation of fetal genetic disease.[2] Formal written consent must be obtained before the procedure.

Indications of Chorionic Villus Sampling

- Abnormal first trimester screen results
- Increased nuchal translucency or other abnormal ultrasound findings
- Family history of a chromosomal abnormality or other genetic disorder
- Parents are known carriers for a balanced translocation or other chromosomal disorder
- Parents are carriers of autosomal recessive disease
- Previous child with nondisjunctional chromosomal abnormality
- Advanced maternal age (maternal age above 35 years at the time of delivery).
- Advanced maternal age (AMA) is associated with increase risk of Down's syndrome and at age 35, risk is 1:400.[3] Screening test is usually carried out first before deciding, if CVS should be done.

Procedure

Chorionic villus sampling can be done by transcervical or transabdominal route.[4-6] The choice of route depends upon position of uterus and placenta and the operator experience. The transcervical route is preferred for those with posterior placenta, while transabdominal is preferred for fundal/anterior placenta.[7] During the procedure in order to reduce risk of infection, probe should be enclosed in a sterile bag and separate sterile gel should be used. Screening tests for blood-borne infections should be carried out and necessary precautions taken in women who test positive.

Transabdominal technique:[8,9] Part is cleaned with antiseptic solution and local anesthesia given in the skin at the site. About 18–20 gauge disposable spinal needle is used and advanced under continuous ultrasound guidance into

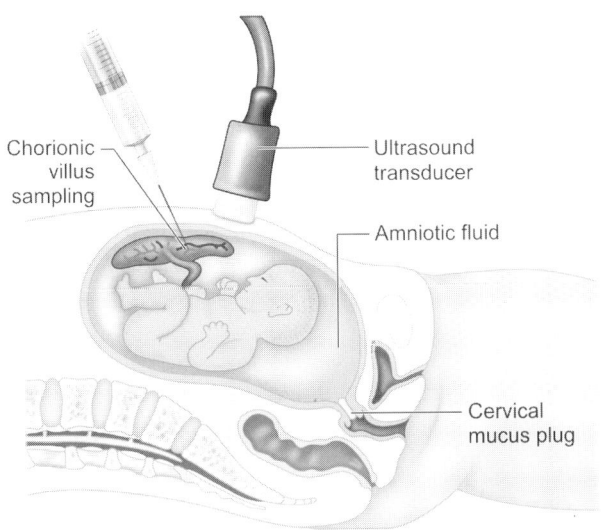

Fig. 7.1: Transabdominal CVS

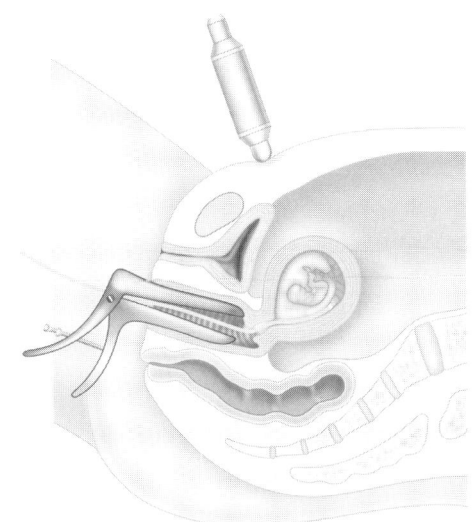

Fig. 7.2: Transcervical CVS

chorion frondosum 10–15 mL of tissue/villi is aspirated in a syringe with 4 mL of medium **(Fig. 7.1)**.

Transcervical CVS technique: A polyethylene catheter with a stylet (diameter < 2 mm) is used to aspirate the villi. The vagina is flushed with saline, the cervix held with tenaculum and polyethylene catheter advanced intracervically till it reaches the lower edge of placenta, the stylet is withdrawn and material aspirated. If the tissue obtained is less the same can be repeated, but no more than 2 attempts should be made as with each extra attempt the risk of abortion doubles, trebles, respectively **(Fig. 7.2)**.

Transcervical CVS	Transabdominal CVS
Large sample size of tissue	Small size of tissue
Less discomfort	More discomfort
Better approach in posterior placenta	Better for fundal placenta
Longer learning curve	Easy to learn

Drawbacks and risks:[10-12] Risk of spontaneous abortion is more for cervical route than abdominal route 2–7% to 2–4% respectively. A causal association has been found in fetal limb defects and early CVS. Its incidence is about 0.3% versus 0.06% in CVS done less than 9 weeks and those done later than 10 weeks. There is some risk of maternal bleeding and abdominal pain. Abortion risk between amniocentesis and early CVS are comparable with trained operators.[13,14]

A high level of expertise in ultrasound scanning is essential for operators undertaking amniocentesis or CVS in multiple, dichorionic pregnancies, because uterine contents have to be 'mapped' with great care. This is essential to ensure that separate samples are taken for each fetus and clearly labelled as such.

Material obtained is subjected to genetic tests: Fluorescence *in situ* hybridization (FISH) and karyotyping.

The result can be obtained as early as 1 to 3 days with cytogenetic diagnosis, but with culture for karyotyping the result takes about 6–12 days. Occasionally, there can be no result, false positive result, and rarely false negative result. Mosaicism can be seen more common in direct preparation testing.[15]

AMNIOCENTESIS

Amniocentesis is one of the earliest guided procedures in use for more than 100 years. It is relatively simple and low risk technique.

Indications of Amniocentesis[16-18]

- To determine fetal karyotype in patients with screen positive prenatal diagnostic tests
- Presence of two or more soft markers for chromosomal abnormalities on USG
- History of child with chromosomal abnormality
- Investigations of Rh-incompatibility/isoimmunization.
- *Testing for lecithin:* Sphingomyelin ratio and phosphatidylglycerol in the third trimester for assessment of lung maturity
- To rule out metabolic disorders
- To diagnose intrauterine infections
- Therapeutic amniocentesis in case of polyhydramnios to relieve maternal distress, prevent preterm labor. In case of twins with poly- and oligoamnios to improve the prognosis of both twins.
- *Amniocentesis for pharmacologic interventions:* Intra-amniotic drugs may be administered for cardiac arrhythmias (digitalis agents) or hypothyroid fetal goiter (thyroxine).

Timing of Amniocentesis

- *Early amniocentesis*: 12 and 14 weeks
- *Conventional amniocentesis*: 15–18 weeks
- *Late ammiocentesis*: 21 weeks

Procedure:[19-21] Conventionally performed between 15 to 18 weeks. At this gestation, there is least risk to vital fetal organs like bladder and bowel and amniotic fluid is in sufficient quantity to have less chance of failed tapping and risk of infection or maximum number of cells can be obtained for cytogenetic diagnosis. True gestational age should be confirmed with sonography, also for correct interpretation of laboratory results. The transducer is applied to the abdomen over sterile ultrasound gel or antiseptic solution, visualizing placenta and cord insertion and using 20 to 22 gauge spinal needle around 20 mL of fluid is aspirated. Continuous ultrasound guidance helps reduce blood staining and other complications of procedure. If a clear pool of amniotic fluid can be reached only by passage through the placenta, then this is the approach of choice. Under these circumstances, placing the needle through the thinnest available part of the placenta is recommended. It is also important to ensure that the placental cord insertion is avoided **(Fig. 7.3)**.

In case of twins both the amniotic cavities should be punctured separately. In earlier times dyes such as methylene blue or more recently indigo carmine have been used to confirm that the sample is being collected from two different sacs. Cytogenetic testing usually obtains result between 8 to 12 days.

Drawbacks and risks of amniocentesis: A small risk of infection such as amnionitis and peritonitis. Rh-isoimmunization can take place in case of Rh-negative pregnancies inadvertently missing on anti-D prophylaxis. The risk to the fetus is comparatively more than maternal risk. A recent systematic review estimated total post-amniocentesis pregnancy loss (background and procedure-related loss combined) to be 1.9%. There is 1% risk of intrauterine death and the chance of spontaneous rupture of membranes is 0.5 to 2%. Early amniocentesis is not a safe alternative to second-trimester amniocentesis because of increased pregnancy loss 7.6% compared with 5.9%. Sometimes there may be continuous leak of amniotic fluid which may close spontaneously in few hours with rest or may be persistent, in which case the monitoring for sepsis is must with clinical signs and symptoms and laboratory parameters such as total leukocyte count or C-reactive protein. Orthopedic deformities have been reported in cases of membrane rupture.[22,23] Occasional abruption followed by bleeding may set in especially in case of transplacental amniocentesis. Compared with mid-trimester procedures, complications including multiple attempts and blood stained fluid are more common in third-trimester procedures.

CORDOCENTESIS (PERCUTANEOUS UMBILICAL BLOOD SAMPLING)

Daffos et al. in 1983 were first to perform modern cordocentesis involving transabdominal access of umbilical cord under ultrasound guidance for diagnostic or therapeutic purposes.[24]

Procedure: In the presence of high resolution ultrasound, umbilical vein or umbilical artery is punctured usually 0.5 to 1 cm from the placental end of the cord as it is least mobile here. Free loops of umbilical cord are more difficult to pierce because it is very mobile, and slips under the needle.[25] Decreasing the fetal movements by injecting sedative like pancuronium bromide in the fetus is helpful and is used usually in therapeutic cordocentesis. Umbilical vein, if preferred more than artery because of its wider caliber and less risk of vasospasm and fetal bradycardia. And 1 mL of fetal blood is enough for testing **(Fig. 7.4)**.

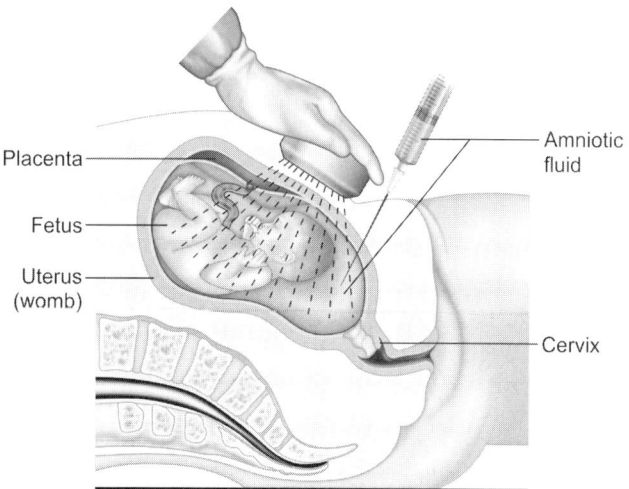

Fig. 7.3: Amniocentesis

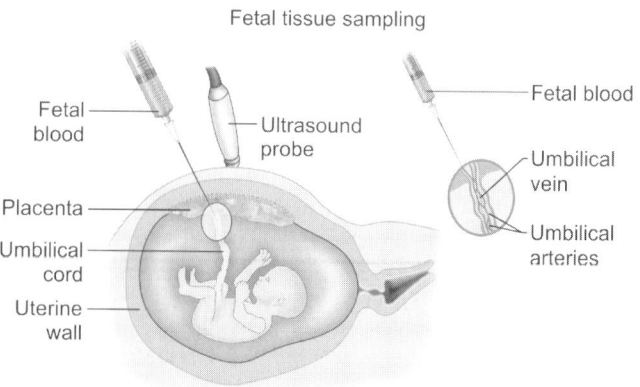

Fig. 7.4: Percutaneous umbilical blood sampling (PUBS) cordocentesis

Indications of Cordocentesis[26]

- Fetal infections such as TORCH, Varicella, Parvo virus.
- Diagnosis of karyotype.
- Diagnosis of fetal anemia.
- Diagnosing Fetal congenital diseases such as coagulopathies, hemoglobinopathies, Immune Deficiency, Thrombocytopenia, SLE and Duchenne muscular dystrophy.
- Diagnosing asphyxia in case of fetal growth retardation by measuring fetal acid-base status or fetal blood gases
- Blood chemistry (measuring thyroxine in fetal goiter).

Risks of cordocentesis: The risks are more than amniocentesis.[27] Fetal loss is approx 1%. They involve, blood vessel lumen narrowing or arterial spasm, cord hematoma, Fetal bradycardia, fetomaternal transfusion or bleeding. The procedure should not be performed, if the mother is HIV or HBsAg positive for the risk of transmitting infection to the fetus.

PLACENTAL BIOPSY

Placental biopsy is done in second or third trimester for indications same as cordocentesis where it cannot be performed due to significant risk. It has the advantage of providing faster result and is performed in the same way as transabdominal CVS in first trimester.[28]

FETOSCOPY

Fetoscopy is an old technique of directly visualizing the fetus, and getting blood samples and skin biopsy. It is rarely performed these days and only for selective hereditary skin diseases such as epidermolysis bullosa and congenital ichthyosis.[29] Recently, it has been used for laser coagulation of placental vessels in fetal twin to twin transfusion syndrome. Fetoscope has a small area of vision and thus needs to be performed on USG guidance. There is 2 to 5% risk of abortion, 4 to 5% risk of premature rupture of membranes and 10% risk of preterm labor.

Ultrasound-guided Therapeutic Procedures in Pregnancy

Therapeutic Amnioinfusion

Therapeutic Amnioinfusion was originally used in prolonged oligoamnios, by infusing normal saline in the amniotic cavity to diagnose potter syndrome.[30] This will aid in improving visualization of stomach and bladder functions.

Fetal Therapy

Fetal therapy was first performed in 1963 by Sir William Liley,[31] who treated fetal anemia in Rh-incompatibility by passing a needle into the fetal abdomen under ultrasound guidance and infusing a donor blood concentrate (0 Rh-negative) into the abdomen.

Advancement in high resolution ultrasonography and more knowledge about fetal diseases have led to further progress in this field. Some interventions in fetus are well established but some have uncertain role and not well established as treatment options. While planning for fetal therapy, we should keep in mind that interventions should be done before irreversible damage has already been caused to fetus and therapy is of use to fetus. At the same time, all therapies involve maternal risk, so that has to be weighed, counseled and minimized against benefit to fetus.[32]

International fetal medicine and Surgery Society consensus has provided prerequisite for doing surgical procedure on fetus.[33] Ethical consideration for fetal therapy has been published by American Academy of Pediatrics.[34]

Fetal therapy can be directly into fetus or indirectly into maternal circulation or amniotic fluid **(Table 7.1)**.

Open fetal surgery is still experimental and new and prognosis is guarded.

Fetal therapy for twin-to-twin transfusion syndrome: Using laser, coagulation of fetal vessels in placenta is done to correct unbalanced flow in donor and recipient fetuses.[35] A trocar is inserted under ultrasound guidance in amniotic cavity of recipient fetus having polyhydramnios, all anastomosis are coagulated using Nd: YAG laser. At the same time, the excess

Table 7.1: Fetal therapy can be directly into fetus or indirectly into maternal circulation or amniotic fluid

Disease	Therapy direct or indirect
Fetal lung maturation	Glucocorticoid
Hyperthyroidism	Propylthiouracil
Hypothyroidism	L thyroxine
Cardiac arrhythmia	Digoxin
Anemia	Red blood cell transfusion
Alloimmune thrombocytopenia	Platelet transfusion
Pleural effusion	Thoracocentesis
Ascites	Aspiration of ascites
Pleural effusion	Thoracic shunt
Hydronephrosis	Renal shunt
Fetofetal transfusion syndrome	Coagulation of communicating placental vessels
Teratoma	Coagulation of tumor feeding teratoma
Congenital diaphragmatic hernia	Repair of defect
Myelomeningocele	Repair of defect

amniotic fluid is drained to normal volume. This is a far superior procedure than serial amniocentesis and improves survival outcome of atleast one twin.[36]

Fetal reduction or selective termination:[37] This may be performed in multiple pregnancies, to selectively reduce fetal number, or to selectively terminate an abnormal fetus. Selective termination can be performed by ultrasound-guided intracardiac lethal injection of potassium chloride. The risks associated with it are miscarriage of remaining fetuses and preterm labor or infection. About 30% of patients lose the entire pregnancy.

Percutaneous procedures in the fetus: Different percutaneous procedures can be performed under ultrasound guidance. Fluid aspiration in diseases such as chylothorax, hydrothorax, renal cyst, ovarian cyst, ascites in nonimmune hydrops.[38] Obstructive uropathies with distended renal pelvis and urinary bladder can be decompressed using percutaneous aspiration, which is both therapeutic and diagnostic at the same time **(Figs 7.5A and B)**.

Intrauterine shunts: Placement of intrauterine shunts is commonly performed procedure for obstructive or non-obstructive conditions leading to large collection of fluid in various body cavities. Shunts are inserted for hydronephrosis in urinary tract obstruction or severe hydrothorax, large pulmonary cyst, chylothorax, hydrocephalus[39-41] Various complications such as infection, obstruction, dislodgement, migration or oligoamnios are reported in many cases. But all shunting procedures should be undertaken when benefits outweigh risks and no irreversible damage has already been reported to the organ.

Fetal therapy for Rh-immunization:[42] Intra-abdominal transfusion of blood for fetal anemia has largely been abandoned in favor of intravenous transfusion in umbilical vein directly under ultrasound guidance in woman suffering from Rh-isoimmunization or fetal hydrops. It is far more rapid and effective procedure.

Ultrasound-guided management of ectopic pregnancy: As many as 2% of pregnancies among women in the general population and 4.5% of pregnancies among women who undergo fertility treatments are ectopic. In cases of tubal pregnancy, US-guided direct chemical injection of the ectopic implant is an important alternative to surgery.[43]

Procedure:[44] After antibiotic prophylaxis is administered and the vaginal vault is cleansed with preparatory solution, a needle (e.g. 20-gauge Chiba type) is inserted with transvaginal US guidance into the amniotic sac. An electronic needle guide is typically used to facilitate planning of the needle route, and color Doppler imaging helps verify the absence of vessels along that route. Typically, the amniotic fluid is aspirated first, and a chemical is then injected into the sac.

Aspiration is performed first (a) to mechanically disrupt the sac and (b) to prevent overdistention of the sac and leakage of the chemical during injection.

Common chemicals that may be injected include methotrexate (1 mg per kilogram of body weight), potassium chloride (1–3 mL in a 2 mEq/mL solution), and hyperosmolar glucose (50% solution).

Potential advantages of injecting methotrexate directly into the amniotic sac are a higher local concentration of the chemical and a lower risk of systemic toxic effects. Potassium chloride or another chemical solution other than methotrexate may be used to allow retention of the intrauterine implant in women with heterotopic pregnancies or in women with severe pulmonary disease, blood dyscrasia, or another contraindication to methotrexate therapy.

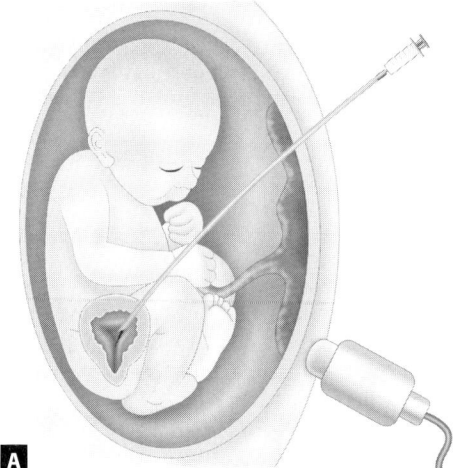
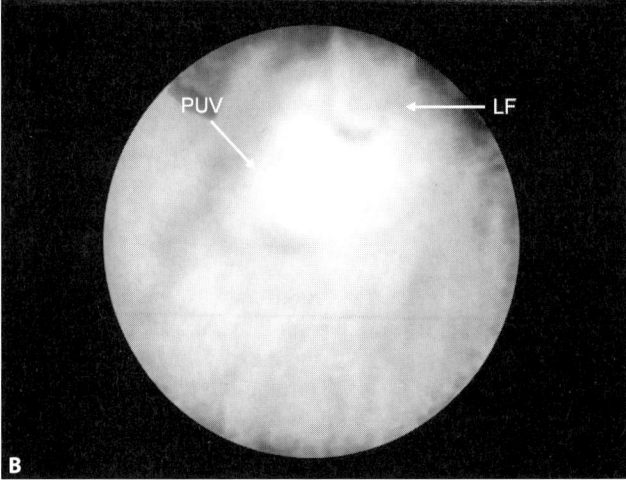

Figs 7.5A and B: (A) Percutaneous endoscopy through the maternal abdomen and uterus into the fetal bladder enabling direct visualization of the fetal bladder neck; (B) Cystoscopic view of a dilated posterior urethra *(For color version of Fig. B, see Plate 1)*

In women with a viable tubal pregnancy indicated by fetal cardiac activity, the injection of potassium chloride may be preferred to increase the probability of cessation of cardiac activity. Follow-up after direct chemical injection of an ectopic sac is similar to that after intramuscular injection of methotrexate.

The primary contraindications to direct injection of an ectopic sac are hemodynamic instability and hemoperitoneum, which are typically considered indications for immediate surgery.

Direct chemical injection is also a potentially effective therapy for an ectopic sac implanted in the cornu, cervix, or cesarean section scar. It is also of use in heterotopic pregnancy, when there is simultaneous ovarian or tubal pregnancy along with viable intrauterine pregnancy.

Some interventional radiologists perform UAE immediately before a cornual sac injection to reduce the risk of postinjection hemorrhage. Some authors also have reported the use of UAE in conjunction with intramuscular methotrexate therapy, or after failed methotrexate therapy, for the successful treatment of cornual and cervical ectopic pregnancies.

REFERENCES

1. Brambati B, Simoni G. Diagnosis of fetal trisomy 21 in first trimester. The Lancet. 1983;1(8324):586. doi:10.1016/S0140-6736(83)92831-3. PMID 6131275
2. Boehm FH, Salyer SL, Dev VG, et al. Chorionic villus sampling: quality control-m-A continuous improvement model. Am J Obstet Gynecol. 1993;168:1766-77.
3. Spencer K, Souter V, Tul N, et al. A screening program for trisomy 21 at 10-14 weeks using fetal nuchal translucency, maternal serum free B-human chorionic gonadotrophin and pregnancy-associated plasma protein A. Ultrasound Obstet Gynecol. 1991;13:231-7.
4. Committee on Genetics. ACOG Committee Opin 1995;160:19. Jackson LG, Zachary JM, Fowler SE, et al. Randomized comparison of transcervical and transabdominal chorionic villus sampling. N Engl J Med. 1992;327:594-8.
5. Silver RK, MacGregor SN, Sholl JS, et al. Initiating a chorionic villus sampling program. Relying on placental location as the primary determinant of the sampling route. J Reprod Med. 1990;35:964-8.
6. Brambati B, Oldrini A, Lanzani A. Transabdominal and transcervical chorionic villus sampling: efficiency and risk evaluation of 2,411 cases. Am J Med Genet. 1990;35:160-4.
7. Liu DT, Agbaje R, Preston C, Savage J. Intraplacental sonolucent spaces: Incidences and relevance to chorionic villus sampling. Prenat Diagn. 1991;11:805.
8. Brambati B, Oldrini A, Lanzani A. Transabdominal chorionic villus sampling: a freehand ultrasound-guided technique. Am J Obstet Gynecol. 1987;157:134.
9. Smidt-Jensen S, Hahnemann N. Transabdominal chorionic villus sampling for fetal genetic diagnosis. Technical and obstetric evaluation of 100 cases. Prenat Diagn. 1988;8:7.
10. Silver RK, MacGregor SN, Sholl JS, Hobart ED, Waldee JK. An evaluation of the chorionic villus sampling learning curve. Am J Obstet Gynecol. 1990;163:917-22.
11. Rhoads GG, Jackson IG, Schlesselman SE, et al. The safety and efficacy of chorionic villus sampling for early prenatal diagnosis of cytogenetic abnormalities. N Engl J Med. 1989;320:609-9.
12. Brambati B, Matarrelli M, Varotto F. Septic complications after chorionic villus sampling. Lancet. 1987;i(8543):1212a.
13. Blakemore KJ, Mahoney MJ, Hobbins JC. Infection and chorionic villus sampling. Lancet. 1985;2:339.
14. Cheng EY, Luth DA, Hickok D, et al. Transcervical chorionic villus sampling and midtrimester oligohydramnios. Am J Obstet Gynecol. 1991;165:1063.
15. Karkut I, Zakrzewski S, Sperling K. Mixed karyotypes obtained by chorionic villi analysis: mosaicism and maternal contamination. In: Fraccaro M, Simoni G, Brambati B (Eds). First Trimester Fetal Diagnosis. Heidelberg: Springer-Verlag. 1985. pp. 144-6.
16. Steele MW, Breg WR Jr. Chromosome analysis of human amniotic fluid cells. Lancet. 1966;1(7434):383-5.
17. Jacobson CB, Barter RH. Intrauterine diagnosis and management of genetic defects. Am J Obstet Gynecol. 1967;99(6):796-807.
18. Valenti C, Schutta EJ, Kehaty T. Prenatal diagnosis of Down's syndrome. Lancet. 1968;2(7561):220.
19. Romero R, Jeanty P, Reece EA, et al. Sonographically monitored amniocentesis to decrease intraoperative complications. Obstet Gynecol. 1985;65(3):426-30.
20. Jeanty P, Rodesch F, Romero R, Venus I, Hobbins JC. How to improve your amniocentesis technique? Am J Obstet Gynecol. 1983;146(6):593-6.
21. Johnson JM, Wilson RD, Singer J, et al. Technical factors in early amniocentesis predict adverse outcome. Results of the Canadian Early (EA) versus Mid-trimester (MA) Amniocentesis Trial. Prenat Diagn. 1999;19(8):732-8.
22. NICHD National Registry for Amniocentesis Study Group. Midtrimester amniocentesis for prenatal diagnosis. Safety and accuracy. JAMA. 1976;236(13):1471-6.
23. Tabor A, Philip J, Madsen M, Bang J, Obel EB, Norgaard-Pedersen B. Randomised controlled trial of genetic amniocentesis in 4606 low-risk women. Lancet. 1986; 1(8493):1287-93.
24. Benecerraf BR, Barss VA, Saltzman DH, et al. Acute fetal distress associated with percutaneous umbilical blood sampling. Am J Obstet Gynecol. 1987;145:1218.
25. Boulot P, Deschamps F, Lefort G, et al. Pure fetal blood samples obtained by cordocentesis: technical aspects of 322 cases. Prenat Diagn. 1990;10:93.
26. Maxwell DJ, Johnson P, Hurley P, et al. Fetal blood sampling and pregnancy loss in relation to indication. Br J Obstet Gynecol. 1991;98:892.
27. Ludomirsky A, Weiner S, Ashmead GG, et al. Percutaneous fetal umbilical blood sampling: procedure safety and normal fetal hematologic indices. Am J Perinatol. 1988;5:264.
28. Holzgreve W, Miny P, Gerlach B, Westendorp A, Ahlert D, Horst J. Benefits of placental biopsies for rapid karyotyping in the second and third trimester (late chorionic villus sampling) in high-risk pregnancies. Amer J Obstet Gynecol. 1990;162:1188-92.

29. Rodeck CH, Nicolaides KH. Fetoscopy. Brit Med Bull. 1986;42: 296-300.
30. Quetel TA, Mejides AA, Salman FA, Torres-Rodriguez MM. Amnioinfusion: an aid in the ultrasonographic evaluation of severe oligohydramnios in pregnancy. Amer J Obstet Gynecol. 1992;167:333-6.
31. Liley AW. Intrauterine transfusion of the fetus in hemolytic disease. Brit Med J. 1963;2:1107-9.
32. Johnsen DE. The creation of fetal rights: conflicts with women's constitutional rights to liberty, privacy, and equal protection. Yale Law Journal. 1986;95:599-625.
33. Harrison MR. Professional considerations in fetal treatment. In: Harrison MR, Golbus MS, Filly RA (Eds). The unborn patient. Philadelphia: Saunders. 1991;pp.8-13.
34. Committee on bioethics, American Academy of Pediatrics: Fetal therapy—ethical considerations. Pediatrics. 1999. pp.1061-3.
35. Ville Y, Hyett J, Vandenbusche FPA, Nicolaides KH. Endoscopic laser coagulation of umbilical cord vessels in twin reversed arterial perfusion sequence. Ultrasound Obstet Gynecol. 1994;4:396-8.
36. Hecher K, Plath H, Bregenzer T, Hansmann M, Hackelöer BJ. Endoscopic laser surgery versus serial amniocenteses in the treatment of severe twin-twin transfusion syndrome. Amer J Obstet Gynecol. 1999;180:717-24.
37. Evans MI, Andriole S, Britt DW. Fetal Reduction: 25 Years' Experience. Fetal Diagn Ther 2014;35:69-82. DOI: 10.1159/000357974.
38. Meagher SE, Fisk NM, Boogert A, Russell P. Fetal ovarian cysts: diagnostic and therapeutic role for intrauterine aspiration. Fetal Diagn Ther. 1993;8:195-9.
39. Harrison MR, Nakayama DK, Noall R, de Lorimier, AA. Correction of congenital hydronephrosis in utero. Decompression reverses the effects of obstruction on the fetal lung and urinary tract. J Pediatr Surg. 1982;17;965-74.
40. Clewell WH, Johnson ML, Meier PR, et al. A surgical approach to the treatment of fetal hydrocephalus. N Engl J Med. 1982;306:1320-5.
41. Nicolaides KH, Azar GB. Thoraco-amniotic shunting. Fetal Diagn Ther. 1990;5:153-64.
42. Agarwal K, Rana A, Ravi AK. Treatment and Prevention of Rh-isoimmunization. J Fetal Med. 2014;1:81. doi:10.1007/s40556-014-0013-z
43. Sivalingam VN, Duncan WC, Kirk E, Shephard LA, Horne AW. Diagnosis and management of ectopic pregnancy. The Journal of Family Planning and Reproductive Health Care/Faculty of Family Planning and Reproductive Health Care, Royal College of Obstetricians and Gynaecologists. 2011;37(4):231-40. *http://doi.org/10.1136/jfprhc-2011-0073*.
44. Monteagudo A1, Minior VK, Stephenson C, Monda S, Timor-Tritsch IE. Non-surgical management of live ectopic pregnancy with ultrasound-guided local injection: a case series. Ultrasound Obstet Gynecol. 2005;25(3):282-8.

SECTION 3: HEMATOLOGICAL DISORDERS DURING PREGNANCY

Chapter 8: Anemia During Pregnancy and New Parenteral Iron

Archana Verma, Pushpa Pandey, Richa Baharani

INTRODUCTION AND MAGNITUDE OF PROBLEM

Anemia is the most common medical disorder during pregnancy. According to the WHO Global Database on Anemia for 1993-2005, children and women of reproductive age are most at risk for Anemia, 47% of children younger than 5 years, 42% of pregnant women, and 30% of non-pregnant women aged 15-49 years are anemic Globally.[1] Africa and Asia account for more than 85% of the absolute anemia burden in high-risk groups, and India is the worst hit. India is one of the countries with very high prevalence of anemia in the world. The National Family Health Survey-3 (NFHS-3) data suggests that anemia is widely prevalent among all age groups, and is particularly high among the most vulnerable viz. pregnant women (nearly 58%), non-pregnant non-lactating women (nearly 50%). In India, National Family Health Survey—4 in 2015-16 shows 23.6–61.7% of women are anemic. The prevalence is higher in urban areas (23.6–61.7%) as compared to rural areas (19.6–58.1%).[2] It is estimated that anemia is the underlying cause for 20–40% of maternal deaths in India. India contributes to about 80% of the maternal deaths due to anemia in South Asia.[3]

DEFINITION

Anemia is defined as a quantitative or qualitative reduction of hemoglobin or circulating red blood cells (RBCs) or decrease in the oxygen carrying capacity of blood. According to WHO, hemoglobin less than 11 g and hematocrit less than 33% in pregnant women constitutes anemia and hemoglobin below 7 g/dL as severe anemia **(Table 8.1)**. The Center for Disease Control and Prevention (1990) defines anemia as less than 11 g/dL in the first and third trimester and less than 10.5 g/dL in second trimester serum ferritin below 15 ug/L is associated with iron-deficiency anemia.

CAUSES AND CLASSIFICATION OF ANEMIA

Etiological classification helps in knowing exact cause of anemia but needs an elaborate panel of investigations.

Table 8.1: WHO/Indian Council of Medical Research Categories of anemia[4,5]

Hb g%	WHO	ICMR
Mild	10–10.9	10–11
Moderate	7–9.9	7–10
Severe	<7	4–7
Very severe		<4

- *Anemia caused by decreased production of RBCs and Hb:*
  - Hypoproliferative anemia
    - Genetic defects such as thalassemias or RBC membrane defects
    - Nutritional deficiency anemia (iron, folate, B_{12} deficiency anemia)
    - Aplastic anemia
    - Infiltrative diseases of bone marrow
    - Chronic inflammatory conditions
    - Others
- *Anemia caused by increased red cell destruction:*
  - Hemolytic anemia
    - Hereditary
    - Acquired
  - Red cell sequestration
- *Anemia caused by blood loss:*
  - Acute
  - Chronic.

Morphological classification: Morphological classification remains most useful in practice, as it requires only peripheral blood smear (PBS) as first-line investigations. Size of red blood cells on microscopic examination of peripheral blood smear is reflected in the mean corpuscular volume (MCV). If the cells are smaller than normal (80 fL) anemia is said to be microcytic. If they are normal size (80–100 fL) normocytic, and if they are larger than normal (over 100 fL) the anemia is classified as macrocytic.[6]

- *Microcytic anemia:*
  - Heme synthesis defect
    - Iron deficiency anemia
    - Anemia of chronic disease (more commonly presenting as normocytic anemia)
  - Global synthesis defect
    - Alpha- and beta-thalassemia
    - Hb E syndrome
    - Hb C syndrome
  - Sideroblastic defects
    - Hereditary sideroblastic anemia
    - Acquired sideroblastic anemia
- *Macrocytic anemia:*
  - Megaloblastic anemia—B_{12}, folic acid deficiency (hypersegmented neutrophils)
    - Pernicious anemia—lack of intrinsic factor
    - Poor absorption of B_{12}
    - Macrocytic anemia due to gastric pass surgery
  - Nonmegaloblastic anemia—alcoholism
    - Normocytic anemia
  - Acute blood loss
  - Anemia of chronic disease, infection, malignancy, collagen disease, rheumatoid arthritis
  - Renal failure
  - Hypothyroidism, hypopituitarism
  - Aplastic anemia
  - Hemolytic anemia.
- *Dimorphic anemia:* Hookworm infestation, B_{12}, folic acid deficiency following blood transfusion
- *Heinz body anemia:* By taking certain medication, it is triggered by eating onion or acetaminophen in cats
- *Specific anemia:*
  - Aplastic anemia—bone marrow fails to produce enough red blood cells
  - Fanconi anemia—hereditary disorder
  - Sickle cell anemia—hereditary disorder
  - Hereditary spherocytosis—defects in RBC cell membrane causing the erythrocytes to be sequestrated and destroyed by spleen
  - Hemolytic causes a separate consideration of symptoms (jaundice and elevated LDH)
  - Myelophthisic anemia—due to replacement of bone marrow or malignant granuloma

In 90% of cases of anemia during pregnancy, the major cause of anemia is insufficient diet, it is prudent to divide anemia in pregnancy in two broad classes:
1. *Nutritional anemia:*
   - Iron deficiency anemia
   - Folate deficiency anemia and B_{12} deficiency anemia
   - Mixed factors deficiency anemia (most common)
2. *Non-nutritional anemia:*
   - Thalassemias
   - Hemolytic anemia
   - Aplastic anemia
   - Anemia caused by blood loss
   - Anemia of chronic diseases
   - Others

In this chapter, details of iron deficiency anemia and megaloblastic anemia have been described.

IRON METABOLISM IN PREGNANCY

- About 1000 mg of iron is required during pregnancy. During the first half of pregnancy, iron requirement is not much and an average balanced diet is enough to provide daily requirement of 1–2 mg in healthy mothers. In the second half, demand is more due to increased red cell mass and rapid fetal growth. Iron requirement increases to 6–8 mg/day in the third trimester. If iron store are already deficient, iron deficiency anemia (IDA) manifests.
- Iron required for fetus and placenta—500 mg
- Iron required for red cell increment—500 mg
- Postpartum loss—180 mg
- Lactation for 6 months—180 mg
- Total requirement—1360 mg
- 350 mg subtracted (saved as a result of amenorrhea)
- So actual extra demand—1000 mg

Fetus derives its iron by active transport through placenta, so the average 4 mg/day requirement of iron is needed. Source of iron is heme and nonheme. Heme iron is found in animal product and nonheme is found in fresh leafy vegetables, lentils, legumes and beans. Iron is mainly absorbed in duodenum and proximal jejunum, added by gastric acid in ferrous form. Absorption is more in deficient state and less in iron overload. Iron absorption increased in presence of ascorbic acid, fermentation, gastric acidity, low iron stores, high attitude hemolysis. Inhibitors of iron absorption are calcium, tannins, tea, coffee, herbal drink, magnesium, bicarbonates, carbonates, oxalates, phosphates, phytates.

The total body iron content is normally about 2.5 g in women and about 6 g in men. About 80% of this is found in hemoglobin while 15–20% remains in storage form. Healthy young females have lower storage in comparison with males because of menstrual blood loss, and are prone to develop anemia whenever extra demand arises as occurs in pregnancy. *Iron is transported in plasma by an iron-binding glycoprotein* called *transferrin*, in normal healthy adult about one-third of transferrin is saturated with iron, yielding average serum iron levels between 60 and 120 µg/dL. Whenever there is an iron deficiency in body saturation of transferrin reduces and its binding capacity to the iron (TIBC) increases.

Iron is further transported to bone marrow to synthesize hemoglobin inside the RBC precursors. Rest of the iron which has not been utilized for Hb synthesis is stored inside the cells attached to *ferritin* which is found at highest level in liver, spleen, and skeletal muscles. Because plasma ferritin is largely derived from storage pool of iron, its levels correlates well with body iron stores.

Stages of Iron Deficiency

- *Prelatent (Negative iron balance):*
  - Stores are depleted without a change in hematocrit or serum iron level
  - Reduced stored iron-serum ferritin with normal hemoglobin.
- *Latent (iron deficient erythropoiesis):*
  - Serum iron drops and the TIBC increases without a change in the hematocrit
  - Reduced stored and transport iron
  - Increased erythrocyte protoporphyrin concentration.
- *Frank IDA:*
  - Stage of reduction of stored, transport and functional iron.
  - Decrease hemoglobin, serum ferritin, erythrocytes are microcytic and hypochromic increased erythrocyte protoporphyrin concentration, increase TIBC (<400).

Erythropoiesis: Erythropoiesis is a Process of Production of RBCs

In adult, bone marrow is the site of erythropoiesis. Proper erythropoiesis requires not only iron but various other factors. These factors are protein, erythropoietin (that stimulates cell formation mainly produced by kidneys), minerals, iron trace elements (including zinc, cobalt, and copper), vitamins particularly folic and vitamin B_{12} (cynocobalamin), vitamin C, pyridoxine, riboflavin and hormones (androgen and thyroxin). It was found recently, that vitamin D_3 also has some role in the erythropoiesis.

Physiological anemia of pregnancy: Hemodilution is a general physiological change which takes place during pregnancy caused by relatively greater expansion of plasma volume compared with increase in red cell mass. In addition to this, there is an increased demand of Iron for compensating extra need generated by pregnancy. This dual effect of hemodilution and negative iron balance results in physiological anemia which can be found in up to 80% of pregnant Indian females.

EFFECT ON ANEMIA ON MATERNAL AND FETAL OUTCOME

Presence of anemia during pregnancy can affect both mother and fetus adversely across all three trimesters and during postpartum period as well.

During Pregnancy

Maternal Complications

- *Hypertensive disorders of pregnancy*: Anemic pregnant females are almost 3-4 times more prone to develop pre-eclampsia and related complications which may be related to folic acid deficiency and hypoproteinemia. Pre-term labor (28.2%) PIH (31.2%) is common in patient with severe anemia.[7] Abruptio placentae is also common in anemia.
- Decreased immunity caused by anemia makes a pregnant lady prone to catch all types of infections.
- *Heart failure*: Load of overall increased circulation on an already compromised heart because of anemia, puts an pregnant lady at risk of developing heart failure, especially during early third trimester (30-32 weeks), when hemodilution is at its peak.

During Labor

- *Heart failure*: With each uterine contraction, there is an extra amount of blood that is pumped into circulatory system which can cause immense stress on already compromised heart.
- *Postpartum hemorrhage (PPH)*: Because of poor reserve even a moderate amount of loss can be labeled as PPH.
- *Sudden collapse*: Because of low intravascular volume, any bleeding which is greater than normal may cause lady to land up in shock and even sudden death.

During Immediate Postpartum Period

- Postpartum hemorrhage
- *Heart failure*: Because of sudden release of uterine pressure from inferior vena cava resulting in increased venous return to heart causing overload.

During Puerperium

- Puerperal sepsis and failure of lactation because of decrease immunity and general weakness
- Subinvolution of uterus
- Deep vein thrombosis because of immobilization
- Pulmonary embolism
- Stages of iron.

SYMPTOMS AND SIGNS

- *Mild anemia*: It may not have any effect on pregnancy and labor except the mother will have low iron store.

- *Moderate anemia*: Patient may complaint of feeling of weakness, loss of appetite, indigestion, exhaustion, restless leg syndrome, lack of contraction, pagophagia (intense desire to eat ice)
- *Severe anemia*: Patient complains palpitation, dyspnea, edema.

On examination: Pallor, koilonychia, glossitis, stomatitis, edema, soft systolic murmur, sign of CCF, may present.

Fetal effects: Irrespective of maternal iron store, fetus gets iron from maternal blood through placenta. Gradually, fetus tend to have decreased iron stores due to depletion of maternal stores.
- Adverse outcome such as preterm and small foredate baby are more common in patient with severe anemia.
- Childhood anemia is more common and due to negative effect on brain. Cognitive behavior problems are more common.
- Delay is psychomotor development with impaired performance in motor and language skills, less coordination and a deficit of intelligent quotient (IQ) by 5–10 points.

LABORATORY INVESTIGATIONS

- *Hemoglobin* concentration and *complete blood count*: Hb, MCV, MCH, and MCHC are simple and inexpensive, rapid to perform and helpful for early prediction of IFA. MCHC being independent of RBC count is the most sensitive index of iron deficiency anemia.
- *Peripheral blood film*: Differentiate iron deficiency anemia, megaloblastic anemia and hemolytic anemia. Iron deficiency anemia there is *microcytes*, hypochromia, anisocytosis and Poikilocytosis, and target cell in blood film. Presence of parasites of malaria and kala-azar and toxic granules of chronic infection give clues for the etiology of anemia.
- *Stool examination*: This should be done as a routine to rule out worm infestation or presence of blood.
- *Serum ferritin*: Ferritin is most useful determinant of iron deficiency level below 15 ug/L is taken as iron deficiency (30 ug/L normal in female). It reflects iron stores accurately and is first abnormal laboratory test in iron deficiency.
- Serum iron and total iron-binding capacity
  - Serum iron varies from 60 to 120 ug/dL and TIBC is 300–350 ug/dL (300–400 ug/dL in pregnancy) TIBC is the indirect measurement that rises as iron concentration declines.
  - Serum iron less than 60 ug/dL, TIBC more than 350 ug/dL indicate deficiency of iron during pregnancy.
- *Free erythrocyte protoporphyrin* (FEP) is the third estimation of iron status rising with defective iron supply to the develop red cell and takes 2–3 weeks to become abnormal after depletion of iron store. It also helps in differentiation between iron deficiency anemia and thalassemia normal (30 ug/dL in iron deficiency, it can rise up to 100 ug/dL or more).
- *Serum transferrin receptor (sTFR)*: It is specific and sensitive marks of iron deficiency in pregnancy. It is a transmembrane protein which transports circulating iron into the RBCs and is expressed on erythrocyte membranes. sTFR and total transferrin concentrations are directly proportional.
- *Reticulocyte hemoglobin content*: Reticulocyte hemoglobin concentration determines the amount of iron presented to the bone marrow for uptake into the new RBCs.[8]
- *Bone marrow iron*: It is invasive method but reliable. The gold standard for diagnosis of IDA is the absence of stainable iron or hemosiderin in marrow **(Table 8.2)**.

Iron deficiency anemia is characterized by microcytic red blood cells. Other conditions causing microcytic RBCs include anemia of chronic disorders, beta-thalassemia, and sideroblastic anemias.

MANAGEMENT

Management of iron deficiency can be achieved at two levels, at the individual patient or at public health level. Prevention strategies comprise, food-based approach, iron supplementation, improvement in health services and sanitation developed by WHO. Prevention of IDA in Indian women, also require control of hookworm, malaria and parasitic infestations.[12]

India, being a high anemia prevalence country, MoHFW has recently introduced concept of *primary prevention* which comprises of empirical treatment of anemia in adolescent girls of 10–19 years with a *weekly dose of 100 mg elemental iron and 500 μg folic acid with biannual de-worming*.

Oral iron prophylaxis during pregnancy: WHO recommends daily 30–60 mg of elemental iron with at least 400 μg of folic acid beyond first trimester till term (Continuing during postpartum period for 3 months)[13] to prevent maternal anemia, puerperal sepsis, low birth weight, and preterm birth along with *deworming using tablet albendazole 400 mg single dose or tablet mebendazole 200 mg twice a day for 3 days*. Intermittent oral iron and folic acid supplementation with 120 mg of elemental iron and 2800 ug (2.8 mg) of folic acid once weekly is recommended for pregnant women to improve maternal and neonatal outcomes if daily iron is not acceptable due to side effects, and in populations with an anemia prevalence among pregnant women of less than 20% (Context-specific recommendation).[14]

In India 2013, Ministry of Health and Family Welfare recommend 100 mg elemental iron and 500 ug of folic acid tablets (IFA) daily during pregnancy for 100 days and 100 days thereafter in postpartum period **(Table 8.3)**.[15]

Table 8.2: Differential diagnosis of various microcytic RBCs etiologies[9-11]

Indicator	IDA	BT	SA	ACI
Hemoglobin	Decreased	Normal or decreased	–	Decreased
MCV (fL)	Decreased	Decreased	Low—normal or slightly decreased	Very low in congenital and raised in acquired
MCH (pg)	Decreased	Decreased	Low—normal or slightly decreased	Very low in congenital and raised in acquired
MCHC (g/dL)%	Decreased	Normal or slightly decrease	Low—normal or slightly decrease	Very low in congenital and raised in acquired
Ferritin	Decreased	Normal increased	Normal or increased	Normal or increased
Serum iron	Decreased	Normal or increased	Normal or increased	Normal or decreased
TIBC	Increased	Normal	Normal	Slightly decreased
TS	Decreased	Normal to increased	Normal to increased	Normal to slightly decreased
sTfR	Increased in severe IDA	>100 mg/L	–	Normal
FEP	Increased	Normal	–	Increased
RDW	Increased	Normal to increased	Increased	Normal
Reticulocytes	Increased	Decreased	–	Normal or decreased

Abbreviations: ACI, acute chronic inflammation; BT, beta-thalassemia; IDA, iron deficiency anemia; FEP, free erythrocyte protoporphyrin; RDW, red cell distribution width; SA, sideroblastic anemia; sTfR, soluble transferrin receptor; TIBC, total iron binding capacity; TS, transferrin saturation

Table 8.3: Recommendations by Ministry of Health and Family Welfare 2013

MoHFW	Daily 100 mg iron+500 µg folic acid—100 days during pregnancy	Mild anemia- 2 IFA tablets/day—100 days	Daily 100 mg iron+500 µg folic acid—100 days in postpartum
		Moderate anemia- IM iron therapy + oral folic acid	
		Severe anemia—IV sucrose, packed red cells	

Therapeutic interventions: Before we start definitive treatment, it is important to establish the cause of anemia. Severe anemia and acute blood loss require immediate red cell transfusion. Anemia becomes recurrent if identified causes are not treated appropriately.[7] Preferred route of iron replacement is oral.

There are three modalities of treating anemia during pregnancy:
1. Oral iron therapy
2. Injectable iron therapy
3. Blood transfusion.

Oral iron therapy: Oral iron is indicated for mild-moderate anemia in first, second and early third trimester. Ideally, tablets should be taken on empty stomach for better absorption. In case of gastritis, nausea, vomiting, etc. advise to take one hour after meal or at night. It is noninvasive, can be used without supervision. Intolerance and noncompliance due to side effects such as nausea, vomiting, gastritis, diarrhea, and constipation are major drawbacks. It takes at least 3 weeks to improve Hb levels, cannot be used in late pregnancy
- Various preparations—ferric pyrophosphate, heme iron, ferrous fumarate, gluconate, succinate, sulfate, carbonate sands sustained release, carbonyl iron, ascorbate
- *Iron sulfate*: Recommended by WHO as side effect profile is not very different yet cheap.

Parenteral iron therapy: Oral iron is preferred way to replace iron, but gastrointestinal side effects make it undesirable for many patients. Most orally consumed iron (without ascorbate) is not absorbed in the gut and even when 100 mg of elemental iron is consumed orally only <10% is absorbed.[16] Thus, replenishment of iron stores with oral iron takes very long time, especially with ongoing blood loss. Parenteral iron is not new but its newer formulation, has a reason for come back, stay and replace oral iron. The main advantage is the certainty to correct the hemoglobin deficit and to build up the iron store. The expected rise in hemoglobin is 0.7–1 g/dL per week. Increase in reticulocyte count within 5–10 days.

Table 8.4: Comparison of the physicochemical properties of different injectable iron[18,25,26]

Property	Ideal	Iron dextran	Iron sucrose C/I in first trimester of pregnancy	Ferric carboxymaltose
Type	I (robust)	I (robust)	II (semirobust)	I (robust)
Molecular weight	>100 kd	>100 kd	34–60 kd	150 kd
Stabiliy	High	High	Moderate	High
Half life	Long	3–4 days	6 hours	16 hours
pH	Neutral	Neutral	High	Near-neutral
Osmolarity	Isotonic	Isotonic	High	Isotonic
Antigenicity	Low	High	Low	Low
Test dose	No	Yes	No	No
Time for injection	Short	4–6 hours for 20 mg/kg	15 minutes for 100 mg	15 minutes for 1000 mg
Maximum dose	High	20 mg/kg	600 mg/week	1000 mg/infusion/week

Parenteral iron may be used from the second trimester and during the postpartum period.[17] Comparison of the physicochemical properties of different injectable iron is shown in **Table 8.4**.

INDICATIONS

- If oral iron is not effective
- Severe anemia with second and third trimester of pregnancy
- Poor absorption of iron
- Noncompliance
- Poor tolerance to oral therapy

Parenteral iron formulations are:
- *Dextran-iron dextran (imferon)*—stable can be given by intramuscular and intravenous route.
- *Iron sorbital* (jectofer) is only given by intramuscular therapy.

Injection site abscess is one of the complication, and test dose is required. Hypersensitivity reactions are also reported. The Ministry of Health and Family Welfare (MoHFW) guidelines for treatment of IDA in pregnancy recommended intramuscular iron following a test dose as treatment of choice for moderate anemia in pregnancy.[15]

Intramuscular administration: Intramuscular iron has been shown to be more effective than oral iron in some RCTs. In two RCTs, IM iron (2 or 3 doses of 250 mg Iron at monthly intervals) significantly improved ferritin compared with oral iron and proposed it as an alternative in patients with poor tolerability to oral iron.[19,20] Similar results were obtained in another study, which used three intramuscular doses of 150 mg each at 4 weekly intervals versus daily 100 mg elemental iron.[21]

Adverse Effects and Test Dose

All new patients planed for dextran should be given a test dose of 25 mg and they should be observed for any adverse event for at least 1 hour. Uneventful test doses do not eliminate a probability of experiencing hypersensitivity reactions later with either the first dose or subsequent doses. A repeat test dose is advised in patients with an interval of no treatment who have been prescribed repeat doses of iron dextran. Mild joint pains and discoloration at the injection site, severe reactions such as allergy, itching, fever, lymphadenopathy, arthralgia, headache, malaise and anaphylaxis.[22]

New Preparations

- Iron sucrose
- Ferric carboxymaltose.

Iron sucrose complex: Iron sucrose is asterile, aqueous complex of polynuclear iron hydroxide in sucrose for intravenous use. Its molecular weight is approximately <60,000 Daltons, prohibiting renal elimination.

Advantages

- No test dose recommended
- Minimum side effect
- Not associated with anaphylactic reaction
- Most preferred in patients under going hemodialysis.

History of repeated blood transfusions have to be asked for excluding hemoglobinopathies, bleeding diathesis. Previous history of any allergic reactions to any drug, bronchial asthma have to be rule out before giving injection iron sucrose and should be avoided in these women.

Dose

- Can be given undiluted @ 1 mL/min maximum dose being 100 mg that is over 5 min. As 5 mL content 100 mg iron (1 amp = 2.5 mL = 50 mg iron)
- Other way is to dilute 5 mL of vial in 100 mL normal saline (1 mg/mL) over at least 15–30 min.
- A maximum of 200 mg dose can be given at a time not more than thrice a week.
- Oral IFA tablets should be discontinued for 48 hours before and after iron sucrose administration.

Calculation of dose of parenteral iron
- Required iron dose (mg) = [2.4 × (target Hb–actual Hb) × prepregnancy weight (kg)] + 1000 mg for replenishment of stores.
- Individual patient's tolerance to high dose of iron vary. The lowest tolerable dose should be used.
- A total dose of 1 g can be given in 4–10 sittings (over a period of one month).
- *Safety aspects emphasized* standard emergency tray should be made available at the bedside for handling any reactions.

Numerous studies in India have evaluated the effectiveness of IV iron as a first-line treatment in moderate-to-severe anemia in the second and third trimester of pregnancy. The requirement for formulating standard protocols and guidelines on IV iron use in pregnancy in India was perceived following an observational study conducted across two states of India by MoHFW in collaboration with WHO.[23] A recent systematic review has shown a significant increase in Hb (mean difference in g/dL 0.85; 95% CI 0.31–1.39; $p = 0.002$) and ferritin levels (mean difference 63.32; 95% CI, 39.46–87.18; $p < 0.00001$), with fewer adverse effects (RR, 0.50; 95% CI, 0.34–0.73; $p = 0.0003$) in the IV compared to oral group. Intravenous iron sucrose was more efficacious with few adverse effects than oral formulation in pregnant women with poor tolerability of oral iron and who required immediate replenishment of iron stores.[24] Various studies Gogienis et al. Tmbhare A, et al. Tripathi S, et al. (2015), Gupta, et al., Mehta MN, et al. Abhilashini GD, et al (2015). etc. found IVIS is safe, more effective in achieving target Hb, in later months of pregnancy.[25]

Ferric Carboxymaltose

Ferric carboxymaltose (FCM) is a new 3rd generation IV iron preparation with high stability and low toxicity. It is mainly used in postpartum anemia, few literatures are available regarding its use in pregnancy.[17] In one prospective study, 65 patients received *ferric FCM between 24 and 40 weeks of pregnancy, Hb values (<0.01) increased from 3 to 6 weeks postinfusion.*[26]

- FCM combines the positive characteristic of iron dextran and iron sucrose, but is not associated with dextran-induced hypersensitivity reactions. It can be administered in much higher dose than iron sucrose or iron gluconate.[27]
- The chemical characteristic of the iron carbohydrate complex in FCM means that iron is released slowly, avoiding toxicity and oxidative stress. It contains iron in stable ferric state as a complex with carbohydrate polymer. It is designed to release utilizable iron to the iron transport and storage protein in the body (ferritin and transferrin) (1 mL contain 50 mg FCM).
- 10 mL contain 500 mg iron as ferric carboxymaltose). Single dose of FCM should not exceed 1000 mg of iron (20 mL) per day. Do not administer 1000 mg of iron (20 mL) more than once a week.

Each vial is intended for single use only. It must only be mixed with sterile 0.9% sodium chloride solution. Preparation for parenteral administration should be used immediately after dilution with sterile 0.9% NaCl solution.

Contraindications

- Known hypersensitivity
- Anemia not attributed to iron deficiency
- Evidence of iron overload
- In pregnancy, especially in first trimester
- Hepatic dysfunction
- Each vial is intended for single use only

Side Effects

- Hypersensitivity—always have backup for anaphylactic reaction treatment
- In case of paravenous leakage, the administration of FCM must be stopped immediately
- Headache—3.3%
- Dizziness/Hypotension/Hypertension/Flushing
- Nausea, abdominal pain, diarrhea (common)
- Myalgia, back pain, arthralgia (uncommon)
- Injection site reaction (common)
- Pyrexia, fatigue, chest pain, malaise.

Indications of blood transfusion in pregnancy:
- Severe anemia first seen in last trimester of pregnancy
- Anemia due to massive hemorrhage—APH and PPH
- Patient not responding to oral or parenteral therapy
- Anemic and symptomatic pregnant women with features of heart failure, irrespective of gestational age **(Flow chart 8.1)**.

The recent RCOG blood transfusion-guideline recommends blood transfusion in labor or immediate post-partum period, if the Hb is < 7 g/dL.[28,29]

Flow chart 8.1: Blood transfusion in anemia during pregnancy[25]

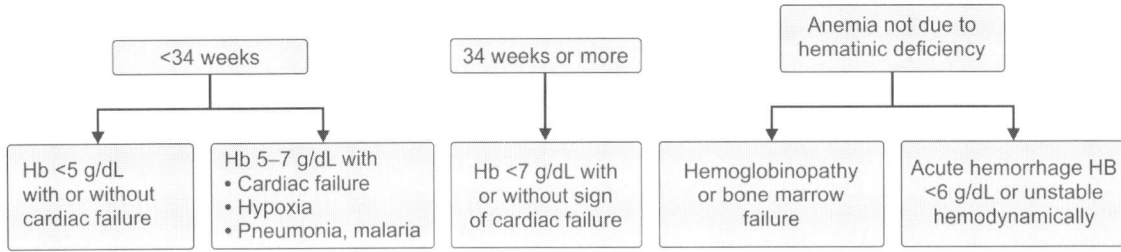

Management During Labor

Women should be delivered in tertiary care hospital with facilities for ICU and blood transfusion.

First stage of labor: In the first stage, patient should be in comfortable position/propped-up position, antibiotic.
- O_2 should be kept ready and given, if there is dyspnea.
- Sedation and pain relief should be given.
- In case of preterm labor, steroids and betamimetics should be given with caution.

Second stage of labor: Second stage is very stressful as patient may go into cardiac failure.

Tendency for prolongation of second stage should be curtailed by forceps/vacuum.

Third stage of labor: Active management of third stage of labor (AMTSL) should be done to decrease postpartum blood loss. Injection methargin should not be given.

Postpartum anemia: Postpartum anemia is defined as hemoglobin level less then 10 g/dL and ferritin level less than 15 ug/L 24–48 hours after delivery, as hemoglobin and ferritin tends to fall during first 24 hrs following delivery, but comes to normal within 7 days.[30] The diagnosis of iron deficiency, anemia relies on a full blood count including hemoglobin, serum ferritin, and serum soluble transferrin receptor, which appear to be reliable indicators of anemia and iron status 1 week postpartum while serum transferrin saturation is an unreliable indicator several weeks after delivery. Some authors defined postpartum anemia as hemoglobin <110 g/L (11 g/dL) at 1 week postpartum and <120 g/L (12 g/dL) at 8 weeks postpartum.[31] WHO recommends postpartum prophylactic iron supplementation of 60 mg elemental iron + 400 µg folic for 3 months.[32,33] Universal iron supplementation was demonstrated to be effective in reducing the prevalence of anemia among low-income postpartum women.[34] MoHFW guidelines recommend daily iron (100 mg elemental iron with 500 µg folic acid) for all nonanemic women in postpartum period for 100 days, whereas the same tablet is advised to be taken twice daily for mild-to-moderately anemic postpartum women.[15]

ADVICE ABOUT FAMILY PLANNING

Pregnant women should have spacing of at least 2 years in between pregnancies and should be advised to avoid frequent child birth by using contraceptive methods. We should tell them about beneficial role of food fortification. It is cost effective component of prevention and control of iron deficiency anemia.

MEGALOBLASTIC ANEMIA

Definition

The megaloblastic anemia is a group of disorders characterized by the presence of distinctive morphologic appearances of the developing red cells in bone marrow. Marrow is usually hypercellular and anemia is based on ineffective erythropoiesis.[35]

Causes of Megaloblastic Anemia

Defect in red cell synthesis is most often due to:
- Hypovitaminosis, especially deficiency of vitamin B_{12} or folic acid. Vitamin B_{12} deficiency alone will not cause the syndrome in the presence of sufficient folate.
- Copper deficiency resulting from an excess of zinc from unusually high oral consumption of zinc containing denture fixation creams has found to be a cause.
- It may occur because of genetic or acquired abnormalities that affect the metabolism of these vitamins or because of defects in DNS synthesis not related to cobalamine or folate.[37]
- Vitamin B_{12} deficiency leading to folate deficiency, e.g. in achlorhydria-induced malabsorption, deficient intrinsic factor (a molecule required for B_{12} absorption), chronic pancreatitis.
- Folate deficiency can occur in alcoholism, deficient intake, increased demand in pregnancy, malabsorption and in certain cases of hypothyroidism.

Symptoms: Common symptoms are fatigue, weakness, shortness of breath on exertion, complaining of looking pale, light headedness, loss of appetite, nausea, diarrhea, sore tongue.

Megaloblastic anemia resulting from cobalamine deficiency may also be associated with neurological symptoms. Initial neurological symptoms may be tingling or numbness in the hands or feet. Additional symptoms develop overtime including balance, gait problems, vision loss due to degeneration (atrophy) of optic nerve, mental confusion, memory loss.

Signs: Pallor, bounding pulse.

Investigations: Complete blood count (CBC), reticulocyte count, mean corpuscular volume (MCV), mean corpuscular hemoglobin (MCH), mean corpuscular hemoglobin concentration (MCHC), serum folate level, serum vitamin B_{12} level, liver function test (LFT), blood sugar test (BSL), urine routine/microscopic (R/M).

Additional tests such as:
- Schilling test which confirms poor absorption as the cause of cobalamin deficiency, may be necessary to diagnose pernicious anemia is not done during pregnancy as it uses contrast.
- Serum homocysteine is elevated in both folate and vitamin B_{12} deficiency.
- Increased formiminoglutamic acid (FIGLU) in urine following a loading dose of histidine is found in folate deficiency.
- Deoxyuridine suppression test can differentiate between vitamin B_{12} and folate deficiency.
- Marrow examination will show a megaloblastic picture, but is rarely required.

Serum B_{12} level may be low in folic acid deficiency anemia and vice versa but a serum level less than 100 pg/mL of vitamin B_{12} is diagnostic of vitamin B_{12} deficiency. A combination of serum folate level of less than 2 ng/mL and a red cell folate less than 150 ng/mL is diagnostic of folate deficiency.[36]

Peripheral blood film may show hypersegmentation of neutrophils, macrocytosis and anisocytosis giant polymorphs, Howell-Jolly bodies.
- MCV > 100 μ^3, MCH is high, MCHC is normal
- Serum folate below 3 ng/mL suggest folate deficiency
- Serum vitamin B_{12} level below 100 pg/mL suggest vitamin B_{12} deficiency (normal 300 pg/mL).

Criteria for Diagnosis of Megaloblastic Anemia[7]

At least two of the following criteria must be present:
1. More than 4% of neutrophil polymorphs have five or more lobes.
2. Howell-Jolly bodies are demonstrated
3. Nucleated red cells
4. Orthochromatic macrocytes must be present with diameter > 12 mm.
5. Macropolycytes may be present.

Effects on Pregnancy[7]

- Abortion
- Growth retardation
- Pre-eclampsia
- Abruptio placantae

Both folate and B_{12} deficiency may mask iron deficiency.

Effect on Fetus[35]

Folic acid supplements at the time of conception and in first 12 weeks of pregnancy reduce neural tube defects by 70%. Most of the protective defect achieved by taking 0.4 mg folic acid daily at the time of conception. Incidence of cleft palate and hare lip also can be reduced by prophylactic folic acid.

Prophylaxis

WHO recommended daily prophylactic folate intake of 400 μg in the antenatal period. Pregnant women should eat more green vegetables (spinach and broccoli).

In over 70 countries (but none in Europe) food is fortified with folic acid (in grain or flour to reduce the risk of NTD). Supplemental folic acid reduces the risk of birth defects in babies born to diabetic mothers. In women who have had a previous fetus with an NTD, 5 mg daily is recommended when pregnancy is contemplated and throughout the subsequent pregnancy.[7,36]

High dose is also advised for women on anticonvulsant drugs.

Treatment

Treatment of established folic acid deficiency by giving 5 mg oral folate per day which should be continued for at least 4 weeks in puerperium. By 4–7 days of therapy, the reticulocyte count is appreciably increased.[7] Hypersegmentation of leukocytes disappears after 2 weeks.

Vitamin B_{12} Deficiency

Patients with established vitamin B_{12} deficiency from any cause, should receive injection cyanocobalamin intramuscularly 1000 μg/week for 1 month and monthly thereafter. Alternatively, hydroxycobalamin given in same dose every 1–3 months intramuscularly is also effective therapy.[37] In cases of deficiency due to inadequate intake, food cobalamin malabsorption and pernicious anemia, oral cyanocobalamin administered at 1000–2000 μg/day for 1 month, followed by 125–500 μg/day is recommended.[38] Reticulocyte count must be checked in a week. Usually hypersegmentation of leukocytes disappear 2 weeks after therapy.

REFERENCES

1. McLean E, Cogswell M, Egli I, et al. Worldwide prevalence of anaemia, WHO Vitamin and Mineral Nutrition Information System, 1993–2005. The prevalence of anaemia in women. 1993–2005.
2. *www.indiaenviormentportal.org.in*/National Family Health Survey 2015-16 (internet) cited on 22-7-2016.
3. Stevens GA, et al. Nutrition impact model study group (Anemia) Global, regional and national trends in haemoglobin concentration and prevalence of total and severe anaemia in children and pregnant and nonpregnant women for 1995–2011. A systemic analysis of population representative data. Lancet Global Health (Internet). 2013;1:16-25 (PubMed).
4. Indian Council of Medical Research. Evaluation of National Nutritional Anemia Prophylaxis Programme, Task Force Studying, New Delhi: ICMR 1989.
5. WHO, iron deficiency anemia, assessment, prevention and control, WHO/NHD/01.3 Geneva; 2001.
6. Gupta A. Iron deficiency anemia. FOGSI Focus. 2008. pp. 5-8.
7. Sharma JB, Shanker M. Anemia in Pregnancy. JIMSA. 2010;23(4):253-60.
8. Wish JB. Assessing iron status: beyond serum ferritin and transferring saturation. Clin J Amsoc Nephrol; 2006;1 (Suppl 1):s4-8.
9. Thomas C, Thomas L. Biochemical markers and hematologic indices in the diagnosis of functional iron deficiency. Clin Chem. 2002;48:1066-76.
10. JW hematologic diseases. Interpretation of Diagnostic Tests. United states: Lippincott Williams and Wilkins. 2006. pp. 385-419.
11. AC anemia. When Is it Iron Deficiency? Pediatr Nurs. 2003;29:2.
12. Rammohan A, Awofeso N, Robitaille Mc. Addressing Female Iron-deficiency Anemia in India: Is vegetarianism the major Obstacle? ISRN Public Health. 2011;2012:1-8.
13. Guideline: daily iron and folic acid supplementation in pregnant women. Geneva: World Health Organization; 2012 (*http://www.who.int/nutrition/publications/micronutrients/ guidelines/daily_ifa_supp_pregnant_women/en/*).
14. Implementation of ANC guideline and recommendations: WHO recommendations on antenatal care for appositive pregnancy experience 2016 [Internet] [cited on 28 nov 2016] (Available from *www.Who.int/reproductivehealth/publications/maternal_perinatal_health/anc-positive-pregnancy-experience/ en/*)
15. National iron plus initiative. Guidelines for Control of Iron Deficiency Anemia, Adolescent Division of Ministry of Health and Family Welfare GOI, 2013.
16. Kaplinsky C. Parental iron therapy. Isr Med Assoc J. 2008;10: 372-3.
17. Pavord S, Myers B, Robinson S, et al. UK guidelines on the management of iron deficiency in pregnancy. Br J Haematol. 2012;156:588-600.
18. Geisser P, Burckhart S. The Pharmacokinetics and Pharmacodynamics of Iron Preparations. Pharmaceutics. 2011;3(11):12-33.
19. Sharma JB, Jain S, Mallika V, et al. A prospective, partially randomized study of pregnancy outcomes and hematologic responses to oral and intramuscular iron treatment in moderately anemic pregnant women. Am J Clin Nutr. 2004;79:116-22.
20. Kumar A, Jain S, Singh NP, et al. Oral versus high dose parenteral iron supplementation in pregnancy. Int J Gynaecol Obstet. 2005;89:7-13.
21. Vijay Z, Swaraj B, Saba AS, et al. Injectable iron supplementation instead of oral therapy for antenatal care. J Obstet Gynecol Ind. 2004;54:37-8.
22. Silverstein SB, Rodgers GM. Parenteral iron therapy options. Am J Hematol. 2004;76:74-8.
23. Devasenapathy N, Singh R, Moodbidri P, et al. An Observational Study on the Use of IV Iron Sucrose Among Anaemic Pregnant Women in Government Healthcare Facilities from Two States of India. J Obstet Gynaecol India. 2015;65:230-5.
24. Shi Q, Leng W, Wazir R, et al. Intravenous iron sucrose versus oral iron in the treatment of pregnancy with iron deficiency Anaemia: A systematic review. Gynecol Obstet Invest. 2015;80:170-8.
25. FOGSI General Clinical Practice Recommendations, Management of Iron Deficiency Anaemia in Pregnancy, Evidence based IFA24 may 2016. Available on Fogsi Website.
26. Frossler et al. Intravenous Ferric carboxymaltose for anemia in pregnancy. BMC Pregnancy and childbirth. 2014;14:115.
27. Herfs R, Fleitmann L, Kocsis I. Treatment of iron deficiency with or without anaemia with intravenous ferric carboxymaltose in gynaecological practices: noninterventional study. Port J Nephrol Hypert. 2009;23(1):11-6.
28. RCOG. Blood Transfusion in Obstetrics, Green-top Guideline No.47, 2015.
29. Candio F, Hofmeyr GJ. Treatments for iron-deficiency anaemia in pregnancy: RHL commentary. The WHO Reproductive Health Library; Geneva: World Health Organization; 2007.
30. Chaudhary SS. Eradication of anaemia during Pregnancy. In: Jaideep Malhotra (Ed) et al. AICOG, Obstetrics and Gynaecology Update; 2016.
31. Milman N., Postpartum anaemia definition prevalence, cause and consequences. Ann Hemato. 2011;90(11):1247-53. doi:10.1007/s00277-1279-zEpub2011 Jun 28.
32. WHO. Recommendations on postnatal care of the mother and newborn; 2013.
33. Stoltzfus RJ, Dreyfuss ML. Guidelines for the use of iron supplements to prevent and treat iron deficiency anaemia. USA: International Nutritional Anemia Consultative Group (INACG), WHO.
34. Mitra AK, Khoury AJ. Universal iron supplementation: a simple and effective strategy to reduce anaemia among low-income, postpartum women. Public Health Nutr. 2012;15:546-53.
35. Hoffbrand AV. Megaloblatic Anemias. In: Karper D, Fauci A, Houser S, et al (Eds). Harrison's Principles of Internal Medicine; New York: McGraw Hill Education; 2015.
36. Koschorke A, Egbor M, Bhide A. Haematological disorders and Red-Cell Alloimmunization in Pregnancy. In: Bhide A, Kumara SA, Damania KR, Daftary SN (Eds). Arias' Practical Guide to High Risk Pregnancy and Delivery. A South Asian Perspective, 4th edition. India: Elsevier; 2015.
37. Shojania AM. Protein Synthesis—Megaloblastic disorders. In: Gross S, Roath S (Eds). Haematology: A Problem-oriented approach. Baltimore: Williams and Wilkins. 1996. pp. 25-54.
38. Nyholm E, Turpin P, Swain D, et al. Oral Vitamin B_{12} can change our practice. Postgrad Med J. 2003;79:218-20.

Chapter 9

Non-nutritional Anemia in Pregnancy

Vasumati S Upadhye, Sheetal K Gujral, Vaishali A Deshpande

INTRODUCTION

Anemia in pregnancy is a major cause of maternal morbidity and mortality and also poses long-term risk to the fetus. As per WHO hemoglobin (Hb) level below 11 g/dL and hematocrit less than 33% in pregnant women is considered as anemia and Hb below 7 g/dL is severe anemia. CDC defines anemia as Hb less than 11 g/dL in first and third trimester and less than 10.5 g/dL in second trimester. WHO estimated prevalence of anemia in pregnant women is 14% in developed and 51% in developing countries and 65–75% in India alone.[1] Prevalence of anemia is highest in South Asia. According to National Institute of Health and Family Welfare, New Delhi. 50% of Indian pregnant women are anemic.[2] There is disproportionate increase in plasma volume as compared to RBC volume so hemodilution occurs and is responsible for physiological anemia in pregnancy. Majority of Indian women are anemic due to nutritional deficiency, faulty dietary habits and low socio-economic status. Although nutritional anemia is very common in pregnancy, non-nutritional causes should not be overlooked as inadvertent treatment with iron may be futile and harmful. At the same time clinician is missing a chance to diagnose thalassemia or major hemoglobinopathies in the fetus. It is always necessary to keep possibility of non-nutritional anemia while managing a patient of anemia with hematinics.

ETIOLOGY OF NON-NUTRITIONAL ANEMIA

Non-nutritional anemia can be congenital or acquired **(Flow chart 9.1)**. In India most common acquired causes are malaria, hookworm infestation, chronic GI blood loss, thyroid disorders and the rare causes are chronic renal disease, malignancies, hemolysis, elevated liver enzymes, low platelet count (HELLP) syndrome and ITP.

There can be congenital defect either in the membrane of the RBCs such as Glucose-6-phosphate-dehydrogenase (G6PD) deficiency, hereditary spherocytosis and sideroblastic anemia or defect in the hemoglobin as in thalassemia and sickle cell anemia.

APPROACH TO THE PATIENT

Elaborate history and detail clinical examination of patient can help the clinician to arrive at the diagnosis of non-nutritional cause for anemia.

- The patients belonging to particular communities such as *Sindhis, Punjabis, Lohanas, Kutchis, Bhanushalis, Jains,* and *Bohris* have a high prevalence of β-thalassemia (4–17%).[3] HbS is prevalent in central India and among the tribal belts in western, eastern and southern India.
- History of menorrhagia and any blood loss related to pregnancy leading to iron-deficiency anemia
- History of bleeding gums, easy bruisability and dark colored urine
- Personal history about addiction, bowel habits to rule out gastrointestinal blood loss.
- Drug history to rule out drug-induced anemia (antiepileptic, antacids, NSAID, etc.)
- Dietary history to rule out nutritional anemia
- Family history of multiple blood transfusion or affected child in family.

CLINICAL EXAMINATION

On physical examination signs suggestive of non-nutritional anemia are:

- Bossing of skull bones (sign of extramedullary hematopoiesis)
- Thyroid swelling
- Hepatosplenomegaly
- Small joint swelling
- Jaundice
- Petechial marks.

LABORATORY EVALUATION OF ANEMIA

The laboratory evaluation of anemia **(Flow chart 9.2)** begins with complete blood count and reticulocyte count. The anemia is then categorized as microcytic, macrocytic

SECTION 3: Hematological Disorders During Pregnancy

Flow chart 9.1: Etiology of non-nutritional anemia

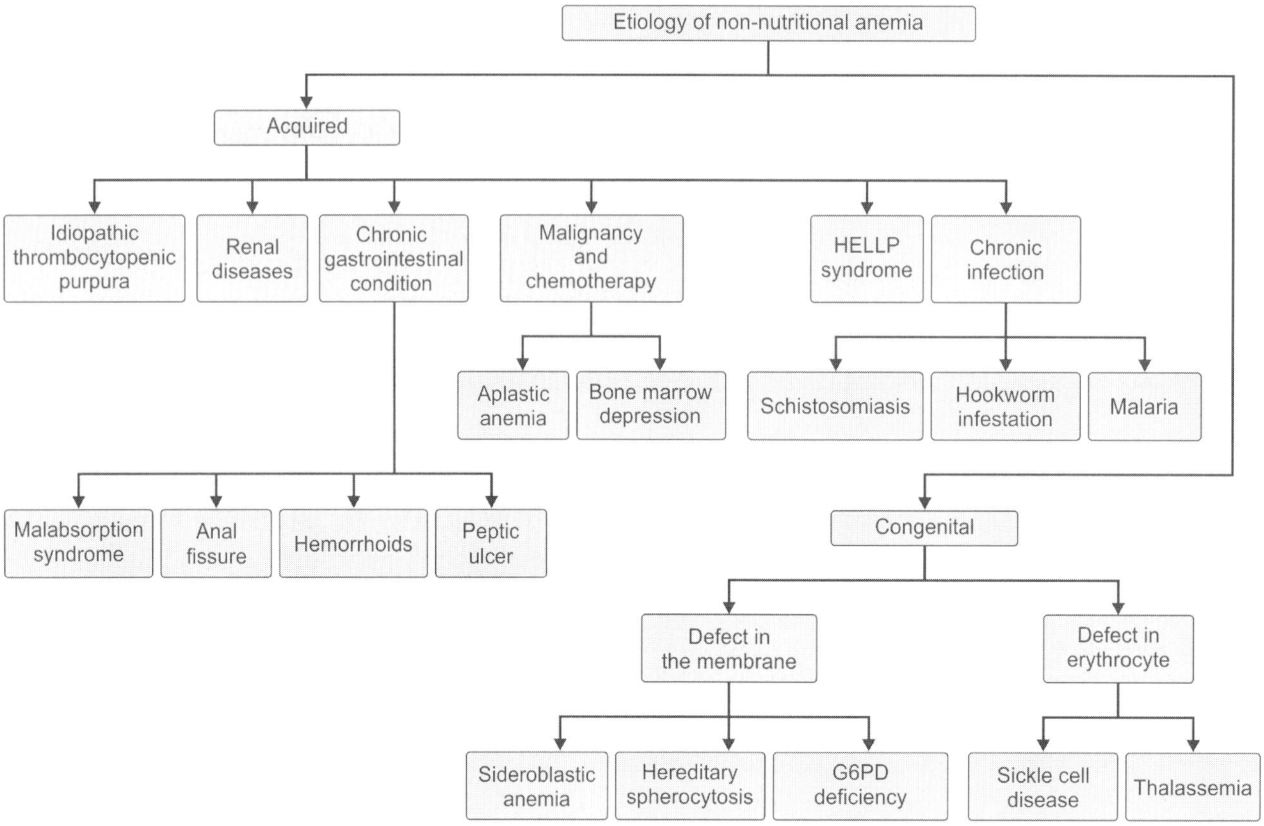

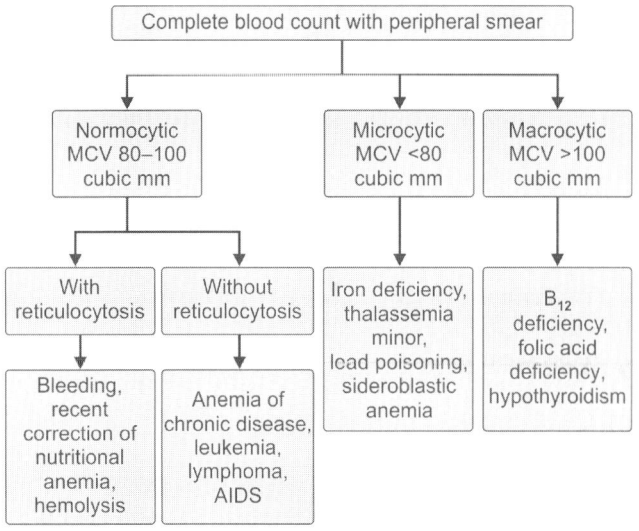

Flow chart 9.2: Laboratory evaluation of anemia

or normocytic with or without reticulocytosis. Examination of peripheral smear and some specific tests confirm the diagnosis. In the vast majority of cases, microcytic anemia can be either iron-deficiency or thalassemia. These can be differentiated by erythrocyte count, RDW, the serum iron level, total iron binding capacity (TIBC), serum ferritin and Hb electrophoresis **(Table 9.1)**. The RDW, a measure of dispersion of erythrocytes, corresponds to clinical assessment of anisocytosis and not poikilocytosis. In thalassemia minor, although there is variation in the cell shape and size, RDW is normal. The body attempts to compensate the anemia with an increase in erythrocytes. Thus in the patient with microcytic anemia, if erythrocyte count is normal or increased, thalassemia is most likely diagnosis.[4]

Evaluation of free erythrocyte protoporphyrin (FEP) helps in differentiating the causes of microcytic anemia. In the final step of heme synthesis iron is inserted into protoporphyrin by enzyme ferrochelatase to form heme. An increase in free FEP content occurs when iron is not available, such as in

Table 9.1: Iron-deficiency anemia or thalassemia can be differentiated by following parameters

Laboratory parameter	Iron deficiency anemia	Thalassemia minor
Poikilocytosis	Increased	Normal
Erythrocyte count	Decreased	Increased
Red cell distribution width (RDW)	Increased	Normal
Serum ferritin level	Decreased	Normal
TIBC	Increased	Normal
Free erythrocyte protoporphyrin (FEP)	Increased	Normal
Mentzer Index (MCV/erythrocyte count)	>13	<13

- Liver function test
- Kidney function test
- Naked eye single tube osmotic fragility test (NESTROFT)
- Sickling test.

Aims of Management

- Treatment of correctable conditions such as worm infestation, malaria, UTI, thyroid disorders, etc.
- Assessment of anemia/hemoglobinopathies to prevent fetal and maternal mortality and morbidity.
- Prevention of complications.

Hemoglobinopathies

Thalassemia and sickle cell disease originally diseases of tropics and subtropics have become worldwide due to migration and represent major group of inherited disorders of Hb synthesis. According to WHO, globally 5% adults are carrier for hemoglobinopathic condition.[6,7] Ineffective bone marrow erythropoiesis and excessive red cell hemolysis together account for anemia in these monogenic disorders. Patient who is affected by sickle cell trait or α-1 thalassemia may not experience any clinical symptoms or be aware of her carrier status but, her fetus may be at risk of *in utero* demise or severe disease after birth. Hb electrophoresis though a definitive test for hemoglobinopathies is too expensive for mass screening. Test such as naked eye single tube osmotic fragility test (NESTROFT) and red cell indices have been found to be very sensitive with high negative predictive value. NESTROFT is an inexpensive test and can be used for mass screening with sensitivity, specificity, positive predictive value and negative predictive value of 91.5, 95.4, 54.6%, and 99.5% respectively, taking HbA$_2$ as the gold standard (ICMR). Molecular genetic test for carrier detection will not be cost effective and should be reserved only for couple desiring prenatal diagnosis.

Bone marrow transplantation (BMT) is the only specific treatment for these disorders. However, the non-availability of HLA identical donors, lack of expertise and high cost of the test and treatment are major prohibitive factors for BMT in India. Cord blood transplantation, though promising is still under trial. Therefore most patients are managed symptomatically. Carrier screening along with prenatal diagnosis and genetic counseling remains of paramount importance in reduction of these diseases worldwide and thereby decreasing the burden on society and family.

ACOG Guidelines for Prenatal Screening

The obstetricians and gynecologists should try to identify couples at increased risk of having offspring with a form of thalassemia or sickle cell disease **(Flow chart 9.3)**.

iron deficiency anemia, anemia of chronic disease or when ferrochelatase is dysfunctional as in lead poisoning. Normal FEP level is 15–85 µg/dL erythrocytes. It is increased to >100 µg/dL erythrocytes in patients with anemia of chronic disease, idiopathic refractory sideroblastic anemia and in iron-deficiency anemia. It is markedly increased to more than 250 µg/dL erythrocytes in patients with Lead poisoning. The FEP value is usually normal in patients with thalassemia and therefore can be used to differentiate thalassemia minor from other causes of microcytic anemia.[5]

If thalassemia is suspected, Hb electrophoresis should be done and quantitative HbA$_2$ and F level measured. HbF level will be increased in many patients with beta thalassemia minor and all patients with delta, beta- and alfa-thalassemia. In patient with hypochromic anemia if iron and HbA$_2$ levels are normal, one is probably dealing with α-thalassemia.

Hemolysis is suggested by elevated bilirubin, elevated lactose dehydrogenase (LDH) level and peripheral smear showing schistocytes or spherocytes. While an elevated LDH level is nonspecific, a normal LDH value is against hemolysis. If there is evidence of intravascular hemolysis and the peripheral smear is normal and Coombs' test is negative one should suspect G6PD deficiency. Heinz body preparation may show oxidized and precipitated hemoglobin during and briefly after an episode of acute G6PD hemolysis.[5]

Other investigations for non-nutritional anemia:
- Stool examination for occult blood and worm infestation
- Urine for occult blood
- Thick blood smear for malaria
- Tests for G6PD deficiency
- Osmotic fragility test
- Coombs' test
- Coagulation profile

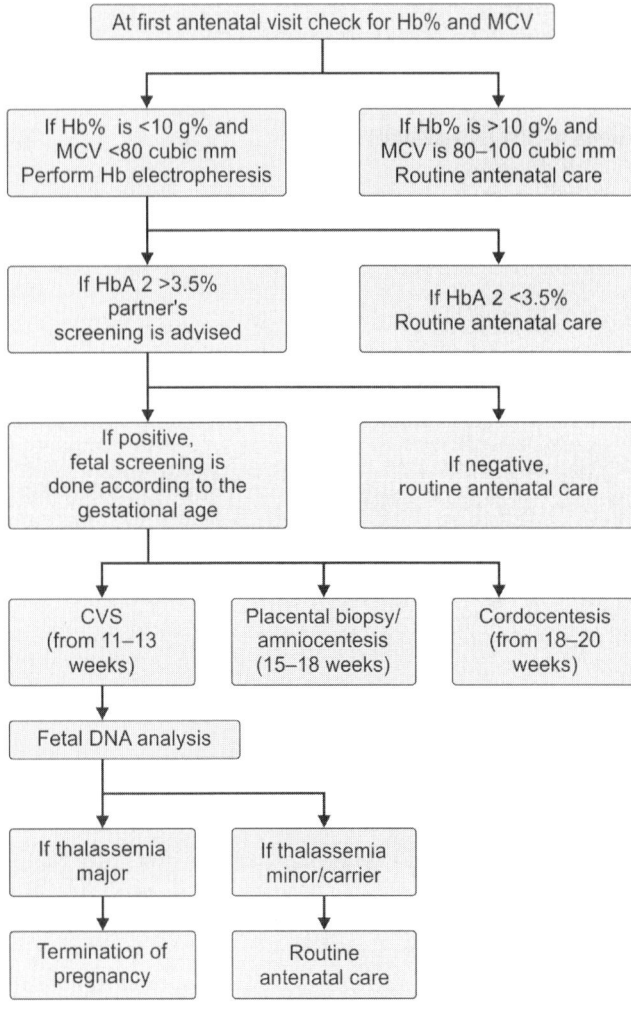

Flow chart 9.3: Diagnosis and management of thalassemia

- *Placental biopsy*: In second trimester, a placental biopsy preferred (13-20 weeks) over amniocentesis as better availability of fetal DNA[9]/Amniocentesis—amniotic fluid is obtained at 15-20 weeks of gestation. The procedure related risk is 0.5-1%.[10]
- Cordocentesis and fetal blood sampling for fetal DNA as well as to analyze globin chain synthesis in Hb Bart's disease is performed at 18-20 weeks of gestation.[11]
- Mutation analysis for diagnosis of sickle cell anemia is done using polymerase chain reaction (PCR) and restriction fragment analysis.

Sickle Cell Disease

It is an autosomal recessive disorder due to sickle gene which results in inherent defect in hemoglobin. Polymerization of abnormal Hb at low oxygen saturation leads to formation of rigid and fragile sickle cells which can cause either hemolysis or vaso-occlusion of small vessels.

There are three types of sickle cell hemoglobinopathies:
1. Sickle cell disease (Hb SS).
2. Sickle cell trait (Hb AS).
3. Sickle cell disease with either thalassemia or Hb C (Hb SC).

Sickle cell disease is least common amongst them. It has high-risk for pregnancy with perinatal mortality of 40 to 60 per 1000 deliveries and maternal mortality rate of 1 to 2%.[12,13] The sickle cell gene is common in tribes of Madhya Pradesh, Maharashtra, Gujarat, Tamil Nadu, and Kerala. The carrier frequency is as high as 30% in some areas.[3] Approximately 5000 babies with sickle cell disease are born each year in India.[14]

Management of Patient with Sickle Cell Disease

Preconceptional Screening

Physician should assess patient's overall health and her potential risk during pregnancy. She is also screened for pulmonary hypertension and renal problems. Patient is counseled about the risks involved in pregnancy and need for frequent visits, monitoring and need for admission. Importance is given to the partner screening to evaluate the risk of transmission in the fetus[15-17]
- Folic acids supplementation 4 mg per day.
- Immunization of patient for *H. influenzae*, pneumococci and meningococci.
- Discontinue any teratogenic drugs such as hydroxycarbamide and ACE inhibitors at least three months prior to pregnancy.
- A woman who has been transfused previously should be tested for RBC allo-antibodies.

- Those who have MCV level less than 80 cubic microns may be a carrier of one of the thalassemia trait and should undergo Hb electrophoresis.
- Elevated HbF and HbA_2 greater than 3.5% are associated with β-thalassemia.
- When an MCV is below normal, iron deficiency anemia has been excluded and Hb electrophoresis is not consistent with β-thalassemia trait, molecular testing should be offered to detect α-globin gene deletions (α-thalassemia).[8]

Prenatal Diagnosis

It should be offered to a couple who are at high-risk of having fetus with a significant hemoglobinopathy.
- Genetic testing of fetal DNA can be performed as after 10 weeks of gestational age by chorionic villous sampling (CVS).

Care During Pregnancy

These patients require multidisciplinary approach with an obstetrician experienced in managing high-risk pregnancies.
- Blood pressure and urine analysis at every visit and midstream urine culture monthly.
- Fortnightly CBC, hematocrit, platelet count, bilirubin, transaminase and lactose dehydrogenase to monitor anemia and hemolysis.
- To start low dose aspirin after first trimester for prevention of pre-eclampsia and thromboembolism.
- Women with history of thromboembolism should receive low molecular weight heparin during pregnancy.
- Early USG for fetal viability.
- Fetal surveillance with serial ultrasound every 3–4 week for fetal growth.
- Plan for mode of delivery according to obstetric indication.
- Painful crisis, chest syndrome during pregnancy can be managed with opioids, rest, fluid therapy and oxygenation and supportive care.

Intrapartum

- Patient should be offered elective birth through induction or cesarean after 38 weeks of gestation.
- Keep adequate cross-matched blood.
- Woman should be kept warm and given adequate fluid.
- Continuous intrapartum electronic fetal heart rate monitorings.
- Use of pneumatic compression devices during labor and at the time of cesarean deliveries.
- Avoid use of pethidine as an analgesic, however, regional anesthesia is preferable for cesarean section.

Postpartum

- Screening of babies for evidence of hemoglobinopathy.
- Maintain O_2 saturation above 94% and adequate hydration.
- Low molecular weight heparin postpartum for seven days following normal delivery and six weeks following cesarean section.
- Contraception–progesterone only pill, injectable contraceptive, LNG IUCD are effective and safe.

Complications of Sickle Cell Disease with Pregnancy

Maternal Complications

- Worsening of anemia.
- Increased risk of infection, particularly UTI and chest infections
- Increased sickle cell crisis particularly in third trimester.
- Chest syndrome is a vaso-occlusive crisis of the pulmonary vasculature commonly seen in patients with sickle cell anemia which presents with fever with or without respiratory symptoms.
- Painful crisis which presents with pain in bone or other part of body due to vaso-occlusion
- Hypertension
- Thromboembolic disease
- Antepartum hemorrhage.

Fetal Complications

- Increased risk of miscarriage
- Intrauterine growth restriction
- Stillbirth
- Iatrogenic and idiopathic prematurity
- Opiate addiction in neonate.

Management of Patient with Sickle Cell Trait

Sickle cell trait is common and frequently goes unnoticed. Partner screening and evaluation of fetus helps in preventing birth of babies with sickle cell disease. In pregnancy sickle cell trait, patient are more prone to UTI, hypertension and thromboembolic episodes. Care should be taken to avoid dehydration, hypoxia, exposure to cold so as to prevent rare episode of sickle cell crisis.

Thalassemia

Normal hemoglobin is a tetramer, composed of two pairs of polypeptide chains designated α, β, γ and δ each of which is covalently linked to heme group. The synthesis of a particular globin subunit is directed by a corresponding gene inherited from each parent. Normal adult Hb is composed of HbA ($\alpha_2\beta_2$) 97%, Hb A2 ($\alpha_2\delta_2$) 3% and fetal hemoglobin (HbF or $\alpha_2\gamma_2$) less than 1%. Normally, α-and β-chain synthesis in erythroid precursor is evenly balanced.

The thalassemias are a diverse group of congenital disorders in which there is quantitative defect in the synthesis of one or more subunits of hemoglobin, mainly α- and β-chains. Thalassemias are designated according to the deficient gene.

α-thalassemia is classified according to number of deletion of the α-chains into following types:
- Deletion of single α-chain gene as silent carrier (α -/α α).
- Deletion of two α-chain genes as α-thalassemia trait (α-/α-) or (- -/α α).
- Deletion of three α-chain genes as HbH disease (- -/α-).
- Deletion of four α chain genes as Hb B art disease (hydrops fetalis) (- - /- -).

β-thalassemia is classified according to varying degrees of ineffective production of β-chains into:
- β-thalassemia minor (thalassemia trait)
- β-thalassemia intermedia
- β-thalassemia major (Cooley's anemia)

β-thalassemia is the most common single gene disorder in India. The mean prevalence of the β-thalassemia gene is 3.3%[3] (varies between 1-17%). It is highest in *Punjabis* (who have migrated from Pakistan), *Sindhis*, *Bengalis* (particularly, β-thalassemia), *Gujratis*, *Bhansualis* and *Jains*. National Institute of Immuno-Hematology has estimated that 7500–12000 β-thalassemia babies are born in India each year.[3] α-thalassemia has not been studied extensively but its frequency is high in India and its interaction with β-thalassemia and sickle cell gene has disease modifying effect.[17]

Antenatal management of pregnancy in thalassemia syndromes:
- *β-thalassemia minor, α-thalassemia silent carrier stage and α-thalassemia trait*: Pregnancy outcome and obstetric complications do not differ from general population. Pregnancy is generally well tolerated in these patients. Periconceptional folic acid 4 mg daily is recommended to avoid fetal neural tube defects due to folate deficiency secondary to increased erythropoiesis. Iron is supplemented only to women with documented iron deficiency. Genetic counseling and screening of partner should be offered to determine the risk of β-thalassemia major. There is 25% chance of fetus having HbH or Hb Bart's, if both the parents are carrier of the heterozygous α-thalassemia-1(- -/ αα).
- *β-thalassemia major and intermedia, HbH disease*: Most cases of pregnancy are limited to β-thalassemia intermedia because of high rate of morbidity and infertility in patient with β-thalassemia major. Aggressive transfusion and iron chelation therapy has improved the possibility of pregnancy in these patients.

  Deletion of three of four α-globin genes results in HbH disease. It is seen primarily in Asian and Mediterranean population.[1] The clinical symptoms range from asymptomatic to severe anemia with hemolysis and splenomegaly. Patients with HbH disease may have hemolytic crisis in response to infection, fever, ingestion of oxidative drugs and pregnancy. HbH disease can also lead to hydrops fetalis and intrauterine demise. Ideally pregnancy management should include interdisciplinary team who is familiar with high-risk pregnancy and care of patient who have thalassemia. Clinician should confirm that patient has completed her hepatitis B and pneumococcal vaccine, if she is asplenic. Patient will require supportive blood transfusion. There are complications and increased risk of pre-eclampsia, prematurity and congestive heart failure.[18] In these patients preconceptional baseline evaluation of hematological indices, iron load status, serology, extent of splenomegaly, cardiac and liver function should be done. It is also recommended to repeat these tests at initial visit and in second and third trimester. Avoidance of medications causing oxidative stress as well as prompt treatment of infection is required. Fetal growth and wellbeing should be followed closely because of increased risk of growth restrictions in these pregnancies. Transfusion therapy should be aimed at keeping hemoglobin level at 10 g/dL.[19-21] Iron chelation therapy with deferroxamine (DFO) is mainstay of the modern management of these patients. Except for the first trimester DFO can be continued throughout pregnancy and is also compatible with breastfeeding.
- *Hemoglobin Bart's disease*: In this disorder, there is absence of functional α-globin chain. This condition is universally fatal.

Delivery

The mode of delivery is individualized. Patient can be delivered vaginally, if she is hemodynamically stable and has no myocardial disease.[19] Cesarean section is reserved for obstetric indications only. Cord blood banking should be considered at delivery which is a source of stem cells for transplant to other family members of the patient who have hemoglobinopathies.

KEY POINTS

- Although nutritional anemia is very common in pregnancy, non-nutritional causes should not be overlooked as inadvertent treatment with iron may be futile and harmful. At the same time, clinician is missing a chance to diagnose thalassemia or major hemoglobinopathies in the fetus.
- In India, most common acquired causes are malaria, hookworm infestation, chronic GI blood loss, thyroid disorders and congenital causes are thalassemia and sickle cell anemia.
- Anemia can be classified as microcytic (MCV<80 cmm), normocytic (MCV 80-100 cmm) and macrocytic (MCV>10 cmm).
- Red cell distribution width (RDW), erythrocyte count, serum ferritin level and free erythrocyte protoporphyrin (FEP) levels help in differentiating iron-deficiency anemia and thalassemia.
- Hemoglobin electrophoresis is confirmative test for thalassemia. Elevated HbF and HbA2 greater than 3.5% are associated with β-thalassemia. Molecular testing is useful to detect α-globin gene deletions (α-thalassemia).
- Advances in management of major hemoglobinopathies with multidisciplinary approach has improved the possibility of successful pregnancy in these patients.

- Patient who is affected by sickle cell trait or thalassemia minor may not experience any clinical symptoms or be aware of her carrier status but, her fetus may be at risk of *in utero* demise or severe disease after birth.
- Carrier screening along with prenatal diagnosis and genetic counseling remains of paramount importance in reduction of these diseases worldwide.
- Naked eye single tube osmotic fragility test (NESTROFT) and red cell indices are inexpensive tests and can be used for mass screening.
- The carrier state has no disadvantage, however, the homozygous state which is very severe and may be fatal can be diagnosed safely in prenatal period. Propagating this message in the community through healthcare professionals is a key step in prevention of major hemoglobinopathies.

REFERENCES

1. DeMayer EM, Tegman A. Prevalence of anaemia in the world. World Health Organization. 1998;38:302-16.
2. K Kalawari. Department of Reprod Medicine, National Institute of Health and Family Welfare, New Delhi, Indian Journal of Medical Research; 2009.
3. Madan N, Sharma S, Sood SK, Colah R, Bhatia HM. Frequency of β-thalassemia and other hemoglobinopathies in northern and western India. Indian J Hum Genet. 2010;16:16-25.
4. Bessman JD, Glimer PR Jr, Gardner FH. Improved classification of anaemia by MCV and RDW. Am J Clin Pathol. 1983;80:322-6.
5. Wallerstein RO Jr. Laboratory evaluation of anaemia. West J Med. 1987;146:443-51.
6. IOSR Journal of Dental and Medicine Sciences (JDMC); 2014;13.
7. Weatherall DJ, Clegg JB. Distribution and population genetics of thalassemia, 4th edn. Oxford Blackwell Science; 2001 Chapter 6.
8. American College of Obstetrics and Gynaecology Committee Opinion. Genetic Screening for Haemoglobinopathies; 2000.
9. Giovanni M, Cristina U, Caoantonia R. Second-Trimester Placental Biopsy versus Amniocentesis for Prenatal Diagnosis of β-Thalassemia N Engl J Med. 1990;322:60-61. DOI: 10.1056/NEJM199001043220115.
10. Old JM. Prenatal diagnosis of the hemoglobinopathies. In: Milunsky A (Ed). Genetic disorders and the fetus. Baltimore (MD): John Hopkins University Press. 1998.pp.581-611.
11. Wanapirak C, Tongsong T, Sirivatanapa P, Sa-nguansermsri T, Sekararithi R, tuggapichitti A. Prenatal strategies for reducing severe thalassemia in pregnancy. Int J Gynaecol Obstet. 1998; 60(3):239-44.
12. Royal College of Obstetricians and Gynaecologists. Management of sickle cell disease in pregnancy, Green-top Guideline No. 2011;61.
13. NHS Screening Programmes. Sickle Cell and Thalassemia. Handbook for Laboratories. London.
14. Verma IC, Bijarnia S. The burden of genetic disorders in India and a framework for community control. Community Genet. 2002;5:192-6.
15. Yaster M, Kost-Byerly S, Maxwell LG. The management of pain in sickle cell disease. Pediatr Clin North Am. 2000;47:699-710.
16. NHS sickle Cell and Thalassemia Screening Programme; 2009 [*http://sct.screenin.nhs.uk/cms.php? folder= 2493 #fileid10756*].
17. Sun PB, Wilburn W, Raynor BD, et al. Sickle cell disease in pregnancy: twenty years of experience at Grady Memorial Hospital, Atlanta, Georgia. Am J Obstet Gynecol. 2001;184: 1127-30.
18. Chui DH, Fuchareon S, Chan V. Hemoglobin H disease: not necessarily a benign disorder. Blood. 2003;101:791-800.
19. Aessopos A, Karabatsos F, Farmakis D, et al. Pregnancy in patients with well-treated β-thalassemia: outcome for mothers and newborn infants. Am J Obstet Gynecol. 1999;180:360-5.
20. Tampakoudis P, Tsatslas C, Mamopoulos M, et al. Transfusion-dependent homozygous beta-thalassemia major: successful twin pregnancy following in five cases. Eur J Obstet Gynecol Reprod Biol. 1997;74:127-31.
21. Kumar RM, Rizk DE, Khuranna A. Beta-thalassemia major and successful pregnancy. J Reprod Med. 1997;42:294-8.

Chapter 10

Rh-incompatibility During Pregnancy

Pragya Dhirawani, Richa Dhirawani

INTRODUCTION

The rhesus blood type was first discovered in 1937 by Karl Landsteiner, Alexander S Wiener and Levine and associates confirmed in 1941 that erythroblastosis was due to maternal isoimmunization against paternally inherited fetal factors Ronald Finn, in Liverpool, England applied a microscopic technique for detecting fetal cells in the mother's blood. It led him to propose that the disease might be prevented by injecting the at-risk mother with an antibody against fetal red blood cells. He proposed this for the first time to the public on February 18, 1960. The first treatment for Rh-disease was an exchange transfusion, which was invented by Alexander S Wiener. Sir William Liley performed the first successful intrauterine transfusion in 1963.

PREVALENCE

In spite of availability of anti-D for prevention of Rh-isoimmunization, it is still prevalent in 0.8–1.5% of pregnancy.[1] In India, a recent perinatal audit found the incidence of perinatal deaths due to Rh-alloimmunization to be between 1 to 2.5%.[2] The incidence of Rh-negative in western countries is about 15%. But its incidence in India varies between 3 and 5.7%.[3] The incidence of Rh-sensitization during pregnancy is about 1.9%[4] and the perinatal loss due to Rh-alloimmunization has been reported to be between 1 and 2.5%.[5]

PATHOPHYSIOLOGY

Rh-incompatibility can occur by two main mechanisms:
1. The most common type occurs when an Rh-negative pregnant mother is exposed to Rh-positive fetal red blood cells secondary to fetomaternal hemorrhage during the course of pregnancy from spontaneous or induced abortion, trauma.[6]
2. Rh-incompatibility can also occur when an Rh-negative female receives an Rh-positive blood transfusion.

Once produced, maternal Rh-immunoglobulin G (IgG) antibodies may cross freely from the placenta to the fetal circulation, where they form antigen-antibody complexes with Rh-positive fetal erythrocytes and eventually are destroyed, resulting in a fetal alloimmune-induced hemolytic anemia.[7] Although the Rh blood group systems consist of several antigens (e.g. D, C, c, E, e), the D antigen is the most immunogenic; therefore, it most commonly is involved in Rh-incompatibility.

During normal pregnancy, fetal red cells cross the placenta in 5% of the cases during the first trimester and in 46% by the end of the third trimester.[8]

Risk of sensitization depends largely upon the following three factors:
1. *Volume of transplacental hemorrhage*: It is found out that greater the number of fetal cells entering the maternal circulation, more is the possibility of maternal sensitization although it has also been found out that some mothers have been immunized with as little as 0.25 mL fetal RBCs.
2. Extent of the maternal immune response.
3. *Concurrent presence of ABO incompatibility*: If the mother is group O and the father is A/B/AB, the frequency of sensitization is decreased by 50–75% because the maternal anti-A or anti-B antibodies destroy the fetal red cells carrying the Rh-antigen before they trigger an immune response. Some are not immunized probably genetically controlled.

Two types of response are elicited during pregnancy in Rh-alloimmunization. *The initial* is the development of anti-Rh IgM antibodies with a molecular weight too large to cross the placenta. This is followed by the synthesis of anti-Rh IgG antibodies that cross the placenta, and hence start the process of destruction in the fetus by sticking to the fetal RBCs. This is followed by the *secondary response* of formation of large amount of antibodies in response to small number of fetal blood leaking through the placenta.

Depending on the severity of hemolysis *during pregnancy*, fetus can suffer in either of the ways:
- Mild anemia, hyperbilirubinemia, and jaundice. The placenta helps in getting rid of some of the bilirubin, but not all.

- Severe anemia with enlargement of the liver and spleen. When these organs and the bone marrow cannot compensate for the fast destruction of red blood cells, severe anemia results and other organs are affected.
- *Hydrops fetalis:* This occurs as the baby's organs are unable to handle the anemia. The heart begins to fail and large amounts of fluid build up in the baby's tissues and organs. A fetus with hydrops is at great risk of being stillborn.

After Birth

- *Severe hyperbilirubinemia and jaundice:* The baby's liver is unable to handle the large amount of bilirubin that results from red blood cell breakdown. The baby's liver is enlarged and anemia continues.
- *Kernicterus:* Kernicterus is the most severe form of hyperbilirubinemia and results from the buildup of bilirubin in the brain. This can cause seizures, brain damage, deafness, and death.

PREVENTION[9]

Antenatal Prophylaxis and Protection

- *First trimester events:*
  - Significant bleeding during threatened abortion
  - Spontaneous miscarriage
  - Medical termination of pregnancy (Anti-D to be given soon after misoprostol administration)
  - Surgical termination of pregnancy
  - Ectopic pregnancy
  - Vesicular mole; particularly of it is a partial mole
  - Chorion biopsy
  - Embryo reduction.
    - In all these events a dose of 50–100 μg should be given, as soon as possible after the sensitizing event. Evidence that women are sensitized after uterine bleeding in the first 12 weeks of pregnancy, where the fetus is viable and the pregnancy continues is scant (threatened abortion), however, it is safer to give an injection of 50 μg anti-D in these cases.
  - *Second trimester events:*
    - *Routine antenatal prophylaxis*: All patients should be tested for Rh-sensitization at the time of registration and again at 28 weeks. All non-sensitized women should be given 100 μg anti-D at 28 weeks and again at 34 weeks or a single dose of 300 μg at 28 weeks. A woman with 'weak D' (also known as Du – positive,) need not receive anti-D. It is desirable to offer antenatal prophylaxis to all Rh-negative women who are nonsensitized, and have a Rh- positive partner.
  - Sensitizing events during second or third trimester.
    - Amniocentesis
    - Abruptio placentae
    - Blunt trauma
    - Intrauterine fetal death
    - External cephalic version
    - Placental pravia with bleeding.
      - All these events should be covered by an anti-D injection of 300 μg at least (This covers 15 mL of fetal RBCs or 30 mL of fetal blood). Ideally, a test for the size of fetomaternal hemorrhage should be done. About 10 μg additional anti-D should be given for every additional 0.5 mL fetal RBCs in maternal circulation.

Postpartum Prophylaxis

All Rh-D negative patients who deliver a Rh-D positive baby either by a normal delivery or a cesarean section should receive 300 μg of Anti D within 72 hours of delivery. If anti-D is not given within 72 hours of delivery or other potentially sensitizing event, anti-D should be given as soon as the need is recognized, for up to 28 days after delivery or other potentially sensitizing event.

Circumstances where routine antenatal anti-D prophylaxis (RADDP) would neither be necessary nor cost effective:
- Has opted to be sterilized after the birth of the baby.
- Is in a stable relationship with the father of the child, and the father is known to be Rh-negative
- Is certain that she will not have another child after her current pregnancy.

The Rh-negative gravid who remains unsensitized (negative anti-D immune globulin antepartum should have her eligibility for postpartum administration determined immediately after delivery and anti-D immune globulin given when the following conditions are fulfilled:
- The infant is Rh-positive.
- The direct Coombs' test reveals whether of not the infant's red cell are covered by irregular antibodies.
- The crossmatch between anti-D immune globulin and their mother's red cells compatible.

INVESTIGATIONS

Prenatal Investigations

- *Paternal Rh-phenotype and genotype*: If the father of the baby is Rh-negative the fetus will not be affected and further tests are unnecessary.
  - If the father is Rh-positive, it is necessary to determine, if he is homozygous or heterozygous for the *RHD* gene.
  - If the father is heterozygous; the fetus has a 50% probabililty of being Rh-negative and determination of their fetal Rh becomes mandatory to avoid unnecessary testing in the 50% fetuses that will be Rh-negative. If the father is homozygous, the fetus will be Rh-positive

and amniocentesis to determine the fetal Rh will be unnecessary.
- *Serum antibody titers*: Manual Rh-titration is universally accepted test because it is simple, cheap and can be easily repeated frequently.
  - A rise in Rh-titer indicates a Rh(D) positive fetus. Several techniques are available to perform this test.
    - Indirect antiglobulin test (IAT)
    - Albumin method
    - Enzyme method.

Quantitation of Anti-D Concentration

Rh-titer, being a semi-quantitative, visual test, results may vary from person to person. Therefore autoanalyzer methods have been developed to quantitate anti-D in microgram amounts.
- Bromelin method
- Bromelin methyl cellulose method
- ELISA.

Critical titer for anti-D antibodies, a titer >1:16 indicates the possibility of severe hemolytic disease.

If alloimmunization is detected and the titer is below critical value, the titer is generally repeated every 4 weekly for the duration of the pregnancy.

If the antibody titer remains under the critical level up to 36 weeks of gestation, the patient with a first sensitized pregnancy should be delivered by elective induction of labor between 38 and 40 weeks, and the birth of a nonaffected (Rh-negative) or mildly affected Rh-positive infant should be anticipated. Women with a first sensitized pregnancy followed with antibody titers that have a sudden antibody titer elevation when they are more than 37 weeks gestation should have amniocentesis and delivered if the fetal lung maturity is adequate.

Spectrophotometric analysis of amniotic fluid: If the fetus is normal, then the amniotic fluid is colorless or pale straw, whereas in severe Rh HDN, it is usually bright yellow because of the transport of fetal bilirubin into maternal circulation.

Liley[10] proposed three zones on the basis of optical density of the amniotic fluid at 450 mm and the gestational age. Values in Zone I (safe zone) indicate mild or no disease. Zone II (intermediate/observation zone) suggests repetition of amniotic fluid examination after a few days and Zone III (dangerous/critical zone) indicates the severely affected fetus. Liley's method is considered reliable only for pregnancies from 27 weeks to term.

Investigations of Fetus

- *Rh-typing*: Prenatal DNA based Rh-typing of the fetus is possible as early as 9th week of gestation, using trophoblasts recovered from the endocervical canal. It can also be done using polymerase chain reaction amplification from the DNA obtained from the fetal cells in maternal peripheral blood or amniotic fluid.
- *Cordocentesis or percutaneous umbilical blood sampling*: Fetal blood sample can be obtained by puncture of the fetal heart, intrahepatic portion of the umbilical vein or by puncture of the umbilical vessel close to its site of insertion and around 1–10 mL of blood can be withdrawn for diagnostic studies.

Postnatal Diagnosis

Immediately after the birth of an infant, blood from the umbilical cord or the infant should be examined for Hb, Rh type and Direct Coombs' test. Cord hemoglobin less than 14 g/dL is abnormal In term neonates. Also a serum bilirubin level in conjunction with the other additional tests may help to assess the degree of hemolysis and risk of kernicterus.

Tests for Determination of Fetomaternal Leak

- *Kleihauer-Betke*: The amount of fetal hemorrhage can be calculated from the results of a Kleihauer-Betke Stain using various formulae:

$$\text{mL of fetal bleed} = \frac{\text{No. of fetal cells} \times 5000}{1000 \text{ adult cells}}$$

$$\text{Fetal blood volume} = \frac{\text{Maternal blood volume} \times \text{maternal hematocrit} \times \% \text{ fetal cells in KB}}{\text{Newborn hematocrit}}$$

- *Rosetting test*: It is based on the principle that Rh-positive fetal cells coated with anti-D form rosettes with Rh-positive indicator cells, thus they look different from Rh-negative maternal cells. It is not reliable when mother is weakly D-positive.
- *Newer tests* such as microscopic Du test and flow cytometry are also available.

Ultrasonography

The middle cerebral artery peak systolic velocity (MCA-PSV) is an accurate noninvasive method for the diagnosis of fetal anemia.[11] The correlation between MCA-PSV becomes stronger as the fetal anemia increases.[12] The Threshold for diagnosis of fetal anemia is a value equal to greater than 1.5 multiples of the median (MoM) for the gestational age. Abnormally elevated MCA-PSV has a sensitivity of 100% and a false positive rate of 2% for the diagnosis of fetal anemia. However, the false positive rate of MCA-PSV is at least 12%. With this approach, we can limit cordocentesis and intravascular transfusion in fetuses showing abnormal MCA PSV values.

Sonographic Features of Hydrops Fetalis

Hydrops fetalis is excessive extravasation of fluid into the third space in a fetus which could be due to heart failure, volume overload, decreased oncotic pressure, or increased vascular permeability. Hydrops fetalis is defined as accumulation of fluid +/- edema involving at least two fetal components, which may manifest as:
- *Fetal pleural effusion*: Pleural effusions can be unilateral or bilateral. Unilateral effusions indicate the presence of a process such as chylothorax. Large effusions can compress the mediastinal vessels, cause upper body edema, and interfere with esophageal functioning to cause secondary polyhydramnios.
- Fetal pericardial effusion
- *Fetal ascites*: Ascites may be small and may be just enough to form a film over the abdominal contents, or ascites may be extensive, with the contents of the abdomen, liver, and gut floating in the fluid. The ascites may extend into the scrotum to form a hydrocele
- *Generalized body edema*: Fetal anasarca/nuchal edema/cystic hygroma edema may be localized to one part of the body, or it may be generalized. Edema is seen most easily over the skull, over which a halo is formed. Edema may be seen in other parts of the body, as well.
- *Placental enlargement*: Placental thickening is a late occurrence, and when affected, the placenta is thicker than 4–5 cm over its entire extent.
- Polyhydraminos
- Hepatomegaly.

REFERENCES

1. Pertl B, Pieber D, Panzitt T, Haeusler MC, Winter R, et al. RhD genotyping by quantitative fluorescent polymerase chain reaction: a new approach. BJOG. 2000;107(12):1498-502.
2. Shah DS, Shroff SA, Ganla K. Perinatal audit: A report produced for the Federation of Obstetric and Gynaecological Societies of India by the Perinatology Committee; 1998.
3. Bhakoo ON. Perinatal problems. In: Krishna menone MK, Devi PK, Bhasker Rao K (Eds). Postgraduate Obstetrics and Gynecology (3rd edn). Hyderabad: Orient Longman; 1986.
4. Salvi V. The clinician's approach to rhesus isoimmunization. In: Shah D, Salvi V (Eds). The Rh Factor. Mumbai: Perinatology Committee FOGSI; 1998:99.
5. Shah D, Shorff S. New approaches in management of rhesus alloimmunization in Saraiya UB, Rao KA, Chettergy A (Eds). Principles and practice of Obstetrics and Gynecology for postgraduates. FOGSI Publication. New Delhi: Jaypee Brothers. 2004:137.
6. Thorp JM. Utilization of anti-RhD in the emergency department after blunt trauma. Obstet Gynecol Surv. 2008;63(2): 112-5. [Medline]. invasive obstetric procedures, or normal delivery.
7. Elalfy MS, Elbarbary NS, Abaza HW. Early intravenous immunoglobin (two-dose regimen) in the management of severe Rh-hemolytic disease of newborn: a prospective randomized controlled trial. Eur J Pediatr. 2011;170(4):461-7.
8. Bowman JM, Pollock JM, Penson LE. Fetomaternal transplacental during pregnancy and after delivery. Vox Sang. 1986;51:117-2.
9. ICOG FOGSI recommendations for good clinical practice, Use of Anti-D Immunoglobulin for Rh Prophylaxis; 2009.
10. Liley AW. Liquor amnil analysis in management of pregnancy complicated by Rhesus sensitisation. Am J Obstet Gynecol. 1961;82:1359-70.
11. Mari G, Adrignolo A, Abuhamad AZ, et al. Diagnosis of fetal anemia with Doppler ultrasound in the pregnancy complicated by maternal group immunization. Ultrasound Obstet Gynecol. 1995;5:400-5.
12. Mari G and the Collaborative Group for diagnosis of fetal anaemia with Doppler ultrasonography. Noninvasive diagnosis by Doppler ultrasonography of fetal anemia due to maternal red-cell alloimmunization. N Engl J Med. 2000;342: 9-14.

Chapter 11

Management of Rh-alloimmunized Pregnancy

Jyotsna Gupta

INTRODUCTION

Introduction of anti-D prophylaxis both antenatal and postnatal have reduced the incidence of Rh-alloimmunization to 6 per 1000 live births. However, every Rh-negative pregnant woman needs her anti-D antibody evaluation at the first prenatal visit itself.

First time sensitized pregnancies need to be monitored by serial ICT titers and when indicated by Doppler ultrasonography of fetal middle cerebral artery for detection of fetal anemia.

When there is history of previous affected infant or neonate, then the maternal ICT titers are no longer predictive of severity of the disease. Fetal middle cerebral artery peak systolic velocity is used to detect fetal anemia and plan transfusion accordingly.

FOLLOW-UP AFTER POSITIVE MATERNAL ANTIBODY SCREENING TEST (ICT POSITIVE MOTHERS)

Maternal Antibody Titer Determination

It is first step in evaluation of a positive antibody screening test. Indirect Coomb's test is used to measure the IgG levels of maternal antibodies against fetal blood cell antigens. IgM levels need not be measured as it does not cross the placenta.

Antibody levels are measured as either serial dilution method or absolute values. A critical titer is defined as antibody levels associated with significant risk of fetal anemia or hydrops. For RhD antigen critical titer is 1:16 or 1:32 depending on the laboratory threshold. For Kell antigen, the critical titer is 1:8 only. Significant risk of fetal anemia or hydrops is present once critical titers are reached or there is four-fold rise in antibody level.[1] Referral to fetal medicine unit should be done for further management in these cases as increased fetal surveillance is required.

Fetal Blood Group and RhD Antigen Determination

Fetal RhD status determination becomes important once maternal antibody titer is at or above critical titer. Paternal zygosity for RhD antigen is useful, as in cases of heterozygous father 50% of fetuses will escape hemolysis and anemia as they will be RhD negative.

Fetal blood group determination in heterozygous paternal genotype helps in filtering those 50% fetuses which are RHD positive and at risk of fetal anemia. So, high risk surveillance can be targeted only to those pregnancies.

Fetal blood group can be determined by invasive fetal testing (Cordocentesis and amniocentesis) and associated with risk of fetomaternal hemorrhage and abortions. Amniocentesis involves studying the amniocytes for fetal antigen detection and tells the fetal genotype. Multiplex PCR is better for this as it helps reduce errors in gene determination. Fetal blood sampling helps determining the fetal blood group phenotyping by serological testing. Fetal blood sampling is associated with significant more fetal loss compared to amniocentesis it should be only done when amniocentesis is not an option. Chorionic villus sampling should not be done, if patient is willing to continue the pregnancy in spite of RhD positive fetus as disruption of chorionic villi during sampling is associated with significant risk of fetomaternal hemorrhage.

Now the fetal RHD status can be determined by a newer non-invasive technique of extracting *cell-free fetal DNA* from maternal plasma known as noninvasive prenatal testing (NIPT). This noninvasive test is available in some countries at present and waiting to be commercially launched in India. Noninvasive analysis of RhD, C, E, Kell antigens can be done. It can reliably determine fetal antigen status (> 97% sensitivity, if done after 11 weeks of gestation).[2] Cell-free fetal DNA is approximately 6–10% of the total DNA pool present in the maternal plasma. The source of this DNA is apoptotic pool of fetal trophoblasts escaping in the maternal circulation.[3,4] The fetal RhD status is determined by doing PCR analysis of the fetal DNA.

Determining Severity of Fetal Anemia

After critical titers of maternal antibodies are reached, fetal surveillance for severe anemia is required. It can be done by fetal Doppler ultrasound study (Noninvasive and preferred method) or by amniocentesis (Optical density method) and cordocentesis (Fetal Hb and hematocrit). Both amniocentesis and cordocentesis are invasive methods for screening and not the preferred route of screening now.

Ultrasound

For noninvasive assessment of fetal anemia Doppler scanning of the fetal middle cerebral artery peak systolic velocity (MCA-PSV) has emerged as the best tool.[5,6] This is based on the principle that in anemic fetus, oxygen delivery to the brain is preserved by increasing cerebral blood flow of this low viscosity blood **(Figs 11.1A and B)**. The correct technique for MCA-PSV measurement needs to be followed for proper and accurate assessment of fetal anemia. The technique used; is to obtain an axial section of the fetal brain including fetal thalamus and sphenoid wings. After proper magnification of the image, color Doppler is applied to identify the circle of Willis and middle cerebral artery. The pulsed wave gate is applied to the proximal third of MCA after its origin from internal carotid with angle of insonation as close to zero as possible and at least three consecutive waveforms are obtained. Peak systolic velocity is then measured and it should be >1.5 MoM for the gestation to be labeled as moderate-to-severe fetal anemia **(Figs 11.2A and B)**.

The sensitivity of an increased MCA-PSV for moderate-to-severe anemia detection is approximately 100% regardless of cause of anemia and with 12% false positiverate.[5,6] Various other ultrasound findings such as hepatic and splenic measurements, placental thickness, aortic Doppler, etc. have been studies but not found consistent in predicting fetal anemia.

Gestation at which MCA-PSV monitoring is initiated depends on the previous pregnancy outcome and maternal antibody titers. In cases of previous fetal or neonatal affection, MCA monitoring is started at 16 weeks of gestation. Whereas in cases of first sensitized pregnancy MCA monitoring is started at 22–24 weeks of gestation. If MCA PSV indicates possible severe anemia, or if a fetal ultrasound indicates signs of hydrops fetalis such as ascites, pleural effusion, skin edema, cardiac biventricular diameter or pericardial effusion, then cordocentesis is done to check the fetal hemoglobin and hematocrit with preparation of fetal blood transfusion in the same setting.

Measurement of MCA-PSV is an excellent noninvasive tool for guiding fetal invasive therapy and is considered standard of care in management of hemolytic disease of fetus and newborn.[7]

Amniocentesis

This is an invasive indirect method to know the fetal bilirubin levels and in-turn know the severity of ongoing hemolysis and anemia. Amniocentesis to monitor fetal anemia is not required after MCA-PSV has been reliably guiding fetal

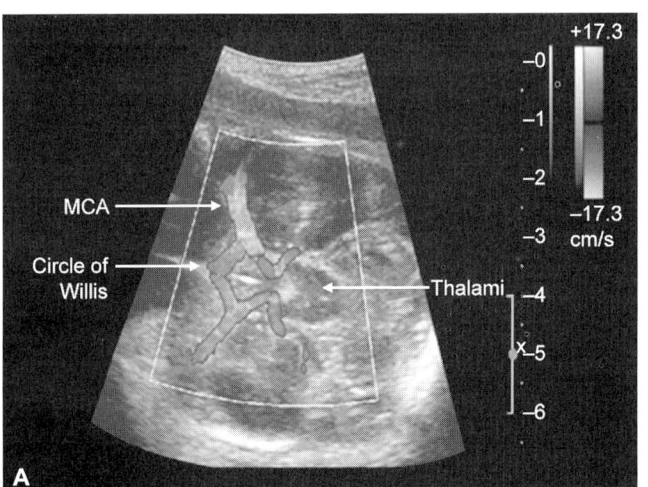
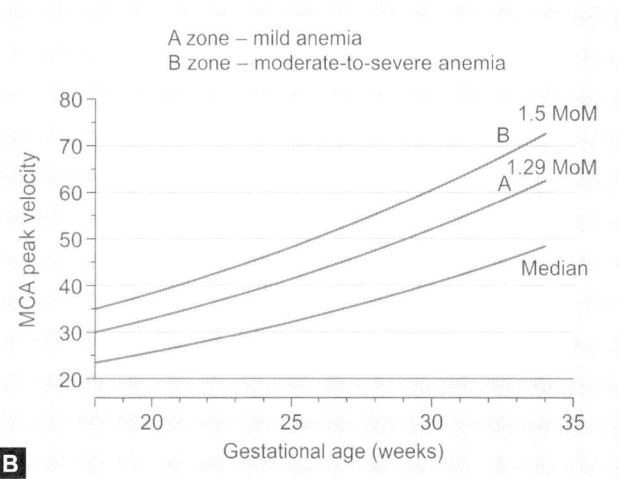

Figs 11.1A and B: (A) Middle cerebral artery; (B) Gestational age-specific middle cerebral artery peak systolic velocity values *(For color version, see Plate 1)*

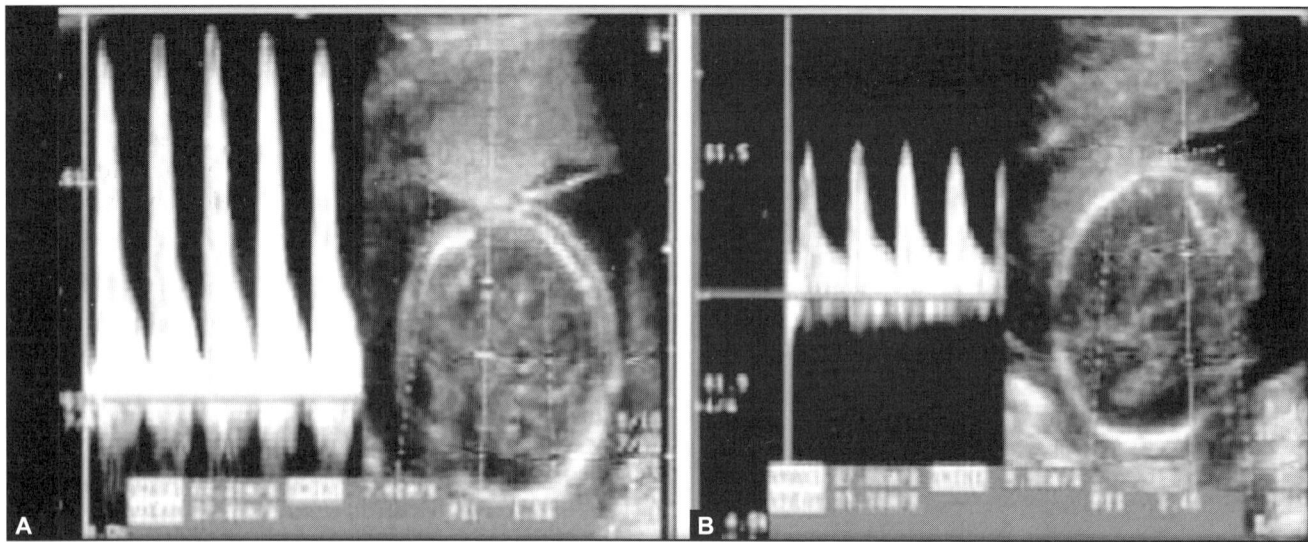

Figs 11.2A and B: (A) Increased fetal MCA-PSV suggesting fetal anemia and (B) Normal MCA-PSV for the gestation

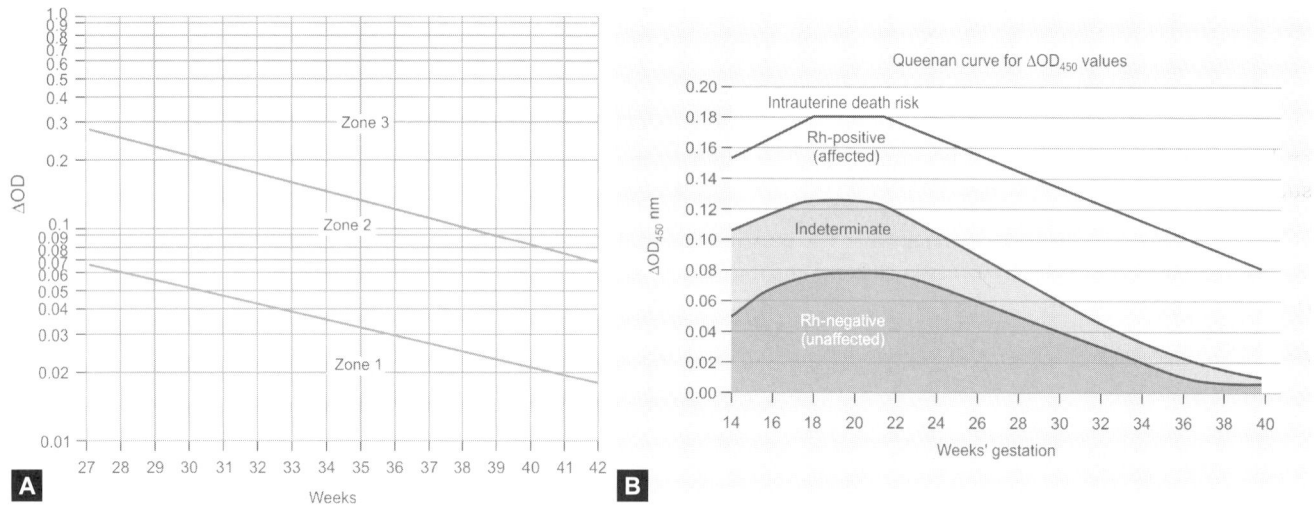

Figs 11.3A and B: (A) Liley's curve for ΔOD$_{450}$ values; (B) Queenan curve for ΔOD$_{450}$ values

moderate-to-severe anemia. Amniocentesis was done when severe fetal anemia was suspected and the level of bilirubin measured to estimate the degree of hemolysis by spectrophotometry. By second trimester, the amniotic fluid contains mainly fetal urine and tracheopulmonary secretions. Amniocentesis is done under ultrasound guidance and sample for spectrophotometry is sent to the laboratory in light resistant container to study the optical density. Same sample portion can be used to determine fetal blood group if not determined yet.

Liley's curves for monitoring and management of fetal hyperbilirubinemia for gestation ages 27–42 weeks had been used for long. Queenan curves were later introduced which had better sensitivity and specificity along with utility at gestations lower than 27 weeks **(Figs 11.3A and B)**. These curves show a declining trend in the optical density as the gestation advances. But if there is increased bilirubin the curve goes up. The graph is divided in three zones 1,2,3. Zone 1 trace suggests no fetal disease while zone 3 suggests severe fetal affection. Management is decided by trend in the serial amniocentesis derived ΔOD_{450} mm values. Serial amniocentesis was done at 10 days –2 weeks interval and continued till delivery to follow the trends in ΔOD_{450} 0 mm. Arising curve or a position on the curve in the upper zone 2 or zone 3 warrants cordocentesis and blood transfusion.

This technique of fetal anemia surveillance though used for long has now lost its touch as it invasive procedure associated with risk of amnionitis, sensitization, rupture of membranes. Also, these graphs can only be used for D antigen associated immunization. In cases of Kell antigen, these curves are not sensitive enough as they have severe fetal anemia even with lower serum bilirubin values. Kell alloimmunization supresses the erythroid blasts in addition to hemolysis, therefore severity of anemia is disproportionate to the degree of hemolysis.[8]

Fetal Blood Sampling

Fetal blood sampling (FBS) is also referred to as percutaneous umbilical blood sampling, cordocentesis, or funipuncture. After MCA-PSV value has reached 1.5 MoM suggesting significant anemia. FBS is done to confirm fetal anemia and samples for fetal Hb, hematocrit, bilirubin, direct Coombs' test, fetal blood type and reticulocyte count are taken to evaluate fetal disease. Fetal blood sampling is associated with 1–2% risk of fetal loss and 50% risk of fetomaternal hemorrhages. Serial FBS are the method of fetal anemia surveillance when MCA PSV > 1.5 MoM. When FBS is planned all preparations for fetal blood transfusion should be kept ready, if the fetal hematocrit (< 30%) or hemoglobin <2 SD of the mean for that specific gestational age.

CLINICAL MANAGEMENT OF FIRST AFFECTED PREGNANCY

In first affected pregnancy ICT test, due RhD alloimmunization the fetal anemia usually develops late in the second or third trimester and sometimes may not develop also. Paternal RhD zygosity is determined as in cases of heterozygosis 50% of fetuses will be RhD positive and 50% negative. In heterozygous paternal Rh status, fetal RhD type is determined by cell-free fetal DNA in maternal plasma.

When ICT titer are at/or above critical value (1:16/1:32), then surveillance for fetal anemia is started by noninvasive Doppler study of fetal middle cerebral artery peak systolic velocity (MCA-PSV) at 1–2 weeks' intervals. Fetal MCA-PSV 1.5 MoM for the gestation correlates well with fetal anemia in moderate-to-severe range.

For pregnancies with MCA-PSV > 1.5 MoM for gestation, fetal blood sampling is planned with all preparations for Intravascular transfusion, if fetal hemoglobin is < 2 SD for the gestation or fetal hematocrit is <30%. Intrauterine transfusions are done, if gestation is less than < 35 weeks because at gestations > 35 weeks induction and delivery is planned and post-natal transfusion is preferred instead of intrauterine transfusion (Flow chart 11.1).[7]

CLINICAL MANAGEMENT OF PREVIOUS FETAL OR NEONATAL AFFECTION

Pregnancies after previous hydrops, intrauterine fetal transfusion therapy, intrauterine fetal demise or neonatal exchange transfusion have earlier onset and severe nature of hemolytic disease in subsequent pregnancies. This is due to repeated entry of fetal RBCs in the maternal circulation at each delivery resulting in anamnestic antibody response.

In these pregnancies, ICT test is not informative enough as predictor for high-risk surveillance. Doppler fetal MCA-PSV monitoring is directly started at 16–18 weeks of gestation.[7]

When MCA-PSV values reach > 1.5 MoM for the gestation, then fetal blood sampling is done with all preparations for transfusion in the same setting if Hb< 2SD from the mean for the gestation. Next transfusion is planned based on final hematocrit after the first transfusion and estimating the rate of fall along with fetal MCA-PSV values. Subsequent transfusion is planned dafter 3–4 week as till now significant fetal erythropoietic suppression takes place and hemolysis is less. In cases of extremely high titers or very early gestation of fetal affection immune-modulator therapy (IVIG and plasmapheresis) need to be considered as fetal blood transfusion earlier than 22–24 weeks is technically difficult and associated with complications (Flow chart 11.2).[7]

FETAL BLOOD TRANSFUSION

Fetal blood transfusion is done to correct significant fetal anemia due to hemolysis. It is done only when fetal hematocrit is below 30% which corresponds to levels of <2.5th percentile for all gestations more than 20 weeks. Fetal transfusion can be done by Intraperitoneal administration of packed RBC or direct intravascular packed RBC transfusion or a combined approach.

Intraperitoneal Transfusion

This is the oldest method used to transfuse packed cells, but now less preferred route due to associated risks and the development of safer technique of intravascular transfusion. This method involves intraperitoneal transfusion (IPT) of packed RBC which are absorbed via lymphatics with fetal respiration. Daily absorption of transfused blood is only 10%. When the fetus is hydropic the absorption is even slower and unpredictable.

Drawbacks of IPT are slow correction of hemoglobin deficit, Higher risk of fetal trauma, risk of excessive blood volume transfusion and obstructing cardiac return as

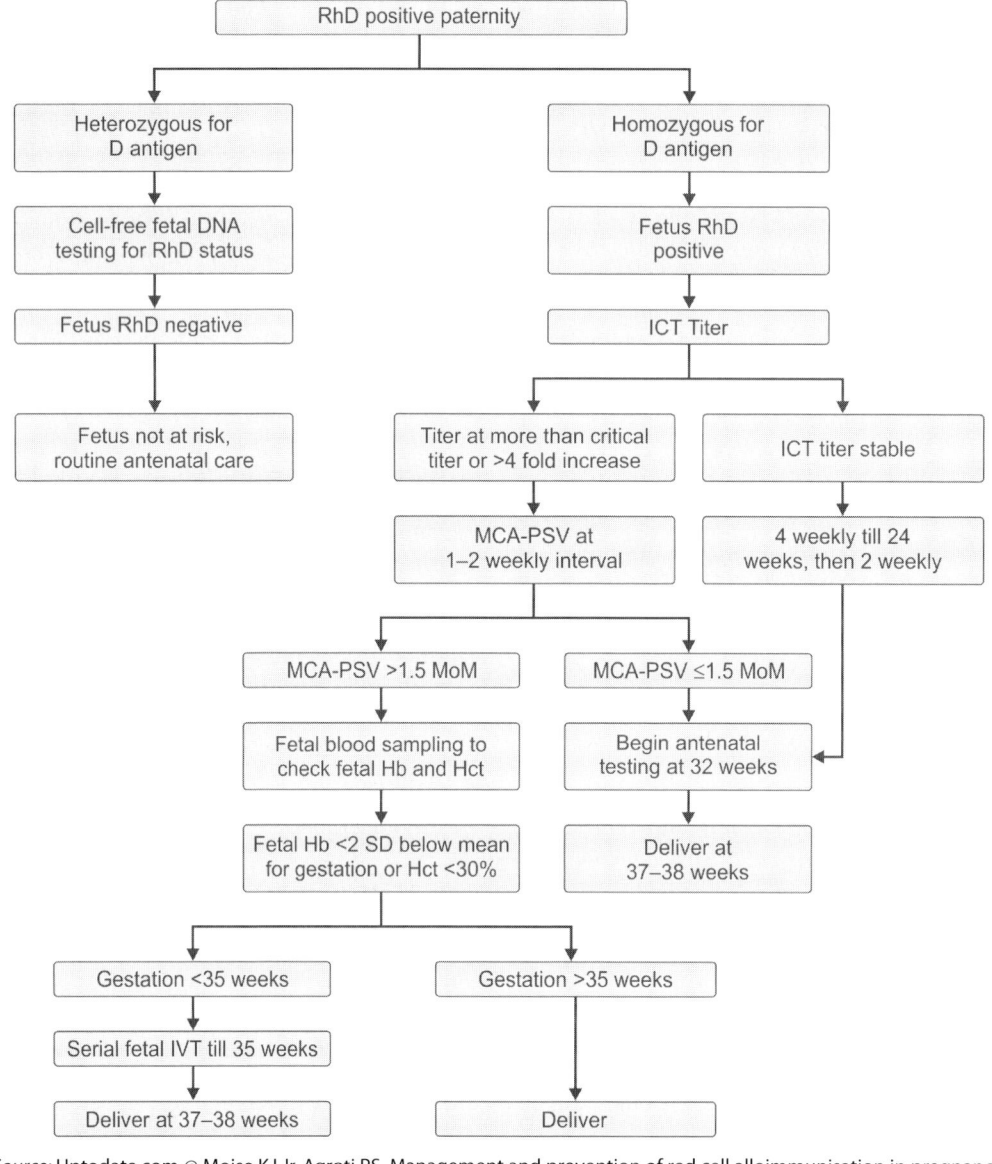

Flow chart 11.1: Clinical management in cases of first affected pregnancy

Source: Uptodate.com @ Moise KJ Jr, Agroti PS. Management and prevention of red cell alloimmunisation in pregnancy: a systematic review. Obstet Gynecol. 2012;120:1132.

the abdominal pressure becomes too high. Incidence of fetal mortality with IPT was six times higher compared to intravascular transfusion.[9]

Transfusion is planned when Hct< 30%. Best site for IPT is fetal abdomen between umbilicus and bladder. Fetus is paralyzed by injecting pancuronium in the fetal buttock. The needle is then placed in the fetal abdomen and blood is then transfused in 1 mL aliquots till the desired amount is transfused. Continuous fetal heart rate monitoring is done till the fetal movements resume. Serial ultrasounds are done to confirm complete absorption of blood. Second transfusion is done after complete absorption of the first one. Subsequent transfusions are planned 4 weeks later.

Intraperitoneal transfusion is now done only in circumstances where early onset severe fetal anemia or hydrops is present and intravascular route is problematic that is at less than 24 weeks of gestation.[7]

Flow chart 11.2: Previously affected fetus/infant

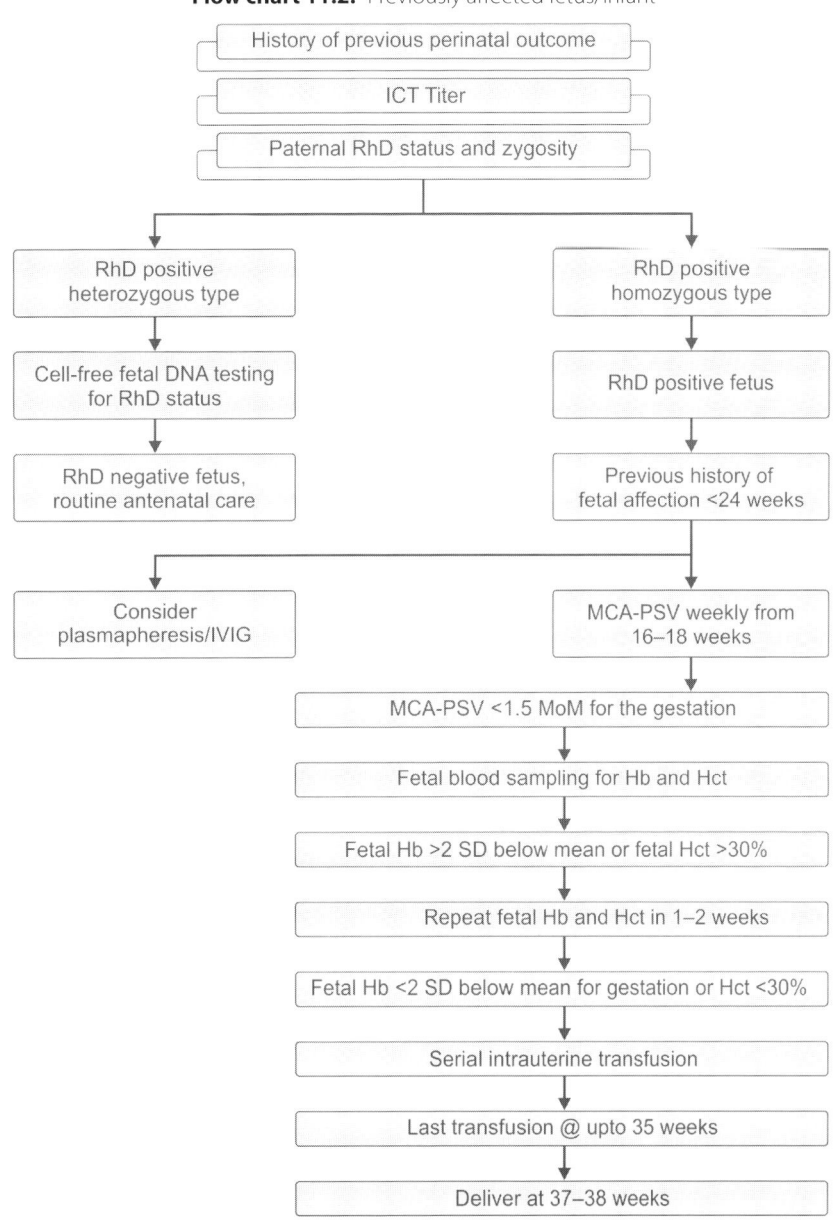

Source: Uptodate.com @ Moise KJ Jr, Agroti PS. Management and prevention of red cell alloimmunisation in pregnancy: a systematic review. Obstet Gynecol. 2012;120:1132.

Intravascular Transfusion

Preferred route of fetal blood transfusion practised now.[10,11] Main aim of intravascular transfusion (IVT) is the delivery of a healthy, non-anemic, neonate at term when it can better tolerate transition to *ex uetro* life and withstand the hyperbilirubinemia. Fetal transfusion is done only when the fetal hematocrit is less than 30%. Transfusion is planned once fetal MCA-PSV is more than 1.5 MoM for the gestation.[5] Percutaneous umbilical blood sampling is done with all preparation of blood transfusion ready, if fetal Hb<2 standard deviation for the gestation or hematocrit less than 30%. Blood to be transfused should be freshly donated O negative blood, compatible with both mother and fetus. It should be leukocyte depleted, gamma irradiated and concentrated blood with hematocrit of 70–80% at least. Blood is gamma irradiated to reduce graft versus host reaction.[12] Fresh blood is preferred as it has a higher concentration of 2,3-diphosphoglycerate. Blood should be subjected to antibody testing for HIV type 1 and 2, CMV, HCV, HTLV 1 and 2, Hep B core antigen, HBsAg, syphilis, p24 antigen of HIV. Nucleic acid amplification for HIV and HCV is done to rule out HIV and HCV.[13]

Four sites can be accessed for sampling and transfusion via fetal umbilical vein:
1. Cord insertion at placental bed
2. Cord insertion proximal to umbilicus
3. Free loop of cord
4. Intrahepatic portion of umbilical vein

Preferred site for fetal blood sampling and transfusion is the placental end of cord insertion. Fetal umbilical vein is the vessel of choice for transfusion as well as fetal blood sampling as arterial puncture leads to vessel spasm and fetal bradycardia. Intrahepatic umbilical vein is another good site to approach in cases where placental end of cord insertion is not accessible. However, it is technically difficult approach and requires fetus to lie in specific position for access into intrahepatic portion of umbilical vein.

Direct cardiac puncture has been described and is not to be considered as it is associated with a high-risk of fetal demise.

Preparation for the transfusion requires freshly donated O negative blood compatible with both mother and the fetus. It should be buffy coat poor, saline washed thrice and irradiated. Diazepam can be given to relax the mother. Abdomen is draped and instruments kept ready for FBS and transfusion later on.

Transfusion starts with umbilical vein site selection for fetal blood sampling. Fetus is paralyzed by injecting pancuronium intramuscularly. First 1–2 mL blood is aspirated for complete blood count, reticount, DCT, hematocrit, blood group, serum bilirubin. Transfuse blood in the vein and after transfusing half the amount do repeat sampling to check Hb and Hct. Check fetal heart rate intermittently to see fetal bradycardia. After transfusing the whole blood before the needle is withdrawn repeat fetal blood samples are taken to get the final hematocrit post-transfusion. Continuous fetal heart rate monitoring is done until fetal movements resume.

Fetal movements need to be suppressed by paralyzing the fetus with pancuronium.[14,15] Post-transfusion the final hematocrit should be in the range of 48–55%. Before finishing the procedure the closing fetal hematocrit sample is withdrawn and checked for accessing optimal therapy and timing of next transfusion.

TIMING OF SUBSEQUENT TRANSFUSION

Fall of hematocrit after IUT falls approximately 1% per day so the next transfusion is guided by combined approach considering rate of fall of hematocrit per day and biweekly assessment of fetal MCA-PSV, which is approximately 10 to 14 days after first transfusion.

After second transfusion, the fetal erythropoiesis is sufficiently suppressed and next transfusion is required approximately 3–4 weeks post last transfusion guided by fetal MCA-PSV determination[8] along with estimating rate of fall in hematocrit from the final value post-transfusion.

FETAL HYDROPS

Hydrops fetalis (fetal hydrops) is a serious fetal condition defined as abnormal accumulation of fluid in 2 or more fetal compartments including ascites, pleural effusion **(Figs 11.4A and B)**, pericardial effusion, and skin edema. It is also

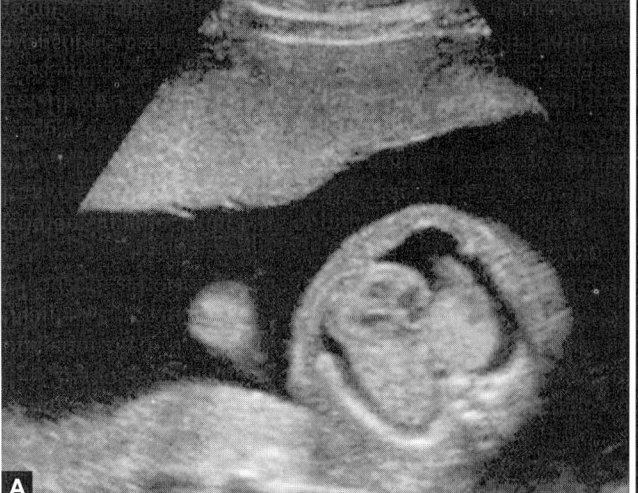 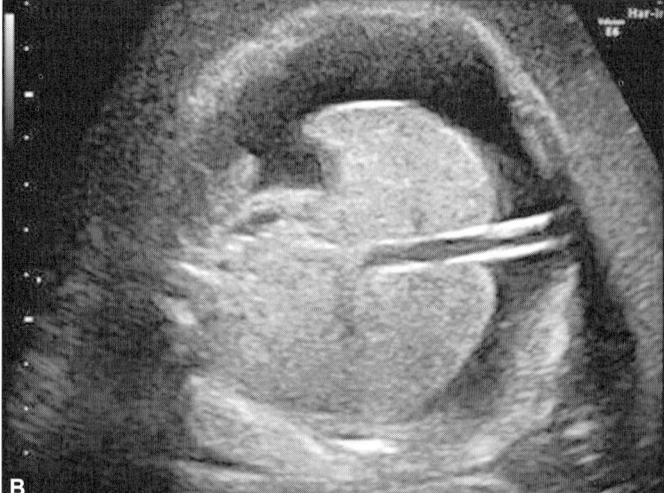

Figs 11.4A and B: (A) Fetal pleural effusion in hydropic fetus, and (B) Ascites in the hydropic fetus

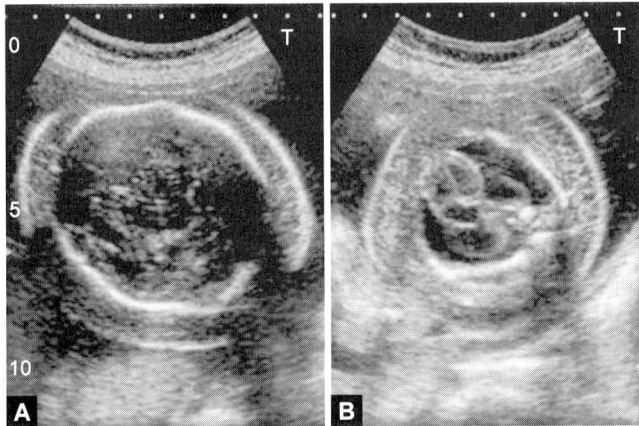

Figs 11.5A and B: (A) Hydropic fetus showing scalp edema on ultrasound and (B) The subcutaneous edema in hydropic fetus

associated with polyhydramnios and placental edema **(Figs 11.5A and B)**. It can be easily detected on antenatal ultrasonography. Untreated hydrops fetalis has poor prognosis. Several hypotheses regarding the pathophysiologic events that lead to fetal hydrops have been suggested. The basic mechanism for the formation of fetal hydrops is an imbalance of interstitial fluid production and the lymphatic return. Fluid accumulation in the fetus can result from congestive heart failure, obstructed lymphatic flow, or decreased plasma osmotic pressure. The fetus is particularly susceptible to interstitial fluid accumulation because of its greater capillary permeability, compliant interstitial compartments, and vulnerability to venous pressure on lymphatic return. Compensatory mechanisms are activated to maintain fetal hemostasis. These mechanisms include increased oxygen extraction by tissues and redistribution of blood to brain, heart and adrenal glands. This leads to renal hypoperfusion leading to activation of renin angiotensin system. This leads to increased venous pressure and in turn increased accumulation of interstitial fluid. Increased venous pressure increases accumulation of fluid, increased capillary leakage of the fluid and impaired return of this fluid to heart. Impaired renal function leads to oliguria and anuria. All these hemodynamic disturbances lead to hydrops fetalis **(Figs 11.6A and B)**.

In hydropic fetus myocardial dysfunction and acidosis makes them less capable of tolerating infusion volume. So the target hematocrit after IVT in these fetuses is 25% only. Second transfusion can be done next day to increase hematocrit up to 50% safely.

In severely anemic hydropic fetuses, there is acidosis and the transfused blood also decreases the blood pH aggravating myocardial failure and fetal death. The fetus needs to be monitored during transfusion. Fetal heart rate is checked intermittently for fetal bradycardia. Umbilical venous pressure measurements is also important as 10 mm Hg rise in umbilical venous pressure is associated with significant perinatal mortality.

SEVERELY ANEMIC EARLY SECOND TRIMESTER FETUS

Fetal anemia due to Rh-alloimmunization occurring at 18–24 weeks is a special challenge to manage. At this gestation, intravascular access for transfusion is technically not possible due to small caliber of fetal vessels and was seen to be associated with 60% mortality rate. In this situation, either immunomodulation therapy or intraperitoneal transfusion is started from 16–18 weeks and after 24 weeks intravascular transfusion is done to manage fetal anemia. IPT are not very helpful, if hydrops is present at this early gestation.

Plasma exchange and administration of intravenous immunoglobulins (IVIG) may maintain the fetal hematocrit above life-threatening levels long enough to achieve a gestational age, when intravascular intrauterine transfusion is technically feasible.[16] The American Society of Apheresis guidelines recommend IVT as the mainstay of treatment, but state that IVIG and/or therapeutic plasma exchange may be indicated, if there is high risk of fetal demise or signs of hydrops prior to 20 weeks.[17]

TIMING OF DELIVERY

When intraperitoneal transfusions were used, the delivery was planned at around 32 weeks of gestation. Delivery at 32 weeks was associated with significant risk of postnatal hyperbilirubinemia and kernicterus as the hepatic enzymatic system is immature before 36 weeks. To avoid permanent brain damage due to high levels of Bilirubin multiple neonatal exchange transfusions were required. Also, the risk of prematurity and hyaline membrane disease add to morbidity for the already anemic and hyperbilirubinemic neonate.

With the introduction of Intravascular transfusions and delivery at 37–38 weeks the risk of prematurity is reduced and the need of neonatal exchange transfusion is drastically reduced.[7]

Advantages of this technique are found to be numerous. Delivery at 37–38 weeks allows the fetal pulmonary and hepatic systems to mature. IVT at 35 weeks gives adequate RBC reserve to fetus lasting for approximately 5 weeks' post-transfusion. Need for neonatal exchange transfusion is decreased as hemolysis is suppressed due to suppressed erythropoiesis in the neonate as a result of multiple intrauterine transfusions replacing fetal RBCs with the Donor blood cells.[7]

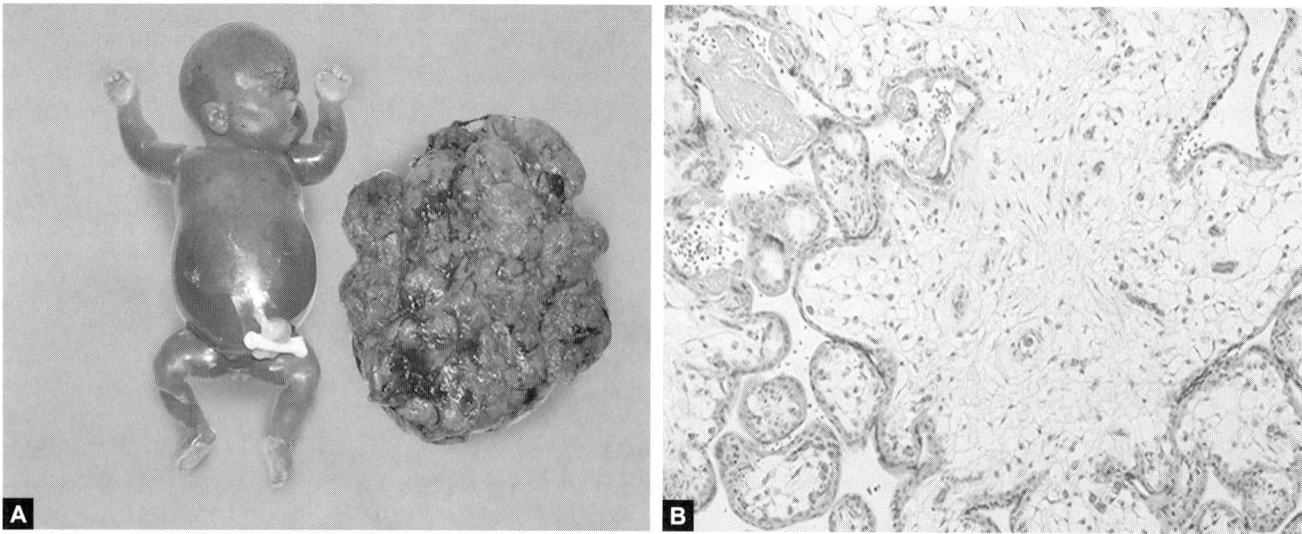

Figs 11.6A and B: (A) Hydropic fetus with large placenta seen in cases of severe fetal affection due to Rh-alloimmunization (*http://accessmedicine.mhmedical.com/content.aspx?bookid=1057&sectionid=59789153*); (B) Histopathology of hydropic placenta showing chorionic villi edema and accumulation of fluid and abundant stroma with intact vessels and no trophoblast proliferation (*http://library.med.utah.edu/WebPath/PLACHTML/PLAC030.html*) (*For color version, see Plate 1*)

POSTNATAL CARE

With IVT at 35 weeks, the postnatal period is good with rare need for exchange transfusion. The hyperbilirubinemia in these neonates can be managed by phototherapy alone. Neonatal follow-up is done by weekly hematocrit and reticulocyte count.

Small top-up transfusions are required to correct anemia due to erythropoiesis suppression from multiple transfusions. The pediatric management involves to keep the neonate asymptomatic but with moderate anemia so that erythropoesis is stimulated.[18]

Recombinant human erythropoietin may be administered to the neonate to accelerate erythropoiesis. The treatment showed early recovery of erythropoiesis and associated reduction in need for blood transfusions postnatal.[19] Iron supplementation is not required as circulating levels of iron are high due to ongoing hemolysis. Folate supplementation 0.5 mg/dL is required for adequate erythropoietic response.

OUTCOME

Outcome is discussed in terms of survival into the postnatal life and long-term sequel associated with increased survival rates. Outcome depends on the presence or absence of hydrops and experience of center performing IUT.

Survival

Overall survival is 84% in cases where intrauterine transfusion was done for Rh-alloimmunization-induced severe fetalanemia. If transfusions are performed in non-hydropic fetuses the survival is much better approximately 92%. If there is presence of hydrops, then survival drops to 70%. The survival rate in hydropic fetus is less, if fetal acidemia is present. If after transfusion in a hydropic fetus, there is resolution of hydrops, the survival rate is better >90%. In cases with persistent hydrops after blood transfusion, the survival is much lower (40%).[15,20]

Long-term Sequelae

Studies regarding the long-term outcomes in anemic fetuses receiving intrauterine transfusions see the neurological status, development delay and hearing loss.

Hearing loss seen in these fetuses is due to the high bilirubin levels in the neonatal life. Prevalence of hearing deficit is increased 5 to 10 folds over general population in infants requiring *in utero* therapy for Rh-alloimmunization. Postnatal evaluation and follow-up is required in these neonates.

A normal neurological outcome can be expected in more than 90% of surviving infants requiring intrauterine transfusions, even if hydrops fetalis was noted at the time of first transfusion.[21,22]

ALTERNATIVE TREATMENT MODALITIES

Alternative treatment modalities aim at suppressing maternal anti erythrocyte antibody concentration or its effects on the fetus. None of these, alternatives have proved to be too efficacious, however, they can be used as an adjunctive therapy in severe cases of early onset alloimmunization.

Plasmapheresis

This technique involves removal of maternal antibodies along with maternal plasma thereby reducing the antibody concentration in maternal serum by 80%. But this reduction is transient and there is rebound increase in antibody titers to more than 200% of the initial levels. Maximum increment (50–80%) in the antibody levels are seen with 48 hours. Plasmapheresis can be used in cases of early onset severe alloimmunization cases where this is started after 12 weeks of gestation and may help delay the fetal transfusion process to up to 22 weeks of gestation, after which the fetal blood transfusions can take over and manage fetal anemia.[17]

Intravenous Immunoglobulins

Intravenous immunoglobulins (IVIG) can be used in management of early onset severe HDFN either alone or as an adjunctive therapy. IVIG therapy when started before 28 weeks showed significant fall in maternal antibody titers, and reduced hemolysis in few studies with favorable fetal and neonatal outcome. This therapy can be used in cases of early onset severe alloimmunization cases and may help delay the fetal transfusion process to up to 22–24 weeks of gestation, after which the fetal blood transfusions can take over and manage fetal anemia.[23]

Chemotherapeutic Agents

Antenatal maternal *phenobarbitone* therapy with 30 mg oral tablet three times daily for atleast 7–10 days before anticipated delivery is shown to reduce the postnatal need for exchange transfusion for hyperbilirubinemia by 75%. This drug enhances the neonatal hepatic enzymatic capacity to conjugate and eliminate Bilirubin by stimulating glucuronyl transferase pathway.[22]

Steroids (Dexamethasone and Betamethasone) cross the placental barrier and were found to decrease the ΔOD_{450} mm. But these drugs do not reduce the severity of HDFN instead alter the bilirubin metabolism, limiting their use.

PRE-PREGNANCY COUNSELING

If a non-pregnant woman is found to have red cell antibodies then she is counseled regarding fetal risk of hemolytic disease depending upon type of maternal antibody and paternal RhD status and zygosity.

In case where previous affection is present, then couple is counseled regarding next pregnancy planning and management options available along with survival rates. Newer alternative options can be discussed to avoid future affection.

PREVENTION OF HDFN FETUS IN FUTURE PREGNANCIES

Prenatal and postnatal Anti-D is best way to prevent HDFN.

In cases where maternal antibody titers are very high or previous. Fetal or neonatal affection is seen, then couple can be given few options as discussed below. But in present era, HDFN is a manageable disease so alternative options discussed for prevention need to be considered with a word of caution.

In vitro fertilization with pre-implantation genetic diagnosis: This can be used only where father is heterozygous for RhD antigen and only RhD negative embryos are selected for transfer in the womb.[24]

Gestational surrogate can be used, if the father is homozygous and maternal antibody titers are high with previous history of fetal or neonatal affection. The embryos from biological parents are prepared by *In vitro* fertilization and transferred in a surrogate who is not alloimmunized.

Use of donor sperm from RhD negative donor can be used for intrauterine insemination of alloimmunized mother. In these cases, the fetus will be RhD negative only, thus avoiding maternal antibody mediated fetal RBC destruction.

REFERENCES

1. Nicolaides KH, Rodeck CH. Maternal serum anti-D antibody concentration and assessment of rhesus isoimmunisation. BMJ. 1992;304:1155-6.
2. Chitty LS, Finning K, Wade A, et al. Diagnostic Accuracy of routine antenatal determination of fetal RHD status across gestation: population based cohort study. BMJ. 2014;349:5243.
3. Lo YM, Tein MS, Lau TK, et al. Quantitative analysis of fetal DNA in maternal plasma and serum: Implications for prenatal diagnosis. Am J Hum Genetics. 1998;62:768-75.
4. Lo YM, Hejlm NM, Fidler C, et al. Prenatal diagnosis of fetal RhD status by molecular analysis of maternal plasma. N Engl J Med. 1998;339:1734-8.
5. Mari G, Deter RL, Carpenter RL, et al. Noninvasive diagnosis by Doppler ultrasonography of fetal anaemia due to maternal red cell alloimmunisation. Collaborative Group for Doppler Assessment of the blood velocity in Anemic foetuses. N Eng J Med. 2000;342:9.
6. Mar G. Middle cerebral artery peak systolic velocity: is it standard of care for diagnosis of fetal anemia?. J Ultrasound Med. 2005;24:697.
7. Moise KJ Jr, Agroti PS. Management and prevention of red cell alloimmunisation in pregnancy: a systematic review. Obstet Gynecol. 2012;120:1132.
8. CP Weiner, et al. Decreased fetal erythropoiesis and hemolysis in Kell hemolytic anemia. Am J Obstet Gynecol. 1996;174 (2): 547-51.

9. Harman MD, Bowman JM, Manning FA, et al. Intrauterine transfusions: intraperitoneal versus intravascular approach. A case control comparison. Am J Obstet Gynecol. 1990;162:1053-9.
10. Bowman JM. Management of Rh-isoimmunization. Obstet Gynecol. 1978;52:1-16.
11. Moise KJ Jr, Carpenter RJ Jr, Kirshon B, et al. Comparison of four types of intrauterine transfusions: effect on fetal hematocrit. Fetal Ther. 1989;4:126-37.
12. Guidelines on Gamma Irradiation of Blood Components for the Prevention of Transfusion Associated Graft versus Host Disease. Transfusion Med. 1996;6:261-71.
13. Brecher ME. Technical Manual of American Association of Blood Banks, 2005.
14. Moise KJ Jr, Carpenter RJ Jr, Deter RL, et al. The use of fetal neuromuscular blockade during intrauterine procedures. Am J Obstet Gynecol. 1987;157:874-9.
15. Schumacher B, Moise KJ Jr. Fetal transfusion for red blood cell alloimmunisation in pregnancy. Obstet Gynecol. 1996;88:137-50.
16. Papantoniou N, Sifakis S, Antsaklis A. Therapeutic management of fetal anemia: review of standard practice and alternative treatment options. J Perinat Med. 2013;41:71-82.
17. Schwartz J, Padmanbhan A, et al. Guidelines on the use of therapeutic apheresis in clinical practise-evidence based approach from the writing committee of the American Society For Apheresis: The seventh Special Issue. 2016;31(3):149-62.
18. Koenig JM, Ashton RD, De Vore GR, et al. Late hyporegenerative anemia in Rh haemolytic disease. J Pediatr. 1989;115:315-8.
19. Shannon KM, Menterz WC, Abels RI, et al. Recombinant human erythropoietin in the anemia of prematurity.: Results of a placebo-controlled pilot study. J Pediatr. 1991;118:949-55.
20. van Kamp IL, Klumper FJ, Bakkum RS, et al. The severity of immune hydrops is predictive of fetal outcome after intrauterine treatment. Am J Ostet Gynecol. 2001;185:668-73.
21. Janssens HM, de Haan MJ, van Kamp IL, et al. Outcome for children treated with fetal intravascular transfusions because of severe blood group antagonism. J Pediatr. 1997;131:373-80.
22. Hudon L, Moise KJ Jr, Hegemeir SE, et al. Long term neurodevelopmental outcome after intrauterine intravascular transfusions because of severe blood group antagonism. Am J Ostet Gynecol. 1998;179:858-63.
23. Margulies MD, Voto LS, Mathet Elena, Margulies Maximo. High-dose intravenous IgG for the treatment of severe rhesus Alloimmunisation. Vox Sanguinis. 1991;61(3):181-9.
24. G Burton, Seeho SKM, Marshall JT. Role of preimplantation genetic diagnosis in cases of severe Rh-alloimmunisation. Human Reprod. 2005;20(3):697-701.

Chapter 12

Disseminated Intravascular Coagulation in Pregnancy

Saroj Singh, Anu Pathak

INTRODUCTION

Disseminated intravascular coagulation (DIC) is characterized by systemic activation of blood coagulation system characterized by microvascular thrombi formation in various organs which can cause multiorgan failure. Consumption causes exhaustion of coagulation proteins and platelets, inducing severe bleeding complications.

EPIDEMIOLOGY

The prevalence of DIC in pregnancy ranges from 0.03–0.35% in population-based studies,[1-3] or 12.5 per 10,000 delivery hospitalizations in one study.[1] Although the overall prevalence of DIC is low in pregnancy, the frequency of DIC in women with specific pregnancy complications can be quite high.

NORMAL COAGULATION CASCADE

Normal intravascular blood coagulation is linked with three different interrelated system (Fig. 12.1):
1. Coagulation system
2. Coagulation inhibitory system
3. Fibrinolytic system.

PHYSIOLOGICAL CHANGES IN PREGNANCY

During pregnancy, there is:
- Increase in concentration of clotting factors II, V, VII, VIII, IX, X, XII.
- Plasma fibrinogen level is significantly increased.
- There is small decrease in platelet count.
- Plasma fibrinolytic activity is suppressed during pregnancy and labor.

Types

- Acute DIC
- Subacute or chronic DIC

TRIGGERING FACTORS FOR DIC

Endothelial Injury

- Pre-eclampsia, eclampsia, HELLP syndrome
- Septicemia
  - Septic abortion
  - Chorioamnionitis
  - Pyelonephritis
- Hypovolemia

Release of Thromboplastin

- Amniotic fluid embolism
- Dead fetus syndrome
- Abruptio placenta
- Hydatidiform mole
- Cesarean section
- Intra-amniotic hypertonic saline
- Shock

Release of Phospholipids

- Fetomaternal bleed
- Incompatible blood transfusion
- Hemolysis
- Septicemia

ETIOLOGY

Acute

- Abruptio placenta
- Endotoxemia
- Amniotic fluid embolism
- Severe pre-eclampsia and HELLP syndrome
- Hydatiform mole
- Intra-amniotic hypertonic saline infusion
- Dextran infusion
- Acute fatty liver of pregnancy
- Hemorrhagic shock

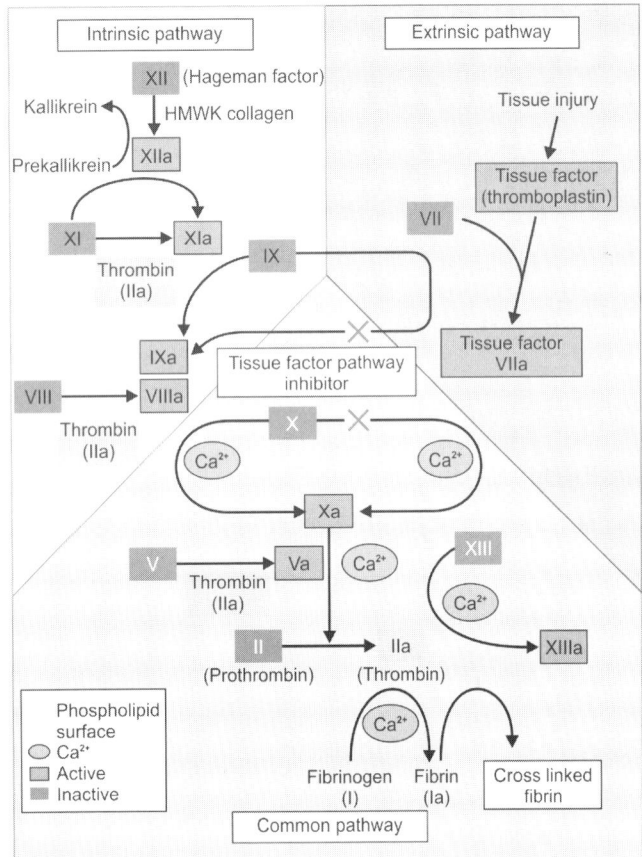

Fig. 12.1: The coagulation cascade. Factor IX can be activated by either factor XIa or factor VIIa. In laboratory tests, activation is predominantly dependent on factor XIa, whereas *in vivo*, factor VIIa appears to be the predominant activator of factor IX. Factors in red boxes represent inactive molecules; activated factors, indicated with a lowercase a, are in green boxes. Note that thrombin (factor IIa) (in light blue boxes) contributes to coagulation through multiple positive feedback loops. The red X's denote points at which tissue factor pathway inhibitor (TFPI) inhibits activation of factor X and factor IX by factor VIIa *(For color version, see Plate 2)*

Abbreviations: HMWK, high-molecular-weight kininogen; PL, phospholipid[4]

Subacute (or Chronic)

- Missed abortion
- Intrauterine death (prolonged)

PATHOPHYSIOLOGY OF DIC

See Flow chart 12.1.

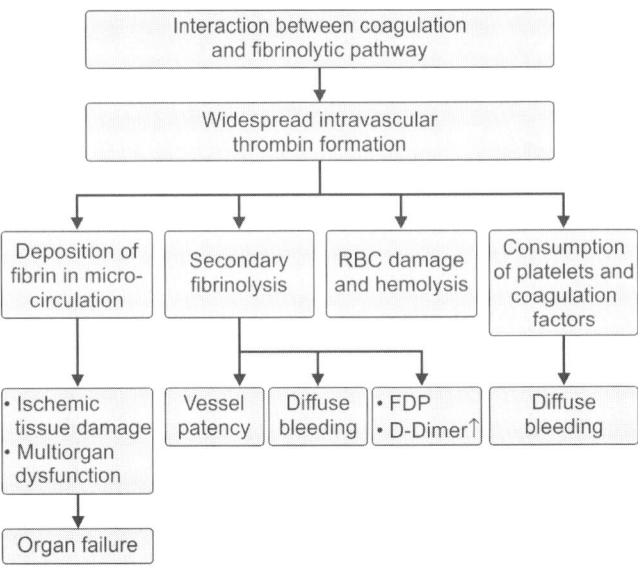

Flow chart 12.1: Pathophysiology of DIC

MECHANISM OF DIC IN DIFFERENT OBSTETRIC CONDITIONS (TABLE 12.1)

- *Abruptio placenta:*
  - *Massive retroplacental clot:* Fibrinogen along with other procoagulants are consumed in the clot
  - Thromboplastin liberated from the clot, damaged decidua and uterine musculature enters the circulation and produces DIC.
- *Amniotic fluid embolism:*
  - Thromboplastin rich liquor amnii containing debris blocks the pulmonary arteries and triggers the complex coagulation mechanism leading to DIC.
  - From the damaged endothelium of pulmonary arteries massive fibrinolytic activators are produced which excite the fibrinolytic system.
- *Dead fetus:* There is gradual absorption of thromboplastin liberated either from the placenta or from amniotic fluid or decidua. This results in depletion of factor VIII and platelets.
- *Cesarean section:*
  - Entry of thromboplastin or amniotic fluid into the circulation through open vessels on uterine wound
  - Excess production of plasminogen activators from the injured uterine site.

Table 12.1: Use of various components of blood and plasma

Blood components	Contents	Amount (mL)	Indications	Dangers	Comments
Whole blood transfusion	All components (fibrinogen: 0.5 g)	500	Massive acute blood loss	Volume overload, allosensitization	Consider component therapy
Packed cells	Red cells	200	Blood replacement	Hepatitis, allosensitization	Hematocrit raised by 3–5%
Fresh-frozen plasma	Clotting factors	200	DIC	Hepatitis	Fibrinogen 10 mg/dL per unit infused
Platelet concentrate	Platelets	50	Hereditary and acquired thrombocytopenia	Rh-isoimmunization	Rise in platelet by 7500/mL per unit (50 mL) infused
Cryoprecipitate	Factor I, V, VIII, XIII	40	DIC, von Willebrand's disease, hemophilia	Hepatitis	Fibrinogen 10 mg/dL per unit infused
Factor concentrates	Factor VIII, IX	20	Hemophilia A; factor IX deficiency	Hepatitis	1 unit = Factor activity in 1 mL of pooled plasma

SYMPTOMS

It occurs due to three pathological processes:
1. *Bleeding from various sites:*
    - *Before delivery:* Petechiae, ecchyomosis, purpuric spots, hematemesis, malena, hematuria.
    - *After delivery:* Postpartum hemorrhage, bleeding from episiotomy site, cesarean section site, vulval hematoma.
2. *Systemic infection and septicemic shock:*
    - High-grade fever
    - Irritability
    - Toxic look
    - Tachypnea
    - Tachycardia
    - Hypotension
3. *Specific organ involvement:*
    - *Brain:* Altered state of consciousness, seizures
    - *Lungs:* Respiratory distress or adult respiratory distress syndrome (ARDS)
    - *Heart:* Hypotension cardiac arrest
    - *Kidney:* Renal failure manifesting as oliguria, anuria, acidosis.

DIAGNOSIS

No single laboratory test is sensitive and specific enough to make a definite diagnosis of DIC.
- Platelet count is reduced.
- Clotting time, especially prothrombin time and activated partial thromboplastin time are prolonged.
- Antithrombin III and protein C levels are reduced.
- Consumption and depletion of coagulation factors such as factor V and factor VII.
- Hypofibrogenemia but single reading may not be useful.
- Fibrin degradation products (FDP) are raised.
- D-dimer levels which detect neoantigens on degraded crosslinked fibrin are raised.

Of all the tests, D-dimer assay has been found to be most useful in diagnosing DIC.

MANAGEMENT

Prophylaxis

Good antenatal care and active management of labor can help in identifying high-risk factors and treating them early and energetically as follow:
- *Abruption placenta:* Adequate blood transfusion, early delivery, liberal and early use of cesarean section.
- Pre-eclampsia eclampsia syndrome
- *Intrauterine death:* Early termination of pregnancy using prostaglandin gel, or oxytocin drip
- Avoidance of use of hypertonic saline for second trimester abortion and using prostaglandin or ethacridine lactate can avoid DIC.
- *Obstetrics shock:* Early and adequate treatment in reversible stage by early administration of fluids and blood transfusion can prevent DIC.

General Management

Treatment of underlying disease is important like use of appropriate intravenous antibiotics in adequate dosage for any infection, timely and appropriate management of hemorrhage and shock.

Specific Treatment

- *Platelets and fresh-frozen plasma transfusion:*
  - Indication—patient with active bleeding, with severe thrombocytopenia (<50000/mm^3), and in those requiring invasive procedure.
  - One unit of FFP (250 mL) raises fibrinogen levels by 10 mg/dL.
- *Cryoprecipitate:*
  - It is prepared from fresh-frozen plasma.
  - It is composed of factor VIII, factor I, factor V, factor XII
  - One unit of cryoprecipitate (40 mL) raises the fibrinogen level by 10 mg/dL.
- *Recombinant activated factor VIIa*: Though approved by US-FDA for hemophilia has been found useful in hemorrhage in dose of 60–100 μg/kg intravenously to control DIC promptly but is very expensive.
- *Anticoagulant therapy*:
  - *Heparin:* Therapeutic doses of heparin (5000 units IV 4–6 hourly)
  - Recombinant tissue factor pathway inhibitor (TFPI)
  - Antifibrinolytic agents such as epsilon aminocaproic acid (EACA), trasylol, aprotinin.

REFERENCES

1. Callaghan WM, Creanga AA, Kuklina EV. Severe maternal morbidity among delivery and postpartum hospitalizations in the United States. Obstet Gynecol. 2012;120:1029.
2. Rattray DD, O'Connell CM, Baskett TF. Acute disseminated intravascular coagulation in obstetrics: a tertiary centre population review (1980 to 2009). J Obstet Gynaecol Can. 2012; 34:341.
3. Erez O, Novack L, Beer-Weisel R, et al. DIC score in pregnant women: a population-based modification of the International Society on Thrombosis and Hemostasis Score. PLoS One. 2014; 9:e93240.
4. Kumar V, Abbas AK, Aster J. Robbins and Cotran: Pathologic basis of disease, 9th edn. Philadelphia: Elsevier, 2014.

SECTION 4: EARLY PREGNANCY COMPLICATIONS

Chapter 13

Recurrent Pregnancy Loss

K Aparna Sharma, Alka Kriplani

INTRODUCTION

Pregnancy loss is one of the most emotionally draining experience of a woman's life. Not just the woman but the partner, family and the caregivers inadvertently go on a journey to find the cause to give it a closure and ensure a better reproductive outcome in future. The repeated occurrence of such a loss (Recurrent pregnancy Loss, RPL) is really traumatic more so because despite extensive efforts by the couples and the physicians, in majority of cases no cause can be found. In such a scenario, the couples and the caregivers are in a turmoil as to how to look upon the future reproductive journey.

To provide an objectivity to the situation, it is imperative to understand the various aspects of RPL:
- *When to investigate:* Defining RPL
- *What is the etiology of RPL:* Evidence-based investigations and treatment
- Managing idiopathic RPL
- *Summary of work-up and diagnosis:* Do's and Don'ts

WHEN TO INVESTIGATE: DEFINING RPL

Providing a definition of RPL is important because the whole battery of investigations available is quite exhaustive and before a couple plunges into the financially and emotionally difficult journey, there should be an agreement that it was required in the first place. Various organizations have given slightly varying definitions of RPL. The recently reviewed French practice guidelines defined RPL by the occurrence of three or more consecutive miscarriages before <14 weeks of gestation.[1]

There also has been an attempt to separately define the early and late pregnancy losses as they have a varied etiology resulting in management implications. So early recurrent pregnancy loss has been defined as 3 consecutive losses <10 weeks gestation and late recurrent losses as >10 weeks < 16 weeks of gestation.[2]

The American Society of Reproductive Medicine has defines RPL as two-failed clinical pregnancies having ultrasound or histopathological diagnosis.[3]

Another dilemma is whether to start investigating after 2 losses or to wait for the third loss to conduct the battery of tests. It has been seen that that women with two losses have identifiable causes as frequently as three losses, so it seems practical to start investigating after 2 losses and not wait for the third.

PREVALENCE AND ETIOLOGY OF RPL: EVIDENCE-BASED INVESTIGATIONS AND TREATMENT

Prevalence

Approximately 15% of pregnant women experience sporadic loss of a clinically recognized pregnancy. Just 2% of pregnant women experience two consecutive pregnancy losses and only 0.4–1% have three consecutive pregnancy losses.[4]

Etiology of RPL

The etiological factors have been associated with recurrent pregnancy losses. Despite extensive research, the definitive association has been proven only with a limited number of causes and almost 50% of cases remain idiopathic. **Figure 13.1** shows the various causes implicated in RPL.

Anatomic Factors Implicated in Pregnancy Losses

Various congenital and acquired uterine abnormalities have been implicated in causing pregnancy losses.

Pathophysiology

Congenital anomalies: The prevalence of uterine anomalies in general population in 4.3% while that in women with RPL has been reported to be 13%.[5]

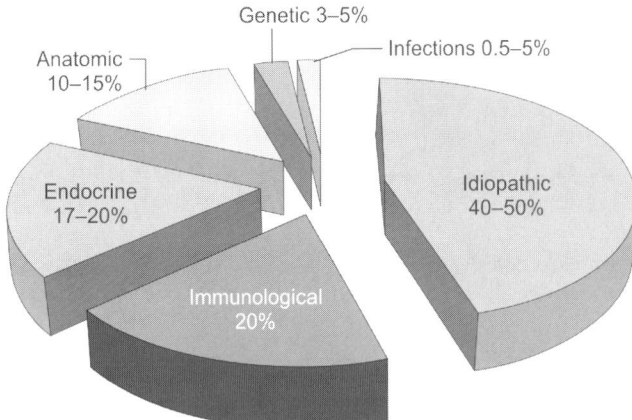

Fig. 13.1: Etiology of recurrent pregnancy loss

The septate uterus is the uterine anomaly associated with the poorest reproductive outcome and the most common uterine abnormality associated with RPL.[6]

A history of first trimester losses was found in 42% of the women with a subseptate uterus and 16% of women with arcuate uterus. A history of second trimester loss was slightly more frequent among women with an arcuate uterus (8% versus 4%).[7,8]

The etiology of pregnancy loss in uterine anomalies has not been clearly established. Uterine cavity distortion, poor implantation or even cervical insufficiency could be the underlying cause but it has not been established.

Acquired causes: Conditions such as intrauterine adhesions, submucous fibroid, endometrial polyp and cervical incompetence are certain conditions that can affect the uterine cavity, and hence can result in pregnancy losses.

Diagnosis

The options for uterine evaluation include techniques such as hysterosalpingography, hysteroscopy, saline infusion sonography, 3D ultrasound and MRI.
- *Sonohysterography:* It shows the internal contours of the uterine cavity and also the provides outer surface and wall of the uterus. It provides information on tubal patency and can distinguish between the septate and bicornuate uterus
- *Hysterosalpingography:* It provides information on the uterine contour and cavity and also tubal patency but does not tell about the outer surface and wall of the uterus, therefore it cannot reliably differentiate between a septate and a bicornuate uterus
- *Hysteroscopy:* Hysteroscopy is the gold standard for diagnosis of intrauterine abnormalities and also provides the option of treatment in the same sitting.
- *Two-dimensional ultrasound:* It can provide information on uterine abnormalities and associated renal abnormalities. It can also delineate the number, size and location of fibroids.
- *Three-dimensional ultrasound:* It can accurately diagnose various uterine anomalies. The availability and cost is an issue.
- *MRI:* MRI is useful for distinguishing between a septate and bicornuate uterus suspected on ultrasonography or HSG. It is less invasive and less costly than laparoscopy for this purpose.

The preferred modality would depend on the availability and access for each provider and the patient. Hysteroscopy remains the gold standard for evaluating the uterine cavity but more invasive than other modalities. Newer techniques such as 3D-USG and MRI are quite sensitive but are expensive.

The logical approach would be a 2-stage procedure in which:
- *Step 1:* 2D-USG, HSG, sonohysterography, hysteroscopy
- *Step 2:* If anomaly suspected: 3D-USG/MRI.

Treatment of Uterine Anomalies

The aspect of treatment of congenital and acquired anomalies has been a matter of debate. Although small individual trials have shown promising results on the benefits of interventions,[9,10] there are no randomized controlled trials:
- A recent review[11] of hysteroscopic metroplasty for septate uterus has concluded that the overall success reported indicates its efficacy and reaffirms the place of minimally invasive treatment such as hysteroscopic metroplasty as the criterion standard and method of choice for treatment of this septate uterus.
- Hysteroscopic polypectomy may be considered for women with RPL, if the polyp is large and no other causes have been found.
- For women with early RPL who have submucosal fibroids, myomectomy should be considered, if no other causes have been identified.
- Although direct evidence is not available, surgical removal of adhesions should be recommended for women with RPL who have no other known causes, with great precaution taken to prevent recurrence.

The paucity of randomized trials should remind practitioners to approach corrective procedures with the knowledge that surgery may not always improve a patient's chances for successful pregnancy.

Genetic Factors Implicated in Pregnancy Losses

Genetic factors are implicated in RPL in 4–5% of cases. The purpose of establishing a genetic etiology in RPL is to be able to predict the chance of recurrence. Genetic abnormalities can be of two types:
1. Aneuploidies
2. Structural chromosomal rearrangements

Aneuploidies: These are implicated as the underlying genetic cause more often in sporadic losses as compared to RPL (70% vs 30%). Of these Trisomy 16, monosomy X and polyploidies are the most frequent causes. Diagnosis requires a karyotype of the conceptus. Cells from chromosomally abnormal abortuses, especially trisomy 7 and triploidies, are less likely to grow in culture, thereby skewing the results of cohort studies of the frequency of aneuploidy in products of conception from spontaneously aborted pregnancies.[12] Array comparative genomic hybridization does not require dividing cells, and therefore can be useful in fetal demise with culture failure.[13] Microarray however, cannot be presently recommended routinely for evaluation of RPL.

Structural chromosomal rearrangements: Parental balanced translocations affect 3% to 4% of couples with RPL. The most common types of balanced translocations are reciprocal translocations, which involve the exchanged of genetic material from one chromosome to another, and robertsonian translocations, whereby the long arms of 2 acrocentric chromosomes erroneously share a centrosome. Carriers of balanced translocations are typically asymptomatic, as they have the normal quantity of genetic material at all loci. However, during gametogenesis, the segregation of chromosomes may result in unbalanced gametes, which can lead to an increased miscarriage rate or ongoing conception with congenital anomalies. Although parental carriers of structural rearrangements have increased reproductive loss rates, similarly to patients with unexplained RPL, most carriers of parental translocation will succeed in having successful pregnancies without intervention.[14]

Practice points:
- Knowledge of karyotype of products of conception allows an informed prognosis for future pregnancy outcome
- Risk of miscarriage due to fetal aneuploidy decreases with an increasing number of pregnancy losses
- If karyotype of miscarried pregnancy is abnormal, there is better prognosis for next pregnancy.

Flow chart 13.1 shows an overview of genetic evaluation of RPL.

Flow chart 13.1: An overview of genetic evaluation in RPL[15]

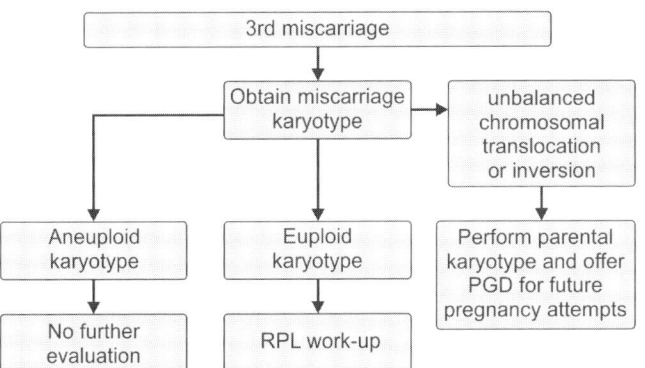

Immunological Factors Implicated in Pregnancy Losses

Antiphospholipid antibody syndrome (APS): Antiphospholipid antibody syndrome (APS) is one of the most established and treatable causes of recurrent pregnancy loss. The presence of antiphospholipid antibodies such as lupus anticoagulant (LAC) and anticardiolipin antibodies (aCL) increase the risk of pregnancy loss. These antibodies lead to various pathophysiological changes such as platelet aggregation, activation of coagulation cascade and complement system, stimulation of proinflammatory cytokines from the endothelial cells and also affect the placental trophoblastic cell growth and invasion.

Diagnosis

The diagnosis of APS can be made on the basis of at least one of the clinical and laboratory criteria as shown:[16,17]

Clinical criteria:
- Vascular thrombosis: ≥1 episodes of arterial, venous and small vessel thrombosis
- Pregnancy morbidity
- ≥1 Unexplained death of morphologically normal fetus as or beyond 10 week
- ≥1 premature births of morphologically normal neonate before 34 weeks due to severe pre-eclampsia recognized failure of placental insufficiency
- ≥3 unexplainable consecutive spontaneous abortions before 10 weeks.

Laboratory criteria:
- Anticardiolipin antibodies IgG or IgM on ≥2 occasions, at least 12 weeks apart (>40 GPL)
- Anti β_2-glycoprotein on ≥2 occasions, at least 12 weeks apart
- Lupus anticoagulant (LAC) on ≥2 occasions at least 12 weeks apart.

Management

Current recommended therapy for women with positive RPL diagnosed with APS and no history of prior thrombosis is prophylactic or intermediate dose unfractionated heparin (UFH) or prophylactic dose low molecular-weight heparin (LMWH) in combination with low-dose aspirin (LDA).[18] The LDA may be started preconceptionally, and the heparin is started once a potentially viable pregnancy is identified (usually around 6 or 7 week gestation). One meta-analysis exploring the use of prophylactic heparin in conjunction with LDA suggested a 50% reduction in pregnancy loss compared with prednisone or LDA alone.[19] In women with APS and a history of a prior thrombosis, full dose (therapeutic) regimens of UFH or LMWH should be used **(Table 13.1)**.

> **Table 13.1:** Suggested protocol for management of APS with RPL
>
> *APS in pregnancy without prior thrombosis*
> - Low dose aspirin (75–150 mg OD):
>   – Start pre-conceptionally
>   – Stopped 4 weeks prior to EDD
> - Heparin:
>   – Start at diagnosis of pregnancy
>   – Stopped when:
>   1. Goes into spontaneous labor
>   2. Night before scheduled induction/LSCS
> - Corticosteroid and intravenous immunoglobulins—not recommended.

Abbreviations: APS, antiphospholipid antibody syndrome; EDD, estimated due date; LSCS, lower segment cesarean section

HEREDITARY THROMBOPHILIAS

Hereditary thrombophilias are a group of inherited conditions which accentuate the naturally procoagulant state in pregnancy and predispose to vascular thrombotic events. Although their association with thrombosis is well established, their role in obstetric mishaps is not yet clearly defined. The common conditions which have been associated with adverse pregnancy outcomes are:

- *Factor V Leiden mutation:* Various studies and meta-analysis have shown that there is a small but increased risk of spontaneous abortion and fetal loss.[20]
- *Prothrombin G20210A mutation (PGA):* Although less common in Asian population the association between PGA and pregnancy loss has not been consistent across studies[20].
- *Protein C deficiency:* The prevalence of protein C mutation is estimated at 0.2% to 0.3% when determined by a functional assay with cutoff between 50% and 60%.[8,13] The mutation may be more common among those of Asian or African descent. Protein C deficiency has not been clearly linked to fetal loss or to RPL.[21]
- *Protein S deficiency:* Free protein S is significantly decreased in pregnancy. Screening is recommended outside of pregnancy, >6 weeks postpartum and in the absence of hormonal contraception. A systematic review indicated an association with stillbirth (defined as unexplained fetal loss over 20 week gestation with no fetal abnormalities) with an OR = 16.2 (95% CI, 5.0–52.3), though it was limited by small study sizes. More robust evidence needs to be generated to assess the association with RPL.[22]
- *Antithrombin III deficiency:* It is the most thrombotic hereditary thrombophilia with a higher prevalence among Asians. The European Prospective Cohort on Thrombophilia (EPCOT) study[23] found a modest increase risk in early fetal loss, as defined by gestational age <28 weeks (OR = 1.7, 95% CI, 1.0–2.8). Presently, there seems to be an association with fetal losses but a definitively causal association still needs to be proven.
- *Methyl tetrahydrofolate reductase deficiency (MTHFR):* Homozygosity for a MTHFR mutation is the most common cause of hyperhomocysteinemia. When homocysteinemia is present, it acts as a procoagulant. However, elevated homocysteine levels remain a weak risk factor for venous thromboembolism (VTE).[24] Similarly, there does not seem to be connection between MTHFR and homocysteinemia with adverse pregnancy outcomes

Treatment of Hereditary Thrombophilias

The use of heparin for prevention of adverse pregnancy outcomes in hereditary thrombophilias has not been validated by large trials (TIPPS trial, 2014).[25] The present evidence does not support screening or treatment of hereditary thrombophilias in women with recurrent pregnancy losses.

Endocrine Factors Implicated in Pregnancy Losses

Thyroid disorders: Severe hypothyroidism and hyperthyroidism in pregnancy are associated with sporadic pregnancy loss[26] and thyroid autoimmunity as documented by the presence of thyroid autoantibodies is specifically associated with RPL.[27,28]

The role of subclinical hypothyroidism (TSH increased with normal T4) is still debated as a causative factor for RPL. In a meta-analysis, an association was found between the presence of antithyroid antibodies (ATAb) in euthyroid women and recurrent pregnancy loss, and also there was an improvement in pregnancy outcome with treatment.

Practice points
- Women with RPL should be screened with TSH and ATAb.
- Overt hypothroidism should be treated to maintain trimester specific TSH levels.
- In women with subclinical hypothyroidism, additional presence of ATAb can be assessed to start treatment with levothyroxine.
- Euthyroid women with ATAb can also be offered treatment to reduce the risk of further miscarriage.

Luteal phase defects: Early pregnancy is supported by the progesterone from the corpus luteum during the luteal phase till the time placenta takes over the function. The definition of abnormalities of the luteal phase known as the luteal phase defect is not standardized and there is no consensus. Studies have estimated the incidence of LPD to be between 17% and 28% in women with RPL.[29] Many treatment options have been proposed for suspected LPD such as ovulation induction, hCG supplementation, and progesterone supplementation alone or in combination, but without any clear effect.

It has been seen that a low progesterone level in early pregnancy does not necessarily justify progesterone supplementation because it might simply reflect an abnormal secretion of hCG by a nonviable or ectopic pregnancy rather than LPD.[30]

Other endocrine factors:
- Obesity, hyperinsulinemia and hyperandrogenism are inherent risk factors for RPL
- The role of metformin in PCOS with RPL is not presently defined
- Treatment with cabergoline/bromocriptine can improve outcome in women with hyperprolactinemia and RPL.

MANAGING IDIOPATHIC RPL

Etiology

Unexplained RPL accounts for a significant proportion of women with RPL. Even this group is a highly heterogeneous group.

In upto 50% of women with RPL no cause can be found. Although, a certain proportion can be attributable to chance and hence a reasonably good prognosis can be expected with tender loving care with a live birth rate of 40–65%.

Possible etiologies could be ovarian aging with resultant decline in oocyte quality, sperm factors such as Y-chromosome microdeletions, oxidative stress and DNA fragmentation, endometrial factors and potential immunological factors such as uterine and peripheral NK cells.[31]

Treatment

Role of Progesterone

There is a large and conflicting data on the role of progesterone in idiopathic RPL. A meta-analysis by Coomarasamy[32] in 2011 and a Cochrane review[33] in 2013 reported that progesterone supplementation reduces the risk of abortion in RPL. However, the recent Prospective Multicenter Imaging Study for Evaluation of Chest Pain (PROMISE) trial[34] has questioned the very role of progesterone in RPL.

The PROMISE study, which included 836 women with idiopathic RPL, found no difference in live birth rate after progesterone supplementation (65.8% for progesterone versus 63.3% for placebo). Currently, the role remains controversial till further evidence becomes available.

Immunotherapy for Unexplained RPL

A Cochrane review[35] in 2014 looked at the evidence of various proposed immunological therapies such as paternal cell immunization, third party donor cell immunization, trophoblast membrane infusion and intravenous immunoglobulin. There was no significant benefit over placebo and these treatments should not be recommended.

Heparin in Unexplained RPL

A review of more than 800 women from 9 studies did not find a benefit of using aspirin, heparin or a combination of both in women with unexplained RPL.[36] Hence, this treatment should not be offered to the women.

SUMMARY OF WORK-UP AND DIAGNOSIS: DO'S AND DON'TS[37]

Evaluating RPL: The Do's
- Test for LAC, aCL, anti-b2-GP1(IgG and IgM)
- Evaluate for uterine malformations with Imaging modality, i.e. SSG, HSG, MRI, hysteroscopy
- Perform karyotype of conceptus should be obtained, if possible. Chromosomal microarray yields better results than conventional karyotype.
- Check for thyroid, prolactin abnormalities and diabetes.

Evaluating RPL: The Don'ts
- Test aPL antibodies other than LAC, aCL and anti B2GP
- Perform endometrial biopsies
- Measure luteal phase progesterone levels
- Test peripheral blood for immunological causes
- Obtain vaginal, cervical, or endometrial cultures
- Perform serological titers TORCH
- Screen for inherited thrombophilias
- Obtain semen analyses in absence of infertility

Treating RPL: The Do's
- Treat APS with heparin low-dose aspirin
- Consider surgically correcting uterine septa/fibroids polyps/adhesions
- Genetic counseling consideration of IVF with PGD
- Treat persistent hyperprolactinemia with dopamine agonist
- Treat thyroid disease and diabetes
- Offer frequent office visits and USG to ensure fetal viability

Treating RPL: The Dont's
- Treat women without APS with heparin
- Treat women with progesterone in unexplained RPL
- Treat with Immunomodulatory agents, i.e. IVIG, intralipids, prednisone, or immunizations

Abbreviations: LAC, lupus anticoagulant; aCL, anti-cardiolipin antibodies; SSG, sonohysterosalpingogram; HSG, hysterosalpingogram; PGD, preimplantation genetic diagnosis

REFERENCES

1. Huchan C, Deffieux X, Beucher G, et al. Pregnancy loss: French clinical practice guidelines. Eur J Obs Gyn Reprod Biol. 2016;201:18-26.
2. Kaiser J, Branch DW. Recurrent pregnancy loss: Generally accepted causes and their management. Clinical Obstetrics and Gynecology. 2016;59(3):464-73.

3. Evaluation and treatment of recurrent pregnancy loss: a committee opinion The Practice Committee of the American Society of Reproductive Medicine. Fertil Steril. 2012;98:1103-11.
4. Salat-Baroux J. Recurrent spontaneous abortions. Reprod Nutr Dev. 1988;28:1555.
5. Branch DW. Clinical practice: recurrent miscarriage. N Engl J Med. 2010
6. Woelfer B, Salim R, Banerjee S, et al. Reproductive outcomes in women with congenital uterine anomalies detected by three-dimensional ultrasound screening. Obstet Gynecol. 2001;98:1099-103.
7. Proctor JA, Haney AF. Recurrent first trimester pregnancy loss is associated with uterine septum but not with bicornuate uterus. Fertil Steril. 2003; 80:1212.
8. Golan A, Langer R, Bukovsky I, Caspi E. Congenital anomalies of the müllerian system. Fertil Steril. 1989;51:747.
9. Mollo A, De Franciscis P, Colacurci N, et al. Hysteroscopic resection of the septum improves the pregnancy rate of women with unexplained infertility: a prospective controlled trial. Fertil Steril. 2009;91:2628.
10. Tomaževič T, Ban-Frangež H, Virant-Klun I, et al. Septate, subseptate and arcuate uterus decrease pregnancy and live birth rates in IVF/ICSI. Reprod Biomed Online. 2010;21:700.
11. Hysteroscopic Metroplasty for the Septate Uterus: Review and Meta-Analysis Valle, Rafael F. et al. Journal of Minimally Invasive Gynecology. 20(1):22-4.
12. Fritz B, Hallermann C, Olert J, et al. Cytogenetic analyses of culture failures by comparative genomic hybridisation (CGH): Re-evaluation of chromosome aberration rates in early spontaneous abortions. Eur J Hum Genet. 2001;9:539
13. ACOG Committee Opinion No. 446: array comparative genomic hybridization in prenatal diagnosis. Obstet Gynecol. 2009;114:1161.
14. Stephenson MD, Sierra S. Reproductive outcomes in recurrent pregnancy loss associated with a parental carrier of a structural chromosome rearrangement. Hum Reprod. 2006;21:1076-82.
15. Kutteh WH. Novel Strategies for the Management of Recurrent Pregnancy Loss. Semin Reprod Med. 2015;33(03):161-8. DOI: 10.1055/s-0035-1552586
16. Wilson WA, Gharavi AE, Koike T, et al. International consensus statement on preliminary classification criteria for definite antiphospholipid syndrome: report of an international workshop. Arthritis Rheum. 1999;42:1309-11.
17. Miyakis S, Lockshin MD, Atsumi T, et al. International Consensus Statement on an Update of the Classification Criteria for Definite Antiphospholipid Syndrome (APS). J Thromb Haemost. 2006;4:295-306.
18. Bates SM, Greer IA, Middeldorp S, et al. VTE, thrombophilia, antithrombotic therapy, and pregnancy: Antithrombotic Therapy and Prevention of Thrombosis, 9th edn. American College of Chest Physicians Evidence-Based Clinical Practice Guidelines. Chest. 2012;141(suppl):e691S-e6736.
19. Empson M, Lassere M, Craig JC, et al. Recurrent pregnancy loss with antiphospholipid antibody: a systematic review of therapeutic trials. Obstet Gynecol. 2002;99:135-144.
20. Rodger MA, Betancourt MT, Clark P, et al. The association of factor V Leiden and prothrombingene mutation and placenta-mediated pregnancy complications: a systematic review and meta-analysis of prospective cohort studies. PLoS Med. 2010;7:728.
21. Rey E, Kahn SR, David M, et al. Thrombophilic disorders and fetal loss: a meta-analysis. Lancet. 2003;361:901-8.
22. Alfirevic Z, Roberts D, Martlew V. How strong is the association between maternal thrombophilia and adverse pregnancy outcome?: a systematic review. Eur J Obstet Gynecol Reprod Biol. 2002;101:6-14.
23. Preston FE, Rosendaal FR, Walker ID, et al. Increased fetal loss in women with heritable thrombophilia. Lancet. 1996;348: 913-6.
24. American Congress of Obstetrics and Gynecology. ACOG practice bulletin no. 138. Practice bulletinno. 138: inherited thrombophilias in pregnancy. Obstet Gynecol. 2013;122: 706-16.
25. Rodger MA, Hague WM, Kingdom J, et al. Antepartum dalteparin versus no antepartum dalteparin for the prevention of pregnancy complications in pregnant women with thrombophilia (TIPPS): a multinational open-label randomized trial. Lancet. 2014;384:1673-83.
26. Stagnaro-Green A, Abalovich M, Alexander E, et al. Guidelines of the American Thyroid Association for the Diagnosis and Management of Thyroid Disease during Pregnancy and Postpartum. Thyroid. 2011;21:1081-125.
27. van den Boogaard E, Vissenberg R, Land JA, et al. Significance of (sub)clinical thyroid dysfunction and thyroid autoimmunity before conception and in early pregnancy: a systematic review. Hum Reprod Update. 2011;17:605-19.
28. Thangaratinam S, Tan A, Knox E, et al. Association between thyroid autoantibodies and miscarriage and preterm birth: meta-analysis of evidence. BMJ. 2011;342:d2616.
29. Li TC, Spuijbroek MD, Tuckerman E, et al. Endocrinological and endometrial factors in recurrent miscarriage. BJOG. 2000;107:1471-9.
30. Practice Committee of the American Society for Reproductive Medicine. Current clinical irrelevance of luteal phase deficiency: a committee opinion. Fertil Steril. 2015;103: e27-e32.
31. Saravelos SH, Reagan L. Unexplained recurrent pregnancy loss. Obstet Gynecol Clin North Am. 2014;41(1):157-66.
32. Coomarasamy A, Truchanowicz EG, Rai R. Does first trimester progesterone prophylaxis increase the live birth rate in women with unexplained recurrent miscarriages? BMJ. 2011;342:d1914.
33. Haas DM, Ramsey PS. Progestogen for preventing miscarriage. Cochrane Database of Systematic Reviews 2013, Issue 10. Art. No.: CD003511. DOI: 10.1002/14651858.CD003511.pub3.
34. Coomarasamy A, Williams H, Truchanowicz E, et al. A Randomized Trial of Progesterone in Women with Recurrent Miscarriages. N Engl J Med. 2015;373:2141-8.
35. Wong LF, Porter TF, Scott JR. Immunotherapy for recurrent miscarriage. Cochrane Database of Systematic Reviews 2014, Issue 10. Art. No.: CD000112. DOI: 10.1002/14651858. CD000112.pub3.
36. de Jong PG, Kaandorp S, Di Nisio M, Goddijn M, Middeldorp S. Aspirin and/or heparin for women with unexplained recurrent miscarriage with or without inherited thrombophilia. Cochrane Database of Systematic Reviews 2014, Issue 7. Art. No.: CD004734. DOI: 10.1002/14651858.CD004734.pub4
37. Branch DW, Silver MR. Practical Work-up and Management of Recurrent Pregnancy Loss for the Front-Line Clinician. Clinical Obstetrics And Gynecology. 2016;59(3):535-8.

Chapter 14

Hyperemesis Gravidarum

Richa Baharani, Pushpa Pandey

INTRODUCTION

Hyperemesis gravidarum means an extreme form of morning sickness that causes severe nausea and vomiting during pregnancy. It can lead to dehydration, weight loss and electrolyte imbalance.

EPIDEMIOLOGY

Nausea and vomiting are common in pregnancy, affecting up to 90% of pregnant women. About 35% of affected women are thought to have clinically significant symptoms. It is more common in primigravidae. Incidence of hyperemesis gravidarum varies from 0.3% to 1.5% of all live births.[1] It is second leading cause of hospitalization in early pregnancy and is more common in nonwhite and Asian populations.

When does it Occur?

Hyperemesis gravidarum starts earlier in the first trimester than usual morning sickness (around 4th or 5th week of pregnancy) and usually starts to rise on its own between weeks 12 and 20 but sometimes it can continue throughout the pregnancy.

SIGNS AND SYMPTOMS[2]

- Severe nausea and vomiting
- Food aversions
- Weight loss of 5% or more of pregnancy weight
- Decrease in urination
- Headache
- Confusion
- Fainting
- Jaundice
- Extreme fatigue
- Low blood pressure
- Rapid heart rate
- Loss of skin elasticity due to dehydration
- Excessive salivation
- Sleep disturbances

RISK FACTORS[3,4]

- 1st pregnancy
- Multiple pregnancy
- Obesity
- Prior or family history of hyperemesis gravidarum
- Trophoplastic disorder
- Eating disorder
- Endocrine imbalances
- PCOD
- Vitamin B deficiencies
- *H. pylori* infection
- Trisomy – 21 (Down Syndrome)
- Triploids
- Hydrops fetalis

DIAGNOSIS

It can be diagnosed when there is protracted nausea and vomiting of pregnancy with triad of more than 5% prepregnancy weight loss, dehydration and electrolyte imbalance.[5] Ketones are present in urine. Other potential causes of the symptoms should be excluded, including urinary tract infection and high thyroid levels.[6]

DIFFERENTIAL DIAGNOSIS[7]

- *Infection*
  - Hepatitis
  - Gastroenteritis
  - Meningitis
  - Urinary tract infection
- *Gastrointestinal disorders*
  - Appendicitis
  - Pancreatitis
  - Cholecystitis
  - Fatty liver
  - Peptic ulcer
  - Small bowel obstruction
- *Metabolic disorders*
  - Diabetic ketoacidosis
  - Hyperthyroidism

- Addison's disease
- Migraine headache
- CNS tumors
- Vestibular lesions
- Drugs
- Gestational trophoblastic diseases

INVESTIGATIONS

- Complete blood count
- Urinalysis, urine for ketones
- Blood sugar level
- Blood urea nitrogen
- Liver function test
- Thyroid function test
- Serum electrolytes
- Serum amylase and lipase
- Ultrasound for wellbeing of fetus and to rule out molar pregnancy
- Upper abdomen sonography to evaluate pancreas, biliary tree, kidney, etc.

COMPLICATIONS

If hyperemesis gravidarum is inadequately treated:

Maternal Complications

- Weight loss
- Dehydration
- Acidosis
- Anemia
- Hyponatremia
- Hypokalemia
- Vitamin deficiencies
- Jaundice
- Hypoglycemia
- Malnutrition
- Kidney failure
- Coagulopathy
- Central pontine myelinolysis
- Wernicke's encephalopathy due to vitamin B_1 deficiency, may be precipitated by high concentrations of dextrose
- Psychological fallout or depression
- Anxiety and social issues
- Economic problems from losing employment.[8]

Fetal Complications

- Low birth weight, small for gestational age, preterm birth

MANAGEMENT

Management depends upon severity of symptoms. Rest and avoidance of sensory stimuli that may provoke symptoms. There should be frequent, small meals and avoiding spicy or fatty foods. Solid foods should be bland tasting, low in fat and high in carbohydrates. High-protein snacks can be given as protein meals more likely to alleviate nausea and vomiting than carbohydrate or fatty meals. Reassurance and psychological support are also needed. Other pathological causes are ruled out by history, examination and investigations. Pyridoxine (vitamin B_6) 10 mg and doxylamine (H_1 receptor antagonist) in combination, can be used which results in fewer admissions.[9]

Hospitalization

It is advised if there is one of the following:[5]
- Continued nausea and vomiting and inability to keep down oral antiemetics.
- Continued nausea and vomiting associated with ketonuria and/or weight loss greater than 5% of body weight, despite oral antiemetics.
- Confirmed or suspected comorbidity such as urinary tract infection and inability to tolerate oral antibiotics.

Antiemetics: If previous therapy fails, antiemetic is warranted

Recommended Antiemetic Therapies[5]

First line: Cyclizine, prochlorperazine, promethazine, chlorpromazine

Second line: Metoclopramide, domperidone, ondansetron

Third line: Corticosteroids: hydrocortisone 100 mg twice daily IV and once clinical improvement occurs, convert to prednisolone 40–50 mg daily PO, with the dose gradually tapered until the lowest maintenance dose that controls the symptoms.

SUMMARY OF TREATMENT (MEDICATION)

Agents	Dosage	Safety and Efficacy (FDA)
Doxylamine	25 mg at night time, oral	Safe and effective* (FDA class A) Reduces nausea and vomiting
Pyridoxine	25 mg every 8 hourly, oral	No known malformations (FDA class A) Reduces nausea and vomiting

Contd...

Contd...

Agents	Dosage	Safety and Efficacy (FDA)
Metoclopramide	5–10 mg every 8 hours orally/ IV/IM maximum 5 days	Less drowsiness, dizziness, dystonia. No known malformations (FDA class B). Reduces nausea and vomiting
Cyclizine	50 mg orally, IM or IV 8 hourly	(FDA class B) Reduces nausea and vomiting
Chlorpromazine	10–25 mg 4–6 hourly orally	(FDA class B) Reduces nausea and vomiting
Ondansetron	4 mg every 8 hours	(FDA class B) Reduces nausea and vomiting after first dose
Promethazine	12.5 mg–25 mg every 8 hours for 24 h	No known malformations (FDA class C) Reduces nausea and vomiting
Droperidol	1.0–2.5 mg over 15 min, then 1.0 mg/hour	No abnormal outcomes (FDA class C) Reduces nausea and vomiting

*Manufacturer recommends against use in pregnancy

- Thiamine supplementation should be given to all women admitted with prolonged vomiting, before administration of dextrose or parenteral nutrition.
- Thiamine should be a routine supplement in patients with protracted vomiting. Pregnant women should ingest a total of 1.5 mg/d. If this cannot be taken orally, 100 mg of thiamine may be diluted in 100 mL of normal saline and infused for 30 minutes to 1 hour weekly. Thiamine reduces the theoretic risk of Wernicke's encephalopathy.[10]
- Intravenous fluids—are given to restore hydration, electrolyte, vitamins, nutrients. Normal saline with additional potassium chloride in each bag, with administration guided by daily monitoring of electrolytes, is the most appropriate intravenous hydration. Dextrose infusions are not appropriate unless the serum sodium levels are normal and thiamine has been administered. Vitamins should be added in intravenous infusion.[5]
- *Complementary therapies:*
  - Ginger, acupressure, acupuncture, may be used.
  - Hypnotic therapies should not be recommended.
- *Thromboprophylaxis* Risk of venous thrombosis is increased due to dehydration and immobility and consideration of prophylactic low molecular weight heparin is required.
- *Monitoring* done with daily clinical examination and investigations. Daily weight chart, urea and serum electrolyte should be checked daily. Urine analysis to rule out infection and to confirm ketonuria, should be done daily. Those women having continued symptoms should be offered serial scans to monitor fetal growth.

REFERENCES

1. Verberg MF, Gillott DJ, Al-Fardan N, Grudzinskas JG. Hyperemesis gravidarum, a literature review. Hum Reprod Update. 2005;11:527-39.
2. Williams Obstetrics 22nd edn. Cunningham F Gary, et al. Ch 49. Her foundation, www.hyperemesis.org
3. Jueckstock JK, Kaestner R, Mylonas I. Managing hyperemesis gravidarum: a multimodal challenge. BMC Medicine. 8: 46.doi:10.1186/1741-7015-8-46. PMC 2913953. PMID 20633258.
4. Ferri Fred F. Ferri's clinical advisor. 5 books in 1 1st ed. Elsevier Mosby. 2012; p. 538.
5. The management of nausea and vomiting of pregnancy and hyperemesis gravidarum. Greentop Guideline No. 69. June 2016.
6. Sheehan P. Hyperemesis gravidarum—assessment and management. Australian Family Physician. 2007;36(9):698-701. PMID 17885701.
7. Bourne Thomas H. Condous, George (eds). Handbook of early pregnancy care. Informa Healthcare. 2006; pp. 149-54.
8. Parikshit dahyalal tank. Early pregnancy complications. In: Amarnath Bhide, Sabaratnam Arulkumaran (eds). Arias Practical Guide to High Risk Pregnancy and Delivery. 4th Edn. India: Elsevier, 2015.
9. Pope E, Maltepe C, Koren G. Comparing pyridoxine and doxylamine succinate-pyridoxine HCl for nausea and vomiting of pregnancy: A matched, controlled cohort study. J Clin Pharmacol. 2015;55:809-14.
10. Lindsey J, Wegrzyniak John T, T Repke, Serdar H Ural. Treatment of hyperemesis gravidarum. Rev Obstet Gynaecol. 2012; 5(2):78-84.

Chapter 15

Early Pregnancy Hemorrhage

Girija Wagh

INTRODUCTION

Hemorrhage is excessive bleeding which is a cause of concern especially during pregnancy. Early pregnancy bleeding is obstetrical hemorrhage before 20 weeks of gestational age (GA).[1] This bleeding can present as vaginal bleeding, uterine bleeding which is concealed or intraperitoneal bleeding as in an ectopic gestation.

Any bleeding during pregnancy is a cause of concern as it can be a marker of abnormality and can result in abnormal outcomes. Early pregnancy, especially before 20 weeks of gestation needs various differential diagnoses to take into account. Out of these, bleeding especially during the first trimester is common and occurs in approximately 25% of clinically recognizable pregnancies.[2]

Etiology of bleeding in early pregnancy is as follows:
- *Miscarriage:* Heavy first trimester bleeding is associated with 24% miscarriage possibility[3]
- Gestational trophoblastic disease
- Ectopic gestations
- Implantation bleeding (physiologic)
- Lower genital tract pathology
- Iatrogenic causes—medications and trauma

Let us deal with them one by one.

MISCARRIAGE

Syn: Spontaneous abortion; it is defined as spontaneous loss of fetus weighing less than 500 g or at gestational age of less than 20 weeks. These are classified as per the gestational age at which they occur **(Table 15.1)**.

Epidemiology

About 30–40% of all conceptions result in miscarriage. The risk of preclinical miscarriage is approximately, 25–30%, especially in women older than 35 years of age. Around 10–15% of clinically recognized pregnancies can miscarry. Miscarriages are commoner before 12 weeks of pregnancy and contribute to 80% of early pregnancy losses **(Table 15.2)**.

Table 15.1: Classification of miscarriages as per the gestational age

Preclinical (biochemical) miscarriage	At or before 5 weeks GA
Clinical miscarriage	Documentation of pregnancy by an appropriate beta-human chorionic gonadotropin (β-hCG) level, ultrasound finding or histopathological evidence
Embryonic miscarriage	6–9 weeks or crown-lump length (CRL) >5 mm without cardiac activity
Fetal miscarriage	10–20 weeks or CRL > 30 mm without cardiac activity

Table 15.2: Risk of miscarriage as per the gestational age and overall incidence as per the age of the mother

GA of miscarriage	Overall incidence	Age of the mother	
Less than 6 weeks	22–57%	<35 years	8–10%
6–10 weeks	15%	>35 years	25–30%
More than 10 weeks	2–3%	>40 years	> 50%

It is noteworthy that advanced maternal age (AMA) is a significant etiological factor contributing to miscarriages.

Etiopathogenesis

Maternal age seems to be having the most profound impact on miscarriage. Many other factors are responsible as mentioned in the **Table 15.3**.

Additionally, factors such as alcoholism, drug abuse, caffeine, obesity and folate deficiency have also been implicated.

Table 15.3: Causes of miscarriage

Chromosomal abnormalities: autosomal trisomies, monosomies or polyploides: 50% of miscarriages	Anembryonic pregnancy	90%
	Embryonic	50%
	Fetal abortions	30%
Maternal conditions	Uterine anomalies	Septate or subseptate uterus
		Cervical insufficiency
	Endocrinopathies	Diabetes
		Thyroid abnormalities
		Luteal phase abnormality
	Autoimmune diseases	APLA (antiphospholipid antibody syndrome)
		SLE (systemic lupus erythematosus)
		RA (Rheumatoid arthritis)
	Hypercoagulability	Hyperhomocysteinemia protein C/S deficiency
	Infection	High-grade fever due to viremia
		Urinary tract infections
		Bacterial vaginosis
	Teratogen exposure	
Previous obstetric performance	Previous risk of miscarriages	
Tobacco	Direct or indirect exposure	

Clinical Presentation

Bleeding per vaginum is the hallmark complaint of women experiencing miscarriage. Pain may or may not be present. Clinically, spontaneous abortions are classified as in **Table 15.4**.

Diagnosis

Careful clinical history suggestive of symptomatology of pregnancy and clinical examination usually confirms the diagnosis. Urine pregnancy test definitively confirms pregnancy but not its location. In any woman presenting in the reproductive age group with abnormal vaginal bleeding, pregnancy should be ruled out. *"Every woman walking in for your consultation is pregnant unless and until proved otherwise"* and this should always be done tactfully. Ultrasonography is the gold standard of diagnosis, especially to rule out if differential diagnoses for cause of bleeding are suspected. Information such as presence or absence of intrauterine pregnancy, viability, number, subchorionic hemorrhage (SCH) or hyperechoic products of conception can be derived from sonography. Additional information such as the status of the cervix (length, internal os), location of the placenta and presence of any fetal congenital anomalies, uterine malformations and adnexal pathology can be identified by sonography. Diagnostic milestones and their correlation with β-hCG levels are important. The viability of the fetus is determined by the presence of the embryonic pole, presence of yolk sac, and cardiac activity (FCA). With the advent of highly evolved ultrasound machines, pregnancy can be diagnosed even at lower β-hCG levels and these ranges are shown in **Table 15.5**.

Criteria for diagnosis of missed abortion are as under (**Box 15.1**).

FCA presence does not always ensure better prognosis of pregnancy, especially in women more than 35 years of age.

Table 15.4: Clinical classification of miscarriages

Threatened	Mostly painless, cervical os is closed, uterine size corresponds to GA
Inevitable	Painful, cervix open, uterine size corresponds to GA
Complete	(Mostly <12 weeks) painful cervix closed, uterus small, contracted and empty
Incomplete	Painful, cervix open with products of conception in the cervix or the vagina, uterine size less than the GA
Missed (delayed miscarriage)	Intrauterine demise of the fetus of less than 20 weeks gestation
Septic abortion/ miscarriage	Neglected spontaneous abortion or unsafe induced abortion can cause additional infection leading to sepsis

Table 15.5: Lowest discriminatory levels with advanced sonography machines and the 99% probability levels for identifying the developmental milestones in early pregnancy

β-hCG levels mIU/mL	Milestone	Diagram
390 to 3,510	G sac	
1,094 to 17,716	Yolk sac	
1,394 to 47,685	Fetal pole	

Box 15.1: Sonographic criteria of missed abortion
- Absence of FCA with a CRL of > 5 mm
- Absence of a fetal pole in the presence of mean sac diameter (MSD) >18 mm transvaginally or > 25 mm transabdominally

Additional Investigations

Complete blood count, blood group, serological tests and other relevant tests such as HbA1c and TSH levels can be done. Testing for serum progesterone and β-hCG levels may be ordered, especially in cases of threatened miscarriage. β-hCG levels normally rise by 55% – 65% in 48 hours in normal pregnancy. Sometimes, the rise may be slower in normal pregnancies and these can help in differentiating molar and ectopic gestations.

Management

Threatened miscarriages are managed expectantly if bleeding is resolved. Bedrest and progesterone treatment do not prevent miscarriage effectively. Many series have used dydrogesterone 10–30 mg daily, natural progesterone 200–400 mg daily transvaginal orally or as injectable and 17 hydroxyprogesterone caproate as injections. Complete abortion needs no intervention except for correction of any underlying causes such as folate or iron deficiency anemia, hypothyroidism, hyperglycemia of pregnancy, etc. Proper documentation of the process of miscarriage should be maintained for better approach in the subsequent pregnancy. Rh-negative mothers should be administered anti-D immunoglobulin to prevent alloimmunization. Incomplete, inevitable or missed miscarriages can be managed by medications or surgical treatment and these choices are usually based on patient's wishes, hemodynamic stability and stage of miscarriage.

Surgical Management

Dilation and evacuation may be necessary in incomplete miscarriage, especially when patient is bleeding and unstable. Early non-viable pregnancy too can be evacuated this way to histopathologically confirm the presence of pregnancy in the uterus. It may also be undertaken for karyotype in cases of recurrent losses. Surgical evacuation is associated with complications such as injury to the myometrium (perforation), the basal layer of the endometrium if too vigorously curetted leading to synechiae and cervical trauma. Preoperative administration of misoprostol 400–600 μg 4–6 hours prior to the procedure helps in softening the cervix and reduces the need of forceful dilatation thus reducing these complications. Anesthesia complications can be added as complications. Preoperative antibiotic prophylaxis can be given as per the hospital antibiotic policy. For this doxycycline 200 mg orally/day prior) or ceftriaxone 1 g IV can be administered half an hour prior or during the procedure.

Medical Management

Septic abortion: Medical management for stabilization and control of infection by antimicrobials guided by the vaginal or blood culture samples are needed. Surgical evacuation of the uterus is needed.

Prevention: Planned pregnancy with correction of anemia and optimizing the maternal condition before conception, prophylactic encirclage in cases of identified cervical insufficiency, progesterone supplements, treatment of vaginal and urinary infections, especially bacterial vaginosis, low molecular weight heparin (LMWH), low dose aspirin in thrombophilias, are some prophylactic measures offered in appropriate situations.

Late miscarriages or second trimester miscarriages: Miscarriages occurring between 13 and 19 weeks of gestation can have slightly a different etiology from the first trimester miscarriages.

Etiology of second trimester miscarriages
- *Cervical insufficiency:* Miscarriage occurs due to the inability of the cervix to hold the growing pregnancy and presents as a painless cervical dilatation and expulsion of the product of conception. Clinical history of previous late abortions. preterm delivery, cervical surgery and cervical shortening on ultrasonography help to diagnose the condition and to offer cervical encirclage
- Thrombophilia
- Maternal infections or exposure
- Placental separation

GESTATIONAL TROPHOBLASTIC DISEASE (GTD)

This group of heterogeneous diseases is neoplasms of the trophoblastic tissue which actually are abnormal conceptions. They are interrelated but distinct and include:
- Premalignant complete and incomplete hydatidiform mole
- Malignant invasive mole
- Choriocarcinoma
- Placental site trophoblastic tumor (PSTT)
- Epithelioid trophoblastic tumor (ETT)

Epidemiology

Higher in Asian and African women and can occur in 1 out of 600 miscarriages and 1 in 1200–1400 pregnancies. Choriocarcinoma is rare while PSTT and ETT can occur in association with any pregnancy condition.

Risk Factors

Race

Asian and African women more at risk.

Extremes of Age

Women with more than 40 years of age have 5.2 times higher risk, while, with age less than 20 years, the risk is 1.2 times. Persistent GTD is commoner in older age group.

Low Socioeconomic Condition

Deficiency of dietary nutrients, especially carotene.

Previous History of Hydatidiform Mole

With one previous molar pregnancy, the risk of GTD is 20 times more while it is 40 times more with previous two molar pregnancies. Live and term pregnancies are protective against subsequent molar pregnancy.

Previous History of Spontaneous Miscarriage

The risk of molar pregnancy is 20 times more.

Etiopathogenesis

Molecular pathogenesis of GTD tumors is an enigma and is related to chromosomal abnormalities. Chromosomally deficient oocytes are fertilized by the paternal sperm, either monospermic with duplication or dispermic. The resultant conceptus will be androgenic and have 46XX,46XY complement and will form the complete mole. The partial mole on the other hand retains the maternal component and is usually triploid, either from dispermic fertilization or due to fertilization with an unreduced diploid sperm.

Clinical Features

Vaginal bleeding is the most common presenting symptom in molar (complete: 97% and partial 75%) pregnancy. Uterine size is greater than the gestational period in complete mole while it is smaller in the partial mole. Reverse association of gestational age and uterine size may be seen in 1/3rd of complete moles and 10% of partial moles and the size can be excessively more. In 91% of partial molar pregnancies, a clinical diagnosis of missed or spontaneous abortions is made. This can be possible due to near normal β-hCG levels and corresponding uterine size and rare association of theca lutein cysts. Theca lutein cysts are commoner in complete moles (25–35%) and β-hCG levels are generally more than 50,000 mIu/mL. Severe hyperemesis (25%) and hyperthyroidism (7%) is associated in complete mole.

Diagnosis

Ultrasound findings: USG usually establishes the diagnosis. Presence of mixed echogenic pattern due to the replacement of the normal placental tissue due to edematous villi and blood clots. The classic "snowstorm appearance" may not always be present. Partial mole may show a coexistent fetus with scattered cystic spaces in the placental tissue.

Histopathological Diagnosis

On gross examination, classical vesicles due to massively enlarged edematous villi and grapelike structures are seen in the complete mole, while in partial mole these, vesicles may be present in focal sites within the placenta. Embryonic and fetal tissue also may not be obvious as early fetal death usually takes place between 8–9 weeks gestation. It is a good practice to carefully examine the products of conception after evacuation in all the spontaneous or missed miscarriages. Microscopically in a complete mole there will be hydropic swelling in majority of the villi along with variable degrees of trophoblastic proliferation. In partial mole, microscopically two sets of chorionic villi are evident; normal and grossly hydropic. Fetal tissue is seen in all partial moles.

Management

In diagnosed cases dilation and evacuation is the treatment accepted. Preoperative work up includes the tests enlisted in **Box 15.2**.

> **Box 15.2:** Preoperative tests in molar pregnancy
> - *Serum β-hCG levels:* Quantitative assay
> - Complete blood count
> - Metabolic panel
> - Renal function and liver function tests
> - Coagulation assessment
> - *Blood typing:* Rh-negative subject to be administered RhD-immunoglobulin
> - Screening for HbSAg and HIV
> - Chest roentgenogram (XRC) for metastasis

> **Box 15.3:** Checklists before and during D and E in vesicular mole
> - Stabilization of medical complications
> - Completely equipped operation room in hospital setting
> - Large bore IV access
> - Induction of regional or general anesthesia
> - Initiation of oxytocin drip after the cervix is dilated and suction is initiated
> - Largest bore suction cannula as can be safely introduced in the cervix

> **Box 15.4:** Postevacuation follow-up of vesicular mole
> - β-hCG levels 48 hours postevacuation and weekly until 3 consecutive levels come negative; then monthly until results are negative for 6 months
> - Regular pelvic examination for involution of pelvic organs and detection of metastasis
> - Repeat XRC if plateau or rise in β-hCG titer is noticed
> - Nonhormonal effective contraceptive method during the follow-up duration
> - Recurrence risk of 1–2% in subsequent pregnancy mandates careful USG evaluation of subsequent pregnancies

The primary treatment for vesicular mole is dilation and evacuation with suction. This procedure should be done carefully and the preoperative checklist should be as per **Box 15.3**.

Appropriate antibiotic is given preoperatively and oxytocin drip continued for a while after evacuation. It is advised not to use prostaglandin cervical preparations, sharp curettage or medical evacuation due to associated concerns of dissemination of the disease. The patient is followed up for 6 months postevacuation to identify residual disease. The components of postevacuation follow-up are as shown in **Box 15.4**.

The GTD prognostic scoring system should be practiced to assess the outcome in molar pregnancy **(Table 15.6)**.

Table 15.6: FIGO/WHO prognostic scoring system for GTD

Scores	1	2	3	4
Age years	≤ 39	≥ 40	-	-
Antecedent pregnancy	Mole	Miscarriage	Term	-
Interval form index pregnancy	< 4	4–6	7–12	>12
Pretreatment β-hCG level (IU/L)	<1000	<10000	<100000	>100000
Largest tumor size including uterus	-	3–4 cm	>5 cm	-
Site of metastases	Ling	Spleen/kidney	GI	Liver/brain
Number of metastases	1	1–4	5–8	>8
Previous failed chemotherapy	-	-	Single drug	3 or more

ECTOPIC GESTATION

Ectopic pregnancy (EP) is a result of implantation of fertilized ovum outside the uterine cavity. Very rarely heterogeneous implantation with concurrent implantation intrauterine as well as extrauterine may occur.

Epidemiology

Ectopic gestation is on the rise due to early diagnostic modalities, increased awareness and changed social structure. Out of all, first trimester pregnancies, 2% are ectopic gestations and 6% of pregnancy-related deaths are attributed to it. Tubal ligation is not a universal protection against ectopic gestation as 2/3rds of all post-ligation conceptions are ectopic pregnancies. Assisted reproductive technologies are associated with 3–5% of occurrence and are detected early. Tubal pregnancy is the commonest type (97%) but implantations can also be within the abdomen, cervix ovary or uterine cornua and rare locations such as previous hysterotomy scar or rudimentary horn. Ectopic pregnancy can rarely occur post-hysterectomy.

Risk Factors for Ectopic Gestations

The following table demonstrates risk factors for primary as well as recurrent ectopic pregnancy **(Table 15.7)**.

Etiology

Multifactorial etiological factors exist and an estimated 40–50% of ectopic gestations have unknown etiology.

Clinical Features

The classic triad of amenorrhea followed by abnormal vaginal bleeding and abdominal or pelvic pain is present in less than 50% of ectopic pregnancies. Vaginal bleeding or spotting is present in 60–80% of patients and is usually scant, altered colored and either intermittent or continuous.

Table 15.7: Ectopic pregnancy: Risk factors

Primary ectopic pregnancy	Recurrent ectopic pregnancy
• Pelvic inflammatory disease	• Previous ectopic pregnancy
• Previous tubal surgery	• Previous spontaneous miscarriage
• Infertility	• Pelvic surgery
• Current or previous use of intrauterine device	
• 2 or more pregnancy terminations	
• Age > 40 years	
• Smoking	
• More than 3 spontaneous abortions	
• ART	

Ectopic pregnancy when ruptured can present as an acute emergency. Pain is usually present in a rupturing EP and is in the lower quadrant but can be anywhere in the abdomen. Clinically, presence of peritonism, adnexal tenderness, mass, or cervical movement tenderness are suspicious signs of ectopic pregnancy. Signs of hemorrhagic shock due to hemoperitoneum secondary to rupture can be present as an acute presentation. Many times the clinical presentation is vague and high index of suspicion is necessary to make a timely diagnosis.

Diagnosis

Transabdominal and transvaginal ultrasound confirms the diagnosis of ectopic pregnancy in addition the serum β-hCG level of more than 1000 IU/mL is suggestive of an ectopic pregnancy. Serum β-hCG level 48 hours apart may show plateauing or suboptimal rise or fall in EP. Ultrasound features are enumerated in **Box 15.5**.

> **Box 15.5:** Ultrasound features of ectopic pregnancy
>
> Heterogeneous adnexal mass
> Empty extrauterine sac with hyperechoic ring (doughnut or bagel sign)
> Extrauterine sac with yolk sac or an embryo with or without heart beat
> Free fluid in Pouch of Douglas
> *Intrauterine pseudosac:* Collection of debris within the uterine cavity

Table 15.8: Clinical presentation of ectopic pregnancy

Hemodynamically unstable (Ruptured)	Hemodynamically stable
Surgical emergency	Generalized tenderness (45%)
Signs of shock: hemorrhagic and neurogenic: tachycardia, hypotension	Bilateral and lower quadrant pain (25%)
Signs of peritonism: guarding, rigidity, rebound tenderness	Unilateral pain (30%)
Shoulder pain (15%) diaphragmatic irritation due to hemoperitoneum	Rebound tenderness and cervical movement tenderness (+/−)
	Palpable adnexal mass and fullness in Pouch of Douglas (40%)

Differential Diagnosis

Salpingitis: Signs and symptoms similar to EP but negative pregnancy test, while fever, leukocytosis and neutrophilia are associated.

Threatened miscarriage: Vaginal bleeding will be heavier, pain will be localized in the lower mid-abdomen and cervical movement tenderness is usually absent.

Ovarian torsion: Initially intermittent pain goes on to a constant excruciating or dull pain. On per vaginal examination, adnexal mass palpable and features of inflammation may be present. Pregnancy test is negative. Torsion can also occur in hyperstimulated ovaries during ART treatment and delayed ovarian hyperstimulation syndrome (OHSS) can present with pain bleeding and positive pregnancy test.

Ruptured ovarian cyst: Corpus luteum cyst or endometriotic cysts or abnormal uterine bleeding can pose diagnostic dilemma

Nongynecological conditions such as appendicitis, gastroenteritis, diverticulitis, urinary tract infection, renal calculus, especially associated with early pregnancy also can be similar in clinical presentation.

Clinical assessment: Commonly two types of presentations are encountered; hemodynamically stable and unstable ectopic pregnancy as per **Table 15.8**.

The progesterone test had a very poor predictive accuracy for diagnosing ectopic pregnancy, for which a low progesterone concentration did not rule in or out an ectopic pregnancy **(Table 15.8)**.

Laboratory evaluation: The mainstay test for diagnosis and management is the quantitative β-hCG test which has to be correctly interpreted. The details of this evaluation is given at the end of this article. Hemoglobin level and hematocrit help in assessment of clinical status of the patient. Metabolic panel is essential in case a conservative approach is planned and baseline hepatic and hematologic dysfunction are to be identified. Progesterone level of more than 20 ng/mL points towards an intrauterine pregnancy and this test is of limited value in diagnosis of ectopic pregnancy.

Management of Ectopic Pregnancy

A ruptured unstable EP should be urgently resuscitated and taken for surgical intervention. Laparoscopic approach is a better option but may not be adopted in absence of technical backup, expertise and unstable patient. A large bore suction cannula placed safely is of great help to quickly aspirate the hemoperitoneum and help in tackling tubal rupture. Laparotomy can be undertaken in such situations. The stable patient is best offered either a surgical or a medical management with methotrexate based on assessment criteria.

IMPLANTATION BLEEDING (PHYSIOLOGIC)

Implantation bleeding is bleeding that occurs when the fertilized ovum implants in the decidua. This happens around the time of the expected menstrual period and is largely physiological needing reassurance.

LOWER GENITAL TRACT PATHOLOGY OR OTHER SITES BLEEDING

Nonobstetrical causes of bleeding can occur during pregnancy causing anxiety and need to be evaluated and treated.

Cervical ectropion is actually the eversion of the cervix due to excessive estrogenic influence during pregnancy and may be associated with genital tract bleeding or postcoital bleeding. Cervical cancer should be ruled out in all patients with cytology especially when suspected. Cervical malignancy is the most common cancers in pregnancy with an estimated incidence of 0.8–1.5 cases per 10,000 live births. Therefore thorough evaluation of cervical pathologies for cancer is important during pregnancy. Cervical polyps may be discovered on per speculum examination and cause bleeding. Many times, they get resolved during delivery or else have to be removed then but not during pregnancy. Assurance and prevention of infection is the treatment.

Vaginal infections such as candidiasis, trichomonal vaginitis and bacterial vaginosis can cause significant tissue damage to cause bleeding and have to be diagnosed and treated appropriately. Herpes simplex infections can also cause bleeding due to excoriation of the vesicles due to scratching or trauma. Such open sores may also alert for screening of other sexually transmitted infections such as syphilis. It is a good practice to take a triple swab test such as the high vaginal swab, endocervical swab for chlamydia, gonorrhea and surface swab for herpes culture.

Vulval trauma due to foreign body, scratching can cause bleeding. Other generalized infections such as allergic dermatitis, lichen planus, psoriasis, etc. should be looked for. Rectal bleeding and urinary tract bleeding due to various etiology can also confuse as genital tract bleeding during pregnancy and should be appropriately evaluated and treated.

IATROGENIC CAUSES—MEDICATIONS AND TRAUMA

Scratching excoriation and some inserts, especially the progesterone suppositories can cause vaginal or cervical bleeding **(Table 15.9)**.

IMPORTANT ISSUES TO BE UNDERSTOOD IN INTERPRETATION OF EARLY PREGNANCY HEMORRHAGE

- *Interpretation of quantitative β-hCG levels:* The serum titers of β-hCG increase in a linear fashion from 2–4 weeks post-ovulation. The titer in normal pregnancy usually doubles every 48–72 hours till it reaches the level of 10,000 IU/mL. For a viable intrauterine pregnancy (IUP), the minimal rise has to be 53% typically in 48 hours. If this rise is less than 50% in 48 hours, it can be considered as an abnormal pregnancy. Slow increase or decrease in the titers when measured serially can be consistent with EP but this should be interpreted in the full clinical context. Single level of β-hCG of 2000 IU/mL with no intrauterine gestational sac on transvaginal sonography mandates a repeat titer in 12–24 hours.

- *Early pregnancy milestones on USG:* Viability of the pregnancy can be determined by the presence of the gestational and /or yolk sac and with the measurement of the CRL. The Gsac should be visible at the β-hCG levels of 1000–2000 mIU/mL (~5 weeks of gestation). A yolk sac is seen at approximately 6 weeks after the LMP. At approximately 7 weeks after the LMP, a fetal pole can be visualized and approximately 8 weeks after the LMP, the fetal heartbeat can be seen. This depends on the ultrasonography machine and the sonologists' expertise.

- *Subchorionic hemorrhage (SCH) (before 12 weeks):* Subchorionic hemorrhage (subchorionic hematoma) collects between the uterine wall and the chorionic membrane and may leak through the cervical canal. SCH in patients with threatened abortion during the first half of the pregnancy increases the risk of miscarriage before 20 weeks gestation. However, the presence of an SCH is not known to increase the adverse pregnancy outcome risk in ongoing pregnancies as observed through some retrospective studies.

- *Interpretation of progesterone levels:* A normal viable pregnancy is associated with serum progesterone levels of 20 ng/mL or greater. A value of less than 5 ng/mL indicates a nonviable pregnancy.

- *Retroplacental hemorrhage (RPH):* RPH is a sonographic entity and occurs when there is perigestational hemorrhage that is restricted to the retroplacental space and may be from the spiral arterioles. Color Doppler imaging is essential to differentiate it from placental thickening, placental abnormality or a myometrial contraction by the elucidation of absence of internal flows.

- *Pregnancy of unknown location (PUL):* Pregnancy of unknown location is defined as the situation when the pregnancy test is positive but there are no signs of intrauterine pregnancy or an extrauterine pregnancy via transvaginal ultrasonography.

- *Pseudosac:* The intrauterine pseudosac of an ectopic pregnancy can be confused with the gestational sac. It is a fluid collection within the endometrial cavity. The fluid, blood and debris in the cavity can induce a heterogeneous appearance. Therefore, it is sensible to make the diagnosis of intrauterine pregnancy only when a yolk sac is seen **(Table 15.10)**.

Table 15.9: Nonobstetric causes of bleeding form the genital tract in early pregnancy

Cervix	Cervicitis, ectropion, cervical polyp, cervical neoplasm
Vagina and vulva	Infection, neoplasm, trauma, varicosities
Gastrointestinal bleeding	Hemorrhoids, rarely malignancy
Urinary tract bleeding	Infection, ureteric or pelvicalyceal stones, rarely malignancy

Table 15.10: Pseudosac and true gestational sac features

True gestational sac	Pseudosac
Usually is slightly off-center	Typically located centrally and may fill the entire endometrial cavity
Detectable double decidual sign	"Double ring" sign absent
Eventually develop an internal yolk sac later followed by an embryo	Will have no yolk sac or embryo eventually

CONCLUSION

Early pregnancy hemorrhage needs to be evaluated carefully as it can be a clinical representation of very innocuous implantation bleed to life-threatening ectopic pregnancy or dreadful malignancy such as cervical cancer and choriocarcinoma.

Also correct correlation of the imaging and the human chorionic gonadotropin levels is essential to avoid unnecessary diagnostic pitfalls.

REFERENCES

1. Carol J Buck. Elsevier Health Sciences, 2013. ISBN 9781455774883. (2014 ICD-10-CM Diagnosis Code O20.9 from 2014 ICD-10-CM/PCS Medical Coding Reference).
2. Pregnancy, Bleeding. eMedicineHealth. URL: *http://www.emedicinehealth.com/pregnancy_bleeding/article_em.htm*. Accessed on: April 12, 2009. Elective Abortion at eMedicine.
3. Hasan R, Baird DD, Herring AH, Olshan AF, Jonsson Funk ML, Hartmann KE. "Association between First-Trimester Vaginal Bleeding and Miscarriage". Obstetrics & Gynaecology. 2009;114(4):860. doi:10.1097/AOG.0b013e3181b79796.

Chapter 16

Unsafe Abortions and its Consequences

Kavita Bapat, Vineeta Ghanghoria

DEFINITION

The World Health Organization (WHO) defines unsafe abortion as "a procedure for terminating an unintended pregnancy carried out either by persons lacking the necessary skills or in an environment that does not conform to minimal medical standards, or both".[1] Unsafe abortions are mostly performed by individuals lacking qualification and skills to perform induced abortions. Some of unsafe abortions are self-induced. They are performed in unhygienic conditions, using dangerous interventions or incorrect medication. Injuries and deaths from unsafe abortions are preventable but still persisting.

MAGNITUDE OF THE PROBLEM

Accurate data of unsafe abortion is not available because of clandestine nature of the procedure. Every year about 56 million induced (safe and unsafe) abortions occur worldwide; out of these, 22 million are estimated unsafe abortion. There are 35 induced abortions per 1000 women aged between 15–44 years. Annual unsafe abortion rate as per 1000 women aged 15–44 years is 4 times higher in developing countries as compared with developed countries (23 and 6 per 1000 women respectively).

Around 47,000 deaths attributed to unsafe abortion worldwide in 2008. It accounts for about 13% of maternal mortality.[2] The mortality rate in safe abortion procedures is less than 1 per 1,00,000 procedures, when it is done in first trimester it is as low as 1 per 10,00,000 procedures. In countries where unsafe abortion is common practice, mortality rate is much higher, i.e. 350 death per 1,00,000 procedures. Morbidity and mortality related to unsafe abortions were higher in developing countries. In Africa, abortion-related deaths are disproportionately higher (about two third of all deaths due to unsafe abortion). In Africa, mortality rate due to unsafe abortion is 680 per 1,00,000 procedures.[3]

Around 5 million women are admitted to hospital as a result of unsafe abortion every year in developing countries. While more than 3 million women who have complications following unsafe abortion do not received post abortion care. Treatment of complication of unsafe abortion results in substantial costs to women, their families and healthcare systems.

CAUSES OF UNSAFE ABORTION

A. Unintended pregnancy: Poor women and adolescents are the high-risk group for unwanted pregnancies and are often at risk of unsafe abortion when they cannot access safe abortion services. Unwanted pregnancy is an extremely common, affecting nearly 80 million women each year. Women may not want a new pregnancy but since they are unable to avoid conception because of insufficient access to or information about contraception, incorrect and inconsistent use of contraceptive. Stigma for use of contraception, inadequate information on sexuality and various cultural factors also affect contraceptive use. Sometimes, pregnancy which was a wanted, may become unwanted because of changes in life circumstances, such as: abandonment by spouse, risk to her life or health, fetal malformation, inability to care for an additional child, etc[3].

B. Lack of access to contraception: Contraceptive use is a critical determinant of abortion. In fact, abortion rate is lowest in region where contraceptive use is high, despite of easily and legally available abortion services.

C. Restrictive abortion law: Unsafe abortion rates are higher in countries where abortion laws are strict, or don't allow abortion at all as compared to nations where abortion is more freely available and abortion laws are liberal. Restrictive laws compel the abortion service provider to provide clandestine services in substandard settings which may result in poor outcome.

D. Safe abortion services inaccessible and nonaffordable: In many countries, limited health infrastructure and shortage of well-trained healthcare providers are big constrain for safe abortion and post-abortion care.

At many centers abortion services are being provided by outdated, risky and expensive techniques. In a study, it was found that the majority of evacuation procedures were done with sharp curettage as well as general anesthesia or sedation.[4]

High cost of safe procedure; social stigma for abortion; unnecessary objection of healthcare providers; and unnecessary requirements such as: mandatory waiting periods, mandatory counseling, provision of misleading information, third-party authorization, medically unnecessary tests also affect the safe abortion services adversely.[5]

E. Economic and geographic barriers: Poverty is associated with women's inability to access safe abortion services. Poor women are likely to be uneducated or less educated. These women are not aware of their rights, law for safe abortion and the resources to pay for safe services. Poor women have difficulty to access safe services because they cannot pay for travel if living in a distant area. Where women work or are primary caregivers, inability to afford the time to seek services is an additional barrier. Raising the funds for an abortion further delays the procedure, which becomes riskier with advancing pregnancy. In fact, poor women usually pay significant sums of money for services, regardless of safety.

F. Cultural constraints: Healthcare provider plays the pivotal role for enhancing the accessibility and availability of safe abortion—both where legal and where restricted. It is important that healthcare provider must be updated with the knowledge, laws and the skills required for safe abortion as these can affect the outcome of abortion services. A Brazilian study revealed that confusion and misperception were widespread about the legal indications for abortion.[6]

Prevailing social ideologies and dynamics shape policies concerning contraceptives, abortion, sexuality, education and women's ability to make independent choices. In male dominant society, the female perspective is absent. The low social status of women leads to low levels of contraceptive use and higher rate of unwanted pregnancy and unsafe abortion. Involvement of women in policy-making decisions and liberalization of abortion laws with easy contraceptive access can reduce the incidence of unsafe abortion.

Abortion is considered a stigma in many societies. As a consequence, both women and provider do not discuss about their experiences. Women hide their pregnancies, seek services without good advice, and may delay seeking treatment for the complications.

Because people do not talk openly about abortion, misinformation is rampant. For example, women who self-induce abortion often use ineffective methods, such as herbal remedies, because they are misinformed about the best way to induce an abortion. These contributing factors affect poor and uneducated women disproportionately (RCOG). Barriers to accessing safe abortion include: restrictive laws, poor availability of services, high cost, and stigma, etc.

Methods of unsafe abortion:[7] Various methods of unsafe abortion are known and can be broadly classified in oral, injectable, vaginal, intrauterine and direct injury over abdomen or vagina.

- Oral
  - *Toxic solutions:* Turpentine, laundry bleach, detergent, acids, cottonseed oil, arak (a strong liquor)
  - *Tea and herbal remedies:* Strong herbal tea or tea made of livestock manure, boiled and ground avocado or basil leaves, wine boiled with raisins and cinnamon; black beer boiled with soap, oregano and parsley; boiled apio (celery plant) water with aspirin, "Tea with apio, avocado bark, ginger, etc; bitter concoction" assorted herbal medications. Absorption of soap water can lead to renal toxicity and death.[8]
  - *Drugs:* Uterine stimulants, such as misoprostol or oxytocin (used in obstetrics), quinine and chloroquine (used for treating malaria), oral contraceptive pills (ineffective in causing abortion).
  - *Treatments placed in the vagina or cervix:* Potassium permanganate tablets, herbal preparations, misoprostol. Potassium permanganate can lead to chemical burns to vagina and, sometimes, bowel injury.[9]
- *Foreign bodies placed into the uterus through the cervix:* Stick, sometimes dipped in oil, lump of sugar, hard green bean, root or leaf of plant, wire knitting needle, rubber catheter bougie (large rubber catheter), intrauterine contraceptive device, coat hanger, ballpoint pen, chicken bone, bicycle spoke, air blown in by a syringe or turkey baster, sharp curette. Foreign bodies can injure the uterus, bowels and other organs.
- *Enemas:* Soap, shih tea (wormwood).
- *Trauma:* Abdominal or back massage, lifting heavy weights, jumping from top of stairs or roof. It can lead to uterine rupture.

CONSEQUENCES OF UNSAFE ABORTION

There are approximately 22 million unsafe abortions occur annually, lead to 47,000 deaths, and more than 5 million complications.[3]

High-risk Group for Complications

Any woman with an unwanted pregnancy, who cannot access safe abortion is at risk of unsafe abortion. Poor women are more likely to have an unsafe abortion than more affluent women. Deaths and injuries are higher when unsafe abortion is performed later in pregnancy. The rate of unsafe abortions is higher where access to effective contraception and safe abortion is limited or unavailable.

Complications and their Management[10]

The major life-threatening complications resulting from unsafe abortion are hemorrhage, infection, and injury to the genital tract and internal organs.

A. Incomplete abortion: Occurs when some tissue remains in the uterus. Symptoms include abdominal pain; vaginal bleeding; and a soft, enlarged uterus. Treatment involves removing the remaining tissue in the uterus with vacuum aspiration or, if that is not available, with dilation and curettage.

B. Infection: Infection of uterine tissue can result from use of contaminated instruments or when tissue remains in the uterus. Symptoms include those of incomplete abortion as well as fever, chills, and foul-smelling vaginal discharge and uterine tenderness. Most often, symptoms appear two to three days after the abortion. Treatment involves antibiotics and vacuum aspiration if needed to remove the remaining tissue in the uterus.

C. Heavy bleeding: Bleeding results when an incomplete abortion is not treated or from some abortion techniques such as dilation and curettage or insertion of sticks or other objects into the cervix. Heavy bleeding also can be triggered by toxic reactions caused by herbs, drugs, or chemicals that are swallowed or placed in the vagina. Treatment may require removing remaining tissue in the uterus and administration of drugs to stop the bleeding, intravenous fluid replacement, and, in severe cases, blood transfusion or surgery.

D. Uterine perforation: It can occur when a sharp object or instrument is inserted into the uterus. Other organs also can be injured, including the cervix, ovaries, bowel, bladder, and rectum. Observation and antibiotics may be all that is needed as treatment, but in more severe cases, surgery may be needed to repair damage to bowel, blood vessels, or other organs.

Untreated, these complications can cause disabilities and chronic conditions like chronic pelvic pain; pelvic inflammatory disease, an infection of the reproductive organs and infertility.

Clinical Assessment of Unsafe Abortion

An accurate initial assessment is essential to ensure appropriate treatment and prompt referral for complications of unsafe abortion. The critical signs and symptoms of complications that require immediate attention include: body temperature of >37.9°C, pulse >119, shock (collapse of the circulatory system), other organ failure, abdominal pain, adnexal or abdominal tenderness or signs of peritonitis, evidence of foreign body or mechanical injury, abnormal vaginal bleeding or offensive vaginal discharge, and signs of tetanus.

Complications of unsafe abortion can be difficult to diagnose. For example, a woman with an extrauterine or ectopic pregnancy (abnormal development of a fertilized egg outside of the uterus) may have symptoms similar to those of incomplete abortion. It is essential, therefore, for healthcare personnel to be prepared to make referrals and arrange transport to a facility where a definitive diagnosis can be made and appropriate care can be delivered quickly.

Late Complications

According to the WHO, approximately 20–30% of unsafe abortions lead to reproductive tract infections and that about 20–40% of these result in upper-genital-tract infection and infertility. In 5% cases the infection becomes chronic.

Unsafe abortion increases the long-term risk of ectopic pregnancy, premature delivery, and spontaneous abortion in subsequent pregnancies. Life-threatening sepsis or hemorrhage may lead to hysterectomy. Consequences of internal organ injury (urinary and stool incontinence from vesicovaginal or rectovaginal fistulas), bowel resections. Gas gangrene and tetanus can be developed.[11]

Other unmeasurable consequences of unsafe abortion include loss of productivity and psychological damage. The burden of unsafe abortion lies not only with the women and families, but also with the public health system. Every woman admitted for emergency post-abortion care may require blood products, antibiotics, oxytocics, anesthesia, operating rooms, and surgical specialists. The financial and logistic impact of emergency care can overwhelm a health system and can prevent attention to be administered to other patients. The cost of post-abortion care is several times that of providing safe abortion.[12]

Post-abortion Care

According to the World Health Organization:
- In some areas of the developing world, as many as half of the admissions to hospital gynecological wards, are women needing treatment after unsafe abortions.
- Studies show that hospitals in some developing countries spend as much as 50 percent of their budgets to treat complications of unsafe abortion.

International health organizations generally recognize post-abortion care to include:
- Emergency treatment for complications of abortion or miscarriage.
- Counseling to identify and respond to women's emotional and physical health needs and other concerns.
- Contraceptive and family planning services to help women prevent an unwanted pregnancy or unsafe abortion or to practice birth spacing.
- Management of sexually transmitted infections.

- Reproductive and other health services that are provided on-site or through referrals to other accessible facilities.

PREVENTION OF UNSAFE ABORTION

- Effective family planning and/or contraception is key to prevent unintended pregnancy and unsafe abortion.
- The safe abortion services should be accessible and affordable to needy women. It will save the huge material and resources that are being utilized in the treatment of unsafe abortion and its complications.
- Health centers should be adequately equipped and health providers should be trained to have requisite skills and knowledge to provide quality abortion-related care to women.
- Implementation of law to promote and support safe abortion services to reduce complications of unsafe abortion. Evidence demonstrates that liberalizing abortion laws to allow services to be provided openly by skilled practitioners can reduce the rate of abortion-related morbidity and mortality.
- Ensure proper circulation of abortion care-related standards and guidelines.
- Sex education to women and adolescent and education regarding contraception and appropriate abortion care is must to reduce safe abortion.
- Educating women regarding their reproductive health should be incorporated in schools.
- Government and nongovernmental organizations need to find effective ways to overcome cultural and social misconceptions that restrict women from receiving necessary health care.

CONCLUSION AND RECOMMENDATIONS

Ministry of Health, Human Rights Commission and Gender Commission should implement new constitution that enables both health providers and women to know all the grounds, wherein abortion is legal to the full extent of the law. Liberalization of abortion laws can have a dramatic impact on reducing mortality and morbidity related to unsafe abortion. Increasing access to and education about effective family planning methods to both men and women. Educating women regarding rights to contraception, safe abortion and post-abortion care.

Training of healthcare providers and ensuring access to high quality care such as appropriate uterine evacuation technologies, including mifepristone and mesoprostol as well as manual vacuum aspiration which are safe and cost efficient. Involving and educating communities about risk of unsafe abortion. Removing misinformation about family planning and contraception.

REFERENCES

1. World Health Organization. The prevention and management of unsafe abortion. Report of a Technical Working Group. Geneva, World Health Organization, 1992 (WHO/MSM/92.5).
2. Unsafe abortion: global and regional estimates of the incidence of unsafe abortion and associated mortality in 2008, sixth edition; 2011. Department of Reproductive Health and Research, World Health.
3. Sedgh G, Henshaw S, Singh S, Ahman E, Shah IH. Induced abortion: estimated rates and trends worldwide. Lancet. 2007;370:1338-45.
4. Brown HC, Jewkes R, Levin J, Dickson-Tetteh K, Rees H. Management of incomplete abortion in South African hospitals. BJOG. 2003;110:371-7.
5. World Health Organization. Preventing unsafe abortion. Fact sheet. Updated; 2016.
6. Goldman LA, Garcia SG, Diaz J, Yam EA, Brazilian obstetrician-gynaecologists and abortion: a survey of knowledge, opinions and practices. Reprod Health. 2005;2:10.
7. Warriner IK, Shah IH (Eds). Preventing unsafe abortion and its consequences. Priorities for research and action. New York: The Guttmacher Institute; 2006.pp.73-91.
8. Burnhill MS. Treatment of women who have undergone chemically induced abortions. J Reprod Med. 1985;30: 610-14.
9. O'Donnell RP. Vesicovaginal fistula produced by potassium permanganate. Obstet Gynecol. 1954;4:122-3.
10. Population reference bureau. Unsafe Abortion facts & figure; 2005.pp.13-4.
11. David A Grimes, Janie Benson, Susheela Singh, Mariana Romero, Bela Ganatra, Friday E Okonofua, Iqbal H Shah. Unsafe abortion: the preventable pandemic. The Lancet Sexual and Reproductive Health Series; 2006.
12. Johnston HB, Gallo MF, Benson J. Reducing the costs to health systems of unsafe abortion: a comparison of four strategies. J Fam Plann Reprod Health Care. 2007;33:250-7.

SECTION 5: MEDICAL DISORDERS DURING PREGNANCY

Chapter 17

Gestational Diabetes

Jigyasa Dengra, Meenu Agarwal

INTRODUCTION

Carbohydrate intolerance with recognition or onset during pregnancy, "irrespective of treatment with diet or insulin whether or not condition persists after pregnancy" is called as gestational diabetes.[1] It is one of the most common medical conditions encountered during pregnancy. Although this definition also puts diabetic patients in pregnancy who were undiagnosed prior to pregnancy into the category of gestational diabetes mellitus (GDM), this is the most commonly used definition.

The prevalence of diabetes in pregnancy has been increasing in the world with India becoming the diabetic capital of the world. The incidence of GDM is also on a rise because the age of onset of diabetes and prediabetes is declining while the age of childbearing is increasing. There is also an increase in the rate of overweight and obese women of reproductive age; thus, more women entering pregnancy have risk factors that make them vulnerable to hyperglycemia during pregnancy.[2,3]

The International Diabetes Federation (IDF) estimates that one in six live births (16.8%) are to women with some form of hyperglycemia in pregnancy. While 16% of these cases may be due to diabetes in pregnancy (either pre-existing diabetes—type 1 or type 2—which antedates pregnancy or is first identified during testing in the index pregnancy), the majority (84%) is due to GDM.

Both pre-gestational type 1 diabetes and type 2 diabetes confer significantly greater maternal and fetal risk than GDM, with some differences according to type.

GDM is associated with a higher incidence of maternal morbidity, including spontaneous abortion, fetal anomalies, intrauterine death, cesarean deliveries, shoulder dystocia, birth trauma, hypertensive disorders of pregnancy (including pre-eclampsia), and subsequent development of type 2 diabetes and obesity. Moreover, hyperglycemia first appearing during pregnancy is associated with a high-risk of developing diabetes and cardiovascular diseases in later life.[4-8]

Perinatal and neonatal morbidities also increase; the latter include macrosomia, birth injury, hypoglycemia, polycythemia, and hyperbilirubinemia. Long-term sequel in offspring with *in utero* exposure to maternal hyperglycemia may include higher risks for obesity and diabetes later in life.

In the upper class setting pregnant women with GDM or pregnancy with diabetes get the benefits of progress made in all areas of medicine and in obstetrics in particular. State-of-the-art tools have been developed for diagnosis, treatment, and follow-up of both mother and fetus, such as fetal heart rate monitors, USG, glucose self-monitors, and insulin pumps. As a result, leading private institutes report a major reduction in maternal and fetal complications of diabetic pregnancies reaching levels similar to those in normal pregnancy due to early diagnosis, adequate treatment, and close follow-up.

However, majority of women in low, lower middle settings especially in the rural areas are not properly screened and treated for diabetes during pregnancy which account for maternal and perinatal deaths and poor pregnancy outcomes.

PATHOPHYSIOLOGY OF GDM

What Leads to Glucose Intolerance in GDM?[9]

In the pathophysiology of GDM, we have to consider two main points:
1. Role of fetoplacental unit
2. Role of the adipose tissue

Insulin resistance and the decrease in insulin sensitivity during pregnancy are mainly attributed to the increase in the levels of pregnancy-associated hormones as estrogen, progesterone, cortisol and placental lactogen in the maternal circulation.

Normally, the insulin resistance of the whole body is increased to about three times of that seen in the non-pregnant state. The increased resistance is caused by post-insulin receptor events and is probably brought about by the cellular effects of the increased levels of one or all of the above hormones.

As pregnancy progresses and the placenta grows larger, hormone production also increases and so does the level of insulin resistance. This process usually starts between 20 and 24 weeks of pregnancy. At birth, when the placenta is delivered, the hormone production stops and so does the condition, strongly suggesting that these hormones cause GDM.

The placenta synthesizes pregnenolone and progesterone from cholesterol. Some of the progesterone enters the fetal circulation and provides the substrate for the formation of cortisol and corticosterone in the fetal adrenal glands. Some of the pregnenolone also enters the fetal circulation and, along with pregnenolone, synthesized in the fetal liver, is the substrate for the formation of dehydroepiandrosterone sulfate (DHEAS) and 16-hydroxydehydroepiandrosterone sulfate (16-OHDHEAS) in the fetal adrenal. Some 16-hydroxylation also occurs in the fetal liver. DHEAS and 16-OHDHEAS are transported back to the placenta, where DHEAS forms estradiol and 16-OHDHEAS forms estriol. The principal estrogen formed is estriol, and since fetal 16-OHDHEAS is the principal substrate for the estrogens, the urinary estriol excretion of the mother can be monitored as an index of the state of the fetus.

HPL, which is the product of the HPL-A and HPL-B genes, is secreted into both the maternal and fetal circulations after the sixth week of pregnancy. The level of HPL in the maternal circulation is correlated with fetal and placental weight, plateauing in the last 4 weeks of pregnancy. Therefore, measurement of HPL level is used as a screening test for fetal distress and neonatal asphyxia, however, there is a large variation in normal range hence it is not an ideal indicator.

Pregnancy induces a progressive change in maternal carbohydrate metabolism. As pregnancy advances, insulin resistance and diabetogenic stress due to placental hormones necessitate compensatory increase in insulin secretion. Progressively increasing insulin levels enables to maintain plasma glucose levels following glucose load and if this compensation is inadequate, which occurs in chronic beta cell dysfunction, GDM occurs.

In the nutshell, *GDM is a stage in the evolution of type 2 DM*.

SCREENING AND DIAGNOSIS

When it comes to screening the main doubt remains is to do selective screen or universal screen. Compared to selective screening, universal screening for GDM detects more cases and improves maternal and neonatal prognosis. Hence, universal screening for GDM is essential, as it is generally accepted that women of Asian origin and especially ethnic Indians are at 11 fold higher risk of developing GDM and subsequent type 2 diabetes, as compared to Caucasians. If one does selective screening 45% of pregnant women will go unscreened and 35–50% of GDM would be missed. IDF guidelines suggests not only do universal screening but almost assume that every woman has diabetes and doing the screening is to reassure her that she does not have diabetes.

Screening is important as diabetes produces serious maternal and perinatal outcomes which are discussed here and screening and subsequent management prevents those complications and improves maternal and infant health.

Screening of GDM is done at booking (first trimester); 24–28 weeks and after 32 weeks.

Early screen is to pick up undiagnosed preexisting diabetes (DIP) and repeat screen is to detect diabetes occurring in pregnancy (GDM).

The various screen tests have been proposed and suggested from time to time along with various criteria. The different screen tests used are:
- Urinary sugars
- Random blood sugar levels
- Fasting and postprandial blood sugar levels
- 50 g glucose challenge test
- 75/100 g glucose tolerance test
- OGTT
- Single-step test.

Urinary Sugars

It is easy to perform in poor resource settings but is unreliable as 73% of glycosuria turn out not to have GDM and a large majority of GDM will not have glycosuria.

Blood Sugars

- Random >200 mg/dL
- Fasting >126 mg/dL
- Postlunch >200 mg/dL

Lack of conclusive data documenting reproducibility and sensitivity. Some GDMs exhibit high glucose levels only after meals, with normal fasting levels.

50 g Glucose Challenge Test

RCOG and ADA recommends GCT. In this, 50 g of glucose is given irrespective of fasting and a 2 hr reading of 140 mg% or more, if positive would require OGTT.

Oral Glucose Tolerance Test

World Health Organization (WHO) recommends using a 2 h 75 g oral glucose tolerance test (OGTT) with a threshold plasma glucose concentration of greater than 140 mg/dL at 2 hours, similar to that of IGT (>140 mg/dL and <199 mg/dL), outside pregnancy.[10]

The International Association of the Diabetes and Pregnancy Study Groups (IADPSG) recommends that diagnosis of GDM is made when any of the following plasma glucose values meet or exceed: Fasting: ≥ 5.1 mmol/L (92 mg/dL), 1-hour: ≥ 10.0 mmol/L (180 mg/dL), 2-hour: ≥ 8.5 mmol/L (153 mg/dL)7 with 75 g OGTT.[11]

The IADPSG also suggests: Fasting plasma glucose (FPG) > 7.0 mmol/L (126 mg/dL)/A1C > 6.5% in the early weeks of pregnancy is diagnostic of overt diabetes.

Disadvantages of the IADPSG suggestions are:
The patient has to be in fasting stage. Most of the time pregnant women do not come in the fasting state because of long distance travel and belief not to fast for long hours. The dropout rate is very high when a pregnant woman is asked to come again for the glucose tolerance test.

Attending the first prenatal visit in the fasting state is impractical in many settings.

In all GDM, FPG values do not reflect the 2-hour post-glucose with 75 g oral glucose [2-hour plasma glucose (PG)], which is the hallmark of GDM.

Ethnically, Asian Indians have high insulin resistance and as a consequence, their 2-hour PG is higher compared to Caucasians. The insulin resistance during pregnancy escalates further and hence FPG is not an appropriate option to diagnose GDM in the Asian Indian women. In this population by following FPG > 5.1 mmol/L (92 mg/dL) as cut-off value, 76% of pregnant women would have missed the diagnosis of GDM made by the WHO criterion.

Asian and South Asian ethnicity are both independently associated with increased insulin resistance in late pregnancy. A diagnostic FPG was present in only 24% of those with GDM in Bangkok and 26% in Hong Kong.

Center to center differences occur in GDM frequency and relative diagnostic importance of fasting, 1 hour and 2-hour glucose levels. This may impact strategies used for the diagnosis of GDM.

WHO Economical Tests

These tests require one blood sample drawn at 2 hours after 75 g oral glucose load for estimating plasma glucose. Even if the test is to be repeated in each trimester, the cost in performing the procedure will be 66% less than the cost of performing IADPSG recommended procedure. Thus, the WHO procedure is feasible, sustainable, cost-effective and high impact best-buy for less resource settings.[12]

Evidence-based: A study performed by Crowther, et al. found that treatment of GDM diagnosed by the WHO criterion reduces serious perinatal morbidity and may also improve the women's health-related quality of life. Diagnosis of GDM with OGTT 2-hour PG ≥ 7.8 mmol/L (140 mg/dL) and treatment in a combined diabetes antenatal clinic is worthwhile with a decreased macrosomia rate and fewer emergency cesarean sections. The treatment of GDM women as defined by the WHO criterion was associated with reduced risk of pregnancy outcome. Wahi, et al. observed in their randomized controlled study, the advantage of adhering to a cut-off level of 2-hour PG ≥ 7.8 mmol/L (140 mg/dL) in diagnosis and management of GDM for a significantly positive effect on pregnancy outcomes, both in relation to mother and the child. Perucchini, et al. also suggest one-step diagnostic procedure (2-hour PG ≥ 7.8 mmol/L) to diagnose GDM.

A long-term outcome study conducted by Franks, et al. documented that when maternal 2-hour PG was ≥ 7.8 mmol/L, the cumulative risk of offspring developing type 2 DM was 30% at the age 24 years.

A Single-test Procedure to Diagnose GDM in the Community (Diabetes in Pregnancy Study Group India)[13-14]

Diabetes in Pregnancy Study Group India (DIPSI diagnostic criteria 2-hour PG ≥ 140 mg/dL is similar to WHO criteria 2-hour PG ≥ 140 mg/dL to diagnose GDM) "A single-step procedure" was developed due to the practical difficulty in performing glucose tolerance test in the fasting state, as seldom pregnant women visiting the antenatal clinic for the first time come in the fasting state. If they are asked to come on another day in the fasting state, many of them do not return. Hence, it is important to have a test that detects the glucose intolerance without the woman necessarily undergoing a test in the fasting state and it is preferable to perform the diagnostic test at the first visit itself.

Procedure

In the antenatal clinic, a pregnant woman after undergoing preliminary clinical examination, is given a 75 g oral glucose load, irrespective of whether she is in the fasting or non-fasting state and without regard to the time of the last meal. A venous blood sample is collected at 2 hours for estimating plasma glucose by the GOD-POD method. GDM is diagnosed if 2-hour PG ≥ 140 mg/dL (7.8 mmol/L). If 75 g glucose packet is not available, remove and discard 5 level teaspoons (not heaped) of glucose from a 100 g packet which is freely available. In hospitals where glucose is supplied in bulk, a cup or container of 75 g may be used. The glucose marketed is in anhydrous form. Performing this test procedure in the non-fasting state is rational, as glucose concentrations are affected little by the time since the last meal in a normal glucose tolerant woman, whereas it will, in a woman with gestational diabetes. After a meal, a normal glucose tolerant woman would be able to maintain euglycemia despite glucose challenge due to brisk and adequate insulin response, whereas, a woman with GDM who has impaired insulin secretion, her glycemic level increases with a meal and with glucose challenge, the glycemic excursion exaggerates further. This cascading effect is advantageous as this would not result in false-positive diagnosis of GDM.

Advantages of the DIPSI procedure are:
- Pregnant women need not be fasting
- Causes least disturbance in a pregnant woman's routine activities
- Serves as both screening and diagnostic procedure.
- Cost effective

This single-step procedure has been approved by the Ministry of Health, Government of India and also recommended by the WHO.

Gestational Weeks at which Screening is Recommended

By following the usual recommendation for screening between 24 and 28 weeks of gestation, the chance of detecting unrecognized type 2 diabetes before pregnancy (DIP) is likely to be missed. If the 2-hour PG is > 200 mg/dL in the early weeks of pregnancy, she may be a DIP and A1C of ≥ 6.5 is confirmatory. So all pregnant women to be screened for diabetes at the first antenatal visit. A pregnant woman found to have normal glucose tolerance (NGT), in the first trimester, should be tested for GDM again around 24th–28th week and again at around 32nd–34th week.

MANAGEMENT OF GESTATIONAL DIABETES MELLITUS

Monitoring Glycemic Control

The success of the treatment for a woman with GDM depends on the glycemic control maintained with meal plan or pharmacological intervention. Studies suggest 1.5 and 2-hour post-meal for monitoring glycemic control. 2-hour post-meal monitoring is preferred as the diagnosis of GDM is also based on 2-hour PG. It is easier to remember this timing, as the time for diagnosis and also for monitoring is the same, i.e. 2 hours. However, whichever time is targeted for monitoring glycemic control and adjusting insulin dose, blood tests must be performed at the same time at each visit. They should be advised to perform self-monitoring of blood glucose (SMBG) on a daily basis, failing which, at least weekly monitoring should be encouraged.[15]

Four times blood sugar tests for diet treated cases, 1 fasting and 3 postmeals once in 15 days.

Six times blood sugar tests in insulin treated cases once in a week or 4 tests on any two days is ideal.

Target is to achieve fasting <90 mg/dL and postprandial <120 mg/dL with mean plasma levels of 105 mg/dL to 110 mg/dL.

If self-monitoring is not possible, laboratory venous plasma glucose has to be estimated for adjusting the dose of insulin.

Treatment targets in maintaining a mean plasma glucose (MPG) level of 105–110 mg/dL is desirable for a good fetal outcome. This is possible if FPG and 2-hour postprandial peaks are 90 mg/dL and 120 mg/dL respectively. The goal is not only to improve perinatal outcome but also to prevent long-term maternal and fetal effects.

HbA1C in Pregnancy

This test reflects the average glucose level in the three months prior to measurement. It is correlated with the risk of congenital malformations, not to any other adverse pregnancy outcomes. It is best used for pregnancy planning and prenatal follow-up in cases of diabetes in pregnancy. HbA1c does not replace the OGTT for the diagnosis of GDM. Due to physiological increases in red blood cell count, HbA1C levels fall during normal pregnancy. Also, as HbA1C represents an integrated measure of glucose, it may not fully capture postprandial hyperglycemia, which drives macrosomia. Thus, while A1C may be useful, it should be used as a secondary measure, after self-monitoring of blood glucose.[16]

Observational studies show the lowest rates of adverse fetal outcomes in association with HbA1C value of 6–6.5% early in gestation. Clinical trials have not evaluated the risks and benefits of achieving these targets, and treatment goals should account for the risk of maternal hypoglycemia in setting an individualized target of 6–7%.

In the second and third trimester, HbA1C, 6% has the lowest risk of large-for-gestational-age infants, whereas other adverse outcomes increase with HbA1C 6.5%. Taking all of this into account, a target of 6–6.5% is recommended but 6% may be optimal as pregnancy progresses. These levels should be achieved without hypoglycemia, which, in addition to the usual adverse sequelae, may increase the risk of low birth weight babies. Given the alteration in red blood cell kinetics during pregnancy and physiological changes in glycemic parameters, HbA1C levels need to be monitored more frequently.

TREATMENT

It starts with psychological support, counseling, medical nutrition therapy, exercise followed by pharmacological management.

Medical Nutritional Therapy:[17] All women with GDM should receive nutritional counseling. The meal pattern should provide adequate calories and nutrients to meet the needs of pregnancy. The expected weight gain during pregnancy is 300–400 grams per week and total weight gain is 10–12 kg by term and if BMI >30 weight gain should be between 5–10 kg. Once diagnosis is made, Medical Nutritional Therapy (MNT) is advised initially for 2 weeks. If MNT fails to achieve control, i.e. FPG >90 mg/dL and/or post-meal glucose >120 mg/dL, insulin may be initiated.

MNT should be individualized with focus on carbohydrate controlled meal plan and overall healthy food choices with good cooking practices and portion control. There should be no fasting or feasting.

Exercise: It is a part of healthy lifestyle which should be continued during pregnancy. The goal of exercise in pregnancy is to improve or maintain overall fitness. Exercise or activities with risks of falling or trauma should be avoided. Even women who were not exercising can start simple exercises like walking. Exercise increases insulin sensitivity and decreases body fat and reduces oxidative stress

Oral antidiabetic drugs: Traditionally, when MNT and exercise was insufficient to maintain normoglycemia in women with GDM, insulin was the only available medical therapy.[18] In the past, oral antidiabetic agents (OAD) were not recommended during pregnancy owing to the fear of potential adverse fetal effects, including teratogenicity and neonatal hypoglycemia. Although neither glyburide nor metformin is approved for use in pregnancy, their use as an adjunct therapy in GDM has been considered by several organizations. For example, glyburide has been acknowledged in the Fifth International Workshop-Conference on Gestational Diabetes Mellitus and both are considered in the NICE guidance.[19] Use of oral agents is increasing, and in some settings, they are the first option when drug treatment is required for women with GDM.

Glibenclamide is being used in a few centers in India and abroad, but not yet approved by drug controller of India. Metformin (alone or with supplemental insulin) was not associated with increased perinatal complications as compared with insulin. Metformin has been found to be useful in women with polycystic ovarian disease (PCOD) where it was prescribed for induction of ovulation and continued thereafter, but use of OADS should be individualized and proper counseling and documentation is a must.

Insulin Therapy in GDM

When blood glucose targets cannot be reached by diet and/or OADs, insulin is required. Insulin is the preferred agent for management of pre-gestational type 1 diabetes and type 2 diabetes that are not adequately controlled with diet, exercise, and metformin. The physiology of pregnancy requires frequent titration of insulin to match changing requirements. In the first trimester, there is often a decrease in total daily insulin requirements, and women, particularly those with type 1 diabetes, may experience increased hypoglycemia. In the second trimester, rapidly increasing insulin resistance requires weekly or biweekly increases in insulin dose to achieve glycemic targets. In general, a smaller proportion of the total daily dose should be given as basal insulin (50%) and a greater proportion (50%) as prandial insulin. In the late third trimester, there is often a leveling off or small decrease in insulin requirements.

Due to the complexity of insulin management in pregnancy, referral to a specialized center offering team-based care (with team members including high-risk obstetrician, endocrinologist, dietitian, nurse, and social worker, as needed) is recommended if this resource is available.

There is no evidence supporting the advantages of any one type of insulin or regimen of insulin over another. Thus, insulin type and regimens should be individualized.[20] It is beneficial to pair rapid-acting with intermediate or long-acting insulin in order to simulate the physiologic insulin secretion throughout the day. In women with diabetes, insulin requirements gradually increase throughout the pregnancy: 0.7 units/kg/day in the first trimester; 0.8 units/kg/day from week 18; 0.9 units/kg/day from week 26; and 1.0 units/kg/day from week 36 until delivery. In some instances, lower doses may suffice. Regular soluble human insulin and neutral protamine Hagedorn (NPH) human insulin are commonly used for treating diabetes during pregnancy. Although NPH is considered as intermediate-acting insulin,[21] its basal insulin action in pregnant women may require 2–3 daily injections increasing the risk of hypoglycemia especially at night. These disadvantages in human insulin can be overcome by the use of combination of short-acting and long-acting insulin analogues, or continuous insulin infusion in a pump. All insulins are pregnancy category B except for glargine, glulisine, and degludec, which are labeled category C.

Insulin during delivery: If labor is to be induced or cesarean to be planned, morning dose of insulin to be avoided and BSL to be monitored every hour and insulin to be given accordingly to maintain target of 80–100 mg/dL blood sugars.

Pregnancy and Insulin Pumps

The conventional treatment for diabetes in pregnancy has been with MDI (multiple doses of insulin). However, the incidence of glycemic variability and ultimate pregnancy outcomes have always been a concern with poor control of blood glucose.

Tight glycemic control results in better outcomes for mother with lesser chances of cesarean delivery and low risk of perinatal mortality. Tight glycemic control also results in lower incidences of neonatal hypoglycemia and macrosomia.[22] Use of pumps has been an alternate way to control blood glucose to targets in pregnancy. Various studies have shown the safety and efficacy of pump use in pregnancy.[23]

Indications for pump use are stronger in the following situations:[24]
- Highly labile diabetes
- Requirement for high doses of insulin when MDI is used
- Frequent hypoglycemia or hypoglycemia unawareness
- Erratic lifestyle, e.g ladies who undertake frequent long distance travel, shift workers where there can be unpredictable insulin delivery
- Significant "Dawn Phenomenon" (early morning rise in blood sugar levels)
- Pregnant ladies reluctant to do frequent blood glucose testing as the newer pumps can display real time continuous blood glucose monitoring graphs

The only drawback in the use of pumps is the training involved and support by a trained center. Also in certain populations, cost involved can be prohibitive. These situations can limit their use to a large extent.

KEY POINTS

Recommendations for Pharmacological Treatment in Women with Gestational Diabetes Mellitus

Insulin, glyburide, and metformin are safe and effective therapies for GDM during the second and third trimesters, and may be initiated as first-line treatment after failing to achieve glucose control with lifestyle modification.

Among OADs, metformin may be a better choice than glyburide however. *It is important to note that there is no long-term evidence on the safety of OADs.*

Insulin should be considered as the first-line treatment in women with GDM who are at high risk of failing on OAD therapy such as:
- Diagnosis of diabetes <20 weeks of gestation
- If gestational age >30 weeks
- Fasting BSL >110 mg/dL
- 1-hour postprandial glucose >140 mg/dL

SURVEILLANCE DURING PREGNANCY

Type 1 Diabetes

Women with type 1 diabetes have an increased risk of hypoglycemia in the first trimester and, like all women, have altered counter-regulatory response in pregnancy that may decrease hypoglycemia awareness. Hypoglycemia education for patients and family members is important before and during early pregnancy and throughout pregnancy to help to prevent and manage the risks of hypoglycemia. Insulin resistance drops rapidly with delivery of the placenta. Women become very insulin sensitive immediately following delivery and may initially require much less insulin than in the prepartum period. Pregnancy is a ketogenic state, and women with type 1 diabetes, and to a lesser extent, those with type 2 diabetes, are at risk for diabetic ketoacidosis at lower blood glucose levels than in the non-pregnant state. All insulin-deficient women need ketone strips at home and education on diabetic ketoacidosis prevention and detection. In addition, rapid implementation of tight glycemic control in the setting of retinopathy is associated with worsening of retinopathy.

Type 2 Diabetes

Pregestational type 2 diabetes is often associated with obesity. Recommended weight gain during pregnancy for overweight women is 6.8–11 kg and for obese women is 4.5-9 kg. Glycemic control is often easier to achieve in type 2 diabetes than in type 1 diabetes but can require much higher doses of insulin, sometimes, necessitating concentrated insulin formulations. As in type 1 diabetes, insulin requirements drop dramatically after delivery. Associated hypertension and other comorbidities often render pregestational type 2 diabetes as high or higher risk than pregestational type 1 diabetes, even if the diabetes is better controlled and of shorter duration, with pregnancy loss appearing to be more prevalent in the third trimester in type 2 diabetes compared with the first trimester in type 1 diabetes.

Examination of the fundus and estimation of microalbuminuria and serum creatinine in every trimester is recommended particularly in women with pregestational diabetes.

Ultrasound fetal monitoring: Ultrasound monitoring is recommended at least every trimester for accurate dating, screening anomalies, monitoring growth.

Doppler should be done to detect pre-eclampsia and IUGR.

Labor and Delivery

Delivery before full term is not indicated unless there is evidence of macrosomia, polyhydramnios, poor metabolic control or other obstetric indications (e.g. pre-eclampsia or intrauterine growth retardation).

With advancing gestation, the risk of macrosomia, shoulder dystocia and stillbirth increased. Management options included expectant management, induction of labor or elective cesarean delivery.

The timing and the mode of delivery was not straight forward as well-controlled prospective studies were lacking. Delayed fetal lung maturation and surfactant production also is of concern particularly if labor is to be induced.

For the timing of delivery, the ADA in 2004 recommended delivery at 38 weeks unless obstetric considerations dictated alternative management, while ACOG did not recommend routine delivery before 40 weeks. The NICE in 2008 recommended pregnant women with diabetes should be offered elective birth through induction of labor after 38 completed weeks. RCOG in 2012 recommended induction of labor at term to reduce the incidence of shoulder dystocia in women with gestational diabetes. One systemic review included one RCT and four observational studies. The RCT suggested that active induction at 38 weeks could reduce birth weight and macrosomia without increasing caesarean delivery. The four observational studies suggested a potential reduction in macrosomia and shoulder dystocia with elective delivery.

They found it difficult to draw conclusions based on the limited evidence. A retrospective cohort study observed that expectant management may increase risk of mortality at

39 weeks when compared with delivery. 1500 deliveries would be needed to prevent one death at 39 weeks. However, the degree of glycemic control of the subjects was not available. For the mode of delivery, cesarean delivery would only be suggested for an estimated fetal weight of 4500 g in mothers with diabetes to prevent brachial plexus injury by a decision analysis study. The delivery option of well-controlled GDM remained uncertain.

A few obstetricians prefer to terminate pregnancy around 38 gestational weeks to reduce the complication rate and labor complications like shoulder dystocia in a bigger baby.

COMPLICATIONS OF GDM

The Mother

GDM is associated with increased maternal morbidities like polyhydramnios, hypertension, preeclampsia and eclampsia, abruption, preterm labor, increased risk of cesarean deliveries, spontaneous abortions, IUD and PPH.[25-29]

Women who have had GDM are much more likely to develop type 2 DM or metabolic syndrome later in life. A systematic review of 28 studies covering 28 years showed the cumulative incidence of type 2 DM to range from 2.6% to 70% of women who had GDM. The cumulative incidence of conversion to type 2 DM increases markedly in the first 5 years after gestational diabetes and increases more slowly after 10 years.

In addition to developing type 2 DM later in life, women who have had GDM with one pregnancy are 30–69% more likely to develop GDM again in future pregnancies. A study involving 651 patients diagnosed with GDM showed that macrosomic births and increased prepregnancy weight after the index GDM pregnancy were both predictive of recurrence. Another smaller study showed that many risk factors are linked to the recurrence of GDM, including a parity of >1, a body mass index of >30 kg/m², and a need for insulin in the index pregnancy.[12] In this study, weight gain of >15 lb (6.8 kg) between pregnancies and an interval of <24 months between pregnancies were found to be the strongest risk factors for future GDM.

Maternal hypertension is often associated with GDM. One retrospective study of 286 Danish women found that 19.6% of GDM patients developed hypertension during pregnancy, versus 10.5% of nondiabetic women ($p = 0.046$). Another study of 874 GDM patients and 61,209 general obstetric patients found hypertension rates of 17% and 12%, respectively ($p < 0.001$).

If a patient is having any pre-existing nephropathy, retinopathy, neuropathy; it may aggravate with pregnancy.

The Fetus and the Neonate

Depending upon the timing of (embryonic–fetal) exposure to the aberrant fuel mixture, different events may develop.

Early in the first trimester, intrauterine growth restriction and organ malformation, described by Freinkel as "fuel-mediated teratogenesis" may occur. During the second trimester, at the time of brain development and differentiation, behavioral, intellectual, or psychological damage may occur. During the third trimester, abnormal proliferation of fetal adipocytes and muscle cells, together with hyperplasia of pancreatic beta cells and neuroendocrine cells may be responsible for the development of obesity, hypertension, and T2DM mellitus later in life.[30]

Fetal death has long been thought to be associated with GDM, but there have been no well-designed trials linking an increase in fetal death to GDM.

The complication that is perhaps the hallmark of GDM is macrosomia, defined as an infant weighing more than 9 lb (4 kg). One study defined macrosomia as a body weight greater than 9.9 lb (4.5 kg) and found a frequency of macrosomia of 14.0% in mothers with GDM and 6.3% in a control group of mothers without GDM ($p = 0.049$). In another large, retrospective study, 23% of infants born to mothers with GDM weighed more than 8.8 lb (4 kg), compared with 8% of infants born to nondiabetic women ($p < 0.001$).

Shoulder dystocia, a complication associated with macrosomia, is defined as impaction of the anterior fetal shoulder behind the maternal pubic symphysis. This can lead to fetal injury or uterine hemorrhage in the mother. The frequency of shoulder dystocia ranges from 0.6% to 2.8% of pregnancies. One study found a 3% rate in patients with GDM, versus 1% in control mothers ($p < 0.001$). The difference was thought to be due to macrosomia in infants secondary to maternal GDM. Another study found a frequency of shoulder dystocia of 35% in macrosomic births, versus 2% of infants born with a body weight of less than 9.9 lb.

Neonatal hypoglycemia occurs more often in pregnancies complicated by GDM, resulting in possible coma or even death if undetected. One study observed a 24% rate of neonatal hypoglycemia in infants born.

Delayed fetal lung maturation and surfactant production also is of concern particularly if labor is to be induced.

Other complications common with GDM include hypocalcemia, hyperbilirubinemia and polycythemia.

Major adverse effects of diabetes detected in first trimester include cardiac, respiratory, CNS, renal and urinary, limb defects, spinal defects and gastrointestinal malformations.

POSTPARTUM CARE

Lactation: All women including those with GDM should be actively encouraged to exclusively breastfeed to greatest possible during the first year. Women on insulin should have meal or snack before feeding to prevent hypoglycemia.

Breastfeeding has been shown to be protective against the occurrence of infant and maternal complications,[31] including reduction in childhood obesity, T2DM, and even T1DM.[32] Moreover, breastfeeding helps postpartum weight loss. Treatment with insulin or commonly used OADs, such as glyburide and metformin, is not a contraindication to breastfeeding as levels of OAD medications in breast milk are negligible and do not cause hypoglycemia in the baby.

Contraception: Choice to be individualized and chosen via cafeteria approach with regular follow-up and checking of glucose tolerance and lipid and other cardiovascular risk as per the standard guidelines.[33]

At each visit, BP should be measured and healthy lifestyle to be reinforced.

Postpartum screening: Patient to be screened 6 weeks postpartum with OGTT with 75 g oral glucose using WHO criteria for nonpregnant population and, if found in diabetic range should be referred to diabetologist or endocrinologist. High-risk women should be screened again at 6 months. Every time importance of diet and exercise should be reinforced.

PRECONCEPTION CARE

It is estimated that 30–90% of women have at least one condition or risk factor, such as anemia, malnutrition, obesity, diabetes, hypertension, and thyroid disorders, etc. that may benefit from an appropriate preconception intervention.[34-35]

We need to increase awareness and the concept of preconceptional counseling which can improve maternal health during pregnancy. Preconceptional counseling in the context of GDM not only rules out pre-existing diabetes but also identifies women who are at risk of GDM.

Only normalizing blood glucose levels in the preconception period and in early pregnancy will reduce the rate of congenital malformations seen with marked maternal hyperglycemia. In this context, postpartum care of GDM women is preconception care for a subsequent pregnancy.

PREVENTION OF GDM

Prevention of GDM can be grouped into three approaches:
1. Lifestyle changes
2. Pharmacological
3. Nonpharmacological

Lifestyle Changes

It seems obvious that lifestyle approaches should prevent GDM. Physical activity and healthy eating interventions, either separately or together, can prevent, or at least delay, type 2 diabetes for >9 months in the majority of women with impaired glucose tolerance, including those with previous GDM.[36-37]

In the Finnish Diabetes Prevention Study (FDPS), the more goals achieved, the greater the reduction in incidence type 2 diabetes, such that for the 20% achieving four to five of the five goals, none progressed to type 2 diabetes over 4 years.[38]

Pharmacological Approaches

The only drug to date that has been used for prevention of GDM is metformin, which has also been used extensively in women with polycystic ovarian syndrome (PCOS) before and during pregnancy.[39] While metformin is known to cross the placenta, there is no evidence of teratogenesis to date.

Nonpharmacological Approaches

Antenatal myoinositol has been proposed as a possible supplement that could increase insulin sensitivity and reduce GDM. Serum 25-hydroxyvitamin D (25OHD) concentration is inversely related to the risk of GDM, and a low vitamin D concentration (serum 25OHD <50 nmol/L) is associated with a 1.61 (95% CI 1.19–2.17) excess risk of GDM.[40]

A recent study examining probiotics in pregnancy suggested a benefit in reducing the incidence of gestational diabetes (Laitinen 2008).

Probiotic supplementation, if beneficial, would be much easier to use in clinical practice.

Key Points

- Prevention of GDM
- Lifestyle changes
- Metformin in PCOS
- Myoinositol
- Vitamin D supplementation
- Probiotics

REFERENCES

1. Proceedings of the 4th International Workshop-Conference on Gestational Diabetes Mellitus. Chicago, Illinois, USA. 14-16 March 1997. Diabetes Care. 1998;21(Suppl 2):B1–B167.
2. World Health Organization. Global status report on noncommunicable diseases 2010. *http://www.who.int/nmh/publications/ncd_report_full_en.pdf*. Published 2011.
3. Matyka KA. Type 2 diabetes in childhood: epidemiological and clinical aspects. Br Med Bull. 2008;86:59-75.
4. Bellamy L, Casas JP, Hingorani AD, Williams D. Type 2 diabetes mellitus after gestational diabetes: a systematic review and meta-analysis. Lancet. 2009;373(9677):1773–9.
5. Ratner RE, Christophi CA, Metzger BE, Dabelea D, Bennett PH, Pi-Sunyer X, et al. Prevention of diabetes in women with a history of gestational diabetes: effects of metformin and lifestyle interventions. J Clin Endocrinol Metab. 2008;93(12):4774-9.
6. Retnakaran R. Glucose tolerance status in pregnancy: a window to the future risk of diabetes and cardiovascular disease in young women. Curr Diabetes Rev. 2009;5(4):239-44.
7. Retnakaran R, Shah BR. Mild glucose intolerance in pregnancy and risk of cardiovascular disease: a population-based cohort study. CMAJ. 2009;181(6-7):371-6.
8. Kessous R, Shoham-Vardi I, Pariente G, Sherf M, Sheiner E. An association between gestational diabetes mellitus and long-term maternal cardiovascular morbidity. Heart. 2013;99(15):1118-21.

9. Mohammed Chyad Al-Noaemi, Mohammed Helmy Faris Shalayel. Pathophysiology of Gestational Diabetes Mellitus: The Past, the Present and the Future, Gestational Diabetes, Prof. Miroslav Radenkovic (Ed.), ISBN: 978-953-307-581-5, 2011.
10. World Health Organization. Diagnostic Criteria and Classification of Hyperglycaemia First Detected in Pregnancy. http://apps.who.int/iris/bit-stream/10665/85975/1/WHO_NMH_MND_13.2_eng.pdf. Published 2013.
11. Colagiuri S, Falavigna M, Agarwal MM, Boulvain M, Coetzee E, Hod M, et al. Strategies for implementing the WHO diagnostic criteria and classification of hyperglycaemia first detected in pregnancy. Diabetes Res Clin Pract. 2014;103(3):364-72.
12. International Association of Diabetes and Pregnancy Study Groups Consensus Panel, Metzger BE, Gabbe SG, Persson B, Buchanan TA, Catalano PA, et al. International association of diabetes and pregnancy study groups recommendations on the diagnosis and classification of hyperglycemia in pregnancy. Diabetes Care. 2010;33(3):676-82.
13. Anjalakshi C, Balaji V, Balaji MS, Ashalata S, Suganthi S, Arthi T, et al. A single test procedure to diagnose gestational diabetes mellitus. Acta Diabetol. 2009;46(1):51-4.
14. Seshiah V, Balaji V, Shah SN, Joshi S, Das AK, Sahay BK, et al. Diagnosis of gestational diabetes mellitus in the community. J Assoc Physicians India. 2012;60:15-7.
15. Hawkins JS, Casey BM, Lo JY, Moss K, McIntire DD, Leveno KJ. Weekly compared with daily blood glucose monitoring in women with diet-treated gestational diabetes. Obstet Gynecol. 2009;113(6):1307-12.
16. Jovanovic L, Savas H, Mehta M, Trujillo A, Pettitt DJ. Frequent monitoring of A1C during pregnancy as a treatment tool to guide therapy. Diabetes Care. 2011;34(1):53-4.
17. Freinkel N. Summary and recommendations of the Second International Workshop-Conference on Gestational Diabetes. Diabetes. 1985;34(Suppl 2):S123–S126.
18. American Diabetes Association. Gestational diabetes mellitus (Position Statement). Diabetes Care. 1998; 21(Suppl 1): S60–S61.
19. National Collaborating Centre for Women's and Children's Health (UK). Diabetes in Pregnancy: Management of Diabetes and its Complications from Preconception to the Postnatal Period. (NICE Clinical Guideline, No. 63). London: RCOG Press; 2008.
20. Pertot T, Molyneaux L, Tan K, Ross GP, Yue DK, Wong J. Can common clinical parameters be used to identify patients who will need insulin treatment in gestational diabetes mellitus? Diabetes Care. 2011;34(10):2214-6.
21. Langer O, Anyaegbunam A, Brustman L, Guidetti D, Levy J, Mazze R. Pregestational diabetes: insulin requirements throughout pregnancy. Am J Obstet Gynecol. 1988;159(3): 616-21.
22. Buchanan TA, Kjos SL. Gestational Diabetes: Risk ot Myth. J Clin Endocrinol Metab. 1999;84:1854-7.
23. Simons D, Thompson CF. Diabetes Care: 2001;24(12): 2078-82.
24. Grunberger G, Abelseth JM. AACE/ACE Consensus Statement on Insulin Pump Management: Endocr Pract. 2014;5:463-89.
25. Rudge MV, Calderon IM, Ramos MD, Peraçoli JC, Pim A. Hypertensive disorders in pregnant women with diabetes mellitus. Gynecol Obstet Invest. 1997;44(1):11-5.
26. Yogev Y, Xenakis EM, Langer O. The association between preeclampsia and the severity of gestational diabetes: the impact of glycemic control. Am J Obstet Gynecol. 2004;191(5):1655-60.
27. Ehrenberg HM, Durnwald CP, Catalano P, Mercer BM. The influence of obesity and diabetes on the risk of cesarean delivery. Am J Obstet Gynecol. 2004;191(3):969-74.
28. Peters RK, Kjos SL, Xiang A, Buchanan TA. Long-term diabetogenic effect of single pregnancy in women with previous gestational diabetes mellitus. Lancet. 1996;347(8996):227-30.
29. Kim C, Newton KM, Knopp RH. Gestational diabetes and the incidence of type 2 diabetes: a systematic review. Diabetes Care. 2002;25(10):1862-8.
30. Freinkel N. Banting Lecture 1980. Of pregnancy and progeny. Diabetes. 1980;29(12):1023-35.
31. Mayer-Davis EJ, Rifas-Shiman SL, Zhou L, Hu FB, Colditz GA, Gillman MW. Breastfeeding and risk for childhood obesity: Does maternal diabetes or obesity status matter? Diabetes Care. 2006;29(10):2231-7.
32. O'Reilly M, Avalos G, Dennedy MC, O'Sullivan EP, Dunne FP. Breastfeeding is associated with reduced postpartum maternal glucose intolerance after gestational diabetes. Ir Med J. 2012;105(5 Suppl):31-6.
33. Skouby SO, Mølsted-Pedersen L, Petersen KR. Contraception for women with diabetes: an update. Baillieres Clin Obstet Gynaecol. 1991;5(2):493-503.
34. Adams MM, Bruce FC, Shulman HB, Kendrick JS, Brogan DJ. Pregnancy planning and pre-conception counseling. The PRAMS Working Group. Obstet Gynecol. 1993;82(6):955-9.
35. Kim C, Ferrara A, McEwen LN, Marrero DG, Gerzoff RB, Herman WH, et al. Preconception care in managed care: the translating research into action for diabetes study. Am J Obstet Gynecol. 2005;192(1):227-32.
36. Knowler WC, Barrett-Connor E, Fowler SE, et al. Diabetes Prevention Program Research Group: reduction in the incidence of type 2 diabetes with lifestyle intervention or metformin. N Engl J Med. 2002;346:393-403.
37. Tuomilehto J, Lindstrom J, Eriksson JG, et al. Prevention of type 2 diabetes mellitus by changes in lifestyle among subjects with impaired glucose tolerance. N Engl J Med. 2001;344:1343-50.
38. Koivusalo SB, Rönö K, Klemetti MM, et al. Gestational diabetes mellitus can be prevented by lifestyle intervention: the Finnish Gestational Diabetes Prevention Study (RADIEL): a randomized controlled trial. Diabetes Care. 2016;39:24-30.
39. Ratner RE, Christophi CA, Metzger BE, et al. Diabetes Prevention Program Research Group: prevention of diabetes in women with a history of gestational diabetes: effects of metformin and lifestyle interventions. J Clin Endocrinol Metab. 2008;93:4774-9.
40. Corrado F, D'Anna R, Di Vieste G, et al. The effect of myoinositol supplementation on insulin resistance in patients with gestational diabetes. Diabet Med. 2011;28:972-5.

Chapter 18
Cardiac Diseases in Pregnancy

Niraj Jadav, Kirtan M Vyas

INTRODUCTION

Cardiac diseases in pregnancy can present challenges to cardiovascular and maternal-fetal management. Around 1–3% of all pregnancies are complicated by maternal cardiac disease, without pre-existing cardiac abnormalities that will result in approximately 15% of all maternal deaths. The heart diseases complicate between 0.25% and 1.0% of pregnancies in Indian population. There is a rising trend of maternal cardiac diseases in recent times because of increased prevalence of advanced maternal age, obesity, diabetes and moreover higher lifespan of patients with *congenital heart diseases* in present era.[1]

Pregnancy and labor inevitably increase cardiac strain and any complication will further add to this burden. So in a patient with cardiac disease preventive measures should be implicated right from preconception period. There are a few causes which can prove disastrous during pregnancy and might result in death for example, sudden arrhythmic death syndrome (SADS), cardiomyopathy, aortic dissection and rheumatic heart disease.

Cardiac diseases in pregnancy are broadly divided into 2 categories, namely congenital and acquired. The acquired group includes rheumatic heart disease, cardiomyopathies and ischemic heart disease. There has been a decrease in the cases of rheumatic heart diseases worldwide but it continues to be a leading cause in India. Rheumatic heart diseases account for the bulk of around 85–90%. The commonest valve involved is the mitral valve and the commonest lesion is mitral stenosis followed by mitral regurgitation and aortic stenosis. Congenital cardiac diseases include pre-existing disorders, those that develop during the course of the pregnancy or the postpartum period, congenital or acquired structural abnormalities and arrhythmias. In developed countries, there is a promising rate survival of newborns affected by congenital heart disease around 80%. As a consequence, the cardiologists and the obstetricians are today facing an increasingly large group of pregnant women with surgically corrected congenital abnormalities. Usually, the regurgitate lesions are better tolerated by patients compared to obstructive lesions.[2]

The medical management of the pregnant cardiac patient is controlled by the cardiologists or the intensive care specialists and anesthesiologists. The obstetrician, however, should have adequate information about cardiac diseases during pregnancy so that he can function effectively while taking care of the patient. Also, he should be able to diagnose and, in many cases, initiate the management of some of the medical complications that may affect the pregnant patient with heart disease.[3]

PRECONCEPTIONAL COUNSELING

Women with adverse cardiac conditions who desire or anticipate pregnancy should ideally be subjected to preconception counseling. The first step in the preconception counseling session is to obtain a thorough history, perform a physical examination, electrocardiograms and echocardiograms. The patient should be classified functionally and to be placed in a risk category as shown in **Tables 18.1 and 18.2**.

There has been a recommendation of the most important risk factors for a primary cardiac event or complication during pregnancy. It is considered to be 5% risk for a significant cardiac event, most commonly pulmonary edema or arrhythmia to pregnant patients with heart disease and none of the risk factors shown in **Table 18.3**. If one of these factors is present, the risk increases to 25%. If more than one of these factors is present, the risk assigned is 75%. This helped in

Table 18.1: New York Heart Association functional classification of cardiac disease

Grade I	Patients have no limitations of physical exercise; ordinary activity does not cause undue fatigue, palpitations, dyspnea, or angina
Grade II	Patients have slight limitations of physical exercise
Grade III	Patients have marked limitations of physical activity less than ordinary activity
Grade IV	Patients have an inability to carry on physical activity without symptoms

Table 18.2: Risk of cardiac events during pregnancy in women with heart disease	

Low risk	• Small left to right shunts such as ASD, VSD, and PDA
	• PDA repaired lesions with normal cardiac function
	• Mild-to-moderate pulmonic or tricuspid lesions
	  – Marfan's syndrome with normal aortic root
	  – Homograft or bioprosthetic valves
	  – Bicuspid aortic valve without stenosis

Intermediate risk	• Uncorrected cyanotic heart disease
	  – Large left to right shunt
	  – Uncorrected, uncomplicated aortic stenosis
	  – Mechanical valve prosthesis
	  – Severe pulmonic stenosis
	  – Moderate to severe left ventricular dysfunction
	  – Previous left ventricular dysfunction now resolved (such as peripartum cardiomyopathy)
	  – Previous myocardial infarction

High risk	• Pulmonary hypertension
	  – Marfan's syndrome with aortic valve involvement
	  – Cardiomyopathy
	  – Complicated aortic coarctation

Table 18.3: Predictors of cardiac events during pregnancy	
N	New York Heart Association Grade > II
O	Obstructive lesions of he left heart • Mitral valve < 2 cm • Aortic valve < 1.5 cm • Gradient peak > 30
P	Prior cardiac event before pregnancy • Heart failure • Arrhythmia • Transient ischemic attack • Stroke
E	Ejection fraction < 40%

explaining to the patient the need for further testing during pregnancy, increased frequency of visits, need for prolonged hospitalization, and in some cases, the need for surgical or medical procedures before pregnancy. Risk assessment is also useful to decide where the patient should be going for labor. Every effort should be made to make the patient deliver in a well-equipped tertiary care center.

The physician must discuss clinical problems that women may develop during pregnancy. The desirability of future conception, the current fitness and status of the patient to embark on a pregnancy and the anticipated complications during pregnancy and delivery and their risks to the mother and the fetus are the important areas to be discussed with patient and her husband. Heart failure, pulmonary edema, fatal arrhythmias, aortic dissection, and any other complications pertinent to their specific cardiac condition and their functional and risk classification should also be discussed openly. The need for induction of labor, shortening of the second stage of labor, methods of anesthesia used during labor and delivery, endocarditis prophylaxis, and anticoagulation therapy should be a part of preconception counseling.

HEMODYNAMIC CHANGES DURING PREGNANCY

The physiology of pregnant woman starts adapting to changes during pregnancy. Multiple changes take place in the circulation. These bear a significant impact on the heart and its functions and have many implications on the management of cardiac diseases for the obstetricians. The marked hemodynamic changes developing during normal pregnancy can mimic signs and symptoms of heart disease. All the changes which happen during pregnancy can lead to decompensation of previously well-tolerated lesions. The most important points are that normal pregnancy significantly increases the workload of the heart, circulation is hyperdynamic, and a high cardiac output is present.[4] The increase in cardiac output starts at about 8–10 weeks, reaches a maximum at about 28–32 weeks and it is high thereafter till the patient delivers. The rise in cardiac output is initially determined by an increase in stroke volume. Later, as pregnancy advances, there is an increase in heart rate of 10–15 beats/minute that will contribute to this change.

Peripheral vascular resistance decreases during pregnancy. Compression of inferior vena cava by the large uterus in the supine position results in a decrease in the venous return to the heart leading to lowering of cardiac output and decrease in blood pressure. It is important to understand that even if there is a fall after 32 weeks, the cardiac output at term is still significantly greater than the basal non-pregnant state. In women with *Marfan's syndrome*, there is an increase in size and compliance of the aortic root. That might contribute aortic dissection, especially those who have dilated aortic roots before they get pregnant. A clinician must be keeping watch on certain warning signs; for example, worsening dyspnea or dyspnea at rest, increasing rales and rhonchi in the chest, worsening chest pain with exertion, syncope preceded by palpitation, loud cardiac murmurs, cyanosis or clubbing, jugular venous distension, cardiomegaly or ventricular heave, increasing edema of the lower limbs or back.

During labor, both the heart rate and blood pressure rise. The cardiac output and oxygen consumption may increase during uterine contractions.[5] There is further increase in cardiac output in the immediate postpartum period. Hemodynamically, a shift occurs from the extravascular space, the decrease in uterine size relieves the pressure on inferior vena cava, thereby increasing venous return and cardiac output. These all changes begin to reverse within one to three days after delivery and the cardiac output falls to non-pregnant levels in two weeks postpartum.

Centre for Maternal and Child Enquiries (CMACE) states that a pregnant woman must be evaluated further if she complains of chest pain which is severe, radiating or associated with breathlessness, vomiting, tachycardia or other features. Obese women or those who have hypertension need a special concern.[6]

EFFECT OF PREGNANCY ON MATERNAL CARDIAC DISEASE

Patients with cardiac disease experience great hemodynamic alterations during the period of pregnancy. The increased circulatory load in pregnancy modifies the cardiac reserve predisposing to decompensation and congestive heart failure. Maternal mortality rises to a profound number in these patients.[7]

There is an increased risk of endocarditis. These patients have a tendency of hypercoagulation. This along with atrial fibrillation increases the risks of thrombosis and embolism. There can be some special phases in pregnancy when the danger of cardiac decompensation is specially great. The first one is between 12 and 16 weeks of gestation when the hemodynamic changes of pregnancy begin. A second critical period is between 28 and 32 weeks of gestation when the hemodynamic changes of pregnancy peak and cardiac demands are at a maximum. Another dangerous time for pregnant cardiac patients is during labor and delivery with a special concern of postpartum period.

EFFECTS OF MATERNAL CARDIAC DISEASE ON PREGNANCY

Pregnancy outcome is affected by the presence of cardiac disease to a major extent. The severity of the underlying lesion and the degree of hypertension and hypoxia are the major determinants. Fetal morbidity is usually secondary to preterm delivery and fetal growth restriction, conditions that frequently occur in pregnant women with heart disease. This is probably due to their relative inability to maintain an adequate uteroplacental circulation. The frequency of these problems is related to the severity of the functional impairment of the heart and severity of the chronic tissue hypoxia. Another fetal risk is that of congenital heart disease. If the mother has congenital heart disease, there is an increased incidence of fetal congenital cardiovascular anomalies.

Adequate prenatal care, hospitalization, and intensive care are what one requires to safeguard the fetus along with the mother.[8] Fetal death still occurs in pregnancy with cardiac disease, mostly in mothers with cyanotic heart conditions.

GENERAL MEASURES FOR THE CARE OF PREGNANT PATIENTS WITH HEART DISEASE

Evaluation of the cardiac status should be done as early in pregnancy as possible. Moreover, preconception advices are of great importance whenever possible. The patient needs to be informed about the risks so that to have a choice of MTP when indicated.[9] The level of antepartum care required by pregnant women with heart disease depends on their risk classification. The role of the primary care physician and the high-risk obstetrics specialist is to monitor the fetal condition and the maternal cardiac function at frequent intervals in order to determine if the physiological changes elicited by pregnancy are exceeding the functional capacity of the heart and, in some cases, to use medications to limit the extent of these changes and improve the outcome. The anesthesiologist should be consulted early in pregnancy to assess the anesthetic risk of the patient and discuss with her the pain control that she will receive during labor and delivery. The cardiologist should be consulted on regular basis. Early in the pregnancy and particularly if the fetus is affected by congenital heart disease, the patient should see the neonatologist and, if necessary, the pediatric cardiologist to discuss possible neonatal outcomes and to find out what to expect when the baby is born. There are a few indications for MTP for heart diseases in pregnancy and they require a consideration. These include Eisenmenger syndrome, *New York Heart Association (NYHA) grades* III and IV, pulmonary hypertension, selected cases with prosthetic valves, patients with critical *mitral stenosis*—who may plan pregnancy postsurgery and heart transplant patients. It is noteworthy that nonsurgical cardiac intervention has improved the prognosis for a better obstetric outcome of patients with pregnancy and co-existing heart diseases.[10]

EVALUATION OF CARDIAC FUNCTION DURING PREGNANCY

Evaluation of the cardiac response of the patient with heart disease is done mainly by clinical observation, ECG and echocardiography. Women with congenital heart diseases can be evaluated with genetic counseling and fetal echocardiography. The NYHA functional classification should be assessed in every visit. Easy fatigability, shortness of breath, orthopnea, and pulmonary congestion are signs and symptoms characteristic of left-sided heart failure. Weight gain, dependent edema, hepatomegaly, and raised JVP are signs and symptoms suggestive of right-sided heart failure.

The women may present with varying degrees of biventricular failure and signs and symptoms of left or right failure may predominate, depending on the defect causing the CHF.[11] Patients with peripartum cardiomyopathy (PPCM) have signs and symptoms of biventricular failure. One thing to mention is that shortness of breath is one of the most common complaints of left-side failure and normal pregnant women may complain the same. The breath hunger that occurs during pregnancy is usually not severe so she has to limit the routine activities. A patient with LVF often complains of limitation of activities or cough. The most important sign of left-sided failure is the presence of bibasilar rales. The signs and symptoms of right-sided heart failure are different from that of the LVF. RVF tends to produce systemic venous congestion. Raised jugular venous pressure, hepatomegaly, and dependent edema are seen in such cases. The first two of these signs are not present in normal pregnancy but the last is normally present.

The physicians taking care of patients are supposed to see at each prenatal visit for clinical evidence suggesting the onset of heart failure. Deterioration of the NYHA functional classification due to increase in body weight, orthopnea, tachycardia, and hepatomegaly and the presence of pulmonary rales may point to CHF and demand further evaluation. In such cases the cardiologist should come into picture and the patient should be admitted to the hospital for further assessment and treatment.

COMPLICATIONS OF CARDIAC DISEASES IN PREGNANCY

Palpitations and arrhythmias are not uncommon during pregnancy. Atrial fibrillation, in particular, can lead to embolism and so is considered as an emergency. Patients with atrial fibrillation must receive prophylactic anticoagulation, even in the absence of other risk factors. Supraventricular tachycardia and ventricular tachyarrhythmia are less common during pregnancy. Mitral Stenosis, the commonest heart lesion during pregnancy, can lead to pulmonary venous hypertension and congestion with pulmonary edema. Radiological features like cephalization of pulmonary vascular markings, Kerley B lines, 'hilar moustache' and eventually frank pulmonary edema and whitening of lung fields are usually seen. The compensatory rise in systemic venous pressure is observed as three 'E's, namely Elevation of jugular venous pressure, Enlarged liver and Edema of ankles. Acute rheumatic carditis might lead to sudden death. Subacute endocarditis mainly occurs due to *Streptococcus viridans* and mainly seen in younger patients with mobile valves. A pregnant patient with heart disease has five times the risk of dying compared to normal pregnant woman and majority of the deaths occur in postpartum. Cardiac failure with or without pulmonary edema account for almost 75% of all deaths. A satisfactory outcome is expected with careful antepartum, intrapartum and postpartum management. Although some patients may not have the hemodynamic capacity to tolerate pregnancy, many have sufficient cardiac reserve to safely carry pregnancy to term.

MANAGEMENT OF WOMEN WITH HEART DISEASE

Antepartum

Bedrest can be regarded as one of the most important measures for attenuating the impact of pregnancy on heart. Bedrest increases the venous return to the heart, improves renal perfusion, induces dieresis, and promotes elimination of water. Bedrest reduces the metabolic needs of several organs, the blood flow to these organs at rest decreases markedly, so is the workload on the heart.

Define limits of activity, diet which should be simple and easily digestible and at the same time nutritious. Dietary salt restriction is a measure which helps to prevent excessive retention of sodium and water. Most pregnant cardiac patients tolerate a moderate sodium dietary restriction (4–6 g daily).[12]

Prophylactic digitalization is commonly used in pregnant patients with severe heart disease who are not in overt CHF. The objective of using prophylactic digitalization is to improve the contractility of the heart and to relieve symptoms such as easy fatigability, orthopnea, and weakness. A secondary benefit is to avoid the production of ventricular tachycardia and rapid atrial rhythms. Digitalis crosses the placenta, but can be used after weighing risk-benefit ratio. There is a risk of preterm labor and decreased uterine flow following the use of inotropic drugs. ACE inhibitors are a strict NO due to their teratogenic effects. Aldosterone antagonists like spironolactone are not used as they may cause feminization of male fetus. Other treatments of heart failure in the form of nonthiazide diuretics or nitrates may be continued depending on disease severity and fetal risk.

Women with congenital heart disease frequently require anticoagulation during pregnancy. The need for anticoagulation is apparent in women with artificial mechanical valve prosthesis and with chronic or recurrent arrhythmias. Various approaches have been attempted for anticoagulation. Either *LMWH* or *Unfractionated Heparin* can be used throughout the pregnancy or they can be used till 13 weeks of pregnancy with *Warfarin* from 13 to 35 weeks and return to heparin thereafter till delivery.

DURING LABOR AND DELIVERY

Preterm labor and growth restriction are the commonest problems faced by obstetricians. Vaginal delivery is advantageous than cesarean section for women with heart disease because of benefits of smaller volume shifts, less hemorrhage and fewer infections. Cesareans are reserved for obstetric indications.[13] Routine oxytocics during the third stage of labor should be avoided. A little extra blood loss during the third stage acts like an exit valve preventing sudden cardiac overload after delivery. Maternal hemodynamic circulation adjustment occurs better during the course of normal labor. However, a long labor and a difficult vaginal delivery are much more morbid than a cesarean and, in many cases, it is preferable to avoid the hemodynamic effects of labor and delivery by performing a quick cesarean section. Lateral decubitus is always preferred in a laboring patient in order to avoid the hemodynamic problems caused by the dorsal decubitus.

The patient should be offered adequate pain relief during labor. Epidural analgesia remains the method of choice. In a low resource setting, application of programmed labor protocols remains effective alternative and preferred. Analgesia is effective in reducing tachycardia, myocardial work, and cardiac output. It has been calculated that pain during labor increases the cardiac output 50% above the elevation normally seen during the second stage of labor.

Moreover, at the same time in a laboring patient, IV fluids should also be restricted. Almost all cardiac patients in labor should be kept on the "dry" side and IV fluids administered to no more than 75 mL per hour.

Pulse oximetry monitoring is mandatory during labor. Mild degrees of desaturation may be corrected by oxygen administration via nasal prongs rebreathing mask. Desaturation during labor that is not corrected by oxygen is suggestive of the development of pulmonary edema.

Antibiotic prophylaxis is given to patients with congenital or acquired heart lesions and with artificial valve prosthesis at the time of delivery in order to avoid subacute bacterial endocarditis.

Cardiac patients who are not anticoagulated might develop thromboembolization in the postpartum period. The factors responsible are relative immobilization, pooling of blood in the lower extremities, and alterations in coagulation and fibrinolysis. Therefore, it is important to initiate ambulation immediately, use pneumatic compression of the lower extremities, and give prophylactic low-dose-heparin during labor, delivery, and the immediate postpartum period. In the postpartum period, the uterus markedly decreases in size and ceases to obstruct the return circulation to the heart. Plus most of the blood contained in the uterine vessels is suddenly infused into the systemic circulation. So these physiological alterations combine to increase the blood volume to a point where it may exceed the ability of the heart to pump effectively, and that might result in acute pulmonary edema. These patients should be placed in the sitting position following delivery.

At the time of delivery, oxytocin is given to make the uterus contract and to avoid intrapartum and postpartum bleeding. In the cardiac patient, it is important not to administer the medication as an intravenous bolus. Also, cardiac patients should not be supplemented with ergotamine for PPH because it can cause significant vasoconstriction and elevation of blood pressure, which can lead to dangerous consequences.

POSTPARTUM

The first 12 hours after the delivery are the most crucial because the right-sided heart suffers some overload with the diversion of blood that normally would have gone to the placenta and the uterus. One has to watch for signs of pulmonary congestion and edema. Cardiomyopathy patients carry a poor prognosis, especially if they have decreased LVEF and if the heart remains dilated after 6 months of therapy. Sedatives are to be given to reduce anxiety tachycardia. Bedrest is advisable for first few days. Infection prevention remains the prime target for the clinician and the patient. *Contraceptive* instructions form a major part and should be offered at the earliest. Barrier contraceptives should be advised in these couples. Depot provera every 3 months or low dose OC pills after 6 weeks form a good choice in patients who are not willing for permanent methods.

IMPORTANT POINTS

1. Obstetricians nowadays are facing increasing number of pregnancies with cardiac diseases. Rheumatic heart disease still remains the leading cause in India.
2. Pregnancies with congenital heart disease in mothers are on a rise because of increased survival of children due to surgical correction in childhood.
3. Preconception counseling and examination should be offered whenever possible. The condition can be defined and the risk assessment is possible with that.
4. There is a marked alteration in hemodynamic circulation during pregnancy. In a patient with heart disease, these changes might prove disastrous at times depending on the pre-existing cardiac condition.
5. MTP is advisable when patient falls into high-risk category according to the classification and guidelines.
6. The patient should be explained regarding the warning signs of worsening the symptoms.
7. There can be some deleterious effects of pregnancy on the existing cardiac disease as well as of the cardiac disease on pregnancy.

8. Multidisciplinary approach by the team of an obstetrician, cardiologist and intensive care specialist should be employed in the management of cardiac disease with pregnancy.
9. Bedrest, salt-restriction in diet, prophylactic digitalization and requirement of anticoagulation are the areas to be taken care in antepartum phase.
10. Labor is stressful but vaginal delivery is preferred except obstetric indications. Programmed labor is a good choice in a low resource setting.
11. Postpartum phase is crucial in terms of hemodynamic adjustments and a close watch is necessary.
12. Contraceptive advice remains an important area in the post-pregnancy period.

REFERENCES

1. Avila WS, Rossi EG, Ramires JA, et al. Pregnancy in patients with heart disease; experience with 1000 cases. Clin Cardiol; 2003.p.26.
2. Bonnow RO, Carabello B, de lanon AC/AHA guidelines for the management of patient with valvular heart disease, 1998.
3. Daftary SN, Desai SV. Heart disease complicating pregnancy selected topics in obstetrics and gynaecology (2nd edition) BI publication, 2006.
4. Presbitero P, Somerville JK, Stone S, et al. Congenital heart disease; outcome of mother and foetus, 1994.
5. Siu S, Colman JM. Cardiovascular problems in pregnancy; an approach to management cleve. Clin J Med, 2004.
6. Saving Mothers Lives. Reviewing Maternal Deaths to make Motherhood Safer: 2006-2008; Centre for Maternal and Child Enquiries (CMACE), BJOG, 2011.
7. Tank DK, Paghadiwalla KP. Maternal and fetal outcome in cardiac disease current concepts FOGSI publication, 2001.
8. ACOG prophylactic antibiotics in labor and pregnancy. ACOG practice bulletin no 47, October 2003.
9. Cardiac disease in pregnancy; practical guide to high-risk pregnancy South Asian perspective, 3rd edition, 2008.
10. Zuber M, Gautschi N, et al. Outcome of pregnancy in women with congenital shunt lesion, 1999.
11. Stout K. Pregnancy in Women with Congenital Heart Disease: The importance of Evaluation and Counseling. Heart. 2005;91(6):713-4.
12. Steer PJ. Pregnancy and Contraception. Adult Congenital Heart Disease: A Practical Guide, Oxford BMJ Publishing. 2005. pp.16-35.
13. Elkayam U. Pregnancy and cardiovascular diseases. Brraunwald's Heart Disease: A Textbook of Cardiovascular Medicine, 7th edn. Philadelphia PA: WB Saunders; 2005. pp.1965-81.

Chapter 19: Specific Cardiac Conditions and Complications During Pregnancy

Tripti Deb, Amit Bharadiya, Richa Baharani

INTRODUCTION

Around 0.2–4% of all pregnancies are complicated by cardiovascular disease (CVD)[1] and these numbers have seen a rising trend because of the increase in prevalence of hypertension, diabetes, obesity and maternal age. Advances in treatment of coronary heart disease (CHD) have resulted in more number of CHD patients attaining the childbearing age and ultimately adding to the number of cases. A working knowledge of the normal physiology of pregnancy and risks associated with specific cardiac conditions during pregnancy and their management is often helpful in the management of pregnant patients with heart disease.

PHYSIOLOGICAL CHANGES IN THE CARDIOVASCULAR SYSTEM DURING PREGNANCY

Pregnancy is a dynamic process associated with significant physiological changes in the cardiovascular system (CVS). These changes (Table 19.1) are mechanisms that the body has adapted to meet the increased metabolic demands of the mother and fetus and to ensure adequate uteroplacental circulation for fetal growth and development. Insufficient hemodynamic changes can result in maternal and fetal morbidity, as seen in pre-eclampsia and intrauterine growth retardation. In addition, maternal inability to adapt to these physiological changes can expose underlying, previously silent, cardiac pathology, which is why some call pregnancy nature's stress test.

Changes in the CVS in pregnancy begin as early as 5 weeks and by eight weeks of gestation, the cardiac output increases up to 20%. The primary event is probably peripheral vasodilatation which is mediated by endothelium-dependent factors, including nitric oxide synthesis, upregulated by estradiol and possibly vasodilatory prostaglandins (PGI). Peripheral vasodilation leads to a 25–30% fall in systemic vascular resistance, and to compensate for this, cardiac output increases by around 40% during pregnancy. This is achieved predominantly via an increase in stroke volume, but

Table 19.1: Cardiovascular changes in pregnancy

Changes System	Parameters	First trimester	Second trimester	Third trimester	Labor	Post-partum
Hemodynamic	Cardiac output	↑	↑↑	↑↑	↑↑↑↑	↓
	Stroke volume	↑	↑	↓	↑	↓
	Heart rate	↑	↑↑	↑↑↑	↑↑↑↑	↓
	Blood pressure	↓	↓	↔	↑	↓
	Systemic vascular resistance	↓	↓↓	↓↓	↑	↓
	Plasma volume	↑↑	↑↑↑	↑↑↑↑	↑↑↑↑↑	↓
	Red blood cell mass	↑	↑↑	↑↑	Autotransfusion	↓
Structural changes in heart	Left ventricle wall mass	↑	↑	↑	–	↓
	Chamber size	All four chamber enlargement				↓
	Aorta	Increased distensibility				↓

also to a lesser extent, an increase in heart rate. The maximum cardiac output (CO) is found at about 20–28 weeks gestation. There is a minimal fall at term.

An increase in stroke volume is possible due to the early increase in ventricular wall muscle mass and end-diastolic volume seen in pregnancy. The heart is physiologically dilated and myocardial contractility is increased. Although stroke volume declines towards term, the increase in maternal heart rate (HR) of 10–20 beats per minute (bpm) is maintained, thus preserving the increased cardiac output. Blood pressure (BP) decreases in the first and second trimesters but increases to non-pregnant levels in the third trimester. There is a profound effect of maternal position towards term upon the hemodynamic profile of both the mother and fetus. In the supine position, pressure of the gravid uterus on the inferior vena cava (IVC) causes a reduction in venous return to the heart and a consequent fall in stroke volume and CO. Turning from the lateral to the supine position may result in a 25% reduction in cardiac output. Pregnant women should therefore be nursed in the left or right lateral position, wherever possible. If the woman has to be kept on her back, the pelvis should be rotated so that the uterus drops to the side and off the IVC, and CO and uteroplacental blood flow are optimized. Reduced CO is associated with a reduction in uterine blood flow and therefore in placental perfusion, which could compromise the fetus. Although both blood volume and stroke volume increase in pregnancy, pulmonary capillary wedge pressure and central venous pressure do not increase significantly. Pulmonary vascular resistance (PVR), like systemic vascular resistance (SVR), decreases significantly in normal pregnancy. Although there is no increase in pulmonary capillary wedge pressure (PCWP), serum colloid osmotic pressure is reduced by 10–15%. The colloid osmotic pressure/pulmonary capillary wedge pressure gradient is reduced by about 30%, making pregnant women particularly susceptible to pulmonary edema. Pulmonary edema will be precipitated, if there is either an increase in cardiac preload (such as infusion of fluids) or increased pulmonary capillary permeability (such as in pre-eclampsia) or both. Labor is associated with further increases in CO, i.e. 15% in the first stage and 50% in the second stage. Uterine contractions lead to an auto-transfusion of 300–500 mL of blood back into the circulation and the sympathetic response to pain and anxiety further elevate the HR and BP. CO is increased between contractions but more so during contractions.

Following delivery, there is an immediate rise in CO due to relief of the IVC obstruction and contraction of the uterus, which empties blood into the systemic circulation. CO increases by 60–80%, followed by a rapid decline to pre-labor values within about one hour of delivery. Transfer of fluid from the extravascular space increases venous return and stroke volume further. Those women with cardiovascular compromise are therefore most at risk of pulmonary edema during the second stage of labor and the immediate postpartum period. CO has nearly returned to normal (pre-pregnancy values) two weeks after delivery, although some pathological changes (e.g. hypertension in pre-eclampsia) may take much longer. The above physiological changes lead to changes on cardiovascular examination that may be misinterpreted as pathological by those unfamiliar with pregnancy.

Changes may include a bounding or collapsing pulse and an ejection systolic murmur, present in over 90% of pregnant women. The murmur may be loud and audible all over the precordium, with the first heart sound loud and possibly sometimes a third heart sound. There may be ectopic beats and peripheral edema. Normal findings on ECG in pregnancy that may partly relate to changes in the position of the heart include atrial and ventricular ectopics, Q wave (small) and inverted T wave in lead III, ST-segment depression and T-wave inversion in the inferolateral leads and left-axis shift of QRS.

ASSESSMENT OF RISK IN PATIENTS WITH CARDIAC DISEASE

Cardiac conditions can be pre-existing (e.g. rheumatic or congenital heart disease) and unmasked by increased volume load in pregnancy, or can be caused by pregnancy [e.g. hypertensive disorders or peripartum cardiomyopathy (PPCM)].[2,3] Physicians are therefore increasingly faced with providing adequate counseling on pregnancy risk to women wishing to conceive who are known to have cardiac disease (e.g. operated congenital heart disease or previous valve replacement because of rheumatic heart disease), or present in the advanced stage of pregnancy (>20 weeks) having heart failure because of pre-existing or newly acquired cardiac disease.

The 2011 ESC guidelines recommend that maternal risk assessment should be carried out according to the modified World Health Organization (mWHO) risk classification.[4] This risk classification integrates all known maternal cardiovascular risk factors including the underlying heart disease and any other comorbidity. It includes contraindications for pregnancy that are not incorporated in the other risk scores/predictors. The general principles of this classification are depicted in **Table 19.2**. A practical application is given in **Table 19.3**. Women in mWHO class I have a very low risk and cardiology follow-up during pregnancy may be limited to one or two visits. Those in mWHO II are at low or moderate risk, and follow-up every trimester is recommended. For women in mWHO class III, there is a high risk of complications and frequent (monthly or bimonthly) cardiology and obstetric review during pregnancy is recommended. Women in WHO class IV should be advised against pregnancy; but if they become pregnant and will not consider termination, monthly

Table 19.2: Modified WHO classification of maternal cardiovascular risk: Principles

Risk class	Risk of pregnancy by medical condition
I	No detectable increased risk of maternal mortality and no/mild increase in morbidity.
II	Small increased risk of maternal mortality or moderate increase in morbidity.
III	Significantly increased risk of maternal mortality or severe morbidity. Expert counseling required. If pregnancy is decided upon, intensive specialist cardiac and obstetric monitoring needed throughout pregnancy, childbirth, and the puerperium.
IV	Extremely high risk of maternal mortality or severe morbidity; pregnancy contraindicated. If pregnancy occurs termination should be discussed. If pregnancy continues, care as for class III.

Table 19.3: Modified WHO classification of maternal cardiovascular risk: Applications

Conditions in which pregnancy risk is WHO I	*Uncomplicated, small or mild* • Pulmonary stenosis • Patent ductus arteriosus • Mitral valve prolapse Successfully repaired simple lesions (atrial or ventricular septal defect, patent ductus arteriosus, anomalous pulmonary venous drainage). Atrial or ventricular ectopic beats.
Conditions in which pregnancy risk is WHO II or III	*WHO II (if otherwise well and uncomplicated)* • Unoperated atrial or ventricular septal defect • Repaired tetralogy of Fallot • Most arrhythmias *WHO II–III (depending on individual)* • Mild left ventricular impairment • Hypertrophic cardiomyopathy • Native or tissue valvular heart disease not considered WHO I or IV • Marfan syndrome without aortic dilatation • Aorta <45 mm in aortic disease associated with bicuspid aortic valve • Repaired coarctation *WHO III* • Mechanical valve • Systemic right ventricle • Fontan circulation • Cyanotic heart disease (unrepaired) • Other complex congenital heart disease • Aortic dilatation 40–45 mm in Marfan syndrome • Aortic dilatation 45–50 mm in aortic disease associated with bicuspid aortic valve
Conditions in which pregnancy risk is WHO IV (pregnancy contraindicated)	• Pulmonary arterial hypertension of any cause • Severe systemic ventricular dysfunction (LVEF <30%, NYHA III–IV) • Previous peripartum cardiomyopathy with any residual impairment of left ventricular function • Severe mitral stenosis, severe symptomatic aortic stenosis • Marfan syndrome with aorta dilated >45 mm • Aortic dilatation >50 mm in aortic disease associated with bicuspid aortic valve • Native severe coarctation

Table 19.4: Maternal predictors of neonatal events in women with heart disease

1. Baseline NYHA class >II or cyanosis
2. Maternal left heart obstruction
3. Smoking during pregnancy
4. Multiple gestation
5. Use of oral anticoagulants during pregnancy
6. Mechanical valve prosthesis

or bimonthly review is needed. Neonatal complications occur in 20-28% of patients with heart disease[5-7] with a neonatal mortality between 1% and 4%.[5-7] Maternal and neonatal events are highly correlated. Predictors of neonatal complications are listed in **Table 19.4**.

Iris van Hagen and colleagues[8] validated the mWHO risk classification in advanced and emerging countries and identified additional risk factors for cardiac events during pregnancy using data from the registry of pregnancy and cardiac disease (ROPAC), which includes more than 2500 pregnant women. The spectrum of cardiac disease differed in advanced versus emerging countries with congenital heart disease being the most prevalent diagnosis in advanced countries and valvular heart disease and cardiomyopathies being the most common diagnoses in emerging countries. There was a substantial difference in cardiac events between regions, occurring in 12.8% of patients in advanced countries versus 36.3% in emerging countries. The mWHO classification showed only a moderate performance in predicting risk between women with or without cardiac events [c-statistic 0.711, 95% confidence interval (CI) 0.686-0.735] with a better performance in advanced countries compared with emerging countries.

SPECIFIC CARDIAC LESIONS

Congenital Heart Disease and Pulmonary Hypertension

The number of adults with congenital heart disease now outnumbers children, reflecting improved surgical outcomes and medical care over recent decades. Young women with uncomplicated secundum type atrial septal defect (ASD) or isolated ventricular septal defect (VSD) usually tolerate pregnancy well. Patent ductus arteriosus (PDA) is not associated with an additional maternal risk for cardiac complications, if the shunt is small to moderate, and if pulmonary artery pressures are normal. Once these shunts are repaired, the risk during pregnancy is minimal. It is unusual for women with such left to right shunts to develop pulmonary hypertension during the childbearing years; however, the presence of pulmonary hypertension with a left to right shunt substantially increases the risk of complications during pregnancy.

Pulmonary hypertension (PHT) is defined at cardiac catheter as a mean pulmonary pressure ≥25 mm Hg at rest or 30 mm Hg on exercise. Pregnancy in the presence of PHT of any cause remains high risk. Fixed pulmonary vascular resistance prevents any increase in pulmonary blood flow to match the increased cardiac output. Pregnancy is poorly tolerated with a risk of worsening cyanosis and hypoxia, arrhythmias, heart failure and death. The majority of complications occur at term or during the first postpartum week. Maternal mortality depends on the underlying cause, with mortality rates of 36% in Eisenmenger's syndrome, 30% in primary pulmonary hypertension and 56% in secondary pulmonary hypertension reported.[9] Patients should be advised of these risks when contemplating pregnancy. Anticoagulation, oxygen therapy and pulmonary vasodilators (sildenafil, nitric oxide or prostacyclins [endothelin antagonists are contraindicated in pregnancy]) may improve outcome.[10] The postpartum period is particularly high risk for maternal mortality and, as such, high dependency care should continue for several days post-delivery.

Valvular Heart Disease

Owing to a fall in peripheral vascular resistance, left-sided valvular regurgitant abnormalities are generally well tolerated in pregnancy. However, the increased stroke volume of pregnancy and delivery can have profound effects in the presence of left-sided stenotic valvular abnormalities.

Mitral Regurgitation

Chronic mitral regurgitation (MR) most commonly is the result of myxomatous degeneration or rheumatic heart disease and usually is well tolerated during pregnancy. However, new-onset atrial fibrillation or severe hypertension can precipitate hemodynamic deterioration. Acute MR (e.g. from rupture of chordae tendineae) may produce flash pulmonary edema and life-threatening cardiac decompensation. Women with severe MR and signs of cardiac decompensation before pregnancy are advised to undergo operative repair before conception. Mitral valve prolapse in isolation rarely causes any difficulties during pregnancy.

Aortic Regurgitation

Aortic regurgitation (AR) may be encountered in women with rheumatic heart disease, a congenitally bicuspid or deformed aortic valve, infective endocarditis, or connective tissue disease. AR generally is well tolerated during pregnancy. Ideally, women with severe AR and signs of cardiac decompensation should undergo operative repair before conception. Women with bicuspid aortic valves, with or without AR, are at increased risk for aortic dissection and should be followed carefully for signs and symptoms of this complication. Congestive heart failure from MR or AR can be treated with digoxin, diuretics, and vasodilators, such as hydralazine. Angiotensin-converting enzyme inhibitors (ACEI) are teratogenic, and therefore contraindicated. Beta-blockers are generally safe during pregnancy, although fetal bradycardia and growth retardation have been reported.

Mitral Stenosis

Mitral stenosis (MS) in women of childbearing age is most often rheumatic in origin. Patients with moderate-to-severe MS often experience hemodynamic deterioration during the third trimester or during labor and delivery. The physiologic increase in blood volume and rise in heart rate lead to an elevation of left atrial pressure, resulting in pulmonary edema formation. Additional displacement of blood volume into the systemic circulation during contractions makes labor particularly hazardous. The development of atrial fibrillation in the pregnant patient with mitral stenosis may result in rapid decompensation. Digoxin and beta-blockers can be used to reduce heart rate, and diuretics can be used to reduce the blood volume and left atrial pressure gently. With atrial fibrillation and hemodynamic deterioration, electrocardioversion can be performed safely. The development of atrial fibrillation increases the risk of stroke, necessitating the initiation of anticoagulation. Mild mitral stenosis can often be managed with careful medical therapy during pregnancy. In contrast, patients with moderate-to-severe mitral stenosis should be referred to a cardiologist. Severe MS is associated with a high likelihood of maternal complications (including pulmonary edema and arrhythmias) or fetal complications (including premature birth, low birth weight, respiratory distress, and fetal or neonatal death), approaching 80% of pregnancies.[11] These women may require correction via operative repair or replacement or percutaneous mitral balloon valvotomy before conception or during pregnancy. During pregnancy, percutaneous valvotomy is usually deferred to the second or third trimesters to avoid fetal radiation exposure during the first trimester. Most patients with MS can undergo vaginal delivery. However, patients with symptoms of congestive heart failure or moderate-to-severe mitral stenosis might require close hemodynamic monitoring during labor, delivery, and for several hours into the postpartum period. In these patients, epidural anesthesia is usually better tolerated hemodynamically than general anesthesia during labor and delivery.

Aortic Stenosis

The most common cause of aortic stenosis (AS) in women of childbearing age is a congenitally bicuspid valve. Mild-to-moderate AS with preserved left ventricular function usually is well tolerated during pregnancy. Severe AS (aortic valve area less than 1.0 cm, mean gradient more than 50 mm Hg), in contrast, is associated with a 10% risk of maternal morbidity, although maternal mortality is rare. Symptoms such as dyspnea, angina pectoris, or syncope usually become apparent late in the second trimester or early in the third trimester. Cardiac surgery is needed in approximately 40% of patients with severe aortic stenosis within 2.5 years of pregnancy.[12] Women with known severe AS should be referred to a cardiologist. Ideally, they should undergo correction of the valvular abnormality before conception. Treatment options include surgical repair, surgical valve replacement, and percutaneous balloon valvotomy. The choice of an appropriate treatment for severe AS before pregnancy is complicated and will likely require a number of discussions. When severe symptomatic AS is diagnosed during pregnancy, maximal medical therapy is preferred over any intervention. However, if a patient has refractory symptoms and hemodynamic deterioration, despite maximal medical therapy, percutaneous balloon valvotomy may be performed. Spinal and epidural anesthesia are discouraged during labor and delivery because of their vasodilatory effects. As with mitral stenosis, hemodynamic monitoring is recommended during labor and delivery.

Prosthetic Heart Valves

Bioprosthetic heart valves in the presence of a normally functioning left ventricle and the absence of PHT are not associated with increased risk during pregnancy. Some reports have suggested that pregnancy accelerates structural degeneration of bioprosthetic valves.[13,14] However, several recent large series have failed to confirm this.[15-17] Patients with mechanical heart valves require lifelong anticoagulation to reduce the risk of thrombotic events. During pregnancy, the risk of thrombosis increases further owing to the hypercoagulable state.

Hypertensive Disorders

Hypertension during pregnancy is defined as a systolic pressure of 140 mm Hg or higher, a diastolic pressure of 90 mm Hg or higher, or both. The definition of hypertension in pregnancy is based on absolute BP values[18,19] and distinguishes mildly (140–159/90–109 mm Hg) or severely (≥160/110 mm Hg) elevated BP, in contrast to the grades used by the European Society of Hypertension (ESH)/ESC or others.[19] Hypertension in pregnancy is not a single entity but comprises:
- Pre-existing hypertension
- Gestational hypertension

- Pre-existing hypertension plus superimposed gestational hypertension with proteinuria.
- Antenatally unclassifiable hypertension.

Pre-existing Hypertension

Pre-existing hypertension complicates 1–5% of pregnancies and is defined as BP ≥140/90 mm Hg that either precedes pregnancy or develops before 20 weeks of gestation. Hypertension usually persists 42 days postpartum. It may be associated with proteinuria. Undiagnosed hypertensive women may appear normotensive in early pregnancy because of the physiological BP fall commencing in the first trimester. This may mask the pre-existing hypertension and, when hypertension is recorded later in pregnancy, it may be interpreted as gestational.

Gestational Hypertension

Gestational hypertension is pregnancy-induced hypertension with or without proteinuria, and complicates 6–7% of pregnancies. It is associated with clinically significant proteinuria (≥0.3 g/day in a 24 hour urine collection or ≥30 mg/mmol urinary creatinine in a spot random urine sample) and is then known as pre-eclampsia. Gestational hypertension develops after 20 weeks gestation and resolves in most cases within 42 days postpartum. It is characterized by poor organ perfusion.

Pre-eclampsia is a pregnancy-specific syndrome that occurs after mid-gestation, defined by the *de novo* appearance of hypertension, accompanied by new-onset of significant proteinuria 0.3 g/24 hour. It is a systemic disorder with both maternal and fetal manifestations. Edema is no longer considered part of the diagnostic criteria, as it occurs in up to 60% of normal pregnancies. Overall, pre-eclampsia complicates 5–7% of pregnancies,[20] but increases to 25% in women with pre-existing hypertension. Pre-eclampsia occurs more frequently during the first pregnancy, in multiple fetuses, hydatidiform mole or diabetes. It is associated with placental insufficiency, often resulting in fetal growth restriction. Additionally, pre-eclampsia is one of the most common causes of prematurity, accounting for 25% of all infants with very low birth weight (1500 g).[21] Symptoms and signs of severe pre-eclampsia include right upper quadrant/epigastric pain due to liver edema, hepatic hemorrhage, headache, visual disturbance (cerebral edema), occipital lobe blindness, hyper-reflexia, clonus, convulsions (cerebral edema) and HELLP syndrome: hemolysis, elevated liver enzymes, low platelet count.

Management of pre-eclampsia focuses essentially on recognition of the condition and ultimately, delivery of the placenta, which is curative. As proteinuria may be a late manifestation of pre-eclampsia, it should be suspected when *de novo* hypertension is accompanied by headache, visual disturbances, abdominal pain, or abnormal laboratory tests, specifically low platelet count and abnormal liver enzymes; it is recommended to treat such patients as having pre-eclampsia.

Pre-existing Hypertension Plus Superimposed Gestational Hypertension with Proteinuria

When pre-existing hypertension is associated with further worsening of BP and protein excretion ≥3 g/day in 24 hour urine collection after 20 weeks gestation, it is classified as pre-existing hypertension plus superimposed gestational hypertension with proteinuria.

Antenatally Unclassifiable Hypertension

When BP is first recorded after 20 weeks gestation and hypertension (with or without systemic manifestation) is diagnosed, it is antenatally unclassifiable hypertension. Re-assessment is necessary at or after 42 days postpartum.

Nonpharmacological management should be considered for pregnant women with systolic BP of 140–150 mm Hg or diastolic BP of 90–99 mm Hg or both. Management depends on BP, gestational age and the presence of associated maternal and fetal risk factors. It includes close supervision, limitation of activities, and some bed rest in the left lateral position. A normal diet without salt restriction is advised, particularly close to delivery, as salt restriction may induce low intravascular volume. Calcium supplementation of at least 1 g daily during pregnancy almost halved the risk of pre-eclampsia without causing any harm. Although it might be beneficial for the mother with hypertension to reduce her BP, a lower BP may impair uteroplacental perfusion and thereby jeopardize fetal development. Women with pre-existing hypertension may continue their current medication except for ACE inhibitors, ARBs, and direct renin inhibitors, which are strictly contraindicated in pregnancy because of severe fetotoxicity, particularly in the second and third trimesters. If taken inadvertently during the first trimester, switching to another medication and close monitoring including fetal ultrasound are advisable and usually are sufficient. Alpha-methyldopa is the drug of choice for long-term treatment of hypertension during pregnancy.[22] The alpha/beta-blocker labetalol has efficacy comparable with methyldopa. If there is severe hypertension, it can be given intravenous (IV) metoprolol is also recommended. Calcium-channel blockers such as nifedipine (oral) or isradipine (IV) are drugs of second choice for hypertension treatment. These drugs can be administered in hypertensive emergencies or in hypertension caused by pre-eclampsia. Potential synergism with magnesium sulfate may induce maternal hypotension and fetal hypoxia. Urapidil can also be selected for hypertensive emergencies. Magnesium sulfate IV is the drug of choice for treatment of seizures and prevention of eclampsia. Diuretics should be avoided for treatment of hypertension because they may decrease blood flow in the placenta. They are not recommended in pre-eclampsia.

Aortopathies

Pregnancy has been associated with an increased risk of aortic dissection in the general population.[23] This is probably due to the combination of an increased cardiac output, blood volume and hormonal changes that weaken the aortic wall. Women with known aortopathy are at increased risk, particularly, near term or postnatally.

Marfan Syndrome

Marfan syndrome is an inherited disorder of connective tissue. A total of 80% of Marfan patients have some cardiac involvement, usually mitral valve prolapse (MVP), MR, aortic root dilatation and/or aortic incompetence. In women with Marfan syndrome, pregnancy increases the risk of thoracic aortic aneurysm leading to aortic dissection, rupture, or both. The risk appears to be dependent on aortic root diameter. With an aortic root less than 4 cm, the overall maternal mortality during pregnancy is 1%. It increases to as much as 25% as the aortic root diameter expands beyond 4 cm.[24] In this situation, pregnancy should be postponed until after aortic arch replacement.[25] In the event of an unplanned pregnancy, the option of termination of pregnancy should be discussed. Aortic root diameter should be monitored throughout pregnancy with serial echocardiograms, and if aortic root dilatation occurs, prophylactic β-blockade is advised. Hypertension should be treated aggressively.

Coarctation of the Aorta

Coarctation of the aorta occurs in 6–8% of patients with congenital heart disease. The majority of cases are diagnosed in infancy or childhood and are either surgically corrected or treated by balloon dilatation or stent implantation. Women with repaired coarctation of the aorta are expected to reach childbearing age. By contrast, native coarctation is encountered much less frequently. Pregnancy is usually well tolerated in adequately repaired coarctation.[26] It is essential to assess cardiac status prior to conception, excluding and appropriately managing complications such as recoarctation, aneurysm at the site of repair, an associated bicuspid aortic valve or systemic hypertension. In both corrected and native coarctation, pregnancy poses the risk of aortic dissection and rupture, and resistant hypertension. Poorly controlled hypertension may lead to pre-eclampsia, hypertensive crisis and rupture of an intracranial aneurysm and, as such, needs to be tightly controlled with β-blockers as the first-line agent.

Bicuspid Aortic Valve Disease

The presence of a bicuspid aortic valve is associated with proximal aortic aortopathy. This can occur in the presence of coarctation of the aorta and/or aortic stenosis (AS). This form of aortic root dilatation during pregnancy is predisposed to aortic dissection; particularly in the third trimester.[27] If the aortic root is dilated at diagnosis, then it should be closely monitored with monthly echocardiograms. Where the aortic root diameter is less than 4 cm, it should be monitored with echocardiograms in each trimester. Symptoms of dissection should be promptly investigated with echocardiogram and computed tomography, accepting that there is a risk of radiation exposure.

Coronary Artery Disease

Acute myocardial infarction (AMI) during pregnancy is rare, occurring in 1 in 35,000 pregnancies. Independent predictors of AMI during pregnancy include chronic hypertension, maternal age, diabetes, and pre-eclampsia. Most myocardial infarctions occur during the third trimester in women older than 33 years who have had multiple prior pregnancies. Coronary spasm, *in situ* coronary thrombosis, and coronary dissection occur more frequently than classic obstructive atherosclerosis. Maternal mortality is highest in the antepartum and intrapartum periods. Recent studies have found a 5–7% case-fatality rate in women with pregnancy-associated AMI, which may reflect improvements in diagnosis and therapy over the past decade.[28] Medical therapy for AMI must be modified in the pregnant patient. Although thrombolytic agents increase the risk of maternal hemorrhage substantially (8%), their use is permitted for situations in which cardiac catheterization facilities are not available. Low-dose aspirin and nitrates are considered safe. Beta-blockers are generally safe. Short-term heparin administration has not been associated with increased maternal or fetal adverse effects. ACEI and statins are contraindicated during pregnancy. Hydralazine and nitrates may be used as substitutes for ACEI. Clopidogrel and glycoprotein IIb/IIIa receptor inhibitors have been used safely in individual pregnant patients. Percutaneous coronary intervention using both balloon angioplasty and stenting has been successfully performed in pregnant patients with AMI, with the use of lead shielding to protect the fetus.[29]

Cardiac Arrhythmias

Pregnancy increases the incidence of cardiac arrhythmia. The risk of both new onset and exacerbation of supraventricular tachycardia (SVT) is increased during pregnancy.[30] Atrial fibrillation and atrial flutter are rare and may be caused by pre-existing congenital or valvular heart disease, thyrotoxicosis or electrolyte imbalance. Owing to the risk of thromboembolism and the potential detrimental effect on the fetus, early treatment is important either with conversion to sinus rhythm or ventricular rate control. Other causes of SVT encountered in pregnancy are re-entrant tachycardia, for example, Wolf–Parkinson–White syndrome and Lown–Levine–Ganong syndrome. Initial treatment in the hemodynamically stable patient to terminate an SVT should involve the vagal maneuver. If this fails, intravenous adenosine may be safely used. Second-line treatments include digoxin, beta-blockers and calcium-channel blockers. Ventricular tachycardia is uncommon in pregnancy. It is usually associated with underlying heart disease, but new onset of ventricular tachycardia without structural heart disease has been reported.[31] Initial therapy with lidocaine or procainamide should be considered in hemodynamically stable patients. Amiodarone is relatively contraindicated, as it is associated with fetal hypothyroidism, growth retardation and prematurity, although it has been recently used to control fetal tachyarrhythmias. Beta-blockers and sotalol are used prophylactically. Electrical cardioversion is safe in pregnancy and necessary in all patients with tachyarrhythmias who are hemodynamically unstable.[31] Attention should be paid to airway management to reduce the risk of aspiration/regurgitation of gastric content and care should be taken to avoid the supine position and thus aortocaval compression.

CARDIOMYOPATHY

Dilated Cardiomyopathy

Increased intravascular volume and cardiac output during pregnancy is poorly tolerated in patients with dilated cardiomyopathy, potentially leading to cardiac decompensation. Moderate/severe left-ventricular dysfunction and NYHA class greater than II are predictive of adverse cardiac events.[32] Patients should be advised of these risks when contemplating pregnancy. In the event of an unplanned pregnancy, a termination of pregnancy should be offered.

Hypertrophic Cardiomyopathy

Clinical and genetic screening of families with hypertrophic cardiomyopathy and the widespread use of echocardiography, has led to the identification of increasing numbers of women with hypertrophic cardiomyopathy, who would have previously been unaware of their condition. Pregnancy in asymptomatic women is usually well tolerated.[33] However, in those women with heart failure or severe symptoms prior to pregnancy, there is a risk of symptomatic progression, atrial fibrillation, syncope and maternal death.

Peripartum Cardiomyopathy

Peripartum cardiomyopathy (PPCM) is defined as the development of idiopathic left ventricular systolic dysfunction (demonstrated by echocardiography) in the interval between the last month of pregnancy up to the first 5 postpartum months in women without pre-existing cardiac dysfunction. It is thought to be caused by the interaction of several factors, including hemodynamic stress, genetics, immune dysregulation and fetal microchimerism. The severity of symptoms varies from catastrophic to subclinical. Recent mortality rates of approximately 30% have been reported.[34,35] Adequate treatment with beta-blockers, diuretics, hydralazine and digoxin reduce mortality rates and improve overall prognosis. Most ACEI can be initiated during the postpartum period, even in women who breastfeed. Anticoagulation can be considered for select patients with severe left ventricular dilation and dysfunction. As with other causes of dilated cardiomyopathy, when conventional medical therapy is unsuccessful, women with PPCM may require intensive intravenous therapy, mechanical assist devices, or even cardiac transplantation. Cardiac transplantation is required for about 4% of women with PPCM. More than half of women with PPCM completely recover normal heart size and function; usually within 6 months of delivery.[36] Complete recovery is more likely in women with a left ventricular ejection fraction of more than 30% at diagnosis.[37] The remainder experience persistent stable left ventricular dysfunction or continue to experience clinical deterioration. Maternal mortality is approximately 9%.

Subsequent pregnancy after a diagnosis of PPCM carries higher risk of relapse, if left-ventricular systolic function is not fully recovered first; and even with full recovery, some additional risk of relapse remains.[38] Recent data suggested a role for prolactin in the pathophysiology of PPCM and a proof-of-concept study has shown that bromocriptine may be of benefit.[39]

Maternal Placental Syndromes

A group of disorders, known collectively as maternal placental syndromes, have been associated with an increased maternal risk of premature cardiovascular disease. In the Childhood and Adolescent Migraine Prevention (CHAMPS) study,[40] a maternal placental syndrome (MPS) was defined as the presence of pre-eclampsia, gestational hypertension, placental abruption, or placental infarction during pregnancy. MPS occurred in 7% of the 1.03 million women who were free from cardiovascular disease before pregnancy. Interestingly, traditional cardiovascular risk factors were more prevalent in women with MPS than in women without

MPS. Women with MPS were twice as likely to experience a hospital admission or revascularization procedure for coronary, cerebrovascular, or peripheral vascular disease compared with women without MPS.[40] The growing body of evidence-linking cardiovascular risk factors, MPS, and future cardiovascular disease may indicate an underlying abnormal vascular health that predates pregnancy and can manifest as MPS during pregnancy or as chronic cardiovascular disease later in life.

EFFECT OF HEART DISEASE ON PREGNANCY OUTCOMES

Obstetric Complications

The presence of heart disease does appear to increase the risk of obstetric complication. In a retrospective study of 112 pregnancies in women with congenital heart disease, Ouyang et al. report a 32.6% rate of adverse obstetric outcomes.[41] Preterm delivery and postpartum hemorrhage were the most frequent complications seen. Preterm delivery was due to preterm premature rupture of membranes and indicated deliveries. The increased rate of postpartum hemorrhage is probably due to an increased rate of planned assisted delivery. However, the use of anticoagulation in the peripartum period and cyanosis are independent predictors of postpartum hemorrhage.[42] The only cardiac lesion with specific increased risks is coarctation of the aorta, which is associated with an increased risk of pregnancy-induced hypertension.[42] If obstetric complications do occur, this can have significant impact on the outcomes of pregnancy. For example, pre-eclampsia increases the risk of cardiac decompensation and death and postpartum hemorrhage can lead to hypovolemic shock, which is often poorly tolerated. The relative immunocompromise state of pregnancy increases the risk of infection (e.g. urinary tract infection). This can increase the heart rate, potentially worsening cardiac function.

Fetal and Neonatal Outcomes

The presence of maternal heart disease impacts on the fetus in a number of ways. First, the risk of spontaneous miscarriage and therapeutic abortion is increased in women with heart disease.[43] The offspring of a mother with congenital heart disease are also at increased risk of inheriting a congenital heart disease. The overall risk of the offspring inheriting polygenic cardiac disease is quoted at 3–5%, compared with a 1% risk in the general population.[44] The risk is, in fact, dependent on the affected parent's condition and there is an increased risk, if a previous sibling has been affected **(Table 19.3)**.[45] Certain cardiac medications can adversely affect the fetus (e.g. ACEI, warfarin and statins). ACE inhibitors are known to have teratogenic effects in the first trimester and should therefore be avoided during this period.[46] Exposure in the second and third trimester can lead to marked fetal hypotension and decreased (fetal) renal blood. Where ACEI must be continued, the lowest possible dose should be used, and amniotic fluid levels and fetal growth should be monitored carefully. Statins have been identified as potential teratogens on the basis of theoretical considerations. However, epidemiological data suggest that statins are not major teratogens. Given the scarcity of available data, it is still advisable to avoid statins during the first trimester.[47] The rate of neonatal complication is significantly increased in women with heart disease. Siu et al. in their prospective longitudinal study of pregnancy outcomes in women with heart disease reported neonatal outcomes in 302 pregnancies.[43] Neonatal complications occurred in 18% of pregnancies. Preterm delivery occurred in 15%, fetal growth restriction in 4%, respiratory distress syndrome or intraventricular hemorrhage in 2% and neonatal death in 3% of pregnancies. Neonatal complications are particularly high in women with cyanotic heart disease and in women with a fontan repair.[48] Pregnancy is associated with a high incidence of fetal loss, stillbirth, fetal growth restriction and preterm delivery.[49] In cyanotic heart disease, the risk increases significantly when maternal oxygen saturations fall below 85%. This should be discussed in advance and the fetus should be monitored carefully throughout pregnancy.

DIAGNOSTIC APPROACH

The risk of inheritance of cardiac abnormalities to the descendants is significantly higher in women with CVD, i.e. between 3% and 50% depending on type of disease, compared to parents without CVD.[45] Genetic testing may be useful in some cases of cardiomyopathies and channelopathies, when other family members are affected and when other genetic malformations associated with CVD are present. All women with congenital heart disease should be offered fetal echocardiography in the 18th to 22nd week of pregnancy. Detailed personal and family history is mandatory. Thorough clinical examination for new or changing murmurs and signs of heart failure is needed. If such findings, echocardiography should be performed. Blood pressure, proteinuria, especially in pregnant women at risk for pre-eclampsia and pulse oximetry in congenital heart disease needs to be taken. Echocardiography for the evaluation of chest pain, 24-hour Holter monitoring in cases of known history of paroxysmal or persistent arrhythmia or palpitations are required. Echocardiography is the preferred diagnostic tool during pregnancy due to absence of radiation exposure, ease of use, bedside availability and ability to evaluate a multitude of CVD (congenital heart disease, cardiomyopathy, aortic disease, etc). Transesophageal electrocardiography, on the other hand, is fairly safe but rarely needed. Submaximal stress testing (80% of max.) could be performed in asymptomatic patients with suspected CVD. Cardiac MRI (without gadolinium) only for congenital heart disease or aortic disease is indicated, if echo is inconclusive. Chest X-ray, CT, cardiac cath, electrophysiological study generally not recommended, may be considered with shielding of the fetus under very strict and vital indications and no alternative.

MANAGEMENT PRINCIPLES

Although strict protocols for the management of heart disease in pregnancy do not exist, a number of basic principles can be applied.

Prepregnancy Counseling

The management of women with heart disease should ideally take place before conception. In women with congenital lesions, this process should begin during adolescence with discussions about family planning, contraception and pregnancy. Women with heart disease contemplating pregnancy should be assessed in a multidisciplinary pre-pregnancy clinic (staffed by an obstetrician, cardiologist, anesthetist and midwife). Echocardiography should assess cardiac hemodynamics including valve areas and pulmonary pressures. In patients with impaired functional capacity an exercise test with maximum oxygen uptake refines risk stratification for pregnancy. These risks should be discussed with the woman and her family and a risk of maternal morbidity and mortality quoted. Patients should be assessed and counseled regarding their need for any medical, interventional or surgical treatment prior to conception. Avoidance of pregnancy should be advised for patients with pulmonary hypertension, Eisenmenger's syndrome or Marfan's syndrome with an aortic root diameter greater than 4 cm. Contraception should also be discussed as a means of delaying or preventing pregnancy.[50] A sensitive yet important issue that should be addressed with the mother and her family is her capacity to care for a child and her overall life-expectancy. The risk of recurrence of heart disease in the offspring should also be considered.

Antenatal Care

Once pregnant, women should be cared for by medical personnel who are experienced in the management of pregnant patients with heart disease. A multidisciplinary approach should be applied including obstetricians, cardiologists, anesthetists and neonatologists. Regular antenatal checks are advised throughout pregnancy. The purpose of antenatal care is to ensure the continued wellbeing of the mother and fetus. Prompt treatment of anemia, urinary tract infection and arrhythmias are important. Intervention before major cardiac decompensation and the early diagnosis and management of pre-eclampsia can prevent significant problems. Medication should be reviewed, teratogenic drugs must be stopped and an alternative used, wherever possible. In general, warfarin should be changed for low-molecular-weight heparin for the duration of pregnancy, except in the case of metallic heart valves. In certain circumstances, specific therapy is required, including avoidance of vasodilators to maintain preload, empirical beta-blockers in Marfan's syndrome and prophylactic heparin in pregnancy complicated by pulmonary hypertension. Admission for bed rest and monitoring may be required and is advised with a NYHA class greater than III. As there is an association between increased nuchal thickness and cardiac defects in both chromosomally abnormal and normal fetuses, fetal assessment should involve a nuchal translucency scan early in pregnancy. A fetal echogram should be performed between 18 and 22 weeks with a routine anomaly scan at 20 weeks. The assessment of fetal growth with serial ultrasound scans is essential in women with heart disease, especially if this is in the form of cyanotic heart lesions.

Anticoagulants

Several conditions require the initiation or maintenance of anticoagulation during pregnancy, including mechanical valves, certain prothrombotic conditions, prior episode of venous thromboembolism, acute deep vein thrombosis or thromboembolism during pregnancy, antiphospholipid antibody syndrome, and atrial fibrillation. The three most common agents considered for use during pregnancy are unfractionated heparin (UFH), low-molecular-weight heparin (LMWH), and warfarin. In women with venous thromboembolism, LMWH has become the anticoagulant of choice. In women with mechanical heart valves, data are more limited and there has been some concern regarding the efficacy of heparins with respect to the prevention of valve thrombosis. In these patients, the maternal and fetal risks and benefits must be carefully explained before choosing one of the aforementioned three strategies. When an UFH or LMWH strategy is selected, careful dose monitoring and adjustment are recommended.

Warfarin freely crosses the placental barrier and can harm the fetus, but it is safe during breast-feeding. The incidence of warfarin embryopathy (abnormalities of fetal bone and cartilage formation) has been estimated at 4–10%; the risk is highest when warfarin is administered during weeks 6 through 12 of gestation. When administered during the second and third trimesters, warfarin has been associated with fetal central nervous system abnormalities. The risk of warfarin embryopathy may be low in patients who take 5 mg or less of warfarin per day. UFH does not cross the placenta and is considered safer for the fetus. Its use, however, has been associated with maternal osteoporosis, hemorrhage, thrombocytopenia or thrombosis (HITT syndrome), and a high incidence of thromboembolic events with older generation mechanical valves. The UFH may be administered parenterally or subcutaneously throughout pregnancy; when used subcutaneously for the anticoagulation of mechanical heart valves, the recommended starting dose is 17,500–20,000 U twice daily. The appropriate dose adjustment of UFH is based on an activated partial thromboplastin time (aPTT) of 2.0–3.0 times the control level. High doses of UFH are often required to achieve the goal aPTT because of the hypercoagulable state associated with pregnancy. Lower doses of UFH may be appropriate for anticoagulation in certain cases, such as the prevention of venous thromboembolism during pregnancy. Parenteral infusions should be stopped 4 hours before cesarean sections. UFH can be reversed with protamine sulfate. Low-molecular-weight heparin (LMWH) produces a more predictable anticoagulant response than UFH and is less likely to cause heparin-induced thrombocytopenia (HIT). Its effect on maternal bone mineral density appears to be minimal. LMWH can be administered subcutaneously and dosed to achieve anti-factor Xa levels of 1–1.2 U/mL around 4–6 hours after injection. Although there is data to support the use of LMWH in pregnant women with deep vein thrombosis, data on the safety and efficacy of LMWH in pregnant patients with mechanical valve prostheses are limited. Experience with these agents is accruing.

In summary, anticoagulation in the pregnant patient can be difficult because of the risk profile associated with each drug regimen. In planned pregnancies, a careful discussion about the risks and benefits of warfarin, UFH, and LMWH will help the patient and physician involved to choose an anticoagulation strategy. Unplanned pregnancies are often diagnosed partway through the first trimester. It is advisable to stop warfarin when the pregnancy is discovered and to use UFH or LMWH, at least until after the 12th week. Dosing regimens for warfarin, UFH, and LMWH may vary by diagnosis; detailed dosing guidelines have been published.[51]

Labor and Delivery

The appropriate timing for delivery is crucial to balance both maternal and neonatal mortality and morbidity. Labor and delivery require careful planning. Vaginal delivery is recommended in most women with heart disease. There is no direct evidence to link vaginal mode of delivery with outcome; however, it is known to be associated with a smaller shift in blood volume, hemorrhage, clotting and infection. In the absence of infection, infective endocarditis prophylaxis is not recommended except in high-risk patients. Labor and delivery are an additional burden on the maternal cardiovascular system and requires continuous monitoring of both mother and fetus. Maternal preload, blood pressure and blood loss should be monitored carefully throughout, with invasive monitoring occasionally required. Low-dose epidural with adequate volume loading does not decrease systemic vascular resistance, and is thus the analgesia of choice. The length of the second stage may be shortened by elective assisted delivery to avoid excessive maternal effort. During the third stage of labor bolus doses of oxytocin should be avoided as they result in an initial fall in arterial blood pressure followed by an increase in cardiac output. Oxytocin also has a direct effect on the heart, causing decreased cardiac contractility and heart rate. If oxytocin is to be used, it should be given by slow intravenous infusion. Ergometrine should also be avoided in most cases as it can cause acute hypertension. The safety of misoprostol is yet to be determined. Mechanical maneuvers to reduce postpartum hemorrhage such as bimanual compression, uterine compression sutures and intrauterine balloons are useful alternatives. Careful hemodynamic monitoring postpartum is typically required for 24–72 hour, but this should be extended to 10–14 days in cases of pulmonary hypertension. Multidisciplinary follow-up should take place 6 weeks after delivery.

KEY POINTS

1. Around 0.2–4% of all pregnancies are complicated by CVD.
2. Changes in the CVS in pregnancy begin as early as 5 weeks and by 8 weeks of gestation, the cardiac output increases up to 20%.
3. The 2011 ESC guidelines recommend that maternal risk assessment should be carried out according to the modified World Health Organization (mWHO) risk classification.
4. The number of adults with congenital heart disease now outnumbers children, reflecting improved surgical outcomes and medical care over recent decades.
5. The presence of heart disease does appears to increase the risk of obstetric complication by around 32%.
6. The overall risk of the offspring inheriting polygenic cardiac disease is quoted at 3–5%, compared with a 1% risk in the general population.
7. Certain cardiac medications can adversely affect the fetus, e.g. ACEI, warfarin and statins should be avoided.
8. All women with congenital heart disease should be offered fetal echocardiography in the 19th to 22nd week of pregnancy.
9. Avoidance of pregnancy should be advised for patients with pulmonary hypertension, Eisenmenger's syndrome or Marfan's syndrome with an aortic root diameter greater than 4 cm.

10. Vaginal delivery is recommended in most women with heart disease as it is known to be associated with a smaller shift in blood volume, hemorrhage, clotting and infection.

REFERENCES

1. Weiss BM, von Segesser LK, Alon E, et al. Outcome of cardiovascular surgery and pregnancy: a systematic review of the period 1984–1996. Am J Obstet Gynecol. 1998;179:1643-53.
2. Sliwa K, Libhaber E, Elliott C, et al. Spectrum of cardiac disease in maternity in a low-resource cohort in South Africa. Heart. 2014;100:1967-74.
3. Naidoo P, Desai D, Moodley J. Maternal deaths due to pre-existing cardiac disease. Cardiovasc J Afr. 2002;13:17-9.
4. Regitz-Zagrosek V, et al. ESC Guidelines on the management of cardiovascular diseases during pregnancy: the Task Force on the Management of Cardiovascular Diseases during Pregnancy of the European Society of Cardiology (ESC). European Society of Gynecology (ESG); Association for European Paediatric Cardiology (AEPC); German Society for Gender Medicine (DGesGM), ESC Committee for Practice Guidelines. Eur Heart J. 2011;32(24):3147-97.
5. Siu SC, Sermer M, Colman JM, et al. Prospective multicentre study of pregnancy outcomes in women with heart disease. Circulation. 2001;104:515-21.
6. Drenthen W, Pieper PG, Roos-Hesselink JW, et al. Outcome of pregnancy in women with congenital heart disease: a literature review. J Am Coll Cardiol. 2007;49:2303-11.
7. Drenthen W, Boersma E, Balci A, et al. Predictors of pregnancy complications in women with congenital heart disease. Eur Heart J. 2010;31:2124-32.
8. Van HI, Boersma E, Johnson M, et al. Global cardiac risk assessment in the registry of pregnancy and cardiac disease: results of a registry from the European Society of Cardiology. Eur J Heart Fail. 2016;18:523-33.
9. Weiss BM, Zemp L, Seifert B, et al. Outcome of pulmonary vascular disease in pregnancy: a systematic overview from 1978 through 1996. J Am Coll Cardiol. 1998;31(7):1650-57.
10. Warnes CA. Pregnancy and pulmonary hypertension. Int. J. Cardiol. 2004;97(Suppl. 1):11-3.
11. Silversides CK, Colman JM, Sermer M, et al. Cardiac risk in pregnant women with rheumatic mitral stenosis. Am J Cardiol. 2003;91:1382-5.
12. Silversides CK, Colman JM, Sermer M, et al. Early and intermediate-term outcomes of pregnancy with congenital aortic stenosis. Am J Cardiol. 2003;91:1386-9.
13. Sbarouni E, Oakley C. Outcome of pregnancy in women with valve prostheses. Br Heart J. 1994;71(2):196-201.
14. Badduke BR, Jamieson WR, Miyagishima RT, et al. Pregnancy and childbearing in a population with biological valvular prostheses. J Thorac Cardiovasc Surg. 1991;102(2):179-86.
15. North RA, Sadler L, Stewart AW, et al. Long-term survival and valve-related complications in young women with cardiac valve replacements. Circulation. 1999;99(20):2669-76.
16. Avila WS, Rossi EG, Grinberg M, et al. Influence of pregnancy after bioprosthetic valve replacement in young women: a prospective five-year study. J Heart Valve Dis. 2002;11(6):864-9.
17. El SF, Hassan W, Latroche B, et al. Pregnancy has no effect on the rate of structural deterioration of bioprosthetic valves: long-term 18-year follow-up results. J Heart Valve Dis. 2005;14(4):481-5.
18. Levine RJ, Ewell MG, Hauth JC, et al. Should the definition of preeclampsia include a rise in diastolic blood pressure of >/=15 mm Hg to a level <90 mm Hg in association with proteinuria? Am J Obstet Gynecol. 2000;183:787-92.
19. Mancia G, De Backer G, Dominiczak A, et al. ESH-ESC Practice guidelines for the management of arterial hypertension: ESH-ESC Task force on the management of arterial hypertension. J Hypertens. 2007;25:1751-62.
20. Steegers EA, von Dadelszen P, Duvekot JJ, et al. Pre-eclampsia. Lancet. 2010;376:631-44.
21. Hiett AK, Brown HL, Britton KA. Outcome of infants delivered between 24 and 28 weeks' gestation in women with severe pre-eclampsia. J Matern Fetal Med. 2001;10:301-4.
22. Cockburn J, Moar VA, Ounsted M, et al. Final report of study on hypertension during pregnancy: the effects of specific treatment on the growth and development of the children. Lancet. 1982;1:647-9.
23. Nolte JE, Rutherford RB, Nawaz S, et al. Arterial dissections associated with pregnancy. J Vasc Surg. 1995;21(3):515-20.
24. Rossiter JP, Repke JT, Morales AJ, et al. A prospective longitudinal evaluation of pregnancy in the Marfan syndrome. J Obstet Gynecol. 1995;173(5):1599-606.
25. Williams A, Child A, Rowntree J, et al. Marfan's syndrome: successful pregnancy after aortic root and arch replacement. BJOG.2002;109(10):1187-8.
26. Vriend JW, Drenthen W, Pieper PG, et al. Outcome of pregnancy in patients after repair of aortic coarctation. Eur Heart J. 2005;26(20):2173-8.
27. Immer FF, Bansi AG, Immer-Bansi AS, et al. Aortic dissection in pregnancy: analysis of risk factors and outcome. Ann Thorac. Surg. 2003;76(1):309-14.
28. James AH, Jamison MG, Biswas MS. Acute myocardial infarction in pregnancy: A United States population-based study. Circulation. 2006;113:1564-71.
29. Dwyer BK, Taylor L, Fuller A, et al. Percutaneous transluminal angioplasty and stent placement during pregnancy. Obstet Gynecol. 2005;106:1162-4.
30. Tawam M, Levine J, Mendelson M, et al. Effect of pregnancy on paroxysmal supraventricular tachycardia. Am J Cardiol. 1992;72:838-40.
31. Cox JL, Gardner MJ. Treatment of cardiac arrhythmias during pregnancy. Prog Cardiovasc Dis. 1993;36:137-78.
32. Grewal J, Siu SC, Ross HJ, et al. Pregnancy outcomes in women with dilated cardiomyopathy. J Am Coll Cardiol. 2009;55(1):45-52.
33. Thaman R, Varnava A, Hamid MS, et al. Pregnancy related complications in women with hypertrophic cardiomyopathy. Heart. 2003;89:752-6.
34. Felker GM, Thompson RE, Hare JM, et al. Underlying causes and long-term survival in patients with initially unexplained cardiomyopathy. N Engl J Med. 2000;342:1077-108.
35. Sliwa K, Skudicky D, Bergemann A, et al. Peripartum cardiomyopathy: analysis of clinical outcome, left ventricular function, plasma levels of cytokines and Fas/APO-1. J Am Coll Cardiol. 2000;35:701-5.
36. Elkayam U, Akhter MW, Singh H, et al. Pregnancy-associated cardiomyopathy: clinical characteristics and a

comparison between early and late presentation. Circulation. 2005;111:2050-5.
37. A cathepsin-D cleaved 16-kD form of prolactin mediates postpartum cardiomyopathy. Cell. 2007;128:589-600.
38. Elkayam U, Tummala PP, Rao K, et al. Maternal and fetal outcomes of subsequent pregnancies in women with peripartum cardiomyopathy. Circulation. 2010;344(21):1567-71.
39. Sliwa K, Blauwet L, Tibazarwa K, et al. Evaluation of bromocriptine in the treatment of acute severe peripartum cardiomyopathy: A proof-of-concept pilot Study. Circulation. 2010;121(13):1465-73.
40. Ray JG, et al. Cardiovascular health after maternal placental syndromes (CHAMPS): a population-based retrospective cohort study. Lancet. 2005;366:1797-1803.
41. Ouyang DW, Khairy P, Fernandes SM, et al. Obstetric outcomes in pregnant women with congenital heart disease. Int J Cardiol. DOI: 10.1016/j.ijcard.2009.04.006 (2009) (Epub ahead of print).
42. Siu SC, Sermer M, Colman JM, et al. Cardiac Disease in Pregnancy (CARPREG) investigators. Prospective multicenter study of pregnancy outcome in women with heart disease. Circulation. 2001;104:515-21.
43. Siu SC, Colman JM, Sorensen S, et al. Adverse neonatal and cardiac outcomes are more common in pregnant women with cardiac disease. Circulation. 2002;105:2179-84.
44. Romano-Zelekha O, Hirsh R, Blieden L, et al. The risk for congenital heart defects in offspring of individuals with congenital heart defects. Clin Genet. 2001;59:325-9.
45. Burn J, Brennan P, Little J, et al. Recurrence risks in offspring of adults with major heart defects: results from first cohort of British collaborative study. Lancet. 1998;351: 311-6.
46. Cooper WO, Hernandez-Diaz S, Arbogast PG, et al. Major congenital malformations after first trimester exposure to ACE inhibitors. N Engl J Med. 2006;354(23):2443-51.
47. Kazmin A, Garcia-Bournissen F, Koren G. Risks of statin use during pregnancy: a systematic review. J Obstet Gynaecol Can. 2007;29(11):906-8.
48. Drenthen W, Pieper PG, Roos-Hesselink JW, et al. ZAHARA investigators. Pregnancy and delivery in women after Fontan palliation. Heart. 2006;92(9):1290-4.
49. Presbitero P, Somerville J, Stone S, et al. Pregnancy in cyanotic heart disease: Outcome of mother and fetus. Circulation. 1994;89:2673-6.
50. Silversides CK, Sermer M, Siu SC. Choosing the best contraceptive method for the adult with congenital heart disease. Curr Cardiol Rep. 2009;11(4):298-305.
51. Bates SM, Greer IA, Hirsh J, Ginsberg JS. Use of antithrombotic agents during pregnancy. Chest. 2004;126:627-44S.

Chapter 20

Peripartum Cardiomyopathy

Anita Singh, Aashita Shrivastava

INTRODUCTION

Peripartum cardiomyopathy (PPCM) is a rare but critical disorder causing heart failure in women in late pregnancy or puerperium.

European Society of Cardiology (ESC) working group on PPCM defines PPCM as "an idiopathic cardiomyopathy presenting with heart failure secondary to left ventricle systolic dysfunction towards the end of pregnancy or in the months following delivery, where no other cause of heart failure is found".

Working committee on PPCM[1] has modified the definition of PPCM and includes following four criteria (three clinical and one echocardiographic):
1. Development of heart failure during last trimester of pregnancy or first six months postpartum.
2. Absence of any identifiable cause for cardiac failure
3. Absence of any recognizable heart disease prior to last trimester of pregnancy
4. *Echocardiographic criteria:* Demonstrable echocardiographic proof of left ventricular systolic dysfunction:
   - Ejection fraction less than 45%
   - Left ventricular fractional shortening less than 30% or
   - Left ventricular end-diastolic dimension >2.7 cm/m^2 of body surface area.

EPIDEMIOLOGY

Peripartum cardiomyopathy is relatively rare condition. The precise incidence in India is not known, an incidence of one case per 1374 live births has been reported from a tertiary care hospital from South India.[2] The disease appears to be more common in African American; in South Africa reported incidence is higher 1 in 1000 live birth.[3] A much higher incidence of I in 300 live births has been reported from Haiti[4] of 1% has been reported from Nigeria.[5] The higher prevalence in developing countries may be attributed to environmental, ecological, and cultural, puerperal and postpuerperal practice besides diagnostic criteria and reporting standards.

Risk Factors

Incidence of peripartum cardiomyopathy has been found to be greater in:
- Multiparous women
- Advanced maternal age
- Multifetal pregnancy (twin and triplets)
- Pre-eclampsia
- Gestational hypertension
- African American race
- Obesity
- Maternal cocaine, alcohol abuse, smoking
- Long-term tocolytic therapy.

ETIOLOGY

The etiology and pathogenesis of PPCM is poorly understood. Multiple etiologies have been proposed for PPCM including inflammation, viral myocarditis, abnormal immune or hemodynamic response to pregnancy, apoptosis, hormonal abnormalities, impaired angiogenesis, increased oxidative stress, malnutrition, cardiomyocyte-specific deletion of the transcription factor signal transducer and activator of transcription 3 (STAT3) protein and genetic factors.

INFLAMMATION

Level of serum markers of inflammation including C-reactive protein (CRP), interferon and interleukin-6, is elevated in PPCM patients.

MYOCARDITIS

Viral infections may cause PPCM. Reported incidence of myocarditis In peripartum cardiomyopathy varies from 9% to 62%.[6-10] Parvovirus B19, human herpes simplex virus, Epstein-Barr virus, and human cytomegalovirus has been implicated in pathogenesis.

Cenac et al. found a correlation between anti-*Chlamydia* pneumonia antibodies and PPCM and suggested that these antibodies were prognostic indicators for PPCM; with higher levels of the antibodies being associated with a poorer prognosis.[11,12]

ABNORMAL IMMUNOLOGIC AND HEMODYNAMIC RESPONSES TO PREGNANCY

Fetal microchimerism refers to the presence of very low numbers of fetal cells in a woman who is, or has been, pregnant. It has been estimated that the number of fetal cells in maternal peripheral blood during the second trimester is around 1-6 cells/mL.

Ansari and colleagues suggested that fetal microchimerism may trigger an exaggerated autoimmune response in the postpartum period.[13] This could explain the higher incidence of PPCM in twin pregnancies and recurrences in subsequent pregnancies.

Physiological changes during pregnancy cause a reversible hypertrophy and dilatation of the left ventricle which resolves shortly after birth in a normal pregnancy. PPCM patients may have an abnormal left ventricular recovery response to physiological changes.[14]

PROLACTIN

STAT3 is thought to be involved in cardiac protection from pregnancy induced oxidative stress by inhibition of the reactive oxygen species. Reduction in STAT 3 leads to increased oxidative stress and activation of cathepsin D, which cleaves prolactin into its antiangiogenic and proapoptotic 16 kDa fragment. The 16 kDa fragment inhibits endothelial cell proliferation and migration, induces endothelial cell apoptosis and impairs cardiomyocyte function.

GENETIC FACTORS

Familial mutation in *MYH7*, *SCN5A*, and *PSEN2* genes and sporadic mutations in *MYH6* and *TNNT2* genes are found in patients of peripartum cardiomyopathy patients.

Pathological Changes

In a patient of PPCM after postmortem the heart specimen appears pale, soft, dilated and heavier in comparison to normal heart. Cardiac chambers show mural thrombi, gray-white patches of endocardial thickening are usually seen at the site of mural thrombi. Heart valves and coronary arteries appear normal, pericardial effusion is occasionally seen.

On histopathological examination, evidence of degeneration, fibrosis, interstitial edema, fatty and mono-nuclear cell infiltration of myocardium is seen. Electron microscopy reveals varying degree of enlargement, destruction or fragmentation of myofibril.

Clinical Features

Patients of PPCM presents with symptoms of systolic dysfunction. New or rapid onset of the following symptoms require prompt evaluation: cough, orthopnea, paroxysmal nocturnal dyspnea, fatigue, palpitations, weight gain, hemoptysis, chest pain, and unexplained abdominal pain.

Physical Examination

Enlarged heart, tachycardia, and decreased pulse oximetry. Blood pressure may be normal, elevated jugular venous pressure, third heart sound, and loud pulmonic component of the second heart sound are usually found, mitral and/or tricuspid regurgitation, and pulmonary rates are also noted.

Worsening of peripheral edema, ascites and hepatomegaly are quite often seen.

Arrhythmias are commonly found which may be responsible for embolic phenomenon peripheral or pulmonary.

In some patients, small-to-moderate pericardial effusion may be found.

Presence of elevated blood pressures (systolic >140 mm Hg and/or diastolic >90 mm Hg) and proteinuria suggests pre-eclampsia.

Overall clinical presentation and hemodynamic changes are indistinguishable from those found in other forms of dilated cardiomyopathy.

Few patients with high output heart failure have also been reported.

DIAGNOSIS

- *ECG*: Resting 12-lead electrocardiogram (ECG) is the first-line diagnostic tool in the assessment of patients with suspected PPCM. Although a normal ECG does not rule out the diagnosis, most women suffering from PPCM have an abnormal ECG. The most common abnormalities on the ECG are ST- or T-wave abnormalities, p-wave abnormality, bundle-branch block, left ventricular hypertrophy, ventricular or supraventricular arrhythmias, and QRS-axis deviation.
- *X-ray*: Cardiomegaly, Kerley B lines, prominent pulmonary vasculature, pulmonary edema, and pleural effusion can be found.
- *Echocardiography* is the most important diagnostic tool in PPCM and is without adverse effects. The finding of left ventricular systolic dysfunction is essential in the diagnosis, and other criteria include a left ventricular ejection fraction less than 45%, fractional shortening of less than 30% on M-mode echocardiography, or both, and a left ventricular end-diastolic dimension of greater than 2.7 cm/m^2 of body surface area.

- *Endomyocardial biopsy*: The endomyocardial biopsy may show features of myocarditis, most beneficial when performed early after the onset of symptoms.
- *Viral and bacterial titer and cultures*: Coxsackie B virus antibody titer should be considered in selected cases.
- *Right heart catheterization*: In women with persistent heart failure, hemodynamic instability or evidence of an organ dysfunction, right heart catheterization to assess the filling pressures and cardiac output should be considered. It will also demonstrate enlargement of all chambers of heart predominantly the left ventricle.
- *Biomarker*: Troponin-T has both diagnostic and prognostic implication. Initial Troponin-T concentration of >0.04 μg/mL predicts persistent left ventricular dysfunction at six months follow-up.
- CRP level are elevated in patients of PPCM. Sliwa and colleagues reported that the baseline levels of C-reactive protein (CRP) correlated positively with baseline left ventricle diameters and inversely with left ventricle ejection fraction and baseline.[15]

Differential Diagnosis

PPCM should be differentiated from other forms of cardiomyopathy.
- The most common and confusing being idiopathic dilated cardiomyopathy (IDCM):
  - PPCM occurs at a younger age and is generally associated with better prognosis, it occur mostly postpartum, whereas IDCM usually manifests by the second trimester.
  - Higher incidence of myocarditis is found in PPCM along with unique sets of antigen and antibodies against myocardium which is not seen in IDCM.
  - Heart size returns to normal after delivery in more number of PPCM patients as compared to IDCM
  - PPCM may lead to rapid worsening of clinical course and poor outcome contrary to IDCM.
- Valvular heart diseases
- Coronary artery disease including acute myocardial infarction
- Pulmonary thromboembolism
- Severe eclampsia and pneumonia.

Treatment (Flow Chart 20.1)

Management of Heart Failure

During Pregnancy: Early diagnosis and prompt treatment are the keys to optimize pregnancy outcome. When considering diagnostic tests or treatment during pregnancy, the welfare of the fetus should always be considered along with that of the mother. Patients with severe forms of heart failure will require ICCU management.

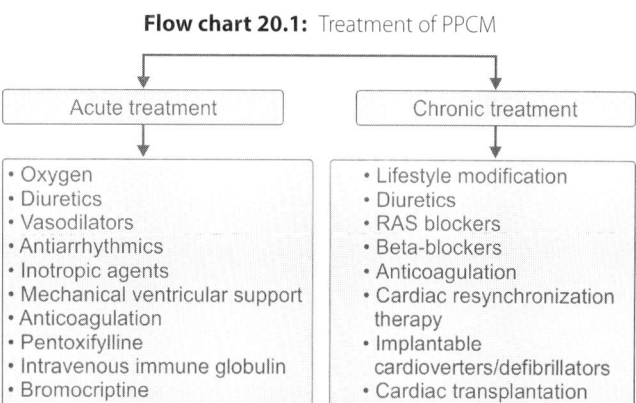

Flow chart 20.1: Treatment of PPCM

Angiotensin-converting enzyme (ACE) inhibitors and ArBs are contraindicated in pregnancy because these can cause birth defects, although remaining the main treatment option for postpartum women with heart failure. The teratogenic effects occur particularly in the second and third trimester, characterized by fetal hypotension, pulmonary hypoplasia, oligohydramnios, anuria, and renal tubular dysplasia.
- Digoxin, loop diuretics, sodium restriction and drugs that reduce afterload such as hydralazine and nitrates have been proven to be safe and are the mainstays of medical therapy of heart failure during pregnancy. Digoxin is effective due to its inotropic and rate-reducing effect.
- Diuretics are useful because of the preload reduction along with salt restriction. They are relatively safe in pregnancy and lactation; however, one should be cautious regarding volume depletion which may result in to dehydration causing uterine hypoperfusion.
- *Calcium-channel blockers:* Amlodipine has been found to improve survival in cardiomyopathy patients.
- Beta-blockers is effective in patients with heart failure, but they have not been tested in peripartum cardiomyopathy. beta-blocker has no known adverse effects on the fetus, and patients taking these agents prior to diagnosis can continue to use them safely.

During postpartum period: Treatment is identical to that for nonpregnant women with dilated cardiomyopathy.
- ACE inhibitors and ArBs are useful. The usual target dose is one half the maximum antihypertensive doses.
- Diuretics are given for symptomatic relief; spironolactone or digoxin is used in patients who have New York Heart Association class III or IV symptoms. The dose of spironolactone is 25 mg/day after dosing of other drugs is maximized.
- The goal with digoxin therapy is the lowest daily dose to obtain a detectable serum digoxin level, which should be kept at less than 1.0 ng/mL.

- Beta-blockers are recommended as they improve symptoms, ejection fraction, and survival. Nonselective beta-blockers (carvedilol) and selective (metoprolol) have shown benefit. The goal dosage is carvedilol 25 mg twice a day or metoprolol 100 mg once a day.

Anticoagulant Therapy

Hypercoagulable state of pregnancy coupled with stasis of blood due to ventricular dysfunction makes PPCM patients prone for thrombus formation. This situation may persists up to six weeks after postpartum, hence use of heparin is advocated in antepartum period and that of heparin or warfarin in the postpartum period, as warfarin is contraindicated in pregnancy because of its teratogenic effect while use of both heparin and warfarin is safe in lactation.

Due to high-risk of venous and arterial thrombosis anticoagulation with subcutaneous heparin should be instituted in these patients more so in:
- Bedridden patients
- Patients with LVEF <35%
- Presence of atrial fibrillation
- Mural thrombi
- Obese patients
- Patients with history of thromboembolism.

Patients with evidence of systemic embolism, with severe left ventricular dysfunction or documented cardiac thrombosis, should receive anticoagulation. Anticoagulation should be continued until return of normal left ventricular function is documented.

Antiarrhythmic Drugs

No antiarrhythmic agent is completely safe during pregnancy quinidine and procainamide should be tried first because of their higher safety profile. Beta-blockers may be useful for atrial arrhythmias and digoxin may also be considered.
- Patients presenting with sudden death or ventricular tachycardia with hemodynamic compromise, strong consideration of an implantable cardioverter defibrillator (ICD) is warranted due to the potential for a fatal recurrence.
- For patients presenting with symptomatic ventricular tachyarrhythmia which are hemodynamically well tolerated, because of the potential transient nature of the myopathy and amiodarone therapy at 200–400 mg orally every six hourly is an alternative. If left ventricular function recovers, the risk of serious arrhythmic event is markedly diminished and amiodarone therapy can be discontinued.
- For patients with asymptomatic non-sustained ventricular tachyarrhythmia amiodarone therapy should not be initiate. Correction of metabolic abnormalities and addition of a beta-receptor antagonist, if not already being utilized is done.

Newer Treatment Modalities

- *Pentoxifylline*: Treatment with pentoxifylline, a xanthine derived agent known to inhibit the production of tumor necrosis factor-alpha, has been shown to improve functional class and left ventricular function in patients with idiopathic dilated cardiomyopathy.
- *Role of bromocriptine and cabergoline:* Prolactin breakdown products has been implicated in the pathology of PPCM. Prolactin secretion can be reduced with bromocriptine which had beneficial effects in a small study. one case study with use of cabergoline which is a strong and long-lasting antagonist of prolactin significant improvement in left ventricular functions were reported.
- *Immune modulating therapy*: Considering the inflammatory nature of peripartum cardiomyopathy and the occasional appearance of myocarditis on endomyocardial biopsy, immunosuppressive and immune modulatory therapy has been utilized. Plasmapheresis has also been utilized effectively for this purpose, and may be an alternative to immune globulin therapy in peripartum cardiomyopathy.
- Other proposed therapies which might be useful are calcium-channel antagonists, statins, monoclonal antibodies and interferon-beta.
- *Other interventions and devices*: PPCM is reversible in good number of patients, the temporary use of an intra-aortic balloon pump or left ventricular assist devices may help in stabilizing critical patients. Extracorporeal membrane oxygenation has been tried successfully in some patients as a bridge to recovery. Ventricular tachycardia leading to cardiac arrest has been reported in PPCM patients, to avoid such situation increasing use of automated implantable cardioverter defibrillator (AICD) is being tried.

  In extreme situations, multiorgan support systems such as ventilator therapy, continuous venovenous hemodialysis may be required besides circulatory assist devices.
- *Cardiac transplantation*: Patients with severe heart failure who does not respond despite maximal drug therapy may be considered for cardiac transplantation to survive because of high-risk of mortality.

Management During Labor

Managing hemodynamic stress of delivery for patients presenting during the late stages of pregnancy, due consideration should be given to limiting the hemodynamic stress of the delivery. Compensated patients may undergo vaginal delivery with appropriate monitoring. For those patients late in pregnancy with more significant hemodynamic compromise, elective cesarean with invasive hemodynamic monitoring of the mother should be considered. Single shot spinal anesthesia is currently not preferred because of severe consequences such as cardiac arrest and pulmonary edema. Controlled epidural analgesia (ER) is a safe and effective method in this situation.

BREASTFEEDING

Breastfeeding is strongly discouraged in more symptomatic patients as pharmacologic therapy to the patient can be passed on to the child. If breastfeeding is considered in these women, it has to be with careful monitoring of the baby.

Follow-up Management

Patients who show normal left ventricular function on echocardiographic evaluation at rest or with low-dose dobutamine stress test can be allowed to tape, and then discontinue heart failure treatment in 6–12 months. They are encouraged to remain as active as their functional status allows, however, aerobic activities and heavy lifting are discouraged for at least the first six months postpartum.

Echocardiogram should be repeated at 6 months post-delivery. For those patients with persistent cardiomyopathy, beta-blockers may be added at this point, if not already on therapy.

Prognosis

PPCM have much higher rate of spontaneous recovery of left ventricular function on echocardiography in postpartum period; nearly half of the women will normalize their ejection fraction during follow-up within six months. Prognosis is directly correlated to recovery of left ventricular function:

- For those women whose LVEF normalizes during follow-up, the prognosis is excellent as without the stimulus of a subsequent pregnancy the chance of development of heart failure or future LV dysfunction is minimal.
- For those women whose left ventricular function does not recover, prognosis remains guarded.

LV size is an important predictor, as women presenting without significant LV dilatation appeared to have a greater chance of spontaneous recovery during follow-up In contrast, women with marked LV dilatation at presentation appeared to have a greater likelihood of developing into a chronic cardiomyopathy.

Initial NYHA class or hemodynamic status does not seem to predict the likelihood of subsequent recovery.

A fractional shortening on echocardiogram less than 20% and a LV end diastolic dimension greater than or equal to 6 cm was associated with a three-fold increase in persistent LV dysfunction.

In patients of PPCM whose left ventricular function fails to normalize during follow-up, subsequent pregnancies carry a high risk of left ventricular deterioration and progressive heart failure, hence pregnancy is strongly discouraged in such patients. Tummala reported mortality in the range of 8–17% in such patients compared to 0–2% in patients with normal left ventricular ejection fraction before the subsequent pregnancy.[16]

Overall recommendation clearly being that pregnancy is avoided in women with persistent poor left ventricular function. Women whose LV function normalizes should still be made aware of the risk of possible recurrence, dobutamine stress test should be performed and due counseling should be done, though majority of these women can have successful pregnancy with appropriate monitoring.

CONCLUSION

Peripartum cardiomyopathy is an uncommon but potential life-threatening cardiac failure of unknown etiology, encountered late in pregnancy or in the postpartum period. Diagnosis of PPCM should essentially include echocardiographic substantiation of left ventricular dysfunction. Benefit of diuretics, vasodilators, digoxin, beta-blockers and anticoagulant in medical management is well established. ACE inhibitors and ArB blockers should be avoided during pregnancy but should be started in postpartum period. In resistant cases, pentoxifylline, immunoglobulin and immunosuppressive drugs may be used. Bromocriptine and cabergoline hold promise for the future. Severe cases might require advanced life-support systems and even heart transplantation. Prognosis is linked to recovery of left ventricular functions. Subsequent pregnancies are associated with a very high mortality more so in those whose LV functions do not improve even six month after puerperium, hence pregnancy should be avoided in this group. In patients with normal cardiac function on echo evaluation subsequent pregnancy may be considered under close supervision and after due counseling.

REFERENCES

1. Pearson GD, Veille JC, rahimttola S, et al. Peripartum Cardiomyopathy. National Heart, Lung and Blood Institute and Office of Rare Diseases (National Institute of Health) Workshop Recommendation and Review. JAMA. 2000;283:1183-8.
2. Pandit V, Shetty S, Kumar A, et al. Incidence and outcome of peripartum cardiomyopathy from a tertiary hospital in South India. Trop Doct. 2009;39:168-9.
3. Desai D, Moodley J, Naidoo D. Peripartum Cardiomyopathy Experience at King Edward VIII Hosp, Durban, South Africa and a review of the literature. Trop Doct. 1995;25:118-23.
4. Fett JD, Christie LJ, Carraway RD, et al. Five year prospective study of the incidence and prognosis of the peripartum cardiomyopathy at a single institution. Mayo Clinic Proc. 2005;80:1602-6.
5. Sanderson JE, Adesanya CO, Anjorin Fi, et al. Postpartum cardiac failure-heart failure due to volume over load? Am Heart J. 1979;97:613-21.

6. Melvin KR, Richardson PJ, Olsen EG, Daly K, Jackson G. Peripartum cardiomyopathy due to myocarditis. Engl J Med. 1982;307(12):731-4.
7. Bultmann BD, Klingel K, Nabauer M, Wallwiener D, Kandolf R. High prevalence of viral genomes and inflammation in peripartum cardiomyopathy. Am J Obstet Gynecol. 2005; 193(2):363-5.
8. Rizeq MN, Rickenbacher PR, Fowler MB, Billingham ME. Incidence of myocarditis in peripartum cardiomyopathy. Am J Cardiol. 1994;74(5):474-7.
9. Midei MG, DeMent SH, Feldman AM, Hutchins GM, Baughman KL. Peripartum myocarditis and cardiomyopathy. Circulation. 1990;81(3):922-8.
10. Felker GM, Jaeger CJ, Klodas E, et al. Myocarditis and long-term survival in peripartum cardiomyopathy. Am Heart J. 2000;140:785-91.
11. Cenac A, Gaultier Y, Devillechabrolle A, Moulias R. Enterovirus infection in peripartum cardiomyopathy. Lancet. 1988;2:968.
12. Cenac A, Djibo A, Chaigneau C, Velmans N, Or Wla J. Are anti- *Chlamydia pneumoniae* antibodies prognosis indicators for peripartum cardiomyopathy? J Cardiovasc Risk. 2003;10: 195.
13. Ansari AA, Fett JD, Carraway RE, et al. Autoimmune mechanisms as the basis for human peripartum cardiomyopathy. Clin Rev Allergy Immunol. 2002;23:301-24.
14. Johnson-Coyle L, Jensen L, Sobey A. American College of Cardiology Foundation; American Heart Association. Peripartum cardiomyopathy: review and practice guidelines. Am J Crit Care. 2012;21(2):89-98.
15. Sliwa K, Forster O, Libhaber E, et al. Peripartum cardiomyopathy: inflammatory markers as predictors of outcome in 100 prospectively studied patients. Eur Heart J. 2006;27: 441-6.
16. Tummala PP, Akhter MW, Hameed AB, et al. Risk of subsequent pregnancies in women with a history of peripartum cardiomyopathy. Circulation. 1999;100:38.

Chapter 21

Respiratory Diseases During Pregnancy

Priyanka Kukrele, Shashi Khare

INTRODUCTION

A variety of physiologic alterations and adaptations occurs to the maternal respiratory system in normal pregnancy. Some level of dyspnea is encountered by almost 70% of pregnant women. This is generally described as "air hunger".[1]

ALTERATION IN RESPIRATORY PHYSIOLOGY DURING PREGNANCY

Upper airway involvement is seen in form of nasal mucosal edema, which is a common finding in normal pregnancy. Symptoms related to rhinitis occurs in around 20% of gravid women,[2] chest wall configuration is altered due to 50% increase in the average costal angle, diaphragmatic position is also elevated by 4–5 cm[3] and functional residual capacity is diminished by about 18% or 300–500 mL.[4] The most striking changes are in the respiratory drive and minute ventilation. Arterial blood gas measurements typically shows the pH ranging from 7.40 to 7.47, with PCO_2 reaching as low as 28–32 mm Hg.

ASTHMA

Asthma in pregnant women is the most common chronic medical disease which is life-threatening. A common reason of asthmatic patient deterioration in pregnancy is poor compliance of patient for medication due to misconception that treatment of asthma is harmful to fetus. Gastro-esophageal reflux disease (GERD) and pregnancy rhinitis are two treatable reasons which worsens the asthma in pregnancy.

Maternal and Fetal Risks

Maternal and fetal risks that are established are an increased risk of preterm delivery, pre-eclampsia, vaginal hemorrhage, complicated labor, neonatal mortality, and placenta previa.[5] The risk of reported complications appears to be greater in women with steroid dependent or poorly controlled asthma.

Management

Patient education is important regarding the use of maintenance and rescue asthma medications. Monitoring the patient with proper use of inhalers, and avoidance of asthma precipitants should be done. The goal of treatment for asthma in pregnancy is to provide optimal therapy to maintain asthma control, defined as minimal or no exacerbations, minimal or no chronic symptoms, no limitation of activity, minimal use of short-acting inhaled $β_2$-agonists and minimal or no adverse effects by treatment.

Asthma Medications in Pregnancy

Asthma medications are classified as either rescue agents or maintenance agents. Rescue agents are the drugs which treat the acute bronchospasm and provide symptomatic relieve, this includes $β_2$-agonists and ipratropium. **Table 21.1**[5] shows the asthmatic medications in pregnancy. Maintenance drugs are those medications that help to control airway hyperactivity and treat the underlying inflammation of the airway.

Management of Asthma in Pregnancy

Treatment of asthma is a stepwise approach:
- Mild intermittent asthma is defined as symptoms upto twice a week and/or, night-time symptoms upto twice a month, peak expiratory flow rate (PEFR) >80% predicted and day-to-day variability. It is treated with inhaled $β_2$-agonists occasionally.[5]
- Mild persistent asthma is defined as symptoms more than twice a week but not daily and/or, night-time symptoms more than twice a month PEFR>80% predicted. Treatment includes inhaled low-dose corticosteroid daily, inhaled $β_2$-agonist, whenever required and alternative drugs such as cromolyn, theophylline and leukotriene-receptor antagonist.[5]
- Moderate persistent defined as night-time symptoms more than once a week, daily symptoms, and PEFR 60–80%. Treatment includes inhaled $β_2$-agonists and, daily inhaled low-dose corticosteroid and salmeterol or daily inhaled

Table 21.1: Asthmatic medications in pregnancy

Class	Agent	Comments
Short-acting inhaled β_2 agonist	Salbutamol, terbutaline	Relieves the respiratory symptoms acutely
Long-acting inhaled β_2 agonist	Salmeterol	Preferred as inhalational route
Inhaled anticholinergic agent	Ipratropium	Usually safe
Inhaled corticosteroids	*Low potency:* beclomethasone *Medium potency:* Triamcinolone *High potency:* Fluticasone, Budesonide	Most important in maintaining asthma control during pregnant and nonpregnant state. Budesonide is safest of all
Mast cell stabilizers	Cromolyn	Less used nowadays
Leukotriene antagonists	Zafirlukast, Montelukast	Not frequently used and helpful in mild cases only
Sustained release methylxanthines	Theophyline Aminophylline	To be used in pregnancy, if patient not relieved by other medications
Systemic steroids	*Oral:* Prednisone *Intravenous:* Methylprednisolone hydrocortisone	It is cornerstone of asthma treatment. It is used when its use overweight the harmful effects in pregnancy
Immunotherapy	Allergen extract used in increasing dose	Much role is not known

medium dose corticosteroid. Alternative treatment with above-mentioned drugs.[5]
- Severe persistent is continual symptoms that limit the patients activity, with frequent night time symptoms and acute exacerbations, and PEFR <60% predicted. Treatment include inhaled β_2-agonists and daily treatment with inhaled high dose corticosteroid, salmeterol, and if needed systemic corticosteroids.[5]

In pregnancy, GERD[6,7] vasomotor rhinitis of pregnancy, and medication noncompliance should always be considered as possible treatable causes of difficult to control asthma.

Treatment of Acute Severe Asthma Exacerbations

Status asthmaticus (acute severe asthma) should be treated in intensive care unit. High doses intravenous steroids are the cornerstone of asthmatic exacerbations requiring hospital admissions.

General guidelines for admission to hospital include a sustained drop in PEFR to less than 60% of baseline, PaO_2 less than 70 mm Hg at sea level, $PaCO_2$ greater than 35 mm Hg, heart rate of greater than 120 bpm or respiratory rate greater than 22/m.[8,9]

Labor and Delivery

Exacerbations occurring at this time should always be approached with a differential diagnosis that includes pulmonary edema, pulmonary embolism and aspiration.

Prostaglandin F-2α and ergot derivatives should not be used in asthmatics.[10] Regional anesthesia is preferred because of lower risk of pulmonary infection and atelectasis. Stress dose of systemic steroids (hydrocortisone) should be given to any women in labor who have received systemic steroids for longer than 2 to 4 weeks in the preceding year.

PNEUMONIA

The incidence of pneumonia in pregnancy is between 0.8 and 2.7 cases per 1000 deliveries,[11,12] respiratory failure develops in upto 10% of pregnant women with pneumonia.[13] The risk factors for the development of pneumonia in pregnancy are maternal diseases including HIV infections, asthma and cystic fibrosis, smoking, cocaine use, alcohol abuse, anemia, maternal corticosteroid administration for fetal lung maturity and tocolytic therapy use. Community-acquired pneumonia in pregnant women presents with typical features such as abrupt onset of fever and rigors, productive cough, tachycardia, tachypnea and localized inspiratory "crackles". Pregnancy associated reduction in cell-mediated immunity leaves pregnant women with an increased susceptibility to viral and fungal pneumonias.

Maternal and Fetal Risks

Severe maternal morbidity and significant mortality from primary varicella (maternal mortality—14%) and influenza pneumonia remain a major concern. A chest X-ray should be obtained in all the patients. A posteroanterior radiograph performed with a grid and a peak voltage of 90 to 120 kV exposes the mother to 5 to 30 Mrad and the fetus to 100 times less, about 300 Urad.[14] Other fetal risks in the setting of maternal pneumonia include an increase risk of miscarriage, preterm labor, prematurity and low birth weight.[15]

Management

Prepregnancy

American College of Obstetricians and Gynecologists (ACOG) have recommended that currently pregnancy or anticipated pregnancy should routinely receive influenza vaccination during the influenza season regardless of gestational age.[16] Pneumococcal vaccine is advised for woman with high-risk condition such as asthma, diabetes mellitus, and chronic pulmonary or cardiac disease.

Prenatal and Postnatal

American Thoracic Society (ATS) has given the treatment guidelines, they include treatment of uncomplicated pneumonia in pregnancy (who do not require hospitalization) with standard therapy of Azithromycin 500 mg PO on day 1 followed by 250 mg daily for 4 days. They also used alternative therapy with Erythromycin 250 mg qid PO for 10-14 days.

ATS mentions that for patients who requires hospitalization therapy given is ceftriazone 2 g IV once daily with azithromycin 500 mg IV daily (or erythromycin 500 mg IV q6h).

Once patient is afebrile and stable switch to azithromycin 500 mg PO daily for 7-10 days (or erythromycin 250-500 mg PO qid for 10-14 days) with cefuroxime axetil 500 mg PO bid for 10-14 days.[17]

Routine collection of sputum and blood culture before initiation of antibiotic therapy is advisable. With the appropriate antibiotic, improvement in clinical course is expected within 72 hours. Antibiotic such as levofloxacin, clarithromycin and tetracycline should not to be used in pregnancy. For symptomatic relief, antipyretic should be given such as acetoaminophen can be used. If exposure to varicella virus occurs in pregnancy in a woman without protective immunity, varicella zoster immunoglobulin (VZIG) should be administered within 96 hours in an attempt to prevent maternal infection. Parenteral acyclovir should be given to all women who develop varicella infection in pregnancy.[18-22]

CYSTIC FIBROSIS

Cystic fibrosis is an autosomal recessive multisystem disorder characterized by recurrent pulmonary infection due to unusual thick bronchial secretions. The incidence of cystic fibrosis is about 1 in 2000 live births.[23] The symptoms and signs of cystic fibrosis include recurrent and persistent pulmonary infections, elevated sweat chloride level and pancreatic exocrine insufficiency. Due to this thick viscous secretion occurs in lungs, pancreas, intestine and reproductive tracts.[24] Around 70% of adult with cystic fibrosis are chronically ultimately infected with *Pseudomonas aeruginosa*. Patient presents with chronic bronchitis and recurrent pneumonia. Cystic fibrosis is characterized by increased cough, sputum production, shortness of breath and fever.

Maternal and Fetal Risks

Women with cystic fibrosis often suffer from reduced fertility due to abnormal cervical mucous and malnutrition-related amenorrhea.[25] Pregnant women who successfully conceive, out of them 70-80% result in live birth. Risk of gestational diabetes mellitus is increased in pregnant women with cystic fibrosis.[26] Fatal risk includes premature labor, chronic hypoxia, malnutrition, IUGR and preterm delivery.[27]

Management

Prepregnancy

Genetic counseling should be done in all women with cystic fibrosis. The nutritional status of the women should be assessed and optimized prior to pregnancy. Pregnant women with cystic fibrosis should undergo pulmonary function test, arterial blood gas analysis and echocardiography. Pregnancy should be discouraged, if FEV_1 is less than 50% of predicted.[28]

Pregnancy and Labor

The main goal of management for women with cystic fibrosis in pregnancy includes optimization of her nutritional and pulmonary status. Chest physiotherapy and postural drainage on daily basis is very essential part of treatment. The use of supplemental oxygen is essential for maternal and fetal wellbeing. Bronchodilator drugs can be used safely in pregnancy. The use of penicillin, cephalosporins, trimethoprim/sulfamethoxazole and aminoglycoside is safe in pregnancy.[29,30] Aerozolized beta-adrenergic agents are used mostly. For women with persistent productive cough are nebulized and endonuclease DNAase1 is often used. During labor, vaginal delivery and regional anesthesia is ideal.

PULMONARY EDEMA AND ACUTE RESPIRATORY DISTRESS SYNDROME

General

Gravid women are at increased risk for pulmonary edema due to physiological changes in pregnancy. There is 50% increase in blood volume and cardiac output, 20% decrease in colloid osmotic pressure and decreased functional residual capacity.[31] The overall incidence of pulmonary edema in pregnancy is approximately 80 in 100, 000 pregnancy.[32]

Cardiogenic Pulmonary Edema

Cardiogenic pulmonary edema is due to elevated pulmonary venous pressure causing hydrostatic pressure gradient that causes the movement of fluid into the alveoli,[33] which is being referred as congestive heart failure. Peripartum cardiomyopathy and pre-eclampsia-associated myocardial dysfunction are the causes specific to pregnancy. Standard therapy for heart failure includes beta-blockers, diuretics, angiotensin-converting enzyme inhibitors.[34]

Noncardiogenic Pulmonary Edema

It is due to result of fluid leakage into alveoli across a leaky pulmonary capillary bed despite normal intravascular pressure. The causes of noncardiogenic edema includes pre-eclampsia, eclampsia, tocolytic therapy, amniotic fluid embolism, sepsis due to any cause, chemical pneumonitis, venous air embolism, aspiration, pancreatitis and severe hemorrhage.[35]

Noncardiogenic pulmonary edema is subclassified as acute lung infection (ALI) and acute respiratory distress syndrome (ARDS). They are diagnosed on the basis of acute onset symptoms, with bilateral chest radiographic infiltrates, pulmonary artery occlusion pressure < 18 mm Hg or no evidence of left atrial hypertension. For diagnosis of ALI impaired oxygenation with PaO_2/FiO_2 of 200–300 mm Hg and ≤200 Hg for ARDS is seen.[36]

Tocolysis-associated Pulmonary Edema

β_2-sympathetic agents administration to premature labor has been associated with 0–4.4% incidence of pulmonary edema.[36] It usually presents after 24 hours of β-adrenergic therapy, with acute onset of dyspnea and pulmonary edema seen on chest radiograph. Discontinuation of the drugs results in acute improvement.

Pulmonary Edema with Pre-eclampsia

Pulmonary edema occurs in 2.9% of patients with pre-eclampsia or eclampsia.[37] Excessive intravenous fluid administration after oliguria is another important factor for pulmonary edema.

Pulmonary Embolism

Pulmonary embolism is one of the leading causes of maternal mortality. Even though the venous thromboembolism is five times increased but still it is relatively infrequent. The risk of thrombosis is increased in pregnancy partly because of the increase in coagulation factors that is V, VIII, X and von Willebrand factor, and due to increase in protein S.[38] Venous stasis is caused by uterine compression of the inferior vena cava. Specific risk factors include patients taking oral contraceptive pills, prolonged bed rest, age and inherited coagulation defects.

The initial diagnosis test should be duplex ultrasonography. The gold standard for detecting lower extremity thrombosis remains venography.[39] Embolism in pregnancy is treated with heparin because warfarin crosses the placenta. If labor begins unexpectedly reversal of the heparin effect with protamine is advisable. Postpartum warfarin can be given safely during lactation.

Amniotic Fluid Embolism

Amniotic fluid embolism (AFE) is a rare but catastrophic complication of pregnancy that typically presents as the abrupt onset of hypotension, dyspnea, and altered mental status proceeding to full blown disseminated intravascular coagulation and ARDS. The diagnosis is critical and should be considered in any women near term who presents with sudden cardiorespiratory failure.

Risk factors for the development of AFE include maternal trauma, increased maternal age, multiparity, prolonged labor, meconium staining of the amniotic fluid, use of oxytocin and cesarean delivery. Some researchers would prefer that the syndrome be called anaphylactoid syndrome of pregnancy.

Presentation of Pulmonary Edema in Pregnancy

Patients of pulmonary edema presents with dyspnea, tachypnea, tachycardia, diffuse crackles, wheezing and cough, chest X-ray with abdominal shielding presents as patchy infiltrates. ABG initially reveal decrease in both PaO_2 and $PaCO_2$, but later $PaCO_2$ begin to rise reflecting respiratory failure. Other laboratory investigations required includes complete blood count (CBC), blood urea nitrogen (BUN) and creatinine, alanine aminotransferase (ALT), uric acid, lactate dehydrogenase (LDH), urine protein to creatinine ratio.

Treatment of Pulmonary Edema in Pregnancy

Immediate goal is to maintain adequate maternal oxygenation (PaO_2 >70 mm Hg, SaO_2 ≥95%)[40] to avoid potential hypoxic injury to the fetus. Next step is to treat the precipitating and underlying course that is sepsis with appropriate antibiotics, stopping the offending drugs and tocolytics, and control of blood pressure.

Gentle diuresis with intravenous doses of furesemide (i.e. 10–20 mg) is very effective in treating pulmonary edema. If oxygenation can not be maintained or the patient shows evidence of respiratory fatigue assisted ventilation is required. Endotracheal intubation is required, if PaO_2 <70 mm Hg or $PaCO_2$ >45 mm Hg on 100% oxygen, pregnant women are at higher risk for aspiration during intubation because of delayed gastric emptying and reduced lower esophageal sphincter tone. The FiO_2 should ideally be kept less than 60% if possible. Excessive levels of PEEP >10 H_2O should be avoided.

OTHER RESPIRATORY DISEASES IN PREGNANCY

Interstitial Lung Disease

In pregnant women when interstitial disease occurs, the reduced diffusing capacity may cause difficulty in meeting the increased oxygen requirements of pregnancy. Usually, restriction lung disease appears reasonably well tolerated in pregnancy.[41]

Pleural Disease

Pleural effusions may accompany obstetric complications such as pre-eclampsia and choriocarcinoma, but many women with normal pregnancies develop small asymptomatic pleural effusion in the postpartum period.[42] Pleural effusion occurs as a result of the increased blood volume and reduced colloid osmotic pressure that occurs in pregnancy. The valsalva maneuver of labor may also produce spontaneous pneumothorax and pneumomediastinum, particularly in patients with predisposing conditions such as asthma.

Obstructive Sleep Apnea

Pregnancy can be complicated by obstructive sleep apnea (OSA) affecting both mother and fetus.[43] And OSA usually occurs in obese patients, precipitated by the airway mucosal edema and vascular congestion that accompany pregnancy. OSA and snoring are more common in woman with pre-eclampsia.[44] Treatment with nasal continuous positive airway pressure is safe and effective.

IMPORTANT POINTS

- Breathlessness in pregnancy should be differentiated from respiratory disease in pregnancy to ensure early diagnosis and treatment.
- A common reason of respiratory disease patient deterioration in pregnancy is poor compliance of patient for medication due to misconception that treatment with medication is harmful to fetus.
- Asthma, pulmonary edema and pneumonia are respiratory diseases whose early diagnosis and treatment can significantly reduce maternal and fetal morbidity and mortality.
- Regular follow-up with physician in patient already having respiratory disease is very important.
- Patient with acute respiratory distress should be urgently managed in ICU settings.

REFERENCES

1. Weinberger S. Dyspnea During Pregnancy. In: Rose BD (Ed). Up to Date. Up to Date Wellesley, MA; 2003.
2. Ellegard EK. Clinical and pathologic characteristics of pregnancy rhinitis. Clin Rev Allergy Immunol. 2004;26(3):149-59.
3. Weinberger SE, Weiss ST, Cohen WR, et al. Pregnancy and the lung: State-of-the art. Am Rev Respir Dis. 1980;121:559-81.
4. Cugell DW, Frank NR, Gaensler EA. Pulmonary function in pregnancy. I. Serial observations in normal women. Am Rev Tuberc. 1953;67:568-97.
5. Powrie RO. Drugs in pregnancy: Respiratory disease. Best Pract Res Clin Obstet Gynaecol. 2001;15:913-36.
6. Theodoropoulos DS, Lockey RF, Boyce HW Jr, Bukantz SC. Gastroesophageal reflux and asthma: A review of pathogenesis, diagnosis, and therapy. Allergy. 1999;54:651-61. PMID: 10442520.
7. Samuelson WM, Kopita JM. Management of the difficult asthmatic. Gastroesophageal reflux sinusitis, and pregnancy. Respir care Clin North Am. 1995;1:287-308.
8. Gordon M, Niswander KR, Berendes H, Kantor AG. Fetal morbidity following potentially anoxigenic obstetric conditions. VII. Bronchial asthma. Am J Obstet Gynecol. 1970;106:421-9. PMID: 5410878.
9. Berendes H, Kantor AG. Fetal morbidity following potentially anoxigenic obstetric conditions. VII. Bronchial asthma. Am J. Obstet Gynecol. 1970;106:421-9. PMID: 5410878.
10. Smith AP. The effects of intravenous infusion of graded doses of prostaglandins F2α and E2 on lung resistance in patients undergoing termination of pregnancy. Clin Sci. 1972;44:17-25. PMID: 4684303.
11. Berkowitz K, LaSala A. Risk factors associated with the increasing prevalence of pneumonia during pregnancy. Am J Obstet Gynecol. 1990;163:981-5. PMID: 2403178.
12. Munn MB, Groome LJ, Atterbury JL, et al. Pneumonia as a complication of pregnancy. J Matern Fetal Med. 1999;8:151-4. PMID: 10406296.
13. Maccato M. Respiratory insufficiency due to pneumonia in pregnancy. Obstet Gynecol Clin North Am. 1991;18:289-99. PMID: 1945256.
14. Lim WS, Macfarlane JT, Colthorpe CL. Pneumonia and Thorax. 2001;56:398-405.
15. Parajani SG, Arun AM, Intrauterine infection with varicella zoster virus after maternal varicella. N Engl J Med. 1986;314:1542-6. PMID: 3012334.
16. Centers for Disease Control and Prevention:Prevention and control of influenza: Recommendations of the Advisory Committee on Immunization Practices [ACIP]. MMWR Morb Mortal Wkly Rep. 1998;47(RR-6):5. PMID: 9450722.
17. Campbell GD, et al. Guidelines for the initial management of adults with community-acquired pneumonia: Diagnosis, assessment of severity, and initial antimicrobial therapy. American Thoracic Society. Medical Section of the American Lung Association. Am Rev Respir Dis. 1993;148:1418-26. PMID: 8239186.
18. Boyd K, Walker E. Use of acyclovir to treat cervical pain in pregnancy. Br Med J. 1988;296:393-4.

19. Glaser JB, Loftus J, Ferragamo V, et al. Varicella-zoster infection in pregnancy. N Engl J Med. 1986;5:1416.
20. Haddad J, Simeoni U, Messner J, Willard D. Acyclovir in prophylaxis and perinatal varicella. Lancet. 1987;1:161.
21. Cox SM, Cunningham FG, Luby J. Management of varicella pneumonia complicating pregnancy. Am J Perinatol. 1990;7:300-1. PMID: 2222616.
22. Chapman SJ. Varicella in pregnancy. Semin Perinatol. 1998;22:339-46. PMID: 9738999.
23. Matthews LW, Drotar D. Cystic Fibrosis: A challenging long term chronic disease. Pediatr Clin North Am. 1984;31:133-52. PMID: 6366714.
24. Katkin JP. Clinical manifestations and diagnosis of cystic fibrosis. Rose BD Uptodate. 2003 Uptodate Wellesley, Mass.
25. Lyon A, Bilton D. Fertility issues in cystic fibrosis. Paediatr Respir Rev. 2002;3:236-40. PMID: 12376060.
26. McMullen AH, Pasta DJ, Frederick PD, et al. Impact of pregnancy on women with cystic fibrosis. Chest. 2006;129:706-11. PMID: 16537871
27. Gilljam M, Antoniou M, Shin J, et al. Pregnancy cystic fibrosis fetal and maternal outcome Chest. 2000;118: 85-91. PMID: 10893364.
28. Edenborough FP. Women with cystic fibrosis and their potential for reproduction Thoram. 2001;56:649-55. PMID: 11462069.
29. Liaschko A, Koren G. Cystic fibrosis during pregnancy. Can Fam Physician. 2002;48:463-67. PMID: 11935708.
30. Koren G, Pastuszak A, Ito S. Drugs in pregnancy. N Engl J Med. 1998;338:1128-37. PMID: 9545362.
31. Powrie RO. Acute lung injury. Lee RV, Rosene-Montella K, Barbour LA, et al. Medical Care of the Pregnant Patient. American College of Physicians. Philadelphia. 2000. pp. 397-411.
32. Sciscione AC, Inester T, Largoga M, et al. Acute pulmonary odema in pregnancy. Obstet Gynecol. 2003;101:511-5. PMID: 12636955.
33. Graves CR. Acute pulmonary complications during pregnancy. Clin Obstet Gynecol. 2002;45:369-76. PMID: 12048396.
34. Murali S, Baldisseri MR. Peripartum cardiomyopathy, Crit Care Med. 2005;33(10 Suppl):S3406.
35. James DK, GonikB, Steer PJ, Weiner CP. High risk pregnancy. Management options. 4th edn, pg. 676.
36. Pisani RJ, Rosenow EC. Pulmonary edema associated with tocolytic therapy. Ann Intern Med.1992;110:714-8.
37. Sibai BM, Mabie BC, Harvey CJ, et al. Pulmonary edema in severe preeclampsia-eclampsia: Analysis of thirty-seven consecutive cases. Am J Obstet Gynecol. 1987;156:1174-9.
38. McColl MD, Walker ID, Greer IA. Risk factors for venous thromboembolism in pregnancy. Curr Opin Pulm Med. 1999;5:227-32.
39. Ginsberg JS, Brill-Edwards P, Burrows RF, et al. Venous thrombosis during pregnancy: Leg and trimester of presentation. Thromb Haemost. 1992;67:519.
40. Meschia G. Safety margin of fetal oxygenation. J Reprod Med. 1985;30:308-11. PMID: 4009545. Supply of oxygen to the fetus. J Reprod Med. 1979;23:160-5. PMID: 513041.
41. Boggess KA, Easterling TR, Raghu G. Management and outcome of pregnant women with interstitial and restrictive lung disease. Am J Obstet Gynecol. 1995;173:1007-14.
42. Heffner JE, Sahn SA. Pleural disease in pregnancy. Clin Chest Med. 1992;13:667-8.
43. Edwards N, Middieton PG, Blyton DM, Sullivan CE. Sleep disordered breathing and pregnancy. Thorax. 2002;57:555-8.
44. Perez-Chada D, Videla AJ, O'Flaherty ME, et al. Snoring, witnessed sleep apnoeas and pregnancy-induced hypertension. Acta Obstet Gynecol Scand. 2007;86:788-92.

Chapter 22

Pregnancy and Chronic Kidney Disease

Rubina Vohra, Shabbir H Husain, Nafisa Husain

There are significant changes in renal anatomy and physiology in normal pregnancy that lead to marked alterations from the non-pregnant physiologic norm. To understand the pathology of normal and compromised pregnancy, it is necessary to learn these changes.

ANATOMICAL AND PHYSIOLOGICAL CHANGES IN KIDNEY DURING PREGNANCY

Anatomy

In normal pregnancy, there is a progressive increase in renal size, maximally 1 to 2 cm by 26 weeks' gestation, and 70% of which is contributed by vascular and interstitial fluid compartments.[1] The most striking anatomic change is dilation of the calyces, renal pelvis, and ureters which is more prominent on right side, and by the third trimester, about 80–90 % of women show evidence of hydronephrosis.[2] A consequence of the ureteral dilation is urinary stasis, which predisposes pregnant women with asymptomatic bacteriuria to development of symptomatic ascending infection (acute pyelonephritis). Rarely, the anatomic changes may be extreme and precipitate the over distension syndrome, with massive dilation, recurrent severe flank pain, increasing serum creatinine, hypertension, or even reversible acute kidney injury.[3]

Physiology

The cause of the dilatation is disputed; some advocate hormonal effects and others, obstruction.[4] There is no doubt that, as pregnancy progresses, the supine or upright posture may cause partial ureteric obstruction as the enlarged uterus compresses the ureter at the pelvic brim, where dilatation terminates as the ureter crosses the iliac artery, and at this point, a filling defect termed the "iliac sign" can be demonstrated. These structural changes have the following important clinical implications:
- Dilatation of the urinary tract may lead to collection errors in tests based on timed urine volume; for example 24-h creatinine clearance and/or protein excretion. Such errors are minimized, if the pregnant woman is sufficiently hydrated to give a high urine flow, and/or if she lies down on her side for an hour before and at the end of the collection.
- Acceptable norms of kidney size should be increased by 1 cm, if radiography is undertaken during pregnancy or immediately after delivery. Dilatation of the ureters may persist until the 16th post-partum week, and elective IVU during this period should be deferred.[5] Ureteric dilation is permanent in up to 11% of parous women with no history of urinary tract infection.[6] Very occasionally, there can be massive dilation of the ureters and renal pelvis (as well as slight reduction in cortical width), but this is without ill-effect.[1] Rarely, the changes may be extreme and precipitate the "overdistension syndrome" and/or hypertension.[3]
- Urinary stasis within the ureters may contribute to the propensity of pregnant women with asymptomatic bacteriuria to develop frank pyelonephritis.

SYSTEMIC HEMODYNAMICS

There are significant alterations in systemic hemodynamics in normal pregnancy. A plasma (and extracellular fluid) volume expansion occurs while red blood cell volume also increases, leading to a large increase in blood volume that correlates with clinical outcome and birth weight. Women with twins and triplets have proportionately greater increments, and those with poorly growing fetuses, as in pre-eclampsia or with a history of poor reproductive performance, have correspondingly poor plasma volume responses. The increase in plasma volume takes place progressively up to 32–34 weeks, after which there is little further change. The plasma volume expansion has a hemodilutional effect, causing decreases in hematocrit: the physiologic anemia of normal pregnancy.[7] Cardiac output is significantly increased by the fifth gestational week, initially caused by a 10–20% increase in heart rate, with stroke volume increased by more than 20% the eighth week. Left atrial and left ventricular end-diastolic dimensions increase, suggesting an associated increase in venous return. Cardiac output increases by 40% to 50% are greatest by the 26th week, despite which systemic blood pressure (BP) substantially decreases in normal pregnancy.[8] The physiologic decrease in BP results from a profound reduction in systemic vascular resistance (SVR) of unknown cause (maximal at 26 weeks), although the loss of responsiveness to vasoconstrictor agents (e.g., angiotensin II, arginine vasopressin) certainly contributes.[9] Inhibition of angiogenic factors in pre-eclampsia causes vasoconstriction, suggesting that these factors, such as vascular endothelial growth factor (VEGF), may contribute importantly to normal gestational vasodilation through stimulation of endothelial nitric oxide and prostaglandins.[10] The combination of increased cardiac output and peripheral vasodilation means that organ blood flow increases in pregnancy, with the most dramatic changes occurring in the kidney and skin circulation throughout gestation and in the uterus in the second part of the pregnancy.[11] Left ventricular mass continues to increase up to 36 weeks, but thereafter, perhaps related to the increasing SVR toward term, systolic and diastolic cardiac function decrease, with increased ventricular wall stress, caused by decrements in both myocardial contraction and relaxation capacity.[12] In the third trimester, the enlarged uterus compresses surrounding tissues and can influence hemodynamic measurements, so that attention should be paid to maternal posture during hemodynamic monitoring. In the supine position, there is partial obstruction of the inferior vena cava and decreased venous return, reducing cardiac output and causing a decrease in BP, the supine hypotensive syndrome of pregnancy. It is important to be aware of these postural effects in measuring BP in late pregnancy.[11]

RENAL HEMODYNAMICS

There are striking changes in renal hemodynamics in normal pregnancy, with an increase in glomerular filtration rate (GFR) and consequent decrease in serum creatinine detectable very early.[11,13] The GFR increases about 25% by 4 weeks after the last menstrual period, and a robust early increase in GFR is associated with a good obstetric outcome. Longitudinal studies in normal pregnant women show that GFR (measured by inulin or 24-hour creatinine clearance) increases by a maximum of about 50% by midpregnancy, which is maintained until the last few weeks of the pregnancy, when values begin to decrease, but remain above the nonpregnant level.[14] These marked increases in GFR mean that serum creatinine decreases to 0.4–0.5 mg/dL (36–45 μmol/L),[15] and values considered normal for nonpregnant conditions, at 0.7–0.8 mg/dL (63–72 μmol/L), can be a cause for concern in normal pregnancy **(Table 22.1)**. In small women, however, whose total muscle mass may be quite low, significantly elevated serum creatinine levels may be absent, even in the presence of renal dysfunction. The increase in renal plasma flow (RPF) of about 60% is slightly more pronounced than the increase in GFR, so that the filtration fraction (FF) decreases (see later discussion). At the end of pregnancy, the RPF decreases proportionally more than the GFR, so that FF returns to the nonpregnant value[14,16] (In pregnant women, there is a decrease in serum protein concentration that contributes slightly to the increased GFR).

Table 22.1: Changes (means) in some common indices during pregnancy

	Non-pregnant	Pregnancy
Hct (vol/dL)	41	33
$P_{protein}$ (g/dL)	7.0	6.0
P_{osm} (mOsm/kg)	285	275
P_{Na} (mEq/L)	140	135
P_{cr} mmol/L (mg/dL)	73 (0.8)	45 (0.5)
P_{urea} mmol/L (mg/dL)	4.5 (27)	3.3 (20)
pH units	7.40	7.44
P_{CO_2} (kPa)	40	30
P_{HCO_3} (mEq/L)	25	20
Serum uric acid (mg/dL, μmol/L)	4.0 (240)	3.2 (190) early 4.3 (260) late
Systolic BP (mm Hg)	115	105
Diastolic BP (mm Hg)	70	60

PREGNANCY IN PATIENT WITH KIDNEY DISEASE

Introduction

In normal pregnancy, significant renal physiological and anatomical changes occur. In women with chronic kidney diseases (CKD), these adaptation may not be optimum and will affect both maternal and fetal outcome.[17] fertility rates are reduced in women with moderate-to-severe CKD. While learning about pregnancy in disease with kidney, two aspects needs to be considered. First is how pregnancy influences underlying kidney disease and second kidney diseases affecting the outcome of pregnancy.

CKD's adverse affects on pregnancy: Upto 3–10% women of child-bearing age have CKD stage 3-5.[18] Pregnancy outcome data are mainly from old studies and probably, they over-estimated the risk compared to outcomes achieved with better perinatal and neonatal care and also now we are using and eGFR rather than creatinine. The key factors which affects the outcome of CKD are:
- Degree of renal impairment
- Control of hypertension
- Degree of proteinuria
- Infection

The gestational increase in GFR seen in normal pregnancies is attenuated in moderate renal impairment and is absent if serum creatinine is >2.3 mg/dL.[17,19,20]

Table 22.2: Maternal renal and fetal outcome according to prepregnancy serum creatinine

Maternal renal outcome	Fetal outcome after accounting 1st trimester miscarriage
Creatinine <1.5 • Permanent loss of GFR in <10% of women • Greatest risk, if GFR <40 mg and proteinuria >1 gm/day • Major determinant is HTN. • Major risk of pre-eclampsia, if baseline proteinuria > 500 mg/dL	• Live births in >90% women • Upto 50% preterm delivery • 60% small for gestational age, if baseline proteinuria >500 mg/day
Creatinine 1.5–2.5 mg/dL • Decline or permanent lose of GFR in 30% women increased to 50%, if uncontrolled HTN • 10% ESRD soon after pregnancy.	• Live births in about 85% women unless uncontrolled HTN (MAP >105) at conception • 60% prematurity
Creatinine >2.5 • Progression to ESRD highly likely during or soon after pregnancy	• High chances of fetal loss

The traditional view was that most women with mild renal impairment (serum creat <1.5 mg/dL) and controlled hypertension have a successful pregnancy outcome.

However, a recent study challenges this view. Perinatal mortality, preterm delivery, small for gestational age rates and development of superimposed pre-eclampsia appear high even in patients with mild renal impairment (**Table 22.2**).[21]

Management Protocols

- Management of HTN for target blood pressure 110–140/80–90 mm Hg.
- Aspirin 75-150 mg daily, if creatinine >1.5 and /or creatinine 0.9-1.5 and proteinuria >1 gm
- *Regular medication review:* Discontinue statins, ACE inhibitors, ARB.
- Correct interpretation of changes in serum creatinine.
- Clinical assessment and maintenance of volume homeostasis
- Correct interpretation and management of proteinuria including nephrotic syndrome
- Identification of superimposed pre-eclampsia
- Identification and management of urinary tract infection
- Consideration of the primary renal disease
- Assessment of for fetal well-being and consider, if delivery is indicated.

Prepregnancy Counseling for Women with CKD

It has long been known that any women with CKD stage 3 to 5 should receive prepregnancy counseling. We now know that this should also apply to women with CKD stage 1 or 2, particularly, if they have associated: HTN, significant proteinuria, a poor obstetric history, recurrent UTI, inheritable renal diseases or other disease (like SLE) likely to worsen during pregnancy.[22-24] **Table 22.3** summarizes the issues which should be covered in counseling.

Table 22.3: Prepregnancy counseling for women with CKD

Maternal Risk:
- Accelerated decline in GFR requiring dialysis during pregnancy or soon after.
- Severe maternal hypertension with risk of stroke
- Superimposed pre-eclampsia with renal hepatic, thrombotic or bleeding with neurological risk
- Nephrotic syndrome with risk of thrombosis or sepsis
- Iron or vitamins deficiency

Fetal Risk:
- Fetal growth restriction
- Intrauterine fetal death from placental insufficiency
- Prematurity with both short- and long-term consequences
- Complications of drug therapy for renal disease during pregnancy
- Inheritance of a renal disorders

Differential Diagnosis of Pre-eclampsia and Pre-existing Renal Disease

Pre-eclampsia is increased significantly in patients with CKD and associated with increased fetal and maternal morbidity. Identification of superimposed pre-eclampsia is important during pregnancy, however, diagnosis of pre-eclampsia in presence of CKD may be difficult. Worsening of hypertension and proteinuria with hyperreflexia favors the diagnosis of pre-eclampsia, and the occurrence of elevated liver enzymes, thrombocytopenia and microangiopathic hemolytic anemia in severe pre-eclampsia makes the diagnosis easy.[25] The distinguishing features between pre-eclampsia and preexisting renal disease are given in **Table 22.4**.

It has been proposed that an increased ratio of soluble fms-like tyrosine kinase 1 (SFlt-1) to placental growth factor PIGF is diagnostic of pre-eclampsia and distinguishing this condition from pregnant women with CKD.[26]

Table 22.4: Differential diagnosis of pre-eclampsia and pre-existing renal disease

During pregnancy	Pre-eclampsia	Pre-existing renal diseases
Proteinuria	After 20 weeks	May occurs before 20 weeks
Hematuria	—	May occur
Cast	Rarely seen	Often seen
HTN	After 20 weeks gestation	May occur before 20 weeks
Thrombocytopenia	Occur in moderate and severe pre-eclampsia	Not usually seen
Elevated hepatic transaminases	Occur in moderate and severe pre-eclampsia	Not usually seen

Indications for Delivery in Women with CKD or Pre-eclampsia

In women with stable CKD and no evidence of fetal compromise, pregnancies should be continued to term and spontaneous labor awaited. The method of delivery is normally determined by other issues such as (previous cesarean section, poor obstetric history, etc) rather than the presence of CKD.

Indications of delivery are:
- Inability to control BP
- Deteriorating GFR
- Neurological abnormalities such as eclampsia, headache with accompanying clonus and hyperreflexia or repeated visual scotomata
- Worsening thrombocytopenia
- Increasing liver transaminase levels
- Failure of fetal growth
- Reversed or absent end diastolic flow or Echo.

RENAL BIOPSY DURING PREGNANCY

It is rare to require renal biopsy in pregnancy after 32 weeks gestation if renal biopsy is indicated it should be done after planning delivery. Complications rates of renal biopsy in pregnancy are similar to nonpregnant patient.[27]

Biopsy may be done during pregnancy in following settings:
- *De novo* onset of nephrotic range proteinuria except pre-eclampsia
- Unexplained decline in GFR with active urinary sediment before fetal viability (<24 weeks gestation)
- Pregnancy <32 weeks and you are planning to prolong pregnancy and want to use immunosuppression or plasmapheresis
- Unexplained decline in GFR in patients with known primary glomerular diseases.
- Acute kidney injury with active urinary sediment
- Worsening of proteinuria or decline in GFR in patients of lupus nephritis or in a patients with lupus without known nephritis
- Deteriorating GFR in patients with renal transplant to rule out acute rejection.

DIALYSIS IN PREGNANCY

There has been significant improvement in the outcome of pregnant women with renal diseases requiring dialysis during pregnancy over the past two decades and also reduction in therapeutic terminations because of more intensive dialysis regimen and advances in neonatal care allowing survival for more premature and growth-restricted infants.[28]

Pregnancies now have one and half to two-thirds chances of fetal survival, although about 80% chance of prematurity.[29,30] **Table 22.5** provides recommendation for managing hemodialysis during pregnancy.

Initializing Dialysis for Progressive CKD

Initiation of dialysis during pregnancy is usually recommended at eGFR <20 mL/minutes or BUN 50 mg/dL and aim for predialysis BUN <45 mg/dL.[31,32]

The available data suggest that dialysis initiated during pregnancy is associated with greater likelihood of successful pregnancy than with continuing conservative treatment

Pregnancy in Patients Already on Dialysis

Pregnancy is uncommon in patients on dialysis and ranges from 0.3 to 1.5%/year in women of child-bearing age.[33] With current management live birth rates (after excluding elective abortion) of 60–70% have been reported. The chances of successful pregnancy to large extent depends on the close cooperation among patient, nephrologist, dialysis staff, obstetrician and neonatologist.[34] Live birth rates of 30–70% have been reported.[35,36]

DIAGNOSIS OF PREGNANCY

Menstruation is irregular in patients on dialysis and up to 42% may have amenorrhea and the diagnosis of pregnancy is often delayed.[37] Moreover levels of human chronic gonadotropin

Table 22.5: Managing hemodialysis during pregnancy

Pre-pregnancy
- Discuss risks of pregnancy (miscarriage, fetal death, fetal growth restriction, prematurity, pre-eclampsia).
- Ensure all medications safe in pregnancy.
- *Aspirin:* 75–150 mg daily
- *Folic acid:* 5 mg daily

During Pregnacy:

Dialysis	20 hour/week in four or more sessions aim for predialysis BUN>40 mg/dL (serum urea 15 mmol/L). Heparin requirement may increase because of hypercoagulability of pregnancy.
Anemia	Intravenous iron to maintain iron stores. Dose ESA to achieve hemoglobin of 10–11 g/dL.
Bicarbonate	Adjust oral and dialysate bicarbonate to achieve normal serum bicarbonate for pregnancy (18–22 mmol/L).
Nutrition	• Dietician advice to ensure adequate protein and nutrient intake • Supplement oral or dialysate phosphate to maintain postdialysis serum phosphate in normal range.
Calcium	Maintain normal serum calcium with additional oral calcium and vitamin D, as well as increased dialysate calcium. Hypercalcemia occasionally provoked by placental PTHrP and vitamin D like substances
Phosphate	Supplement oral or dialysate phosphate to maintain postdialysis serum phoshate in normal range.

After Pregnancy:
- Return to usual dialysis schedule immediately.
- Readjust dry weight and antihypertensive weekly for 6 weeks.

Table 22.6: Outcome of pregnancy

Frequency of abortion	18–17%
IUGR	20–77
Preterm delivery	54–100%
Polyhydramnios	41–61
Cesarean section	14–7%

Abbreviation: IUGR, intrauterine growth restriction

Table 22.7: Management of pregnancy in women with chronic kidney disease

Prepregnancy
- Advise increased risk of adverse pregnancy outcome (preterm labor, IUGR, and pre-eclampsia)
- Discontinue ACE inhibitors, ARBs

Antenatal
- After first trimester increase dialysis regimen to almost daily (20–24 hours/week)
- To keep predialysis BUN <50 g/dL
- Increase EPO and iron to keep Hb 10–11 g/dL
- Recognize gestational weight gain, approximately 0.5 kg/week in 2nd and 3rd trimester
- Give aspirin 75 mg and folic acid 5 mg daily throughout
- Aim for protein intake 1.2–1.8 g/kg/day

Labor and delivery
- Cesarean section most likely
- Women on PD will need temporary HD

Postnatal
Gradually return to nonpregnant dialysis regimen over 2 weeks.

are high in patients with CKD and not reliable for diagnosis of pregnancy.[33] The time of diagnosis (generally by ultrasound) may vary from 14 weeks to 16.5 weeks.[36,37]

Outcome of Pregnancy in Dialysis Patients

Overall rate of successful delivery was around 70% in patients on HD and 64% in patients on peritoneal dialysis **(Table 22.6)**.[38]

The mean age of delivery varied from 30 weeks to 32 weeks.[36,39-42]

MATERNAL COMPLICATIONS

Approximately, 80% of dialysis patients have hypertension. In more than half blood pressure exceeds 170/40 mm Hg requiring intensive care admission.[39]

Principles of Management

Improvements by dialysis management and the use of erythropoietin have increased the chances of conception in dialysis patients **(Table 22.7)**.

Dialysis: Fetal outcome is improved with more frequent hemodialysis sessions, generally 4-6 sessions or 20 hours per week to keep BUN under 50 mg/dL.[43,44] The aim is to avoid hydramnios, control hypertension and improve maternal nutrition. Metabolic acidosis and hypocalcemia should be corrected and hypotension during dialysis avoided. Heparin dose is kept at minimum. Heparin does not cross the placenta and is not teratogenic.[45] Continuous ambulatory peritoneal dialysis (PD) and continuous cycling PD with small volumes and frequent exchanges can be used successfully.[44]

Reduction in hemoglobin occurs in pregnant patients on dialysis and in increased doses of erythropoietin (50-100%) may be needed and has been used safely in pregnant patients on dialysis.[33,36,46] Serum iron and ferritin levels are reduced in pregnancy; intravenous iron may be needed and has been safely used in pregnancy.[47]

REFERENCES

1. Brown MA. Urinary tract dilatations in pregnancy. American Journal of Obstetrics and Gynecology. 1990;164:641-3.
2. Cietak KA, Newton JR. Serial qualitative nephronosonography in pregnancy. British Journal of Radiology. 1985;58:399-404.
3. Khauna N, Nguyn H. Reversible acute renal failure in association with bilateral ureteral obstruction and hydronephrosis in pregnancy. American Journal of Obstetrics and Gynecology. 2001;184,239-40.
4. Croce JF, Signorelli P, Chapparini I. Hydronephrosis in Pregnancy. Ultrasonographic Study (Ital). Minerva Ginicologica. 1994;46:147-53.
5. Rasmussen PE, Nielsen FR. Hydronephrosis during pregnancy: a literature survey. European Journal of Obstetrics, Gynaecology, and Reproductive Biology. 1988;27:249-59.
6. Fried AM, Woodring JH, Thompson DS. Hydronephrosis in pregnancy: A prospective sequential study of course of dilatation. Journal of Ultrasound and Medicine. 1982;2:255-9.
7. Brown M, Gallery EDM. Volume homeostasis in normal pregnancy and preeclampsia: physiology and clinical implications. Clin Obstet Gynecol. 1994;8:287-310.
8. Ogueh O, Brookes C, Johnson MR. A longitudinal study of the cardiovascular adaptation to spontaneous and assisted conception pregnancies. Hypertens Pregnancy. 2009;28:273-89.
9. Magness RR, Gant NE. Normal vascular adaptations in pregnancy: potential clues for understanding pregnancy induced hypertension. In: Walker JJ, Gant NF (Eds). Hypertension in Pregnancy. London: Chapman and Hall Medical; 1997. pp. 5-26.
10. Maynard SE, Min JY, Merchan J, et al. Excess placental soluble fms-like tyrosine kinase may contribute to endothelial dysfunction, hypertension and proteinuria in preeclampsia. J Clin Invest. 2003;111:649-58.
11. Ogueh O, Clugh A, Hancock M, Johnson MR. A longitudinal study of the control of renal and uterine hemodynamic changes of pregnancy. Hypertens Pregnancy. 2011;30:243-59.
12. Zentner D, duplessis M, Brennecke S, et al. Deterioration in cardiac systolic and diastolic function late in normal human pregnancy. Clin Sci. 2009;116:599-606.
13. Lindheimer MD, Davison JM, Katz AI. The Kidney and hypertension in pregnancy: Twenty exciting year. Nephrol. 2001;21:173-89.
14. Baylis C, Davison JUM the renal system. In: Chamberlain G, Broughton Pipkin F (Eds). Clinical physiology in obstetrics. 3rd edn. Oxford: Blackwell Science, 1998:263-307.
15. Larsson A, Palm M, Hansson LO, Axelsson O. Reference values for clinical chemistry tests during normal pregnancy. Br J Obstet Gynaecol. 2008;115:874-81.
16. Roberts M, Lindheimer MD, Davison JM. Altered glomerular perm selectivity to neutral dextran and heteroporous membrane modeling in human pregnancy. Am J Physiol. 1996;270:338-43.
17. Wiliams D. Pregnancy with pre-existing kidney disease. In: Feehally J, Floege J, Johnson RJ (Eds). Comprehensive Clinical Nephrology, Mosby. 2007:495-504.
18. Imbasciati E, Gregorini G, Cabiddu G, et al. Pregnancy in CKD stages 3 to 5: fetal and maternal outcomes. Am J Kidney Dis. 2007;49:753-62.
19. Villar MA, Sibai BM. Clinical significance of elevated mean arterial blood in second trimester and threshold increase in systolic or diastolic pressure during third trimester. Am J Obstetric Gynecol. 1989; 60:419-23.
20. Jungers P, Chauvean G, Choukroun G, et al. Pregnancy in women with impaired renal function. Clin Nephrol. 1997;47:281-8.
21. Bramham K, Briley AL, Seed PT, et al. Pregnancy outcome in women with chronic kidney disease: A prospective cohort study. Reprod Sci. 2011;18:623-30.
22. Picoli GB, Attini R, Vasario E, et al. Pregnancy and chronic kidney disease: A challenge in all CKD stages. Clin J Am Soc Nephrol. 2010;5:844-55.
23. Piccoli GB, Fassio F, Attini R, ET AL. Pregnancy in CKD: whom should we follow and why? Nephrol Dial Transplant. 2012;27(Suppl 3):111-8.
24. Nevis IF, Reitsma A, Dominic A, et al. Pregnancy outcomes in women with chronic kidney disease: A systematic review. Clin J Am Soc Nephrol. 2011;6:2587-98.
25. Hou S. The Kidney in pregnancy. In: Greenberg A (Ed). Primer on kidney Diseases Academic Press. 1998;388-94.
26. Rolio A, Attini R, Nuzzo AM, et al. Chronic kidney disease may be differentiallly diagnosed from preeclampsia by serum biomarkers. Kidney Int. 2013,83;177-181.
27. Brunskill N. Renal biopsy in pregnancy. In: Davison JM, Nelson-Piercy C, Kehoe S, Baker P (Eds). Renal Disease in Pregnancy. London: RCOG Press; 2008. pp. 201-6.
28. Hiadunewich M, Hercz AE, Keunen J, et al. Pregnancy in end stage renal diseases. Semin Dial. 2011;24:634-9.
29. Piccoli GB, Conijn A. Consiglio V, et al. Pregnancy in dialysis patients: is the evidence strong enough to lead us to change our counseling policy? Clin J Am Soc Nephrol. 2010;5:62-71.
30. Hou S. Historical perspective of pregnancy in chronic kidney diseases. Adv Chron Kidney Dis. 2007;14:116-8.
31. Asamiya Y, Otsubo S, Matsuda Y, et al. The importance of low blood urea nitrogen levels in pregnant patients undergoing hemodialysis to optimize birth weight and gestational age. Kidney Int. 2009;75:1217-22.
32. Lindheimer MD, Davison JM. Renal disorder. In: Barron WM (Ed). Medical Disorders in Pregnancy. St Louis: Mosby; 2000 pp. 39-70.

33. Hou S. Pregnancy in chronic renal insufficiency and end stage renal diseases. Am J Kidney Dis. 1999;33:235-25.
34. Reddy SS, Holley JL. Management of the pregnant chronic dialysis patient. Adv Chronic Kidney Dis. 2007;14:146-55.
35. Souqiyyeh MZ, Huraib SO, Saleh AGM, Asward S. Pregnancy in chronic hemodialysis patients in the Kingdom of Saudi Arabia. Am J Kidney Dis. 1992;19:235-8.
36. Malik GH, Al Harbi A, Al-Mohaya S, et al. Pregnancy in patients on dialysis: Experience at a Referral center. J Assoc Physicians India. 2005;53:937-41.
37. Confortini P, Galanti G, Ancona G, et al. Full term pregnancy and successful delivery in a patient on chronic hemodialysis. Proc Eur Dial Transplant Assoc. 1971;8:74-80.
38. Chou Cy, Ling IW, Lin TH, Lee CN. Pregnancy in patients on chronic dialysis: A single center experience and combined analysis of reported results. Eur J Obstet Gynecol Reprod Biol. 2008;136:165-70.
39. Chao AS, Huang JY, Leu R, et al. Pregnancy in women who undergo long term hemodialysis. Am J Obstet Gynecol. 2002;187:152-6.
40. Bagon JA, Vernaeve H, De Muylder X, et al. Pregnancy and dialysis. Am J Kidney Dis. 1998;31:756-65.
41. Romao JE, Luders C, Kahhale S, et al. Pregnancy in women in chronic dialysis: A single center experience with 17 cases. Nephron. 1998;78:416-22.
42. Nakabayashi M, Adachi T, ITAH S, et al. Perinatal and infant outcome of pregnant patients undergoing chronic hemodialysis. Nephron. 1998;82:27-31.
43. Hou SH. Pregnancy in women on hemodialysis and peritoneal dialysis. Baillieres' Clin Obstet Gynecol. 1994;8481-500.
44. Krane K, Hamrahian M. Pregnancy: Kidney diseases and hypertension. Am J Kidney Dis. 2007;49:336-45.
45. Ginsberg JS, Kowalchuk G, Hirsh J, et al. Heparin therapy during pregnancy. Arch Intern Med. 1989;149:2233-6.
46. Mitwali A, Malik GH, Fayed H, et al. Erythropoietin therapy in a pregnant woman on maintenance hemodialysis. Saudi J Kidney Diseases and Transplantation. 1994;5:489-92.
47. Okundaye I, Abrinko P, Hou S. Registry of pregnancy in dialysis patients. Am J Kidney Dis. 1998:31;766-73.

Chapter 23

Thyroid Disorders During Pregnancy

Shreya Goenka, Sarita Agrawal

INTRODUCTION

Thyroid diseases affect up to 5% of all pregnancies.

The normal physiological changes in thyroid function during pregnancy have been well characterized:[1] the concentrations of thyroid binding globulins increase up to mid-pregnancy due to high estrogen levels; thyroid-stimulating hormone (TSH) levels decrease in early pregnancy due to direct thyroidal stimulation by human chorionic gonadotropin; thyroid size and thyroid hormone production increase throughout pregnancy and iodine requirements increase due to increased renal clearance and losses to the feto-placental unit. Pregnancy can be considered as a stress test of maternal thyroid function where women with limited thyroid reserve may develop hypothyroidism.[2] Production of thyroxine (T4) and triiodothyronine (T3) increases by 50%, along with a 50% increase in the daily iodine requirement. Ten percent to twenty percent of all pregnant women in the first trimester of pregnancy are thyroid peroxidase (TPO) or thyroglobulin (Tg) antibody positive and euthyroid. Sixteen percent of the women who are euthyroid and positive for TPO or Tg antibody in the first trimester will develop a TSH that exceeds 4.0 mIU/L by the third trimester, and 33-50% of women who are positive for TPO or Tg antibody in the first trimester will develop postpartum thyroiditis. Although it is well accepted that overt hypothyroidism and overt hyperthyroidism have a deleterious impact on pregnancy, studies are now focusing on the potential impact of subclinical hypothyroidism and subclinical hyperthyroidism on maternal and fetal health, the association between miscarriage and preterm delivery in euthyroid women positive for TPO and/or Tg antibody, and the prevalence and long-term impact of postpartum thyroiditis.[3]

Diagnosing thyroid diseases during pregnancy can be difficult as the clinical signs and symptoms mimic those of pregnancy. Current recommendations suggest targeted TSH screening for women at high-risk for thyroid disease before or during early pregnancy with other thyroid function tests used to confirm the diagnoses and disease severity.[2,4] However, reference ranges of TSH or free thyroxine (fT4) obtained from nonpregnant populations do not reflect normal values in pregnant women because of their physiologic changes in thyroid function.[2,4] Several studies have attempted to create trimester- and population-specific reference intervals for TSH concentrations in healthy pregnant women.[5-7] When population and trimester specific reference ranges are not available, women with serum TSH over 2.5 mIU/L in the first and over 3.0 mIU/L in the second and third trimesters of pregnancy are diagnosed with hypothyroidism.[2,4] The magnitude of TSH elevation and measurements of fT4 are used to distinguish between subclinical and overt hypothyroidism.[2,4] Notably, the lower reference limit of TSH concentrations is also decreased in pregnant women, so euthyroid women can be diagnosed as hyperthyroid if nonpregnant reference ranges are used.[2]

The gold standard in measuring fT4 concentrations during pregnancy is equilibrium dialysis coupled with mass spectrometry,[8] but such assays are not readily available in all clinical laboratories. Commonly employed immunoassays often give biased estimates of fT4 concentrations due to interference by the high concentrations of thyroid binding globulins,[9] although fT4 concentrations measured with most immunoassays exhibit the typical pattern related to pregnancy with elevations in early pregnancy and decreases thereafter. However, although results within an assay are valid, the results between assays are generally not comparable and therefore it is recommended to establish assay- and trimester-specific reference values for fT4.[2,4,9] Some recommended overcoming this problem by measuring total thyroxine.[4] However, total thyroxine reference range is wider than that of fT4 due to the underlying variability of thyroid binding globulin, which may lead to reduced diagnostic accuracy especially among subjects with borderline test results.[10] Additionally, although the nonpregnant reference range of total thyroxine can be adapted to the second and third trimesters of pregnancy by multiplying the range by 1.5,[4] there are no total thyroxine reference ranges for the first trimester of pregnancy when the thyroid binding globulin concentrations increase. Measuring fT4 might therefore be more useful in pregnant patients when trying to distinguish between overt and subclinical thyroid diseases. However, clinical decision on diagnosis and treatment of hypothyroidism or hyperthyroidism should mostly be based on serum TSH concentrations and overall clinical picture and symptoms.[2,4]

Hypothyroidism complicates up to 3% of pregnancies, of which 0.3–0.5% is overt and 2.0–2.5% is subclinical hypothyroidism.[2,4]

DEFINITION OF THYROID DYSFUNCTION[3]

- Overt hypothyroidism (OH)
  - Elevated TSH >2.5 with decreased FT4.
  - TSH ≥10.0 m IU/L or above, irrespective of their FT4 level.
- Subclinical hypothyroidism (SCH)
  - TSH – 2.5–10 mIU/L with normal FT4.
- Isolated hypothyroxinemia
  - Normal TSH with FT4 in lower range (5th or 10th percentile of the reference range)
- *Hyperthyroidism:* TSH less than trimester specific lower limit of normal (0.1 in 1st T, 0.2 in second and 0.3 m IU/L in 3rd trimester).

CAUSES OF HYPOTHYROIDISM IN PREGNANCY

The most common cause of hypothyroidism during pregnancy is:
- Iodine deficiency
- Chronic autoimmune thyroiditis
- Iatrogenic causes including surgery to treat thyroid cancer or nodules, or
- Radioactive iodine ablation to treat hyperthyroidism.

Normal Limits of TSH in Pregnancy

According to the American Thyroid Association Taskforce on Thyroid Disease during Pregnancy and Postpartum trimester-specific range of TSH is depicted in **Table 23.1**.[3]

Testing

Given that pregnant women are at increased risk of TSH elevations, tests for thyroid function should begin early in pregnancy, continuing every 4 weeks until mid-gestation and at least once between 26 and 32 weeks among those with

Table 23.1: Trimester-specific range of TSH

	TSH (normal range)
First trimester	0.1–2.5 U/dL
Second trimester	0.2–3 U/dL
Third trimester	0.3–3 u/dL

levothyroxine treatment to ensure euthyroidism throughout pregnancy.[2,4] Monitoring thyroid function tests every 4 weeks during pregnancy detected over 90% of abnormal values in one study.[11]

COMPLICATIONS OF HYPOTHYROIDISM IN PREGNANCY

Overt and subclinical hypothyroidism as well as increases in maternal TSH concentrations have been associated with
- Increased risk of miscarriages/fetal losses,[12-19]
- Hypertensive disorders of pregnancy,[17,20-23]
- Placental abruptions,[22,24] preterm birth[18,19,24-27] and
- Poor neurological development in the offspring.[20,28,29]

Overt hypothyroidism has also been associated with
- Maternal anemia and postpartum hemorrhage,[21] and
- Subclinical hypothyroidism with cesarean sections,[19]
- Gestational diabetes,[24,30]
- Breech presentation,[31,32]
- Infants being small for gestational age,[18]
- Fetal distress,[19]
- Neonates needing intensive care treatment[24,26] and
- Respiratory distress syndrome.[26]

However, some studies have found no association between adverse perinatal outcomes and hypothyroidism.[33-38]

Due to the well-established associations between overt hypothyroidism and adverse pregnancy outcomes, overt hypothyroidism should be promptly treated to attempt to mitigate these known risks.[2,4] However, there is debate about whether to treat all women with subclinical hypothyroidism. Two different strategies are proposed: to treat everyone[4] or to treat women with subclinical hypothyroidism and positive thyroid antibodies.[2] Up to 40% of women with positive thyroid antibodies develop hypothyroidism during or immediately after pregnancy,[39] but most studies evaluating the association between subclinical hypothyroidism and pregnancy outcomes have been cross-sectional and based on first trimester measures of thyroid function. Therefore, more information is needed to determine whether hypothyroidism detected in the first trimester will progress, which factors predict disease progression, and if some women switch from hypothyroidism to euthyroidism as pregnancy continues. In a study evaluating treatment for subclinical hypothyroidism, 44% of women with initially high TSH had normal thyroid function tests in a repeat sample taken 1 week later.[40]

Isolated hypothyroxinemia should not be treated in pregnancy. Level C recommendation, United States Preventive Services Task Force (USPSTF).[3]

Women who are positive for TPOAb and have SCH should be treated with LT4. Level B-USPSTF.[3]

Women with SCH in pregnancy who are not initially treated should be monitored for progression to OH with a serum TSH and FT4 approximately every 4 weeks until 16–20 weeks gestation and at least once between 26 weeks and 32 weeks gestation. This approach has not been prospectively studied. Level I-USPSTF.[3]

Following delivery, LT4 should be reduced to the patient's preconception dose. Additional TSH testing should be performed at approximately 6 weeks postpartum. Level B-USPSTF.[3]

TREATMENT

Levothyroxine is the treatment of choice for hypothyroidism with the goal of normalizing serum TSH concentrations, using the pregnancy-specific reference intervals.[2] In pregnancy, treatment should be started with a dose as close to the final estimated dose as possible to minimize time with hypothyroidism.[19,41]

The current recommendation is for women to increase their levothyroxine dose by 25–30% upon missed periods.[2]

Women with overt hypothyroidism should receive levothyroxine replacement therapy with the dose titrated to achieve a thyrotropin concentration within the trimester-specific reference range. Serial serum thyrotropin levels should be assessed every 4 weeks during the first half of pregnancy in order to adjust levothyroxine dosing to maintain thyrotropin within the trimester specific range. Serum thyrotropin should also be reassessed during the second half of pregnancy. For women already taking levothyroxine, two additional doses per week of the current levothyroxine dose, given as one extra-dose twice weekly with several days separation, may be started as soon as pregnancy is confirmed.[42]

Among women with subclinical hypothyroidism during pregnancy, those with baseline TSH up to 4.2 mIU/L required smaller levothyroxine doses (1 μg/kg/day) than those with baseline TSH 4.2–10 mIU/L (1.42 μg/kg/day) to achieve euthyroidism.[41] When treating women with subclinical hypothyroidism with steady doses of levothyroxine based on their baseline TSH levels, 79, 82 and 90% of women with baseline TSH 2.5–5.0 mIU/L, 5.0–8.0 mIU/L and higher than 8.0 mIU/L, respectively, reached euthyroidism with respective levothyroxine doses of 50, 75 and 100 μg/day.[40] Either weight-based starting dose or a steady starting dose based on the severity of newly diagnosed hypothyroidism determined by baseline TSH concentration seem to be appropriate in reaching euthyroidism.

Effectiveness of Levothyroxine Treatment

Treatment of clinical hypothyroidism was shown to reduce risk of miscarriage and preterm birth.[43] Only about 62–82% of all ingested levothyroxine is absorbed, with concurrent ingestion of food, caffeine and iron and calcium supplements decreasing the absorption further.[44]

Because coadministration of food and levothyroxine is likely to impair levothyroxine absorption, we recommend that, if possible, levothyroxine be consistently taken either 60 minutes before breakfast or at bedtime (3 or more hours after the evening meal) for optimal, consistent absorption. Delay intake of iron and calcium preparations by 4 hours.

In patients in whom levothyroxine dose requirements are much higher than expected, evaluation for gastrointestinal disorders such as *Helicobacter pylori*—related gastritis, atrophic gastritis, or celiac disease should be considered.[42]

Treatment of Hypothyroidism During the Postpartum Period

Most women with hypothyroidism can reduce their dose of levothyroxine postpartum, with assessment of TSH levels 6 weeks following the dose reduction to ensure euthyroidism.[2,45,46] Women with positive thyroid antibodies are at higher risk of exacerbation of autoimmune thyroid dysfunction postpartum, and over 50% of women with Hashimoto's thyroiditis continued to require increased doses of levothyroxine in the postpartum period.[47] Women with subclinical hypothyroidism during pregnancy may not require levothyroxine treatment during the postpartum period, unless postpartum thyroiditis ensues or the woman is planning to conceive again soon. These women are at high-risk for thyroid dysfunction in their subsequent pregnancies and require adequate preconception consultation and management. They are also at higher risk of developing permanent thyroid disease later in life.[36]

Isolated Hypothyroxinemia

Isolated hypothyroxinemia is characterized by low fT4 concentrations with normal serum TSH levels.[2] Hypothyroxinemia can be due to relative iodine deficiency where the thyroid produces triiodothyronine instead of thyroxine to preserve iodine as raw material, but, it is a condition also observed in populations with iodine sufficiency.[48] Notably, by definition of reference intervals, 2.5% of healthy women will also have fT4 concentrations below the lower reference limit.

Isolated hypothyroxinemia was associated with preterm birth, infants weighing more than 4000 g and gestational diabetes in one study,[49] but, these associations were not seen in another cohort.[24] Some association has also been seen with neonatal intraventricular hemorrhage, but this association was based on a very limited sample size.[24] Like hypothyroidism, hypothyroxinemia has been associated with poorer neuropsychological development in the offspring.[50,51] However, as it is unclear whether the association between adverse outcomes and hypothyroxinemia are due to iodine deficiency or maternal thyroid disease,[48] levothyroxine treatment for isolated hypothyroxinemia cannot be recommended.[2] Adequacy of iodine nutrition should be ensured in women with isolated hypothyroxinemia.[48]

HYPERTHYROIDISM

Hyperthyroidism occurs in 0.1–1.0% of all pregnancies and is diagnosed when TSH concentrations are low or suppressed along with elevated fT4 or free triiodothyronine (in overt disease) or with normal thyroid hormone levels (in subclinical disease).[2]
- Graves' disease, an autoimmune condition characterized by stimulation of the thyroid gland by TSH receptor antibodies (TRAbs), is the most common cause of hyperthyroidism among fertile-aged women.[2]
- Toxic multinodular goiter,
- Toxic adenoma,
- Thyroiditis or
- Struma ovarii.[2,4]

As untreated Graves' disease can lead to ovulatory dysfunction and infertility, a new-onset of Graves' is thought to be rare in pregnancy.[2,4] A more common condition, gestational (transient) hyperthyroidism, occurs in up to 1–3% of all pregnancies and is probably due to the physiologic thyroidal stimulation by high human chorionic gonadotropin levels in early pregnancy.[2,4] Notably, up to 50% of women with hyperemesis gravidarum (severe nausea and vomiting in early pregnancy) have transient hyperthyroidism.[2,4]

Distinguishing between new-onset or recurring Graves' disease in pregnancy and gestational hyperthyroidism may be difficult. Symptoms associated with Graves' disease (goiter or eye symptoms) as well as previous history of thyroid disease help in differentiating between Graves' disease and gestational hyperthyroidism, as gestational hyperthyroidism is more common among women without history of thyroid diseases.[2,4] Elevated TRAb titers are rarely present in gestational hyperthyroidism, so their presence can help confirm Graves' disease in pregnancy.[2,4]

In the presence of a suppressed serum TSH in the first trimester (TSH <0.1 mIU/L), a history and physical examination are indicated. FT4 measurements should be obtained in all patients. Measurement of TT3 and TRAb may be helpful in establishing a diagnosis of hyperthyroidism. Level B-USPSTF.[3]

If the patient has a past or present history of Graves' disease, a maternal serum determination of TRAb should be obtained at 20–24 weeks gestation. Level B-USPSTF.[3]

Hyperthyroidism is associated with increased risk of pregnancy complications, including:
- Miscarriages,
- Pre-eclampsia,[52]
- Low birth weight or
- Preterm birth

- Neonatal respiratory distress syndrome
- Sepsis[53,54]
- Fetal growth restriction[52,55] and
- Maternal cardiac dysfunction,[56] with risks increasing with poorer hyperthyroidism control.[52,55]

Treatment of Hyperthyroidism During Pregnancy

As the associations between untreated persistent hyperthyroidism and adverse pregnancy outcomes are well established, hyperthyroidism should be adequately managed before and during pregnancy.[2,4] Treatment options are:
- Radioactive iodine ablation results in a long latency of 2–6 months before development of hypothyroidism as well as in an increase in TRAb titers. As such, this treatment option is not generally recommended for hyperthyroid women planning pregnancy in the near future (within 6 months of the treatment) as it is unlikely that they would have achieved a stable euthyroid state during that time.[2,57]
- Surgery is an option for patients hoping to conceive soon after the operation, but even then, the optimal management of hypothyroidism after total or near total thyroidectomy should be reached before conception to reduce risk of adverse pregnancy outcomes.[2,57] However, as anesthetic agents are teratogenic in the first trimester and surgery is associated with increased fetal loss in the third trimester, the late second trimester is thought to be the safest period to perform thyroidectomy in a pregnant woman.[57]
- Antithyroid drugs can also be used to control hyperthyroidism in women planning pregnancy or among those with newly discovered Graves' disease during pregnancy.[2,4]

The antithyroid drugs are :
- Methimazole (and its prodrug carbimazole) is associated with teratogenity, including aplasia cutis and choanal or esophageal atresia.[58] However, these specific malformations are very rare on a population level.
- Propylthiouracil, is not associated with teratogenicity but in rare instances propylthiouracil may increase the risk of hepatotoxicity in the mother.[2,4]

Current recommendations suggest using propythiouracil during preconception and in the first trimester of pregnancy to reduce teratogenity and switching to methimazole after the first trimester to reduce maternal hepatotoxicity.[2,4] However, if one antithyroid drug is not available or there are tolerance issues, either prophyltiouracil or methimazole can be used throughout pregnancy as the neonatal and maternal risks of untreated maternal hyperthyroidism outweigh the small risks of malformations or liver toxicity.[2,4] Women with gestational hyperthyroidism generally do not require treatment as the condition is transient and not associated with adverse pregnancy outcomes.[2,34,35,59]

- Propranolol, a beta-blocker, can be used in short-term symptom management as it has some direct antithyroid activity by blocking iodide transport to the thyroid.[2] However, if women do not reach euthyroidism as pregnancy progresses or there are other symptoms, Graves' disease should be suspected and a treatment trial with antithyroid drugs may be useful.[2]

The appropriate management of women with gestational hyperthyroidism and hyperemesis gravidarum includes supportive therapy, management of dehydration, and hospitalization if needed. Level A-USPSTF.[3]

ATDs are not recommended for the management of gestational hyperthyroidism. Level D-USPSTF.[3]

CAVEATS AND GOALS OF ANTITHYROID DRUG TREATMENT

All antithyroid drugs cross the placenta and may have deleterious impacts on the fetal thyroid function.[2] When treating pregnant women with antithyroid drugs, the treatment goal is to maintain fT4 values at or above the upper nonpregnant reference limit or high-normal within the pregnant reference limit (preferred approach) using the lowest possible dose of the drug.[2] Upon treatment initiation, thyroid function tests should be measured every 2-4 weeks and every 4 weeks after treatment goals are reached.[2] Maternal TSH levels may remain suppressed or low throughout pregnancy in spite of adequate antithyroid drug treatment.[2] Overtreatment with antithyroid drugs may lead to goitrogenesis and hypothyroidism in the fetus, the risk of which is thought to be lower by maintaining high-normal maternal fT4 levels.[2]

Graves' disease typically exacerbates in the first trimester of pregnancy and gradually improves afterward.[2] Consequently, up to 20-30% of all women with hyperthyroidism may discontinue antithyroid drug therapy in late pregnancy.[2] However, women with high TRAb titers continue to be at high-risk of recurrence and require antithyroid drug treatment throughout pregnancy.[2]

Besides the fetal hypothyroidism risk inflicted by maternal antithyroid drug therapy, untreated maternal hyperthyroidism may lead to transient central hypothyroidism in the fetus.[2] Maternal TRAbs pass through the placenta and can lead to fetal or neonatal hyperthyroidism.[2] Women with past or present history of Graves' disease should have their TRAb titers checked in mid-pregnancy to estimate this risk as fetal hyperthyroidism is associated with increased neonatal morbidity and mortality.[2] Fetal surveillance with serial ultrasounds is required to diagnose fetal thyroid dysfunction and follow fetal growth and well-being if a woman has uncontrolled hyperthyroidism and/or positive TRAb during pregnancy.[2] Similarly, evaluation for thyroid dysfunction is required in neonates of women with Graves' disease or positive TRAb during pregnancy.[2] Signs of potential fetal hyperthyroidism that may be detected by ultrasonography include fetal tachycardia (bpm >170, persistent for over 10 minutes), intrauterine growth restriction, presence of fetal goiter (the earliest sonographic sign of fetal thyroid dysfunction), accelerated bone maturation, signs of congestive heart failure, and fetal hydrops.

A combination regimen of LT4 and an ATD should not be used in pregnancy, except in the rare situation of fetal hyperthyroidism. Level D-USPSTF.[3]

Treatment of Hyperthyroidism During the Postpartum Period

Women with a history of Graves' disease or hyperthyroidism treated during pregnancy are at a higher risk of relapse during the postpartum period.[2]

MMI in doses up to 20-30 mg/d is safe for lactating mothers and their infants. PTU at doses up to 300 mg/d is a second-line agent due to concerns about severe hepatotoxicity. ATDs should be administered following a feeding and in divided doses. Level A-USPSTF.[3]

Moderate use of antithyroid drugs is safe during lactation and has not been shown to affect thyroid hormone levels or the development of the infant.[2] However, as a safety precaution, infants of mothers taking antithyroid drugs during lactation need to be followed with thyroid function tests and antithyroid drugs should be taken in divided doses immediately after feeding.[2]

AUTOIMMUNE THYROIDITIS AND POSTPARTUM THYROIDITIS

Approximately 11-15% of all fertile aged women have positive thyroid antibodies, either thyroid peroxidase antibodies (TPO-Abs) or thyroglobulin antibodies (TG-Ab), which act as a marker of silent autoimmune thyroiditis. Up to 20-40% of all women with positive thyroid antibodies develop hypothyroidism during pregnancy or immediately postpartum.[39,60]

Thyroid antibody positivity has been associated with increased risk for:

- Miscarriages,[61-64]
- Perinatal mortality[35]
- Preterm birth[63]
- Neonatal respiratory distress[65]
- Externalizing problems, for example, attention problems and aggressive behavior, in children.[66]

However, most of these studies evaluated thyroid function only once during pregnancy, so the effect of hypothyroidism as the underlying reason for these associations cannot be ruled out.

Postpartum thyroiditis is a new-onset thyroid dysfunction during the 12 months following pregnancy in a previously euthyroid woman.[2] The risk of postpartum thyroiditis is higher in women with positive thyroid antibodies or other autoimmune diseases.[2,67] Up to 50% of all women with TPO Ab or TG-Ab positivity in the first trimester of pregnancy develop postpartum thyroiditis.[2,67] In its classical form, postpartum thyroiditis manifests with an episode of thyrotoxicosis followed by transient hypothyroidism and subsequent euthyroidism, but the clinical course varies.[2,67] The thyrotoxic phase generally does not require or respond to antithyroid drugs but symptomatic women may be treated with a low dose of propranolol. Treatment of the hypothyroid phase of postpartum thyroiditis with levothyroxine depends on the symptom severity, if a woman is breastfeeding, if she plans to conceive again in the near future and her preference to receive treatment.[2,67] Treatment for postpartum thyroiditis is usually transient, with discontinuation of treatment 6–12 months after the initiation, unless the patient is pregnant, breastfeeding or trying to become pregnant.[2,67] Postpartum thyroiditis can lead to permanent hypothyroidism in over 50% of all women and annual TSH tests are indicated to those with postpartum thyroiditis history.[2,67]

The strength of each recommendation was graded according to the United States Preventive Services Task Force (USPSTF) Guidelines outlined below:[3]

- *Level A:* The USPSTF strongly recommends that clinicians provide (the service) to eligible patients. The USPSTF found good evidence that (the service) improves important health outcomes and concludes that benefits substantially outweigh harms.
- *Level B:* The USPSTF recommends that clinicians provide (this service) to eligible patients. The USPSTF found at least fair evidence that (the service) improves important health outcomes and concludes that benefits outweigh harms.
- *Level C:* The USPSTF makes no recommendation for or against routine provision of (the service). The USPSTF found at least fair evidence that (the service) can improve health outcomes but concludes that the balance of benefits and harms is too close to justify a general recommendation.
- *Level D:* The USPSTF recommends against routinely providing (the service) to asymptomatic patients. The USPSTF found at least fair evidence that (the service) is ineffective or that harms outweigh benefits.
- *Level I:* The USPSTF concludes that evidence is insufficient to recommend for or against routinely providing (the service). Evidence that (the service) is effective is lacking, or poor quality, or conflicting, and the balance of benefits and harms cannot be determined.

- US Preventive Services Task Force Ratings: Strength of Recommendations and Quality of Evidence. 2003 Guide to Clinical Preventive Services, Third Edition: Period Updates, 2000–2003. Available at: *www.uspreventiveservicestaskforce.org/3rduspstf/ratings.htm* (accessed June 13, 2011).

REFERENCES

1. Glinoer D, De Nayer P, Bourdoux P, et al. Regulation of maternal thyroid during pregnancy. J Clin Endocrinol Metab. 1990;71(2):276-87.
2. Stagnaro-Green A, Abalovich M, Alexander E, et al. Guidelines of the American Thyroid Association for the diagnosis and management of thyroid disease during pregnancy and postpartum. Thyroid. 2011;21(10):1081-125.
3. Stagnaro-Green A, Abalovich M. Guidelines of the American Thyroid Association for the diagnosis and management of thyroid disease during pregnancy and postpartum. Thyroid. 2011;21(10):1081-96.
4. De Groot LJ, Abalovich M, Alexander EK, et al. Management of thyroid dysfunction during pregnancy and postpartum: an endocrine society clinical practice guideline. J Clin Endocrinol Metab. 2012;97(8):2543-65.
5. Boas M, Forman JL, Juul A, et al. Narrow intra-individual variation of maternal thyroid function in pregnancy based on a longitudinal study on 132 women. Eur J Endocrinol. 2009;161(6):903-10.
6. Larsson A, Palm M, Hansson LO, Axelsson O. Reference values for clinical chemistry tests during normal pregnancy. BJOG. 2008;115(7):874-81.
7. Männistö T, Surcel HM, Ruokonen A, et al. Early pregnancy reference intervals of thyroid hormone concentrations in a thyroid antibody-negative pregnant population. Thyroid. 2011;21(3):291-8.
8. Van Houcke SK, Van Uytfanghe K, Shimizu E, et al. IFCC international conventional reference procedure for the measurement of free thyroxine in serum: international federation of clinical chemistry and laboratory medicine (IFCC) working group for standardization of thyroid function tests (WG-STFT)(1). Clin Chem Lab Med. 2011;49(8):1275-81.
9. Sapin R, D'Herbomez M. Free thyroxine measured by equilibrium dialysis and nine immunoassays in sera with various serum thyroxine-binding capacities. Clin Chem. 2003;49(9):1531-5.
10. Midgley JE, Hoermann R. Measurement of total rather than free thyroxine in pregnancy: the diagnostic implications. Thyroid. 2013;23(3):259-61.
11. Yassa L, Marqusee E, Fawcett R, Alexander EK. Thyroid hormone early adjustment in pregnancy (the THERAPY) trial. J Clin Endocrinol Metab. 2010;95(7):3234-41.
12. Abalovich M, Gutierrez S, Alcaraz G, et al. Overt and subclinical hypothyroidism complicating pregnancy. Thyroid. 2002;12(1):63-68.
13. Allan WC, Haddow JE, Palomaki GE, et al. Maternal thyroid deficiency and pregnancy complications: implications for population screening. J Med Screen. 2000;7(3):127-30.

14. Ashoor G, Maiz N, Rotas M, Jawdat F, Nicolaides KH. Maternal thyroid function at 11 to 13 weeks of gestation and subsequent fetal death. Thyroid. 2010;20(9):989-93.
15. Benhadi N, Wiersinga WM, Reitsma JB, Vrijkotte TG, Bonsel GJ. Higher maternal TSH levels in pregnancy are associated with increased risk for miscarriage, fetal or neonatal death. Eur J Endocrinol. 2009;160(6):985-91.
16. Negro R, Schwartz A, Gismondi R, et al. Increased pregnancy loss rate in thyroid antibody negative women with TSH levels between 2.5 and 5.0 in the first trimester of pregnancy. J Clin Endocrinol Metab. 2010;95(9):E44-E48.
17. Sahu MT, Das V, Mittal S, Agarwal A, Sahu M. Overt and subclinical thyroid dysfunction among Indian pregnant women and its effect on maternal and fetal outcome. Arch Gynecol Obstet. 2010;281(2):215-20.
18. Schneuer FJ, Nassar N, Tasevski V, Morris JM, Roberts CL. Association and predictive accuracy of high TSH serum levels in first trimester and adverse pregnancy outcomes. J Clin Endocrinol Metab. 2012;97(9):3115-22.
19. Su PY, Huang K, Hao JH, et al. Maternal thyroid function in the first twenty weeks of pregnancy and subsequent fetal and infant development: a prospective population-based cohort study in China. J Clin Endocrinol Metab. 2011;96(10):3234-41.
20. Ashoor G, Maiz N, Rotas M, Kametas NA, Nicolaides KH. Maternal thyroid function at 11 to 13 weeks of gestation and subsequent development of pre-eclampsia. Prenat Diagn. 2010;30(11):1032-8.
21. Davis LE, Leveno KJ, Cunningham FG. Hypothyroidism complicating pregnancy. Obstet Gynecol. 1988;72(1):108-12.
22. Leung AS, Millar LK, Koonings PP, Montoro M, Mestman JH. Perinatal outcome in hypothyroid pregnancies. Obstet Gynecol. 1993;81(3):349-53.
23. Wilson KL, Casey BM, McIntire DD, Halvorson LM, Cunningham FG. Subclinical thyroid disease and the incidence of hypertension in pregnancy. Obstet.Gynecol. 2012;119(2 Pt 1):315-20.
24. Casey BM, Dashe JS, Spong CY, et al. Perinatal significance of isolated maternal hypothyroxinemia identified in the first half of pregnancy. Obstet Gynecol. 2007;109(5):1129-35.
25. Jones WS, Man EB. Thyroid function in human pregnancy. VI. Premature deliveries and reproductive failures of pregnant women with low serum butanol-extractable iodines. Maternal serum TBG and TBPA capacities. Am J Obstet Gynecol. 1969;104(6):909-14.
26. Casey BM, Dashe JS, Wells CE, et al. Subclinical hypothyroidism and pregnancy outcomes. Obstet Gynecol. 2005;105(2):239-45.
27. Stagnaro-Green A, Chen X, Bogden JD, Davies TF, Scholl TO. The thyroid and pregnancy: a novel risk factor for very preterm delivery. Thyroid. 2005);15(4):351-7.
28. Haddow JE, Palomaki GE, Allan WC, et al. Maternal thyroid deficiency during pregnancy and subsequent neuropsychological development of the child. N Engl J Med. 1999;341(8):549-55.
29. Williams F, Watson J, Ogston S, et al. Mild maternal thyroid dysfunction at delivery of infants born ≤34 weeks and neurodevelopmental outcome at 5.5 years. J Clin Endocrinol Metab. 2012;97(6):1977-85.
30. Tudela CM, Casey BM, McIntire DD, Cunningham FG. Relationship of subclinical thyroid disease to the incidence of gestational diabetes. Obstet Gynecol. 2012;119(5):983-8.
31. Kooistra L, Kuppens SM, Hasaart TH, et al. High thyrotrophin levels at end term increase the risk of breech presentation. Clin Endocrinol (Oxf). 2010;73(5):661-5.
32. Kuppens SM, Kooistra L, Wijnen HA, et al. Maternal thyroid function during gestation is related to breech presentation at term. Clin Endocrinol (Oxf). 2010;72(6):820-4.
33. Cleary-Goldman J, Malone FD, Lambert-Messerlian G, et al. Maternal thyroid hypofunction and pregnancy outcome. Obstet Gynecol. 2008;112(1):85-92.
34. Männistö T, Vääräsmäki M, Pouta A, et al. Perinatal outcome of children born to mothers with thyroid dysfunction or antibodies: a prospective population-based cohort study. J Clin Endocrinol Metab. 2009;94(3):772-9.
35. Männistö T, Vääräsmäki M, Pouta A, et al. Thyroid dysfunction and autoantibodies during pregnancy as predictive factors of pregnancy complications and maternal morbidity in later life. J Clin Endocrinol Metab. 2010;95(3):1084-94.
36. Ashoor G, Maiz N, Rotas M, Jawdat F, Nicolaides KH. Maternal thyroid function at 11–13 weeks of gestation and spontaneous preterm delivery. Obstet Gynecol. 2011;117(2 Pt 1):293-8.
37. Karagiannis G, Ashoor G, Maiz N, Jawdat F, Nicolaides KH. Maternal thyroid function at eleven to thirteen weeks of gestation and subsequent delivery of small for gestational age neonates. Thyroid. 2011;21(10):1127-31.
38. Williams FL, Watson J, Ogston SA, et al. Maternal and umbilical cord levels of T4, FT4, TSH, TPOAb, and TgAb in term infants and neurodevelopmental outcome at 5.5 years. J Clin Endocrinol Metab. 2013;98(2):829-38.
39. Glinoer D, Riahi M, Grun JP, Kinthaert J. Risk of subclinical hypothyroidism in pregnant women with asymptomatic autoimmune thyroid disorders. J Clin Endocrinol Metab. 1994;79(1):197-204.
40. Yu X, Chen Y, Shan Z, et al. The pattern of thyroid function of subclinical hypothyroid women with levothyroxine treatment during pregnancy. Endocrine doi:10.1007/s12020-013-9913-2 (2013) (Epub ahead of print).
41. Abalovich M, Vazquez A, Alcaraz G, et al. Adequate levothyroxine doses for the treatment of hypothyroidism newly diagnosed during pregnancy. Thyroid doi:10.1089/thy.2013.0024 (2013) (Epub ahead of print).
42. Guidelines for the treatment of hypothyroidism prepared by the American Thyroid Association Task Force on Thyroid Hormone Replacement thyroid. 2014;24(12).
43. Vissenberg R, van den Boogaard E, van Wely M, et al. Treatment of thyroid disorders before conception and in early pregnancy: a systematic review. Hum Reprod Update. 2012;18(4):360-73.
44. Liwanpo L, Hershman JM. Conditions and drugs interfering with thyroxine absorption. Best Pract Res Clin Endocrinol Metab. 2009;23(6):781-92.
45. Alexander EK, Marqusee E, Lawrence J, et al. Timing and magnitude of increases in levothyroxine requirements during pregnancy in women with hypothyroidism. N Engl J Med. 2004;351(3):241-9.
46. Mandel SJ, Larsen PR, Seely EW, Brent GA. Increased need for thyroxine during pregnancy in women with primary hypothyroidism. N Engl J Med. 1990;323(2):91-96.
47. Galofre JC, Haber RS, Mitchell AA, Pessah R, Davies TF. Increased postpartum thyroxine replacement in Hashimoto's thyroiditis. Thyroid. 2010;20(8):901-8.

48. Morreale de EG, Obregon MJ, Escobar del RF. Is neuropsychological development related to maternal hypothyroidism or to maternal hypothyroxinemia? J Clin Endocrinol Metab. 2000;85(11):3975-87.
49. Cleary-Goldman J, Malone FD, Lambert-Messerlian G, et al. Maternal thyroid hypofunction and pregnancy outcome. Obstet Gynecol. 2008;112(1):85-92
50. Pop VJ, Kuijpens JL, van Baar AL, et al. Low maternal free thyroxine concentrations during early pregnancy are associated with impaired psychomotor development in infancy. Clin Endocrinol (Oxf). 1999;50(2):149-55.
51. Pop VJ, Brouwers EP, Vader HL, et al. Maternal hypothyroxinaemia during early pregnancy and subsequent child development: a 3-year follow-up study. Clin Endocrinol (Oxf). 2003;59(3):282-8.
52. Millar LK, Wing DA, Leung AS, et al. Low birth weight and preeclampsia in pregnancies complicated by hyperthyroidism. Obstet Gynecol. 1994;84(6):946-9.
53. Männistö T, Mendola P, Grewal J, et al. Thyroid diseases and adverse pregnancy outcomes in a contemporary US cohort. J Clin Endocrinol Metab. 2013;98(7):2725-33.
54. Männistö T, Mendola P, Reddy U, Laughon SK. Neonatal outcomes and birth weight in pregnancies complicated by maternal thyroid disease. Am J Epidemiol. 2013;178(5):731-40.
55. Phoojaroenchanachai M, Sriussadaporn S, Peerapatdit T, et al. Effect of maternal hyperthyroidism during late pregnancy on the risk of neonatal low birth weight. Clin Endocrinol (Oxf). 2001;54(3):365-70.
56. Sheffield JS, Cunningham FG. Thyrotoxicosis and heart failure that complicate pregnancy. Am J Obstet Gynecol. 2004;190(1):211-7.
57. Bahn RS, Burch HB, Cooper DS, et al. Hyperthyroidism and other causes of thyrotoxicosis: management guidelines of the American Thyroid Association and American Association of clinical endocrinologists. Endocr Pract. 2011;17(3):456-520.
58. Yoshihara A, Noh J, Yamaguchi T, et al. Treatment of graves' disease with antithyroid drugs in the first trimester of pregnancy and the prevalence of congenital malformation. J Clin Endocrinol Metab. 2012;97(7):2396-403.
59. Casey BM, Dashe JS, Wells CE, et al. Subclinical hyperthyroidism and pregnancy outcomes. Obstet Gynecol. 2006;107(2 Pt 1):337-41.
60. Negro R, Formoso G, Mangieri T, et al. Levothyroxine treatment in euthyroid pregnant women with autoimmune thyroid disease: effects on obstetrical complications. J Clin Endocrinol Metab. 2006;91(7):2587-91.
61. Lepoutre T, Debieve F, Gruson D, Daumerie C. Reduction of miscarriages through universal screening and treatment of thyroid autoimmune diseases. Gynecol Obstet Invest. 2012;74(4):265-73.
62. Stagnaro-Green A, Roman SH, Cobin RH, et al. Detection of at-risk pregnancy by means of highly sensitive assays for thyroid autoantibodies. JAMA. 1990;264(11):1422-5.
63. Thangaratinam S, Tan A, Knox E, et al. Association between thyroid autoantibodies and miscarriage and preterm birth: meta-analysis of evidence. BMJ. 2011;342:d2616.
64. Negro R, Mangieri T, Coppola L, et al. Levothyroxine treatment in thyroid peroxidase antibody-positive women undergoing assisted reproduction technologies: a prospective study. Hum Reprod. 2005;20(6):1529-33.
65. Negro R, Schwartz A, Gismondi R, et al. Thyroid antibody positivity in the first trimester of pregnancy is associated with negative pregnancy outcomes. J Clin Endocrinol Metab. 2011;96(6):E920-E924.
66. Ghassabian A, Bongers-Schokking JJ, de Rijke YB, et al. Maternal thyroid autoimmunity during pregnancy and the risk of attention deficit/hyperactivity problems in children: the generation R study. Thyroid. 2012;22(2):178-86.
67. Stagnaro-Green A. Clinical review 152: postpartum thyroiditis. J Clin Endocrinol Metab. 2002;87(9):4042-7.

Chapter 24

Jaundice in Pregnancy

Sangeeta Shrivastava, Richa Dhirawani

INTRODUCTION

Jaundice in pregnancy can result either because of conditions specific to pregnancy or because of causes which can occur in the general population. It is important to correctly diagnose the etiology, as different causes have different maternal and fetal outcomes and the management also differs. The clinical picture, mainly nonhepatic manifestations along with biochemical evaluation, may help in arriving at a diagnosis; however, sometimes the clinical picture may be confusing and difficult to diagnose correctly.[1]

Though severe liver disease is only an occasional complication during pregnancy, it has disproportionately high rates.[2]

OBSTETRIC CHOLESTASIS[3,4]

(*Synonyms:* Intrahepatic cholestasis, icterus gravidarum, recurrent jaundice of pregnancy).

Introduction

Obstetric cholestasis is a multifactorial condition of pregnancy characterized by pruritus in the absence of a skin rash with abnormal liver function tests (LFTs), neither of which has an alternative cause and both of which resolve after birth. *It is the second most common cause of jaundice in pregnancy after hepatitis.*

Prevalence

The prevalence is about 0.7–1% being more common in Indian subcontinent.

Etiology

The etiology of obstetric cholestasis is unknown but relates to a genetic predisposition. The basic pathology is stasis of bile in the bile canaliculi with increased conjugated bilirubin levels. It is related to high circulating estrogen levels as the condition recurs in subsequent pregnancies and during oral pill use **(Table 24.1)**.

Table 24.1: Various liver diseases in pregnancy[3,5]

Group I	Liver disorders caused by pregnancy
	• Obstetric cholestasis (Intrahepatic cholestasis)
	• Acute fatty liver of pregnancy
	• Hyperemesis gravidarum-induced hepatic damage
	• Liver damage due to severe pre-eclampsia, eclampsia and HELLP syndrome
Group II	Pregnancy associated liver diseases (Liver disease coincidental to pregnancy)
	• Acute viral hepatitis
	– Hepatitis A, B, C, D, E, G
	• Drug-induced liver damage
	– Isoniazid
	– Rifampicin
	– Phenothiazine
	• Hemodialysis-induced liver damage and jaundice including mismatched blood transfusion, malaria, severe septicemic infection
Group III	Chronic liver diseases preceding (antedating) pregnancy
	• Chronic hepatitis
	• Liver cirrhosis
	• Budd-Chiari syndrome
	• Congenital hyperbilirubinemia
	• Autoimmune hepatitis
	• Liver tumors
	• Liver transplantation
Group IV	Diseases of gallbladder
	• Cholecystitis
	• Cholelithiasis

Clinical Features

Obstetric cholestasis is diagnosed when otherwise unexplained pruritus occurs in pregnancy and abnormal liver function tests (LFTs) and/or raised bile acids occur in the pregnant woman and both resolve after delivery. Pruritus that involves the palms and soles of the feet is particularly suggestive. Commonly present in the third trimester at around 30–32 weeks gestation but there can be associated weakness, nausea and vomiting with slight jaundice. Liver function tests demonstrate mild elevated hepatic transaminases (ALT and AST), moderate elevated serum alkaline phosphatase and serum bilirubin (up to 5 mg%). Although not performed in all cases, there are raised bile acids in most of them with levels at least thrice than normal. There may be associated dark urine, pale stools, steatorrhea and malaise.

Differential diagnosis is from acute or chronic viral hepatitis, gallstones, chronic active hepatitis and primary biliary cirrhosis.

Effect on Pregnancy

Obstetric cholestasis has been linked with an increased incidence of passage of meconium, premature delivery, fetal distress, delivery by cesarean section and postpartum hemorrhage and rarely fetal death. The exact cause of adverse fetal effects is not known and it does not correlate with severity of symptoms and liver function tests abnormalities.

Management

The woman should be counseled about the various risks of intrahepatic cholestasis. Liver function tests (LFTs) and clotting time should be regularly monitored. Control of symptoms should be regularly monitored. Topical emollients are safe but their efficacy is unknown. Antihistamines such as chlorphenamine may provide some welcome sedation at night but do not have a significant impact on pruritus. There is insufficient evidence to demonstrate whether S-adenosyl methionine (SAMe) is effective for either control of maternal symptoms or for improving fetal outcome, and it is not recommended. The drug ursodeoxycholic acid (UDCA) is the drug of choice in dose of 300 mg twice daily for rapid reduction in abnormalities in LFT and for better fetal outcome (American College of Obstetricians and Gynaecologists, ACOG 2006). Ursodeoxycholic acid (UDCA) improves pruritus and liver function in women with obstetric cholestasis. Women should be advised that where the prothrombin time is prolonged, the use of water-soluble vitamin K (menadiol sodium phosphate) in doses of 5–10 mg daily is indicated. Women should be advised that when prothrombin time is normal, water-soluble vitamin K (menadiol sodium phosphate) in low doses should be used only after careful counseling about the likely benefits but small theoretical risk.

Regular fetal surveillance with ultrasound and non-stress test should be done.

Labor should be induced at 38 weeks gestation to avoid fetal adverse outcome and sudden intrauterine death. Vitamin K should be given to the mother to reduce the risk of postpartum hemorrhage. Vaginal delivery is the aim but cesarean delivery is performed for fetal indications.

After delivery, LFTs return to normal and there is no permanent deleterious effect on maternal liver functions. However, symptoms can recur with menstruation and with combined oral pills which should be avoided in them. *Recurrence risk of cholestasis in subsequent pregnancies is 90%.*

ACUTE FATTY LIVER OF PREGNANCY

Acute fatty liver of pregnancy was also previously called acute yellow atrophy of liver. *Acute fatty liver of pregnancy (AFLP) is a rare life-threatening complication of pregnancy* that occurs in the third trimester or the immediate period after delivery. It is closely related to pre-eclampsia sharing many features and pathophysiology with it. It is more common in primigravidas and in twin pregnancies. If not diagnosed and treated promptly, AFLP can result in high maternal and neonatal morbidity and mortality.

Symptomatology

Patient usually presents with nausea, vomiting, malaise, loss of appetite and weight, pain in the epigastrium and right upper quadrant with worsening jaundice. Many women (about 50%) have hypertension and pre-eclampsia. Patients can progress to overt hepatic failure with jaundice, hepatic encephalopathy, ascites, hypoglycemia, lactic acidosis, adult respiratory distress syndrome, hyperuricemia, acute tubular necrosis, and pancreatitis. Although symptoms and signs are similar to those of pre-eclampsia and HELLP syndrome, aminotransferase levels tend to be much higher and hypoglycemia more severe in acute fatty liver of pregnancy.

Investigations

- Hyperbilirubinemia (up to 10 mg/dL)
- Elevated hepatic transaminases to 300–500 u/L
- Prolonged prothrombin time (PT)
- Increase in ammonia and uric acid are suggestive of liver failure
- Renal impairment on renal function tests
- Hypoglycemia
- Coagulopathy (abnormal coagulation profile)
- Ultrasound and computerized tomography (CT scan) are not very sensitive
- Magnetic resonance imaging helps in diagnosis
- Liver biopsy confirms the diagnosis but should be done carefully after ruling out derangement of coagulation system. Histology shows edematous hepatocytes with their cytoplasm filled with microvesicular fat with central nucleus with minimum hepatocellular necrosis.

Etiology

The AFLP is a serious disease but is self-limiting with symptoms subsiding immediately after delivery and recovering in several days in puerperium. It is an important cause of hepatic coma and precoma and is associated with high fatality rate due to multiorgan failure. Perinatal and maternal mortality and morbidity are increased.

Treatment

Such women should be treated in intensive care unit by an obstetrician, hepatologist or physician, anesthetist and an intensivist. Initial treatment involves supportive management with intravenous fluids, intravenous glucose and blood products, including fresh frozen plasma and cryoprecipitate to correct DIC. The fetus should be monitored with cardiotocography. After the mother is stabilized, arrangements are usually made for delivery. Vaginal delivery is preferred. Epidural anesthesia can be given for cesarean delivery, if coagulation profile is normal. The patients should be carefully watched for any hepatic encephalopathy and should be treated in a liver unit. In absence of improvement in LFTs after delivery, liver transplantation may be considered.

VIRAL HEPATITIS IN PREGNANCY

Viral hepatitis is the most common form of liver disease worldwide, and it frequently affects women of childbearing age, either as an acute infection or as a chronic disease. Incidence is 1:1000 clinical jaundice. Liver has dual blood supply by hepatic A and portal vein so it is most vulnerable to viral infection. Malnutrition, poor socioeconomic background and inadequate antenatal care are responsible for high prevalence. Overview of different types of viral hepatitis is shown in **Table 24.2**.

Table 24.2: Overview of the different types of viral hepatitis[1,3,4,5]

Hepatitis A	Hepatitis B	Hepatitis C	Hepatitis D	Hepatitis E
Epidemiology: • Hep A virus • RNA enterovirus (picornavirus) • Resistant to environmental factors	*Epidemiology:* • Hep B virus • DNA virus, Hepadnaviridae • Endemic in India • 4–6% in India	*Epidemiology:* • Hep C virus • SS RNA Flaviviridae • 0.6% of population • Predisposing factors in Hep B	*Epidemiology:* • Hep D • Incomplete virus • Requires Hep B to replicate so Hep D develops only in HbsAg +ve patients	*Epidemiology:* • Hep E • Endemic in India • Primary cause of NANB hepatitis • Maternal mortality high
Transmission: • Feco-oral route • Contaminated food and water • Infected serum	*Transmission:* • Body fluids/blood, semen, vaginal secretions, saliva, breast milk • Mother to infant transmission accounts for 40% of all chronic HB virus carrier	*Transmission:* • Parenterally, perinatally, sexually tattooing • Maternal feto-transmission • Blood transfusion	*Transmission:* • Body fluids/blood, semen, vaginal secretions, saliva, breast milk	*Transmission:* • Contaminated food and water • Vertical transmission has been reported
Incubation period: • 2–7 weeks (average 28 days) • Virus is in blood, bile and stools, therefore patient remain infective during this period	*Incubation period:* • 30–180 days	*Incubation period:* • 15–150 days	*Incubation period:* • 35 days	*Incubation period:* • 2–9 weeks (45 days)
Lab diagnosis: • Detection of anti-HAV IgM in serum	*Lab diagnosis:* • All pregnant women should be routinely screened for HBV antenatally. • High risk should be screened at 28 weeks	*Lab diagnosis:* • Anti-HCV abs. • Molecular tests for diagnosis virus particles • 3rd generation assays for anti-HCV	*Lab diagnosis:* • D antigen in serum or hepatic tissue • IgM antibody to Hep D virus in serum	*Lab diagnosis:* • Demonstration of virus specific antibodies • IgM by ELISA (1 week to 2 months and infection disappear after 4–5 months

Contd...

Contd...

Hepatitis A	Hepatitis B	Hepatitis C	Hepatitis D	Hepatitis E
	• High risk includes – Asians, patient at occupational risks, those exposed to HBV carriers, mentally challenged patients, hemodialysis, history of multiple blood transfusions, multiple sexual partners, Intravenous drugs users	• PCR assay for viral particles (most specific) • E2 particle by ELISA		• IgG appear shortly after IgM • HEV-RNA detected by reverse transcriptase PCR
Clinical features presenting symptoms and clinical course: • General weakness, fatigue, malaise fever • Nausea/vomiting, anorexia, loose motions *Long-term consequences:* • No carrier state • Chronic infection does not occur	*Clinical features:* • Prodormal/preicteric phase: – Gradually increasing anorexia, malaise and fatigue • *Icteric phase:* Right upper quadrant pain, fever, arthralgia, urticaria and rash, jaundice evident, nausea, vomiting, pruritus, darkening urine, stools, lightening in color – Can lead to chronic persistent hepatitis, hepatic failure and death	*Clinical features:* • Similar to hepatitis • 80% asymptomatic and fail to develop jaundice • Acute fulminant infection can lead to hepatic failure and aplastic anemia • 50–80% are chronic infected with HCV • 29–76% chronic active hepatitis/cirrhosis • Chronic infection is strongly linked with the development of hepatocellular malignancy over time about 30 years	*Clinical features:* • 1/3 patients develop fulminant hepatitis • 15–30% of HBV +ve individuals progress to cirrhosis—portal hypertension • Hepatic failure	*Clinical features:* Similar to HAVirus • Self-limiting disease • Fulminating in 10% cases • Mortality rate of 10–18% • Does not result in a chronic carrier state • Vertical transmission reported
Prevention: • Improved sanitation • Strict personal hygiene • Frequent hand washing with soap and water • Active immunization of health workers, day-care providers, waste water workers, vets • Passive postexposure immunization Immunoglobulin (0.02 mL/µg) within 48 hours of exposure up to 2 weeks also • Patients at risk should be given immunization with HAV vaccine	*Prevention:* • Active immunization with 3 doses of recombinant DNA-HBV vaccine • Booster of 5–10 years is recommended • Neonates born to HBV positive mother should receive HBV-Ig in addition to active immunization	*Prevention:* • No vaccine available • Immunoglobulin not effective to prevent infection • Immunoglobulin administration has been associated with HCV infection • Prevents infected blood, organs, semen from entering the donor pool	*Prevention:* • Hep D affects only HBsAg +ve patients so effective immunization against HBV holds the key to Hep D patients	*Prevention:* • No vaccine available • Immunoglobulin does not prevent development of clinical disease

Contd...

Contd...

Hepatitis A	Hepatitis B	Hepatitis C	Hepatitis D	Hepatitis E
Pregnancy: • Incidence 1:1000 • Not transmitted to fetus • May be transmitted to neonate during delivery postpartum period via feco-oral route • Infants born to mothers with HAV infection during 3rd trimester should receive postexposure prophylaxis with immunoglobulins	*Pregnancy:* • Incidence 1–2/1000 • 0.5–10.5% are carrier • No evidence of transplacental transmission	*Pregnancy:* • No vertical transmission • HIV +ve with HCV, there is high risk of vertical transmission • Mother-to-child transmission risk is 5% but 15%, if HIV with HCV is present	*Pregnancy:* • HBV • Perinatal transmission rare	*Pregnancy:* • Disease more severe during pregnancy • Associated with high mortality rate (10–18%) • Vertical transmission known to occur • Perinatal transmission undetermined
	Effects on mother: • GI symptoms are more pronounced • Chronic carrier likely to suffer from cirrhosis, esophageal varices, liver failure	*Effects on mother:* • May be symptomatic • May have clinical features similar to HBV • Fulminant infections may lead to hepatic failure and death		*Effects on mother:* • More severe during pregnancy • Preterm birth common • Risk of PPH high due to prothrombin deficiency • High risk of fatality
	Effects on fetus: • No increased risk of abortion preterm, IUGR, IUD, malnutrition present • No teratogenic effects on fetus • Avoid using scalp electrodes • Gentle resuscitation after birth, avoid mucosal trauma to the pharynx • Breastfeeding poses no risk	*Effects on fetus:* • Generally none • Risk of transmission – 5% • If HIV + HBV—risk of transmission rises 3 fold • Most infected children remain well but are at high risk of developing chronic liver problem of adulthood		*Effects on fetus:* • Vertical transmission known • Perinatal transmission also likely to occur • Prematurity • Low birth weight • Increased perinatal mortality and morbidity
Management: • Routine ANC care • Generalized supportive measures • Nutrition and correct anemia • Avoid exposure to infected individual • Strict personal hygiene	*Management:* • Screen for liver involvement • Family members screen and immunize • Neonates—passive + active immunization within 12 hours of delivery	*Management:* • Similar to Hep A • Monitor fetal growth • No HCV vaccine available • Obstetric intervention should be undertaken for obstetric indications only	*Management:* • Similar to HBV • Treatment with interferon produced improvement in 28–46% patients with chronic HCV 50% showed relapse within 6 months of cessation of therapy	*Management:* • Similar to HAV

Contd...

Contd...

Hepatitis A	Hepatitis B	Hepatitis C	Hepatitis D	Hepatitis E
• Give neonate postexposure prophylaxis • If severely ill (encephalopathy, jaundice, coagulopathy) hospitalize the patient • All precautions—Nursing • Correct fluid and electrolyte imbalance • Fresh blood transfusion, cryoprecipitate blood component therapy • Inactivated virus vaccine, if available administer	• HbsAg negative mother—active immunization after delivery • At high-risk mother—passive immunization • Arrange blood, fresh-frozen plasma • Active management of 3rd stage of labor • Avoid morphine/hepatotoxic drugs • Dispose placenta with incineration	• Elective LSCS is recommended • No HCV vaccine available		

Clinical Features

Viral hepatitis presents in 2 forms:
1. Acute viral hepatitis (AVH)
2. Fulminant hepatic failure (FHF).

Acute Viral Hepatitis: Clinical Features

Those cases which have acute self-limiting disease and serum asymptotic. Aminotransferase is increased up to 5 fold or clinical jaundice or both. It has three phases:
1. Prodormal phase:
   - No surgery, mildest attack; influenza-like symptoms
   - Usually digestive symptoms, anorexia, nausea, mild pyrexia
   - Increased serum transaminases.
2. Icteric phase:
   - Darkening of urine and lightening of feces
   - Development of jaundice; pruritis is there transiently
   - Liver palpable—smooth, tender in 70% cases, spider angioma may develop.
3. Recovery phase:
   - After 1–4 weeks, uneventful recovery
   - Stool regain color, lassitude and fatigue persist.

Fulminant Hepatic Failure: Clinical Feature

Hepatic coma/hepatic failure: Within 4 weeks—encephalopathy may develop.
- Mental change—stupor, coma, confusion; generalized edema + ascites
- Altered mental status, flapping tremors present
- Violent behavior is noted in patients
- S. bilirubin increased
- S. transaminases increased
- Best marker—prothrombin time
- More common in hep B, hep D, hep E

Diagnosis

- To confirm liver involvement—LFT, PT, USG abdomen
- Diagnosing pathology—liver markers, liver biopsy
- Identifying complications—KFT, coagulation profile, upper GI endoscopy
- S. bilirubin >15 mg
- Transaminases >1000 units
- PT prolapsed
- Specific viral markers—HAV, HbsAG, IgM, anti-HBc type, PCR of Hep C and E, anti-Hb-IgM.

Management

Follow universal precautions:
- Safe drinking water, improved sanitation, personal hygiene are the basic steps for prevention of hepatitis.
- Using disposable syringe, screening blood donors for HBsAg and Hep C.

Acute Viral Hepatitis Management

- Conservative treatment is mainstay, rest SOS
- Nutrition 3000 Kcal/day, no specific drugs, high carbohydrate low fat diet

- Avoid fatty food, restricted physical activity
- Hospitalize with severe—anorexia, vomiting or raised prothrombin time.

Fulminant Hepatic Failure Management

- ICU admission, avoid morphine, pethidine, diuretics
- Discontinue oral protein
- Fluid, electrolytes, calorie—3000 Kcal/day
- Steroids have no role, rarely required
- If ICT raised—give mannitol
- IV fluids such as—D10 should be administered
- Oral neomycin 18-6 hourly to prevent toxic nitrogenous compounds
- Lactulose 15–30 mL thrice a day
- Control of severe pruritis by ursodeoxycholic acid 300 mg BD
- Liver transplantation may be life saving
- Interferon therapy is given in selected patients
- Fetal surveillance and monitoring is a must
- During labor, vaginal delivery should be the aim
- Avoid fetal scalp electrodes and fetal blood sampling
- Complications such as hypokalemia, hypoglycemia, hypocalcemia may occur, treat accordingly
- Blood and fresh-frozen plasma be used in cases of PPH
- Breastfeeding is not contraindicated.

Hep B IG: Give immediate prophylaxis in:
- a. Needle stick injuries
- b. Newborn to carrier mother
- c. Sexual contacts of Hep B patients
- Give as soon as possible after accidental inoculation
- Ideally should be given within 6 hours, preferably 48 hours 0.005–0.007 mL/kg
- Simultaneously draw blood to test for viral markers.

CONCLUSION[2-4]

The occurrence of hepatobiliary disease with or without jaundice during pregnancy provides both the physician and obstetrician with an interesting and urgent diagnostic challenge. Advances in our understanding and management of liver disorders unique to pregnancy and hepatobiliary disease in general have resulted in a significant improvement in the outcome for both mother and fetus. The management of jaundice in pregnancy has to be a multispecialty approach with involvement of obstetrician, physician and an intensivist, if required. A careful clinical history, physical examination, appropriate laboratory tests and radiological investigations should allow a diagnosis within 24–48 hours of presentation.

It is imperative for the clinician to diagnose these liver disorders in a timely manner, and to institute appropriate management as maternal and fetal outcome are affected in an adverse manner, if these conditions are left untreated.

REFERENCES

1. Daftery SN, Desai SV. Selected topics in Obstetrics and Gynecology-3, for postgraduates and practitioners; 2007.
2. Reily CA. Hepatic disease in pregnancy. Am J Med. 1994;96:18-22.
3. Sharma JB. Textbook of Obstetrics; 2012.
4. Green-top Guideline No. 43 April 2011.
5. Practical guide to high risk pregnancy and delivery. A south Asian Perspective, Fernando Arias.

SECTION 6: OBSTETRIC COMPLICATIONS

Chapter 25

Prediction and Prevention of Pre-eclampsia

Beenu Kushwaha, Neha Khatik, Swaraj Naik

INTRODUCTION

Pre-eclampsia (PE) is a hypertensive disorder of pregnancy that is diagnosed after the 20th week of gestation, if left untreated, it progresses to eclampsia. It is defined by the American College of Obstetrics and Gynecology as *de novo* hypertension of at least 140/90 mm Hg in a pregnant woman. Proteinuria with the hypertension is sufficient but not required for the diagnosis, especially if a woman displays severe symptoms such as headache, blurry vision, right upper quadrant pain, and low platelet count. PE continues to be a leading cause of maternal and perinatal morbidity and mortality affecting approximately 3% of all pregnancies and 5% of healthy women in their first pregnancy.[1] WHO estimates the incidence of PE to be seven times higher in developing countries (2.8% of live births) than in developed countries (0.4%).[2] Despite significant research and advancements, PE continues to kill 29, 000 mothers per year worldwide.[3] PE contributes to approximately 10% of stillbirths and 15% of preterm births.[4,5] It also causes short- and long-term consequences such as future metabolic and cardiovascular events for the mother and the child born during a pregnancy affected by pre-eclampsia.

PE is a multisystem disorder of pregnancy basically triggered by poor placentation. This condition is commonly divided into early onset (diagnosed and requiring delivery <34 weeks' gestation) and late onset disease.[6,7] Early onset PE occurs less frequently (0.4–1%) than late onset PE but is responsible for a more significant burden of disease, with its associated prematurity and fetal growth restriction, in addition to increased long-term maternal cardiovascular morbidity.[8] Late onset PE, including PE at term, also poses significant health burden and contributes to maximum cases of PE.

A delay in diagnosis and delayed access to appropriate care is a core cause of the PE-related morbidity and severe mortality worldwide. The complex pathogenesis of PE has challenged the ability to effectively predict pre-eclampsia to decrease the delay in its diagnosis. Consequently, early intervention or triage to higher level obstetric care is hindered. In present scenario, there is enough data that provides information on how and when various predictive tests can be best utilized in predicting PE.[9]

ETIOPATHOGENESIS OF PRE-ECLAMPSIA

Although the cause of PE remains elusive, a combination of abnormal placentation and predisposing maternal factors contribute to the development of widespread endothelial dysfunction which leads to the entire syndrome.[10] Early in normal pregnancy, the cytotrophoblastic cells of the developing placenta invade the uterine wall, disrupting the endothelium and tunica media of the spiral arteries. The vascular wall of the spiral arteries is remodeled; this, in turn, leads to a transformation of the spiral arteries from low-flow, highly resistant vessels into the high-flow, low-resistance vessels, which are vital for normal placental development. There are thought to be two stages to cytotrophoblastic invasion: the first involves invasion of the decidual segments of the spiral arteries, at around 10–12 weeks gestation; the second involves invasion of the myometrial segments at 15–16 weeks. In PE, the cytotrophoblastic invasion of the myometrial segments is impaired: the spiral arteries remain narrow, and blood supply to the fetus is restricted **(Fig. 25.1)**. Placental ischemia is thought to develop as a result of this abnormal cytotrophoblastic invasion; this has been proposed as leading to release of placental factors and imbalance of angiogenic factors, causing the widespread endothelial dysfunction which leads to the syndrome clinically of multiorgan involvement.[11]

It is the predisposition of a mother caused by; immunological maladaptation (First pregnancy, short duration of sperm exposure), genetic factors (increased risk-if first degree relatives are affected), preexisting vascular diseases, diabetes, hypertension, obesity, history of renal disease and/or thrombophilia (due to factor V Leiden heterozygosity, antiphospholipid syndrome or prothrombin gene mutations),[12] which eventually play an important role in initiation and progression of disease.

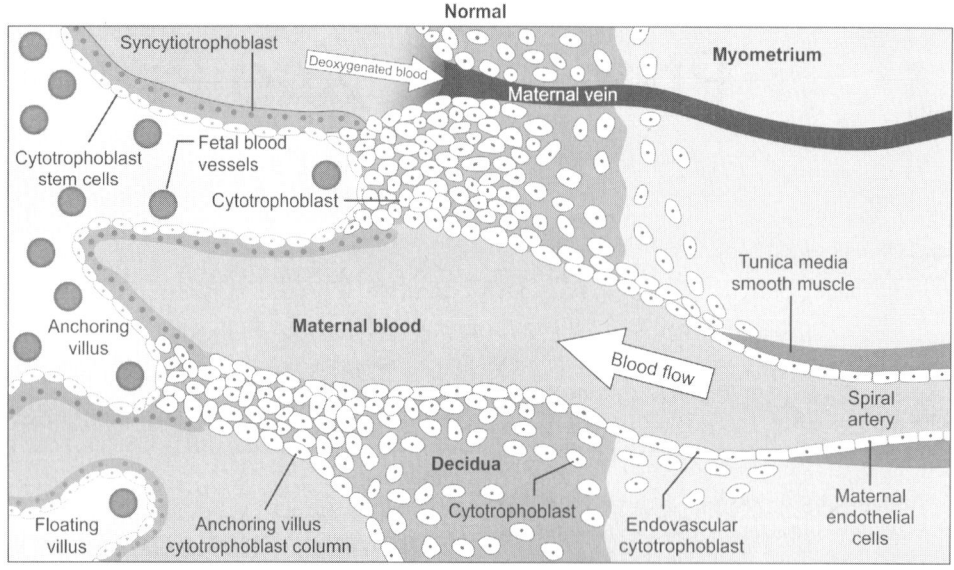
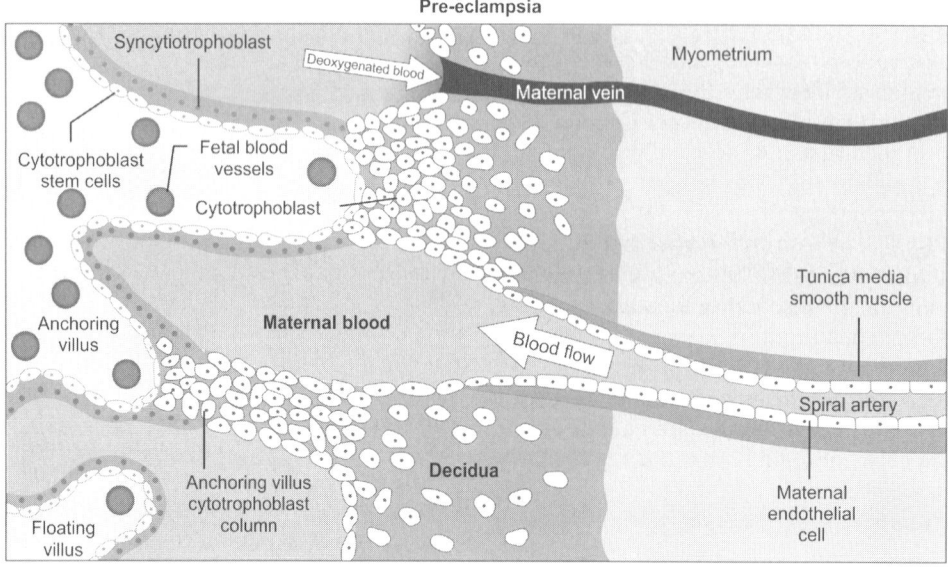

Fig. 25.1: Normal and abnormal placentation

THE RATIONALE FOR PREDICTION

Early prediction of PE would make it possible to offer timely prophylaxis and enhanced surveillance of women at risk, thereby reducing the risk of development of complications such as severe hypertension, cerebrovascular accident, eclampsia, pulmonary edema, renal or liver impairment, placental abruption and fetal death.

A recent meta-analysis reported that the prevalence of PE can potentially be halved by the administration of low-dose aspirin started at 16 weeks or earlier, especially early and severe cases of PE.[13-15] Therefore, if the disease is identified early, prophylactic use of aspirin could very well prevent progression to a severe disease, which justifies exploring a good predictor for the disease.

WHICH SHOULD BE A GOOD PREDICTIVE TEST?

Although there has not been a single screening test till date, apart from identifying clinical risk factors and continuous surveillance with regular measurement of blood pressure and proteinuria throughout pregnancy, which has been adopted into clinical practice, but because of extensive research in

Table 25.1: Predictive tests for development of the pre-eclampsia syndrome	
Testing related to	Name of tests
1. Biophysical markers (Placental perfusion and vascular resistance)	Roll-over test, isometric handgrip or cold pressure test, pressure response to aerobic exercise, angiotensin-II infusion test, mid-trimester mean arterial pressure, platelet angiotensin-II binding, renin, 24-hour ambulatory blood pressure monitoring, uterine artery or fetal transcranial Doppler velocimetry
2. Biochemical markers	
A. Fetal-placental unit endocrine dysfunction:	Human chorionic gonadotropin (hCG), alpha-fetoprotein (AFP), estriol, pregnancy-associated protein A (PAPP A), inhibin A, activin A, placental protein 13, corticotropin-releasing hormone, A disintegrin, ADAM-12, kisspeptin
B. Renal dysfunction:	Serum uric acid, microalbuminuria, urinary calcium or kallikrein, microtransferrinuria, N-acetyl-β-glucosaminidase, cystatin C, podocyturia
C. Endothelial dysfunction/oxidant stress:	Platelet count and activation, fibronectin, endothelial adhesion molecules, prostaglandins, prostacyclin, MMP-9, thromboxane, C-reactive protein, cytokines, endothelin, neurokinin B, homocysteine, lipids, insulin resistance, antiphospholipid antibodies, plasminogen activator inhibitor (PAI), leptin, p-selectin, angiogenic factors such as placental growth factor (PlGF), vascular endothelial growth factor (VEGF), soluble fms-like tyrosine kinase receptor-1 (sFlt-1), soluble endoglin
D. Others:	Antithrombin-III (AT-3), atrial natriuretic peptide (ANP), β_2-microglobulin, haptoglobin, transferrin, ferritin, 25-hydroxyvitamin D, genetic markers, cell-free fetal DNA, serum and urine proteomics and metabolomic markers, hepatic aminotransferases

Abbreviations: ADAM12, ADAM metallopeptidase domain 12; MMP, matrix metalloproteinase

the last 20 years and mainly as a consequence of the shift in screening for aneuploidies from the second- to the first-trimester of pregnancy, researchers have identified a series of early biophysical and biochemical markers of impaired placentation.[16,17]

Based on the pathogenesis of the disease a combination of maternal demographic characteristics including medical and obstetrics history, biophysical markers; uterine artery blood flow characteristics in the form of uterine artery pulsatility index (PI), mean arterial pressure (MAP) and biochemical markers for screening of PE[18-20] have been identified. **Table 25.1** summarizes the name of various biophysical and biochemical markers test, which have been mentioned in literature for predicting PE depending on the basic pathogenesis of PE, followed by a brief discussion of various methods.

MATERNAL CHARACTERISTICS AND OBSTETRIC HISTORY

There are several factors including demographic characteristics and components of obstetric history which are associated with an increased risk for development of PE. **Table 25.2** shows various maternal characteristics and their relative risk of causing PE in a pregnant female, a practical approach would be to estimate individual patient-specific risk by combining maternal characteristics and obstetric history into an algorithm derived by multivariate statistical analysis.[20] The multivariate analysis generates odds ratios for each individual maternal characteristic based on the strength of association with PE which can then be used to generate individual patient-specific risks for early (requiring delivery before 34 weeks) and late onset PE (requiring delivery after 34 weeks) **(Fig. 25. 2)**.

NICE and ACOG Guidelines

Based on evidences[21-23] available on various high-risk factors for causing PE, the National Institute for Health and Care Excellence guideline identifies women with history of hypertensive disease during a previous pregnancy, chronic kidney disease, autoimmune disease such as systemic lupus erythematosus or antiphospholipid syndrome, type 1 or type 2 diabetes or chronic hypertension to be at increased risk of PE and requiring prophylactic treatment with aspirin. In addition, the guideline recommends that women with more than one moderate risk factor (defined as nulliparity, age 40 years or older, pregnancy interval of >10 years, BMI of 35 kg/m² or more at booking, family history of PE or multiple pregnancy) are offered aspirin prophylaxis.

The American College of Obstetricians and Gynecologists does not recommend routine screening to predict PE beyond taking an appropriate medical history to evaluate for risk factors.[24]

Table 25.2: Maternal characteristics and history-based risk factors for developing PE

Risk factor	Unadjustable relative risk (95%CI)
• Race (Africo-Carribean, South Asian)	Increased*
• Nulliparity	2.91 (1.28–6.61)
• Multiparous women	
– Pre-eclampsia in any previous pregnancy	7.19 (5.85–8.83)
– 10 years or more since last baby born	Increased*
• Age 40 years or older	
– Nulliparous women	1.68 (1.23–2.29)
– Multiparous women	1.96 (1.34–2.87)
• Body mass index of 35 kg/m² or higher	1.55 (1.28–1.88)
• Family history of pre-eclampsia (mother or sister)	2.90 (1.70–4.93)
• Diastolic blood pressure of ≥80 mm Hg at booking	Increased*
• Proteinuria at booking appointment (≥+ on dipstick testing on more than one occasion or quantifies at ≥300 mg /24 hours)	Increased*
• IVF conception	Increased*
• Multiple pregnancy	2.93 (2.04–4.21)
• Underlying medical disorders	
– Pre-existing hypertension	Increased*
– Pre-existing renal disease	Increased*
– Pre-existing diabetes	3.56 (2.54–4.99)
– Presence of antiphospholipid antibodies	9.72 (4.34–21.75)

*Risk for pre-eclampsia increased, but by how much is unknown

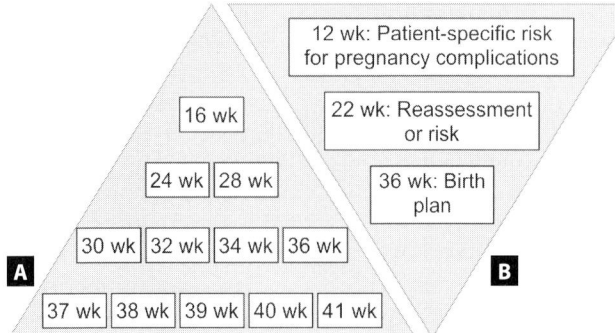

Fig. 25.2: Pyramid of care. (A) An 80-year-old model of prenatal care; (B) Proposed new inverted pyramid model of prenatal care (wk, week)

BIOPHYSICAL MARKERS

Mean Arterial Pressure and Ambulatory BP Monitoring

Mean arterial pressure (systolic + 2 (diastolic)/3) (MAP) in the second trimester of pregnancy, more or equal to 90 mm Hg was proposed long time ago as a predictor of pre-eclampsia. Along with detailed assessment of maternal history at the booking visit to identify risk factors for PE, the measurement of BP during antenatal visits also constitutes the basis of screening for PE throughout pregnancy. The BP measurement is not only increased in the second trimester in those women destined to develop PE but there is evidence suggesting that this increase can be observed from as early as the first-trimester of pregnancy.[25] In current clinical practice, although the use of mercury sphygmomanometers remains the gold standard for noninvasive BP monitoring, but there are concerns for both the clinical performance and safety of these instruments.[26,27] These problems have been largely overcome by the use of automated BP devices measuring mean arterial pressure (MAP), but so far only one of these has been validated for use both in pregnancy and in PE.[28] Despite the lack of randomized trials showing the benefit of ambulatory blood pressure monitoring (ABPM) in predicting PE, some authors recommend serial BP measurement by this method, based on various observational studies and small trials. A study published in *Arquivos Brasileiros de Cardiologia* concluded that certain data from ABPM can predict PIH, particularly diastolic pressure load during wakefulness, diastolic and systolic pressure load during sleep, and pressure variability and maximum diastolic pressure during sleep. Specifically a maximum diastolic arterial pressure on ABPM during sleep of ≥64 mm Hg presented an odds ratio of 6 for PIH with a sensitivity of 80% and a specificity of 60%.[29]

Uterine Artery Pulsatility Index (PI)

As stated earlier, in pregnancies with PE, there is impaired trophoblastic proliferation of maternal spiral arteries, which leads to a state of high-resistance in uteroplacental circulation. This leads to increased impedance to blood flow in the uterine arteries, which can be assessed non-invasively by Doppler ultrasound examination. In women with established PE, this results in increased PI in the uterine arteries, these alterations in the uterine artery PI predate the onset of the disease and in fact are increased from as early as the first trimester of pregnancy.[30,31] Doppler uterine artery analysis is unable in isolation to predict PE risk, as it identifies only 40–60% of those who subsequently develop PE and 20% of those who develop fetal growth restriction.[32] However, when combined with assessment in the first trimester of serum markers associated with the pathophysiology of PE, particularly placental protein 13, placental growth factor, vascular endothelial growth factor (VEGF) and soluble tyrosine kinase-1, it may predict up to 90% of cases of severe preeclampsia for a false positive rate of 9%.[33] Studies reported more accurate prediction by this technique when performed in the late second trimester which can be combined with the routine anomaly scan at around 18–20 weeks.[34,35]

BIOCHEMICAL MARKERS

A series of biochemical markers which could be hormonal (Secreted from placenta mainly), hematological or renal functions based tests, are thought to be involved in placentation or in the cascade of events leading from impaired placentation (basic pathogenesis of PE) to development of clinical symptoms of PE **(Table 25.1)**, have been examined in maternal blood out of which soluble endoglin (sEng), soluble fms-like tyrosine kinase-1 (sFlt-1), serum PAPP-A, placental protein-13 (PP13) and PlGF are extensively studied.[36-39] PAPP-A, PlGF and sFlt-1/PlGF ratio need a special mention as they are the only one which seem to be promising in clinical practice.

Pregnancy-associated Plasma Protein-A (PAPP-A)

Increased level of maternal serum PAPP-A has been observed in established PE.[40,41] PAPP-A is a syncytiotrophoblast derived metalloproteinase which enhances the mitogenic function of the insulin-like growth factors. As insulin-like growth factor system is believed to play an important role in placental growth and development, it is therefore not surprising that low serum PAPP-A is associated with a higher incidence of PE.

Placental Growth Factor

Placental growth factor (PlGF), a glycosylated dimeric glycoprotein, is a member of the vascular endothelial growth factor subfamily. It binds to vascular endothelial growth factor receptor-1 which has been shown to rise in pregnancy. PlGF is synthesized in villous and extravillous cytotrophoblast and has both vasculogenic and angiogenic functions. It is believed to contribute a change in angiogenesis from a branching to a non-branching phenotype controlling the expansion of the capillary network. There is considerable evidence suggesting that in pregnancies with established PE, there is a reduced placental production of PlGF.[19] There are studies suggesting that the maternal serum levels of PlGF are decreased not only in the clinical phase of the disease but also in the first trimester of pregnancy, several weeks prior to the onset of clinical disease. Similar to serum PAPP-A, there is a linear relationship between serum PlGF MoM and gestation at delivery earlier the gestation at delivery, lower the PlGF MoM.

sFlt-1/PlGF Ratio

In the decade since Maynard et al.[42] reported that excessive placental production of sFlt-1, an antagonist of vascular endothelial growth factor and PlGF contributes to the pathogenesis of PE, extensive research has been published demonstrating the usefulness of angiogenic markers in both diagnosis and the subsequent prediction and management of PE and placenta-related disorders. Increased serum levels of sFlt-1 and decreased levels of PlGF, thereby resulting in an increased sFlt-1/PlGF ratio, can be detected in the second half of pregnancy in women diagnosed to have not only PE but also IUGR or stillbirth, i.e. placenta-related disorders. These alterations are more pronounced in early-onset rather than late-onset disease and are associated with severity of the clinical disorder. Whereas studies on the predictive efficacy of the sFlt-1/PlGF ratio in the first trimester have yielded contradictory, reports on the use of this marker as an aid in prediction from the mid trimester onwards have led to its suggested use as a screening tool, especially for identifying all women developing PE and requiring delivery within the subsequent 4-6 weeks.[43]

WHAT IS THE MOST EFFECTIVE METHOD?

The most commonly followed current approach to prenatal care involves visits at 16, 24, 28, 30, 32, 34 and 36 weeks and then weekly until delivery, seems an obsolete practice in today's scenario. The high concentration of visits that were recommended earlier in the third trimester implied, firstly, most complications occur at this late stage of pregnancy and, secondly, that most adverse outcomes are unpredictable during the first or even the second trimester. In the last 20 years, it has become apparent that an integrated first hospital visit at 11–13 weeks combining data from maternal characteristics and history with findings of biophysical and biochemical tests can define the patient-specific risk for a wide spectrum of pregnancy complications, including fetal abnormalities, miscarriage and stillbirth, pre-eclampsia, preterm delivery, gestational diabetes, fetal growth restriction and macrosomia. Each visit would have a predefined objective and the findings would generate likelihood ratios that can be used to modify the individual patient- and disease-specific estimated risk from the initial assessment at 11–13 weeks, that is why there has been a reversal in antenatal care pyramid, where more focus is being put on more number of early trimester visits (*see* Fig. 25.2).

In an appropriately selected pregnant female, on the basis of available evidences, more effective and scientifically proven screening for PE can only be achieved by a combination of maternal characteristics and history, which constitutes the a priori risk, combined with biophysical and biochemical markers. In screening for PE requiring delivery before 34 weeks the detection rate, at a false positive rate of 10%, was about 50% by maternal characteristics and this was improved to about 90% by the addition of biophysical markers and to about 75% by the addition of biochemical markers. The detection rate improved to more than 95% in screening by an algorithm combining maternal factors, biophysical markers and biochemical markers.[12,18]

Therefore, if we adopt inverted pyramid of antenatal care, prediction of PE can be combined with aneuploidy screening in first trimester itself in those pregnant females who are found to be at high-risk from history and personal characteristics and later on from mid trimester onwards sflt/PlGF ratio can be added to further identify those patients who would need early delivery amongst these high-risk females. This approach has been mentioned in a flow chart form in **Figure 25.3**.

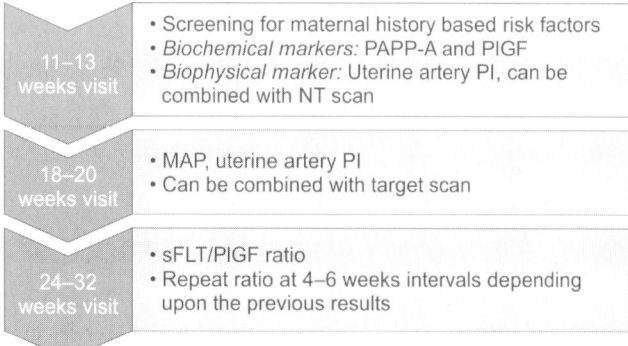

Fig. 25.3: Algorithm for predicting PE, starting from I trimester

RECENT ADVANCES

Genomics and Proteomics

A number of gene polymorphisms have been found to be associated with the risk of developing pre-eclampsia. Further advances are expected from proteomic research. Proteomics has been defined as "knowledge of the structure, function, and expression of all proteins in the biochemical or biological contexts of all organisms". Comparing protein patterns between healthy patients and those with a disease has been increasingly used in recent years to discover markers of disease (biomarkers), which have a number of important roles in medical research.

Metabolomics

Metabolomics is a further area that has the potential to contribute significantly to future research in pre-eclampsia. In complement to studies examining the human genome and proteome, metabolomics can be defined as a "systematic study of the unique chemical fingerprints that specific cellular processes leave behind".

In common with proteomics, studies of the human metabolome can be carried out on routine samples of urine, plasma, or serum requiring minimal specialist preparation of samples.

Cell-free Fetal DNA

The immune-stimulatory properties of cell-free DNA have been known for over 50 years. Cell-free fetal DNA quantification is a promising marker for prediction of PE. However, because of the heterogeneity in published studies, a precise conclusion about the statistical and clinical relevance of this potential marker cannot be made.[44]

PREVENTION OF PRE-ECLAMPSIA

There are many strategies which have been proposed to prevent or modify pre-eclampsia severity. Some are listed below. In general, none of these has been found to be convincingly and reproducibly effective except the initiation of aspirin as early as from 16 weeks, based on a pregnant lady's risk to develop PE.

A. Dietary manipulation — Low-salt diet, calcium or fish oil supplementation
B. Exercise — Physical activity, stretching
C. Cardiovascular drugs — Diuretics, antihypertensives
D. Antioxidants — Ascorbic acid (vitamin C), α-tocopherol (vitamin E), vitamin D antithrombotic
E. Other — Low-dose aspirin, aspirin/dipyridamole, aspirin + heparin, aspirin + ketanserin

Various Methods Used for Preventing PE

- *Dietary and lifestyle modifications:* There are many misconceptions regarding the role of diet in PE but none is proven so far.
  - *Low-salt diet:* One of the earliest research efforts to prevent pre-eclampsia was salt restriction. It is the result of randomized trial that showed that a sodium-restricted diet was ineffective in preventing PE, therefore guidelines from the United Kingdom National Institute for Health and Clinical Excellence (NICE-2010) recommend against salt restrictions.
  - *Calcium supplementation:* Calcium supplementation has been studied in several trials, including one by the National Institute of Child Health and Human Development (NICHD), in one recent meta-analysis, it was reported that increased calcium intake lowered the risk for pre-eclampsia in high-risk women. In aggregate, most of these trials have shown that unless women are calcium deficient, supplementation has no salutary effects.
  - *Fish oil supplementation:* Randomized trials conducted thus far have shown no such benefits.
- *Exercise:* There are a few studies done to assess the protective effects of physical activity on pre-eclampsia. In their systematic review, Kasawara and associates (2012) reported a trend toward risk reduction with exercise. More research is needed in this area.
- *Drugs:*
  - *Antihypertensive drugs:* Because of the putative effects of sodium restriction, diuretic therapy became popular with the introduction of chlorothiazide. Studies found that women given diuretics had a decreased incidence of edema and hypertension but not of PE. Because women with chronic hypertension are at high-risk for PE, several randomized trials—only a few placebo-controlled—have been done to evaluate various antihypertensive drugs to reduce the incidence of superimposed PE. A critical analysis of these trials by failed to demonstrate salutary effects.
  - *Antioxidants:* There are inferential data that an imbalance between oxidant and antioxidant activity may play an important role in the pathogenesis of PE. Thus, naturally occurring antioxidants—vitamins C, D, and E—might decrease such oxidation. Indeed, women who developed pre-eclampsia were found to have reduced plasma levels of these antioxidants. There have now been several randomized studies to evaluate vitamin supplementation for women at high risk for. None of these studies showed reduced PE rates in women given vitamins C and E compared with those given placebo. The recent meta-analysis likewise showed no benefits of vitamin D supplementation.

The rationale for the use of statins to prevent PE is that they stimulate hemoxygenase-1 expression that inhibits sFlt-1 release. There are preliminary animal data that statins may prevent hypertensive disorders of pregnancy.
  - *Antithrombotic agents:* There are sound theoretical reasons that antithrombotic agents might reduce the incidence of PE.
    - *Low-dose aspirin:* In oral doses of 50 to 150 mg daily, aspirin effectively inhibits platelet thromboxane A2 biosynthesis but has minimal effects on vascular prostacyclin production. Recent meta-analysis has shown clear-cut benefits.[14] The 2013 Task Force recommended the use of low-dose aspirin in some high-risk women to prevent pre-eclampsia.
    - *Low-dose aspirin plus heparin:* In women with lupus anticoagulant (LA), treatment with low-dose aspirin and heparin mitigates thrombotic sequel. Because of the high prevalence of placental thrombotic lesions found with severe pre-eclampsia, observational trials have been done to evaluate such treatments for affected women. Benefits have been reported for pregnancy outcomes in women given low-molecular-weight heparin plus low-dose aspirin compared with those given low-dose aspirin alone in cases with LA. Similar findings were reported in a trial that included women with thrombophilia and a history of early-onset pre-eclampsia.

WHO RECOMMENDATIONS FOR PREVENTION OF PRE-ECLAMPSIA[45]

- Advice to rest at home is not recommended as an intervention for the primary prevention of pre-eclampsia and hypertensive disorders of pregnancy in women, considered to be at risk of developing those conditions. (Low quality evidence. Weak recommendation)
- Strict bed rest is not recommended for improving pregnancy outcomes in women with hypertension (with or without proteinuria) in pregnancy (Low-quality evidence, weak recommendation).
- Restriction in dietary salt intake during pregnancy with the aim of preventing the development of pre-eclampsia and its complications is not recommended (Moderate quality evidence, weak recommendation).
- In area where dietary calcium intake is low, calcium supplementation during pregnancy (at doses of 1.5–2.0 g elemental calcium/day) is recommended for the prevention of pre-eclampsia in all women, but especially in those at high risk of developing pre-eclampsia (Moderate quality evidence, strong recommendation).
- Vitamin D supplementation during pregnancy is not recommended to prevent the development of

pre-eclampsia and its complications (Very-low quality evidence. Strong recommendation).
- Individual or combined vitamin C and vitamin E supplementation during pregnancy is not recommended to prevent the development of pre-eclampsia and its complications (high quality evidence, strong recommendation).
- Low-dose acetylsalicylic acid (aspirin 75 mg/day) is recommended for the prevention of pre-eclampsia in women at high-risk of developing the condition (moderate quality evidence, strong recommendation)
- Low-dose acetylsalicylic acid (aspirin 75 mg/day) for the prevention of pre-eclampsia and its related complications should be initiated before 20 weeks of pregnancy (low quality evidence, weak recommendation).
- Diuretics, particularly thiazides, are not recommended for the prevention of pre-eclampsia and its complications (low quality evidence, strong recommendation).

CONCLUSION

Pre-eclampsia is a multi-systemic disorder that originates in early pregnancy and leads to considerable maternal morbidity and mortality. Early detection of PE would allow for planning of appropriate monitoring and for clinical management, following early identification of complications. Recent meta-analyses have suggested that, provided treatment is started at an early (<16 weeks') gestation, there is a significant reduction in early-onset PE and that this is associated with a reduction in prevalence of perinatal death and morbidity and on the basis of these evidences only various national and international agencies currently recommend that women deemed to be at high-risk of PE should be offered aspirin therapy. This reinforces the need for early identification of high-risk women with the objective of implementing targeted interventions for improving perinatal and maternal outcomes.

No single test has demonstrated a sufficient predictive value for PE to be of clinical use.

These tests appear to be most useful in combination with other parameters instead. Because of the heterogeneous nature of PE, a combination of two or more independent biomarkers, each reflecting a different pathophysiological process, should potentially increase the likelihood to derive suitable predictive algorithms. The most promising strategies for the prediction of PE involve multiparametric approaches, which use a variety of individual parameters in combination (e.g. as established in first-trimester aneuploidy screening). A combination of maternal risk factors, the uterine artery pulsatility index (PI), mean arterial pressure (MAP), and maternal serum pregnancy-associated plasma protein-A (PAPP-A), placental growth factor (PlGF), at 11–13 weeks' gestation can be used to identify a high proportion of pregnancies at high-risk for early-onset PE, and those who are found to be at risk can further be subjected to II trimester uterine artery PI measurement and mid-trimester onwards sequential sFlt/PlGF ratio depending upon the results.

REFERENCES

1. Steegers EA, Von Dadelszen P, Duvekot JJ, et al. Lancet. 2010;376: 631-44.
2. WHO, Make every mother and child count in The World Health Report 2005, World Health Organization, Geneva, Switzerland, 2005.
3. Kassebaum NJ, Bertozzi-Villa A, Coggeshall MS, et al. Global, regional, and national levels and causes of maternal mortality during 1990-2013: a systematic analysis for the Global burden of disease study 2013. Lancet. 2014;384:980-1004.
4. Gardosi J, Kady SM, McGewon P, et al. Classification of stillbirth at death (ReCoDe): population-based cohort study. BMJ. 2005;331:1113-7.
5. Iams JD, Goldenberg RL, Mercer BM, et al. The preterm prediction study: recurrence risk of spontaneous preterm birth. National Institute of Child Health and Human Development Maternal-Fetal Medicine Units Network. Am J Obstet Gynecol. 1998;178:1035-40.
6. Crispi F, Dominguez C, Llurba E, et al. Placental angiogenic growth factors and uterine artey Doppler findings for characterization of different subsets in pre-eclampsia and in isolated intrauterine growth restriction. Am J Obstet Gynecol. 2006;195:201-7.
7. Valensise H, Vasapollo B, Gagliardi G, et al. Early and late preeclampsia: two different maternal hemodynamic states in the latent phase of the disease. Hypertension. 2008;52:873-80.
8. Lisonkova S, Joseph KS. Incidence of pre-eclampsia: risk factors and outcome associated with early- versus late- onset disease. Am J Obstet Gyanecol. 2013;209:544.e1-544.e12.
9. Smith GC. Researching new methods of screening for adverse pregnancy outcome: lessons from pre-eclampsia. PLoS Med. 2012;9:el001274.
10. Redman CW, Sargent IL, Staff AC. IFPA Senior Award Lecture: making sense of pre-eclampsia two placental causes of preeclampsia? Placenta. 2014;(Suppl 35):S20-S25.
11. Sargent IL, Smarason AK. Immunology of pre-eclampsia; current views and hypothesis. In: Kurpisz M, Fernandez N (Eds). Immunology of Human Reproduction. BIOS Scientific Publishers Ltd; Oxford. 1995;355-70.
12. Akolekar R, Syngelaki A, Sarguis R, et al. Prediction of early, intermediate and late pre-eclampsia from maternal factors, biophysical and biochemical markers at 11-13 weeks. Prenat Diagn. 2011;31:66-74.
13. Bujold E, Roberge S, Lacasse Y, et al. Prevention of preeclampsia and intrauterine growth restriction with aspirin started in early pregnancy: a meta-analysis. Obstetrics and Gynecology. 2010;116(2):402-14.
14. Roberge S, Villa P, Nicolaides K, et al. Early administration of low-dose aspirin for the prevention of preterm and term preeclampsia: a systematic review and meta-analysis. Fetal Diagnosis and Therapy. 2012;31(3):141-6.
15. Roberge S, Giguère Y, Villa P, et al. Early administration of low-dose aspirin for the prevention of severe and mild preeclampsia: a systematic review and meta-analysis. American Journal of Perinatology. 2012;29(7):551-6.

16. Wright D, Akolekar R, Syngelaki A, Poon LC, Nicolaides KH. A competing risks model in early screening for preeclampsia. Fetal Diagnosis and Therapy. 2012;32:171-8.
17. Akolekar R, Syngelaki A, Poon L, Wright D, Nicolaides KH. Competing risks model in early screening for preeclampsia by biophysical and biochemical markers. Fetal Diagnosis and Therapy. 2013;33(1):8-15.
18. Poon LC, Kametas NA, Maiz N, Akolekar R, Nicolaides KH. First-trimester prediction of hypertensive disorders in pregnancy. Hypertension. 2009;53:812-8.
19. Giguere Y, Charland M, Bujold E, et al. Combining biochemical and ultrasonographic markers in predicting preeclampsia: a systematic review. Clin Chem. 2010; 56:361-75.
20. Poon LC, Kametas NA, Chelemen T, Leal A, Nicolaides KH. Maternal risk factors for hypertensive disorders in pregnancy: a multivariate approach. J Hum Hypertens. 2010;24:104-10.
21. National Institute for Health and Care Excellence (NICE). Hypertension in pregnancy: the management of hypertensive disorders during pregnancy, CG1 07. London; NICE, 2010.
22. Duckitt K, Harrington D. Risk factors for pre-eclampsia at antenatal booking: systematic review of controlled studies. BMJ. 2005;330:565.
23. North RA, McCowan LM, Dekker GA, et al. Clinical risk prediction for pre-eclampsia in nulliparous women: development of model in international prospective cohort. BMJ. 2011;342:d1875.
24. American College of Obstetricians and Gynecologists, Task Force on Hypertension in Pregnancy. Hypertension in pregnancy. Report of the American College of Obstetricians and Gynecologists' Task Force on Hypertension in Pregnancy. Obstet Gynecol. 2013;122:1122-31.
25. Poon LC, Kametas NA, Pandeva I, Valencia C, Nicolaides KH. Mean arterial pressure at 11(+0) to 13 (+6) weeks in the prediction of pre-eclampsia. Hypertension. 2008;51:1027-33.
26. Mion D, Pierin AM. How accurate are sphygmomanometers? J Hum Hypertyens. 1998;12:245-8.
27. Markendu ND, Whitcher F, Arnold A, Carney C. The mercury sphygmomanometer should be abandoned before it is prescribed. J Hum Hypertyens. 2000;14:31-36.
28. Reinders A, Cuckson AC, Lee JT, Shennan AH. An accurate automated blood pressure device for use in pregnancy and pre-eclampsia: the Microlife 3BTO-A.BJOG. 2005;112:915-20.
29. Carvalho R, Campos H, Bruno Z, et al. Predictive factors for pregnancy hypertension in primiparous adolescents: analysis of prenatal care, ABPM and microalbuminuria. Arq Bras Cardiol. 2006;87:487-95.
30. Plasencia W, Maiz N, Bonino S, Kaihura C, Nicolaides KH. Uterine artery Doppler at 11+0 to 13+6 weeks in the prediction of preeclampsia. Ultrasound Obstet Gynecol. 2007;30:742-9.
31. Velauthar L, Plana MN, Kalidindi M, et al. First-trimester uterine artery Doppler and adverse pregnancy 1outcome: a meta-analysis involving 55,974 women. Ultrasound Obstet Gynecol. 2014;43:500-7.
32. Papageorghiou AT, Yu CK, Cicero S, et al. Second-trimester uterine artery Doppler screening in unselected populations: a review. J Matern Fetal Neonatal Med. 2002;12:78-88.
33. Papageorghiou AT, Campbell S. First trimester screening for preeclampsia. Curr Opin Obstet Gynecol. 2006;18:594-600.
34. Yu CK, Khouri O, Onwudiwe N, Spiliopoulos Y, Nicolaides KH, Fetal Medicine Foundation Second-Trimester Screening Group. Prediction of pre-eclampsia by uterine artery Doppler imaging: relationship to gestational age at delivery and small-for-gestational age. Ultrasound Obstet Gynecol. 2008;31:310-3.
35. Cnossen JS, Morris RK, ter Riet G, et al. Use of uterine artery Doppler ultrasonography to predict pre-eclampsia and intrauterine growth restriction: a systematic review and bivariable meta-analysis. CMAJ. 2008;178:701-11.
36. Kleinrouweler CE, Wiegerinck MM, Ris-Stalpers C, et al. Accuracy of circulating placental growth factor, vascular endothelial growth factor, soluble fms-like tyrosine kinase '1 and soluble endoglin in the prediction of pre-eclampsia: a systematic review and meta-analysis. BJOG. 2012;119:778-87.
37. Andraweera PH, Dekker GA, Roberts CT. The vascular endothelial growth factor family in adverse pregnancy outcomes. Hum Reprod Update. 2012;18:436-57.
38. Odibo AO, Zhong Y, Goetzinger KR, et al. First-trimester placental protein 13, PAPP-A, uterine artery Doppler and maternal characteristics in the prediction of pre-eclampsia. Placenta. 2011;32:598-602.
39. Odibo AO, Patel KR, Spitalnik A, at al. Placental pathology, first-trimester biomarkers and adverse pregnancy outcomes. J Perinatol. 2014;34:186-91.
40. Myatt L, Clifton RG, Roberts JM, et al. First-trimester prediction of preeclampsia in nulliparous women at low risk. Obstet Gynecol. 2012;119:1234-42.
41. Smith GC. Researching new methods of screening for adverse pregnancy outcome: lessons from pre-eclampsia. PLoS Med. 2012; 9:el 001274.
42. Maynard SE, Min JY, Merchan J, Lim KH, Li J, Mondal S, Libermann TA, Morgan JP, Sellke FW, Stillman IE, Epstein FH, Sukhatme VK, Karumanchi SA. Excess placental soluble fms-like tyrosine kinase 1 (sFlt1) may contribute to endothelial dysfunction, hypertension, and proteinuria in preeclampsia. J Clin Invest. 2003;111:649-58.
43. Gómez-Arriaga PI, Herraiz I, López-Jiménez EA, Gómez-Montes E, Denk B, Galindo A. Uterine artery Doppler and sFlt-1/PlGF ratio: usefulness in diagnosis of preeclampsia. Ultrasound Obstet Gynecol. 2013;41:530-7.
44. Martin A, Krishna I, Martina B, Samuel A. Can the quantity of cell-free fetal DNA predict pre-eclampsia: A systematic review. Prenat Diagn. 2014;34:685-91.
45. World Health Organization. WHO Recommendations for prevention and treatment of preeclampsia. Geneva: Switzerland: *http://www.ncbi.nlm.nih.gov/books/2001/NBK140560*.

Chapter 26

Management of Pregnancy-induced Hypertension

Richa Baharani, Bharti Sahu

INTRODUCTION

Hypertensive disorders of pregnancy are an important cause of severe morbidity, long-term disability and death among both mothers and their babies. The majority of deaths due to pre-eclampsia and eclampsia are avoidable through the provision of timely and effective care to the women presenting with these complications. Optimizing health care to prevent and treat women with hypertensive disorders is a necessary step towards achieving the Millennium Development Goals. It complicates up to 15% of pregnancies and accounts for approximately a quarter of all antenatal admissions.

PHYSIOLOGICAL CHANGES IN BLOOD PRESSURE DURING PREGNANCY

Early in the first trimester there is a fall in blood pressure caused by active vasodilatation, achieved through the action of local mediators such as prostacyclin and nitric oxide. This reduction in blood pressure primarily affects the diastolic pressure and a drop of 10 mm Hg is usual by 13–20 weeks gestation. Blood pressure continues to fall until 22–24 weeks when a nadir is reached. After this, there is a gradual increase in blood pressure until term when pre-pregnancy levels are attained. Immediately after delivery blood pressure usually falls, then increases over the first five postnatal days.[1]

CLASSIFICATION OF HYPERTENSIVE DISORDERS DURING PREGNANCY

- Gestational hypertension
- Pre-eclampsia
- Eclampsia
- Chronic hypertension
- Superimposed pre-eclampsia.

Gestational Hypertension

Gestational hypertension is usually defined as having a blood pressure higher than 140/90 measured on two separate occasions, more than 6 hours apart, without the presence of protein in the urine and diagnosed after 20 weeks of gestation.[2]

Pre-eclampsia

Pre-eclampsia is defined as BP ≥140/90 mm Hg, with two readings taken at least 15 min apart with proteinuria (>300 mg of protein in a 24 hours urine sample) beyond 20 weeks of gestation.

Eclampsia

- When tonic-clonic seizures appear in a pregnant woman with high blood pressure and proteinuria.
- Pre-eclampsia and eclampsia are sometimes treated as components of a common syndrome.

Chronic Hypertension

Chronic hypertension in pregnancy is defined as BP ≥140/90 mm Hg before 20 weeks of pregnancy.

Superimposed Pre-eclampsia

Superimposed pre-eclampsia is new occurrence of pre-eclampsia in pregnant patient with chronic hypertension.[3]

Women with hypertension in pregnancy have a higher risk of complications such as:
- Abruptio placentae
- Cerebrovascular accident
- Disseminated intravascular coagulation

The fetus has an increased risk of:
- Intrauterine growth restriction
- Prematurity
- Intrauterine death.

WHEN TO TREAT HYPERTENSION DURING PREGNANCY?

Antihypertensive treatment should be commenced when the systolic blood pressure >140–170 mm Hg or diastolic pressure > 90–110 mm Hg. Treatment is mandatory for severe hypertension when the blood pressure is >170/110 mm Hg. Once treatment is started, target blood pressure is also controversial, but many practitioners would treat to keep the mean arterial pressure < 125 mm Hg—for example, a blood pressure 150/100 mm Hg. Overzealous blood pressure control may lead to placental hypoperfusion, as placental blood flow is not autoregulated, and this will compromise the fetus. Unfortunately there is no evidence that pharmacological treatment of chronic or gestational hypertension protects against the development of pre-eclampsia. Changes in diet or bed rest have not been shown to provide maternal or fetal benefit.[4]

High-risk or Low-risk [5]

- Women at high-risk are those with any of the following:
  - Hypertensive disease during a previous pregnancy
  - Chronic kidney disease
  - Autoimmune disease such as systemic lupus erythematosus or antiphospholipid syndrome
  - Type 1 or type 2 diabetes
  - Chronic hypertension.
- Factors indicating moderate risk are:
  - First pregnancy
  - Age 40 years or older
  - Pregnancy interval of more than 10 years
  - Body mass index (BMI) of 35 kg/m² or more at first visit
  - Family history of pre-eclampsia, multiple pregnancy.

Management [6]

Management depends on the woman's BP, gestational age and blood flow in the placenta. Nonpharmacological management is recommended for many women but is not recommended when there is the presence of associated maternal and fetal risk factors. Nonpharmacological management includes close supervision, limitation of activities, and some bed rest in the left lateral position.[7] All pregnant women should receive antenatal education so that they are aware of the symptoms associated with pre-eclampsia, its importance, and the need to obtain medical advice. Such symptoms include:[6,8]
- Severe headache
- *Visual problems*: Blurred vision or flashing before the eyes
- Severe epigastric pain
- Vomiting
- Sudden swelling of the face, hands or feet.

Control of High Blood Pressure

Antihypertensive treatment should be started in women with a systolic blood pressure over 150 mm Hg or a diastolic blood pressure over 100 mm Hg. In women with other markers of potentially severe disease, treatment can be considered at lower degrees of hypertension. Labetalol, given orally or intravenously, nifedipine given orally or intravenous hydralazine can be used for the acute management of severe hypertension. In moderate hypertension, treatment may assist prolongation of the pregnancy. Clinicians should use agents with which they are familiar. Atenolol, angiotensin converting enzyme (ACE) inhibitors, angiotensin receptor-blocking drugs (ARB) and diuretics should be avoided. Chronic hypertensive women already on these medications should be switched to safer antihypertensive during pregnancy. Nifedipine should be given orally not sublingually.[9] The medical provider must be familiar with the dose to be used and potential side effects of each of these medications. Reduction in blood pressure should be gradual in first 60 minutes of therapy. Nifedipine and hydralazine can cause tachycardia. They are not recommended to be used in patients with heart rate above 100/min. Labetalol is appropriate drug in such patients. Labetalol should be avoided in patients with bradycardia (heart rate <60 bpm), asthma, and in those with congestive cardiac failure. Here, Nifedipine is the drug of choice. $MgSO_4$ is recommended to prevent eclampsia and not as an antihypertensives. Diuretics are not recommended for routine use except some conditions like fluid challenge in oliguria and pulmonary edema. In severe pre-eclampsia, Inj. $MgSO_4$, Pritchard regimen is recommended till 24 hours post delivery. Antihypertensive treatment should be continued throughout labor and delivery to maintain systolic BP at <160 mm Hg and diastolic BP at <110 mm Hg.[3]

Assessment of the Woman

Women should be Assessed at Initial Presentation

Although the classification of severity is primarily based on the level of blood pressure and the presence of proteinuria, clinicians should be aware of the potential involvement of other organs when assessing maternal risk, including placental disease with fetal manifestations.

Gestational Hypertension

- *Assess severity*:
  - *Mild:* 140–149/90–99 mm Hg. For patients presenting before 32 weeks (or at high-risk of pre-eclampsia), measure BP twice a week; otherwise, measure BP no more often than weekly. Check urine for protein at each visit.
  - *Moderate:* 150–159/100–109 mm Hg. Monitor BP twice a week—start labetalol (alternatives are methyldopa or nifedipine) to keep systolic BP <150 mm Hg and diastolic BP between 80–100 mm Hg. Dip urine for protein at each visit. Arrange initial blood tests for full

blood count (FBC), electrolytes, renal function and liver function tests (LFTs). Subsequent blood tests are not necessary if there is no proteinuria.
- *Severe:* ≥160/110 mm Hg. Admit to hospital and treat as for moderate (above) to keep systolic BP <150 mm Hg and diastolic BP between 80–100 mm Hg. Measure BP at least four times a day and check urine for protein daily. Weekly blood tests for FBC, electrolytes, renal function and LFTs. Check BP and urine twice weekly (and continue weekly blood tests) when discharged (once BP is in the target range). Perform ultrasound examination at 34 weeks to assess fetal growth and amniotic fluid volume (with umbilical artery Doppler velocimetry.

Maternal and Fetal Monitoring

During expectant management, maternal and fetal. Conditions should be frequently monitored as follows:

Maternal Assessment

- Vital signs, fluid intake, and urine output should be monitored at least every 8 hours
- Symptoms of severe pre-eclampsia (headaches, visual changes, retrosternal pain or pressure, shortness of breath, nausea and vomiting, and epigastric pain) should be monitored at least every 8 hours
- Presence of contractions, rupture of membranes, abdominal pain, or bleeding should be monitored at least every 8 hours
- Laboratory testing (CBC and assessment of platelet count, liver enzyme, and serum creatinine levels) should be performed daily. These tests can then be spaced to every other day if they remain stable and the patient remains asymptomatic.

Fetal Assessment

Kick count and NST with uterine contraction monitored daily:
- Biophysical profile twice weekly
- Serial fetal growth should be performed every 2 weeks and umbilical artery. Doppler studies should be performed every 2 weeks if fetal growth restriction is suspected.

Surveillance of Fetal Well-being

More frequent prenatal visits are recommended for pregnant women with chronic hypertension compared with healthy women. Such visits are designed to evaluate women for complications of chronic hypertension in pregnancy by following blood pressures, urine protein, fundal height, and maternal symptoms. Because these pregnancies are more likely to be complicated by growth abnormalities, The American College of Obstetricians and Gynecologists (ACOG) indicates that "evaluation of fetal growth by ultrasound in women with chronic hypertension is warranted.[10]

Antenatal Corticosteroids

Antenatal corticosteroid therapy is recommended for all women who present with gestational hypertension/pre-eclampsia before 34 weeks' gestation.
- Inj. Betamethsone 12 mg IM 24 hours apart two doses or
- Inj. Dexamethsone 6 mg IM 12 hours apart four doses.

In case of severe pre-eclampsia/eclampsia where delivery is imperative, total dose of 24 mg of either drug can be given within 24 hours.

TIMING OF DELIVERY OF WOMEN WITH PRE-ECLAMPSIA/ECLAMPSIA

The womb actually is the best neonatal intensive care unit but in certain few condition the uterine environment is not beneficial for the baby or maternal condition is such that it would be hazardous for the pregnancy to carry on and delivery is then expedited.

It is the gestational age which has the maximum impact on the outcome of the baby more than any other various measurements. However, it is utmost impertinent that the mothers condition is stable so that prolongation of pregnancy does not endanger her life. In these condition pregnancy may be stretched for a few hours, which permits transportation of patient to a unit better equipped and facilitated higher center or which allows pediatric unit to be organized to take the baby. If pregnancy can be prolonged by few days or weeks, it may be possible to use steroids to mature fetal lungs. if pregnancy is going to be continued, close monitoring of both mother and baby is required.

The definitive treatment of hypertensive disorders of pregnancy (HDP) is delivery. Attempts to prolong pregnancy in order to improve fetal maturity are unlikely to be of value. However, it is unsafe to deliver the baby of an unstable mother even if there is fetal distress, severe hypertention to be controlled and hypoxia corrected, and delivery to be expedited In women with gestational hypertension, induction of labor between 38 and 39 weeks balances the lowest maternal and neonatal morbidity/mortality.

Patients with controlled mild of moderate hypertension may be allowed to await spontaneous labor at term, but should not be allowed to go beyond 40 weeks. In controlled mild to moderate hypertension induction can be planned between 38–40 weeks. If there is IUGR or fetal distress then early induction of labor is advised. One RCT[126] showed that induction of labor in women with gestational hypertension statistically significantly lowered the risks of progression to severe hypertension compared with women who received expectant management. There appear to be no advantages to immediate birth for women with gestational hypertension, other than the prevention of progression to severe hypertension. However, the GDG's view is that if gestational hypertension becomes severe (160/110 mm Hg or higher), even with antihypertensive treatment, then the woman should be offered immediate birth after a course of corticosteroids. The decision on timing of birth should involve consideration of blood pressure and its treatment, potential complications associated with induction of labor, health of the fetus, other obstetric complications, and the woman's preferences. The GDG's view is that senior obstetric involvement is, therefore, required in the decision-making process.

Recommendations

- Do not offer birth before 37 weeks to women with gestational hypertension whose blood pressure is lower than 160/110 mm Hg, with or without antihypertensive treatment.
- For women with gestational hypertension whose blood pressure is lower than 160/110 mm Hg after 37 weeks, with or without antihypertensive treatment, timing of birth, and maternal and fetal indications for birth should be agreed between the woman and the senior obstetrician.
- Offer birth to women with refractory severe gestational hypertension after a course of corticosteroids (if required) has been complete.

Mode of Delivery in HDP

- Vaginal delivery is preferred for women with any type of HDP.
- Cesarean section is required for obstetric indications.

Choice of anesthesia for women undergoing cesarean section should be regional provided there are no contraindications such as thrombocytopenia (<75,000/mm^3) or altered coagulation profile.

Intrapartum Care

The objective of care are as follows:
- Delivery of baby with least possible trauma to the mother and fetus.
- Prevention of maternal complications like cerebrovascular accidents, renal failure pulmonary edema and placental abruption.
- Prevention of convulsions to avoid further maternal, perinatal mortality.
- Complete maternal health restoration.

Postnatal Management

After birth, measure BP daily for the first two days after birth, at least once between day three and day five, then as clinically indicated. Continue on antihypertensive medication but reduce or stop if BP is seen to be falling—particularly if it falls below 130/80 mm Hg. Switch women from methyldopa to an alternative within two days of delivery. Women with mild hypertension not requiring treatment during pregnancy should be started on antihypertensive medication postnatally if their BP is ≥150/100 mm Hg. Lifestyle modifications, regular BP control, and control of metabolic factors are recommended after delivery, to avoid complications in subsequent pregnancies and to reduce maternal cardiovascular risk in the future.[11]

KEY POINTS

- Women with gestational hypertension or pre-eclampsia without severe features should have planned delivery at 37 weeks' gestation.
- Magnesium sulfate is the treatment of choice to prevent eclamptic seizures
- Intravenous labetalol or hydralazine or oral nifedipine may be used to treat severe hypertension during pregnancy.

REFERENCES

1. Sibai BM. Treatment of hypertension in pregnancy. N Engl J Med. 1996;335:257-65.
2. Jump up Lo, JO Mission, JF Caughey, AB. Hypertensive disease of pregnancy and maternal mortality. Current opinion in obstetrics and gynecology. 2013;25(2):124-32. doi:10.1097/gco.0b013e32835e0ef5. PMID 23403779.
3. Submitted for web upload by Chairman GCPR committee Dr Sanjay Gupte, 26, September, 2014.
4. Cockburn J, Moar VA, Ounsted M, et al. Final report of study on hypertension during pregnancy: the effects of specific treatment on the growth and development of the children. Lancet. 1982;i:647-9. [PubMed].
5. Hypertension in pregnancy: diagnosis and management. Clinical guideline [CG107] Published date: August 2010 Last updated: January 2011.
6. Hypertension: management of hypertension in adults in primary care; NICE Clinical Guideline (August 2011).
7. Management of cardiovascular diseases during pregnancy; European Society of Cardiology (2011).
8. Antenatal care for uncomplicated pregnancies; NICE Clinical Guideline (March 2008).
9. RCOG Guideline No. 10(A) 4 of 11 Evidence level III Evidence level Ia P B B A C A C C B 5 of 11 RCOG Guideline No. 10(A).
10. Committee on hypertension in pregnancy. Hypertension in Pregnancy. Washington, DC: American College of Obstetricians and Gynecologists; 2013.
11. Mosca L, Benjamin EJ, Berra K, et al. Effectiveness-based guidelines for the prevention of cardiovascular disease in women - 2011 update: a guideline from the American Heart Association. Circulation. 2011;123(11):1243-62. doi: 10.1161/CIR.0b013e31820faaf8. E pub 2011 Feb.

Chapter 27

Maternal Assessment in Hypertensive Disease of Pregnancy

Suchitra N Pandit, Gorakh G Mandrupkar, Rana Khan Chowdhry

INTRODUCTION

Hypertensive disorders of pregnancy (HDP) is one of the major causes of maternal and perinatal morbidity and mortality. Hypertensive disorders of pregnancy (HDP) comprises of chronic hypertension, gestational hypertension, pre-eclampsia, superimposed pre-eclampsia in chronic hypertensive and eclampsia. These conditions range from mild disease to multiorgan failure causing significant harm. The Society of The Obstetricians and Gynaecologists of Canada (SOGC) Clinical Practice Guideline No. 206 state that despite extensive research, the onset of hypertension during pregnancy has proven difficult to predict.[1]

Hypertension in pregnancy is defined by South Australian Perinatal Practice Guidelines as:[2]
- Systolic blood pressure greater than or equal to 140 mm Hg and/or
- Diastolic blood pressure greater than or equal to 90 mm Hg.

These measurements should be confirmed by repeated readings. Seligman S states that elevations of both systolic and diastolic blood pressures have been associated with an adverse fetal outcome and therefore both are important.[3] There is supporting evidence also as:
- Perinatal mortality rises with diastolic blood pressures above 90 mm Hg[4]
- Readings above these levels were beyond two standard deviations of mean blood pressure.[5]

Previously, a rise in blood pressure from preconception or first visit by more than 30/15 mm Hg was considered for the diagnosis of pre-eclampsia.

Available evidence does not support increased incidence of adverse outcomes.[6,7]

Severity of Hypertension

Brown MA, et al. 2001 consider hypertension in pregnancy is considered to be severe when systolic blood pressure is ≥160 mm Hg and/or diastolic blood pressure ≥100 mm Hg. These levels represent cut-off levels of overcoming cerebral autoregulation. The severe hypertension should be lowered promptly and carefully to prevent cerebral hemorrhage and hypertensive encephalopathy.[8]

CLASSIFICATION

Accurate classification of women having either pre-existing hypertension or pre-eclampsia or gestational hypertension is very important. The management and prognosis are very different in each condition as well as the impact on maternal and perinatal outcomes is also different. It facilitates the action plan, vigilant care and early detection of complications thereby reducing maternal and perinatal morbidity and mortality.

Gestational Hypertension

It is a new onset of hypertension after 20 weeks gestation without proteinuria. It returns to normal within 3 months postpartum.

Pre-eclampsia

Preeclampsia is hypertension after 20 weeks gestation with proteinuria.[9]

It is a multisystem disorder. It is considered severe with either of the following:
- *Significant proteinuria (more than 2+):* Renal involvement
- *Thrombocytopenia, hemolysis, DIC:* Hematological involvement
- *Epigastric pain, elevated liver enzymes:* Liver involvement
- *Hyperreflexia, headache, visual disturbances:* Neurological involvement
- *Pulmonary edema:* Cardio respiratory involvement
- *Abruption, intrauterine growth restriction (IUGR), oligohydramnios:* Placental involvement

Chronic Hypertension

It is defined as a blood pressure more than 140/90 mm Hg confirmed before pregnancy or before 20 weeks of pregnancy.

These women are at high-risk of superimposed pre-eclampsia than with normotensive women.

Pre-eclampsia Superimposed on Chronic Hypertension

It is diagnosed when pre-eclampsia develops in a woman with chronic hypertension after 20 weeks. In such women significant increases in blood pressure, proteinuria and other systemic features will be helping in diagnosis.

Eclampsia

It is characterized by generalized tonic-clonic convulsions in patients with pre-eclampsia.

MEASUREMENT OF BLOOD PRESSURE

- It is measured with arm at heart level with woman seated at 45°.
- It is better to avoid supine position.
- First Korotkoff sound (K1) is systolic and disappearance of sound (K5) is diastolic reading.[10,11]
- The correct method as well as correct cuff size of apparatus minimizes over-diagnosis.[12]

Measurement Devices

- Mercury manometers are the gold standards.
- Newly designed automated devices may give similar mean blood pressure.
- Calibration of devices must be done regularly.

There is a wide intraindividual error and their accuracy may be further compromised in women with pre-eclampsia.

Twenty-four Hours Ambulatory Blood Pressure Monitoring

- Normal blood pressure values by ambulatory blood pressure monitoring (ABPM) are established for pregnancy.
- It is useful in evaluation of early (< 20 weeks gestation) hypertension.
- It is less useful in such a screening in the second half of pregnancy.[13]
- It has also been helpful in prediction of hypertension in high-risk women, but its sensitivity and specificity is low.[9]

Investigation of New-onset Hypertension in Pregnancy

Any pregnant woman with hypertension should be thoroughly investigated for assessment of type of HDP, etiology, severity and fetal well-being. Investigations may be carried out on outpatient basis but if there are premonitory symptoms such as vomiting, headache, epigastric pain or established complications, admission becomes necessary.

The following investigations should be performed in all patients:
- Urine dipstick testing for proteinuria
- Complete blood count (CBC)
- Urea, creatinine, electrolytes
- Liver function tests (LFTs)
- Ultrasound assessment of fetal growth, amniotic fluid volume and umbilical artery flow.

Measurement of Proteinuria

All pregnant women should be assessed for proteinuria testing by dipstick method. It is done for screening.

Though, it is not an accurate method, approximate measurements are done as:

1+ corresponds to 0.3g/L
2+ corresponds to 1 g/L
3+ corresponds to 3 g/L

More definitive testing is advocated when pre-eclampsia is suspected. A protein creatinine ratio more than 30 mg/mmol corresponds with a 24 hours urine excretion of more than 300 mg. This is used to check for significant proteinuria.

- One Canadian study was done in which many parameters were studied including CBC, uric acid and creatinine levels along with coagulation profile, LFTs and urinary dipstick proteinuria, and 24 hours urinary protein.[14]

Higher levels of proteinuria were not always associated with increased maternal or perinatal morbidity/mortality[15,16] and have not predicted short term maternal renal failure **(Table 27.1)**.[16]

Complete Blood Count

It gives idea about anemia status, thrombocytopenia which is one of the worsening signs of pre-eclampsia. Total leukocyte count will identify current infections which may aggravate the condition.

Table 27.1: Normal values of blood investigations

Test	Normal values	Test	Normal values
Creatinine	0.4–1.2 mg/dL	SGOT	Up to 40 IU/L
Blood urea	20–40 mg/dL	SGPT	Up to 40 IU/L
Serum Na+	135–145 mmol/L	Albumin	3.8–5 g/dL
Serum K+	3.5–5.0 mmol/L	Globulin	2.3–3.5 g/dL
Uric acid	3–6.5 mg/dL	LDH	80–460 U/L

Liver Function Tests

Elevated liver enzymes—SGOT, SGPT and LDH are the markers for severity of underlying HDP. Approximately, 12% women with severe pre-eclampsia may develop HELLP syndrome consisting **H**emolysis, **E**levated **L**iver enzymes and **L**ow **P**latelets.

Renal Function Tests

Though acute renal failure is a rare complication in pre-eclampsia these tests not only indicate the severity but also help in diagnosis of causes of chronic hypertension during pregnancy. One must not forget the following causes of chronic hypertension—chronic kidney disease, e.g. glomerulonephritis, reflux nephropathy, and adult polycystic kidney disease. Serum electrolytes help in fluid management.

Frequency of any investigations is individualized as per need in that case.

There are no strict guidelines for the same.

Special Investigations

- Patients with severe early onset pre-eclampsia warrant investigation for associated conditions, e.g. systemic lupus erythematosus, underlying renal disease, antiphospholipid syndrome or thrombophilias.
- Undiagnosed pheochromocytoma, though rare, in pregnancy is potentially fatal and may present as pre-eclampsia.[17]
- 24-hour urinary catecholamines should be undertaken in the presence of very labile or severe hypertension.
- If there is thrombocytopenia or a falling hemoglobin investigations for disseminated intravascular coagulation (coagulation studies, peripheral blood smear, LDH, fibrinogen, D-Dimer) are to be done.

Monitoring

- Monitoring is individualized depending upon case situation.
- Blood pressure is to be measured every 15 minutes initially and then half hourly.
- Foley's catheter should be inserted.
- Detailed input and output records are kept.
- Oxygen saturation, respiratory rate and temperature should be measured.
- Neurological assessment should be performed hourly.
- Fetal well-being should be assessed carefully.

A Need of the Hour

Uterine artery Doppler study is a poor predictor of pre-eclampsia as it has limited test accuracy. But, the trials should be compare a policy of revealed with unrevealed uterine artery Doppler. The studied outcomes should be consequences of pre-eclampsia including need for high dependency units, perinatal mortality and morbidity.

Fetal Surveillance

Perinatal outcome is compromised in many cases of hypertensive disease in pregnancy as compared to normotensive women.

Fetal surveillance is commonly recommended and performed in women with hypertensive disease in pregnancy.[8] There are no definitive guidelines on how it should be performed.[18]

Frequency, intensity, and modality of evaluation will differ in each case.

RECOMMENDATIONS FOR MEASUREMENT OF BP

- BP should be measured with the woman in the sitting position with the arm at the level of the heart (II–2A).
- An appropriately sized cuff (i.e., length of 1.5 times the circumference of the arm) should be used (II–2A).
- Korotkoff phase V should be used to designate diastolic BP (I–A).
- If BP is consistently higher in one arm, the arm with the higher values should be used for all BP measurements (III–B).
- BP can be measured using a mercury sphygmomanometer, calibrated aneroid device, or an automated BP device that has been validated for use in pre-eclampsia (II–2A).
- Automated BP machines may underestimate BP in women with pre-eclampsia, and comparison of readings using mercury sphygmomanometer or an aneroid device is recommended (II–2A).
- Ambulatory BP monitoring (by 24-hour or home measurement) may be useful to detect isolated office (white coat) hypertension (II–2B).
- Patients should be instructed in proper BP measurement technique, if they are to perform home BP monitoring (III–B).

RECOMMENDATIONS FOR DIAGNOSIS OF HYPERTENSION

- The diagnosis of hypertension should be based on office or in-hospital BP measurements (II–2B).
- Hypertension in pregnancy should be defined as a diastolic BP of > 90 mm Hg, based on the average of at least two measurements, taken using the same arm (II–2B).
- Women with a systolic BP of >140 mm Hg should be followed closely for development of diastolic hypertension (II–2B).

- Severe hypertension should be defined as a systolic BP of >160 mm Hg or a diastolic BP of 110 mm Hg (II–2B).
- For non-severe hypertension, serial BP measurements should be recorded before a diagnosis of hypertension is made (II–2B).
- For severe hypertension, a repeat measurement should be taken for confirmation in 15 minutes (III–B).
- Isolated office (white coat) hypertension should be defined as office diastolic BP of >90 mm Hg, but home BP of < 135/85 mm Hg (III–B).

RECOMMENDATIONS FOR MEASUREMENT OF PROTEINURIA

- All pregnant women should be assessed for proteinuria (II–2B).
- Urinary dipstick testing may be used for screening for proteinuria when the suspicion of preeclampsia is low (II–2B).
- More definitive testing for proteinuria (by urinary protein: creatinine ratio or 24-hours urine collection) is encouraged when there is a suspicion of pre-eclampsia, including in hypertensive pregnant women with rising BP or in normotensive pregnant women with symptoms or signs suggestive of pre-eclampsia (II–2A).

RECOMMENDATIONS FOR DIAGNOSIS OF CLINICALLY SIGNIFICANT PROTEINURIA

- Proteinuria should be strongly suspected when urinary dipstick proteinuria is > 2+ (II–2A).
- Proteinuria should be defined as > 0.3g/d in a 24 hours urine collection or > 30 mg/mmol urinary creatinine in a spot (random) urine sample (II–2B).
- There is insufficient information to make a recommendation about the accuracy of the urinary albumin: creatinine ratio (II–2 I).

RECOMMENDATIONS FOR CLASSIFICATION OF HDP

- Hypertensive disorders of pregnancy should be classified as pre-existing or gestational hypertension on the basis of different diagnostic and therapeutic factors (II–2B).
- The presence or absence of pre-eclampsia must be ascertained, given its clear association with more adverse maternal and perinatal outcomes (II–2B).
- In women with pre-existing hypertension, pre-eclampsia should be defined as resistant hypertension, new or worsening proteinuria, or one or more of the other adverse conditions (II–2B).
- In women with gestational hypertension, pre-eclampsia should be defined as new-onset proteinuria or one or more of the other adverse conditions (II–2B).
- Severe preeclampsia should be defined as preeclampsia with onset before 34 weeks' gestation, with heavy proteinuria or with one or more adverse conditions (II–2B).
- The term PIH (pregnancy-induced hypertension) should be abandoned, as its meaning in clinical practice is unclear (III–D).

RECOMMENDATIONS FOR INVESTIGATIONS TO CLASSIFY HDP

- For women with pre-existing hypertension, serum creatinine, serum potassium, and urinalysis should be performed in early pregnancy if not previously documented (II–2B).
- Among women with pre-existing hypertension, additional baseline laboratory testing may be based on other considerations deemed important by health care providers (III–C).
- Women with suspected pre-eclampsia should undergo the maternal laboratory (II–2B) and fetal (II–1B) testing described in respected table.
- If initial testing is reassuring, maternal and fetal testing should be repeated, if there is ongoing concern about pre-eclampsia (e.g. change in maternal and/or fetal condition) (III–C).
- Uterine artery Doppler velocimetry may be useful among hypertensive pregnant women to support a placental origin for hypertension, proteinuria, and/or adverse conditions (II–2B).
- Umbilical artery Doppler velocimetry may be useful to support a placental origin for intrauterine fetal growth restriction (II–2B).

RECOMMENDATIONS FOR PROGNOSIS (MATERNAL AND FETAL) IN PRE-ECLAMPSIA

- Serial surveillance of maternal well-being is recommended, both antenatally and postpartum (II–3B).
- The frequency of maternal surveillance should be at least once per week antenatally, and at least once in the first three days post partum. (III–C)
- Serial surveillance of fetal well-being is recommended. (II–2B)
- Antenatal fetal surveillance should include umbilical artery Doppler velocimetry. (I–A)
- Women who develop gestational hypertension with neither proteinuria nor adverse conditions before 34 weeks should be followed closely for maternal and perinatal complications (II–2B). [All recommendations are by National Institute for Health and Clinical Excellence (NICE) Clinical Guideline 107. Hypertension in pregnancy: The management of hypertensive disorders during pregnancy (August 2010)]

REFERENCES

1. Society of Obstetricians and Gynaecologists of Canada (SOGC) Clinical Practice Guideline No. 206: Diagnosis, Evaluation, and Management of the Hypertensive Disorders of Pregnancy.
2. Hypertensive disorders in pregnancy; South Australian Perinatal Practice Guidelines, 28 June 2004, Last reviewed: 16 August 2010.
3. Seligman S. Which blood pressure? Br J Obstet Gynaecol. 1987;94(6):497-8.
4. MacGillivray I. Pre-eclampsia: The hypertensive diseases of pregnancy. London: WB Saunders; 1983.pp.174-90.
5. Stone P, Cook D, Hutton J, Purdie G, Murray H, Harcourt L. Measurements of blood pressure, edema and proteinuria in a pregnant population of New Zealand. Australian and New Zealand Journal of Obstetrics & Gynaecology. 1995;35(1):32-7.
6. North RA, Taylor RS, Schellenberg JC. Evaluation of a definition of pre-eclampsia. Br J Obstet Gynaecol. 1999;106:767-73.
7. Levine RJ. Should the definition of preeclampsia include a rise in diastolic blood pressure =15 mm Hg? (abstract) Am J Obstet Gynecol. 2000;182:225.
8. Report of the National High Blood Pressure Education Program Working Group on High Blood Pressure in Pregnancy. Am J Obstet Gynecol. 2000;183:1-22.
9. Brown MA, Lindheimer MD, de Swiet M, Van Assche A, Moutquin JM. The classification and diagnosis of the hypertensive disorders of pregnancy: statement from the International Society for the Study of Hypertension in Pregnancy (ISSHP). (Review). Hypertens pregnancy. 2001;20(1):9-14.
10. Brown MA, Mangos G, Davis G, Homer C. The natural history of white coat hypertension during pregnancy. BJOG. 2005;112(5):601-6.
11. Shennan A, Gupta M, Halligan A, Taylor DS, de Swiet M. Lack of reproducibility in pregnancy of Korotkoff phase IV as measured by mercury sphygmomanometry. Lancet. 1996;347:139-42.
12. Brown MA, Reiter L, Smith B, Buddle ML, Morris R, Whitworth JA. Measuring blood pressure in pregnant women: a comparison of direct and indirect methods. Am J Obstet Gynecol. 1994;171:661-7.
13. Brown MA, Davis GK, McHugh L. The prevalence and clinical significance of nocturnal hypertension in pregnancy. [Journal Article. Research Support, Non- U.S. Gov't] Journal of Hypertension. 2001;19(8):1437-44.
14. Caetano M, Ornstein MP, von Dadelszen P, Hannah ME, Logan AG, Gruslin A, et al. A survey of Canadian practitioners regarding diagnosis and evaluation of the hypertensive disorders of pregnancy. 2004;23:197-209.
15. Newman MG, Robichaux AG, Stedman CM, Jaekle RK, Fontenot MT, Dotson T, et al. Perinatal outcomes in pre-eclampsia that is complicated by massive proteinuria. Am J Obstet Gynecol. 2003;188:264-8
16. Hall DR, Odendaal HJ, Steyn DW, Grove D. Urinary protein excretion and expectant management of early onset, severe pre-eclampsia. Int J Gynaecol Obstet. 2002;77:1-6.
17. Hudsmith JG, Thomas CE, Browne DA. Undiagnosed phaeochromocytoma mimicking severe preeclampsia in a pregnant woman at term. International Journal of Obstetric Anesthesia. 2006;15(3):240-5.
18. Sibai BM. Diagnosis and management of gestational hypertension and preeclampsia. Obstetrics and Gynecology. 2003;102(1):181-92.

Chapter 28

Eclampsia and HELLP Syndrome

Gorakh G Mandrupkar

INTRODUCTION

- Eclampsia is occurrence of convulsions in association with pre-eclampsia.
- Pre-eclampsia is a multisystem disorder that is associated with raised blood pressure (>140/90) taken 4-6 hours apart and with proteinuria beyond 20 weeks of pregnancy.
- It ranks second to hemorrhage as a specific, direct cause of maternal death.
- The risk that a woman in a developing country will die of pre-eclampsia or eclampsia is about 300 times that for a woman in a developed country.
  It may be due to:
  - Delay in making a decision to seek treatment.
  - Delay in getting the woman to the healthcare center.
  - Delay in receiving quality treatment.
  - Delay in identifying a complication.

INCIDENCE

- The incidence in our country varies from 1 to 5%.
- More than 50% cases are antepartum and almost 20% are postpartum.
- Maternal mortality is 4-6%.
- Perinatal loss is 45%.
- Possibly the incidence is lower in booked cases verses unbooked cases.[1]

PATHOPHYSIOLOGY

- It is defective trophoblastic invasion of endothelium which triggers these events.
- Cerebral vasospasm, high middle cerebral artery (MCA) perfusion pressure, endothelial damage, ischemic damage, barotraumas, hypertensive encephalopathy along with loss of auto-regulation of cerebral blood flow and cerebral edema are the pathophysiological events in etiology of eclampsia.

EVENTS

Usually, these are the generalized tonic clonic convulsions. Duration of coma varies after convulsions. There can be temporary blindness due to varying degrees of retinal detachments and occipital lobe ischemia or edema. Respiratory rate is increased. Pulmonary edema may occur due to aspiration pneumonitis or volume overload.[2]

MANAGEMENT

Unless proved otherwise the first diagnosis of convulsions in pregnancy beyond 20 weeks of gestation should be eclampsia.

Principles of Management

- Call for help must be given as multiple responsibilities are to be shared.
- Team leader for management should be decided immediately to avoid confusions.
- *Minimizing aspiration*: By giving lateral decubitus position and doing suction.
- *Avoidance of injury*: By the use padded bed rails, restraints.
- *Maintenance of oxygenation:* By nasal O_2 and monitoring by pulse oximetry.
- Initiation of *magnesium sulfate* to control and prevent convulsions
- Control of blood pressure with suitable antihypertensives.
- Corticosteroids, if <34 weeks and stable condition.
- Once stabilized, proceed to delivery (LSCS for obstetric indications only).

INVESTIGATIONS AND TREATMENT

- 16/18 no. IV cannulas—preferably at two places
- Through it only lab should be collected…
  - Complete blood count (CBC)
  - Liver function test (LFT) along with LDH

- Renal function tests (RFT)
- Coagulation profile (Prothrombin time and D-dimer, if available)
- Urine for albumin (Dipstick) taken while doing Foley's catheterization.
- Depending on condition of patient other tests can be added.
- Blood and blood components must be kept cross-matched, if readily available.
- Without waiting for any results magnesium sulfate regimen must be started.

MAGNESIUM SULPHATE

- It is the safe and recommended drug over phenytoin and diazepam.[3]
- Pritchard regimen is preferred regimen worldwide.
- Zuspan regimen is more popular in developed countries.

Mechanism of Action

- It is not clear but proposed action is to cause vasodilatation by relaxation of smooth muscle with subsequent reduction of cerebral ischemia (Belfort 1992).[4]
- It blocks some of the neuronal damage associated with ischemia.
- Also it blocks N-Methyl-D-Aspartate (NMDA) receptors in the brain which are activated in response to asphyxia, leading to calcium influx into neurons, which causes cell injury.

Side Effects

- The most common side effect is flushing.[5]
- Nausea, vomiting, muscle weakness, thirst, headache, drowsiness and confusion.
- With unmonitored doses, it can lead to respiratory depression and arrest (rare).

PRITCHARD REGIMEN[6]

Loading dose: (14 g = 4 g slow IV + 5 g IM in each buttock)

Intravenous: 4 g (as 20 mL 20% solution) slow IV at 4 mL/5 min, i.e. 1 g/min rate
Use 20 mL syringe.
(4 ampules of 50% w/v $MgSO_4$ + 12 mL normal saline or sterile water)
or
(8 ampules of 25% w/v $MgSO_4$ + 04 mL normal saline or sterile water)

Intramuscular: 5 g (as 10 mL 50% solution) deep intramuscular in each buttock.
Use 10 mL syringe
[5 ampules of 50% w/v $MgSO_4$ + 1 mL 2% Lignocaine* (To avoid pain at Injection site)] (*Government of India recommendation)
25% w/v ampules cannot be used for intramuscular injections as it will increase the volume.

Maintenance dose: 5 g deep IM in alternate buttock 4 hourly

Intramuscular: 5 g (as 10 mL 50% solution) deep intramuscular in each buttock.
Use 10 mL syringe
{5 ampules of 50% w/v $MgSO_4$ + 1 mL 2% Lignocaine* (To avoid pain at Injection site)} (*Government of India recommendation)
25% w/v ampules cannot be used for intramuscular injections as it will increase the volume.

Maintenance dose will be given *only if* following parameters are present:
- Respiratory rate > 16/min
- Patellar reflexes present
- Urine output > 100 mL in last 4 hours.
(Serum magnesium monitoring is not superior to clinical one; so it is not recommended)

Maintenance dose is to be delayed until above parameters are returned as specified.

Maintenance dose is given till 24 hours past delivery or 24 hours beyond the last convulsion, whichever is late.

Dose for Recurrence of Convulsion

After loading dose, if convulsions do not stop or/recur repeat 2 g $MgSO_4$ slow IV or alternatively IV diazepam or IV thiopentone sodium are given.

One has to administer the full magnesium sulfate loading dose before transferring patient to higher level when required.

ZUSPAN IV REGIMEN

Loading Dose

4 g (4 ampules of 50% w/v $MgSO_4$ +12 mL normal saline or sterile water) slow IV using 20 mL syringe is given at a rate not to exceed 1 g/min.

Maintenance Dose

It is given as an infusion of 1 g per hour till 24 hours past delivery or last convulsion whichever is late.

OTHER REGIMENS

- Lazard (1925)
- Eastman (1945)
- Sibai (1990)
- Dhaka Regimen
- Dr Sardesai, Solapur—This is low dose regimen.

Loading dose of magnesium sulphate 4 g IM or IV in 20 cc 25% dextrose is given. Following this 2 g IM/IV given 3 hourly. More sustained levels of Mg^{2+} are achieved, with better control and low dose. This regime is well followed in rural and interior southern Maharashtra with good outcome.

WHICH REGIMEN TO USE?

Regimens suggested by Pritchard and Zuspan are the two that have been evaluated in randomized trials of anticonvulsants for women with eclampsia and pre-eclampsia so are recommended and followed worldwide.[7]

ANTIHYPERTENSIVE MEDICINES

Either IV labetalol or oral nifedipine can be used to treat severe hypertension. Alpha dopa has still role in cases of pre-eclampsia with moderate hypertension.

- Since nifedipine is associated with tachycardia, it is recommended that it should not be used in patients with tachycardia (heart rate >100). In these patients, Labetalol is the appropriate drug to use.
- On the other hand, Labetalol should be avoided in patients with bradycardia (heart rate <60), in those with asthma, and in those with congestive heart failure. In these patients, nifedipine is the appropriate drug to use.
- Nifedipine and magnesium sulfate can be used together.
- Alpha-dopa is not given in postpartum period as is associated with increased incidence of postpartum depression.

Drug	Dose and route	Concerns
Labetolol	10–20 mg IV, then 20–80 mg every 20–30 min, max dose 300 mg for infusion: 1–2 mg/min	Less incidence of hypotension CCF, asthma, DM, bradycardia Use if pulse >100/min
Nifedipine	Tabs only: 10–30 mg PO, repeat in 45 m, if needed	Long acting preparations safe Use if pulse <100/min

Delivery Decision

It is the most definite management.

Once patient is settled, we must move towards delivery of patient.

Induction of labor: Dinoprostone can be used based on Bishops score.
Even Misoprostol may be used, if patient is remote from term.
Mechanical dilatation may be done by Foley's catheter or hygroscopic cervical dilators
Aggressive induction for delivery with 24 hours should be aim.

Augmentation of labor: Only oxytocin is to be used for and no PGs.

Vaginal delivery: It is not a contraindication for eclampsia.

Cesarean section: It is done for obstetric indications only.

$MgSO_4$ *is to be continued 24 hours postdelivery or last convulsion whichever is late.*

IV FLUIDS

- In pre-eclampsia and eclampsia, IV fluid management is like double-edged sword.
- More fluids will cause pulmonary edema[8] and less fluid may lead to dehydration.
- Fluid restriction is advisable to reduce the risk of fluid overload.
- No use of plasma expanders or diuretics is recommended.
- Total fluid restriction to 80 mL/hr or 1 mL/kg/hr is beneficial.
- Oliguria is quite common and does not need aggressive treatment but attention.

Conclusion

- Early quality treatment will save every mother of eclampsia.
- No one should hesitate to use magnesium sulphate.
- Timely transfer of woman to higher center to be done after first loading dose of $MgSO_4$ where otherwise facilities are not available to handle the case.
- Early identification of a complication can save the life.

HELLP SYNDROME

Introduction

The HELLP syndrome is one of the serious complications in pregnancy characterized by **H**emolysis, **E**levated **L**iver enzymes and **L**ow **P**latelets occurring in 0.5–0.9% of all pregnancies and in 10–20% of cases with severe pre-eclampsia.[9]

In 1982, Weinstein described this entity as separate from severe pre-eclampsia and named the condition as HELLP.[10]

Sibai has great amount of work in this field and he noted that hypertension may be mild in 30% cases and severe in almost 50% women diagnosed with HELLP syndrome while 20% cases were normotensive indicating even normotensive patients with signs and symptoms of pre-eclampsia without hypertension may be in HELLP.

Criteria for HELLP

Hemolysis: Abnormal peripheral smear
Total bilirubin >/=1.2 mg/dL
Reduced serum haptoglobin
Elevated liver enzymes: AST >70 U/L
LDH: 2 × upper limit of normal
Low platelets: <100,000/mm^3

There are two types of classification systems till date for HELLP.

Classification

HELLP class	Tennessee classification	Mississippi classification
1	Platelets </= 100000/mm^3 AST >/= 70 U/L LDH >/= 600 U/L	Platelets < 50000/mm^3 AST or ALT >/= 70 U/L LDH >/= 600 U/L
2		Platelets 50000-1 lakh/mm^3 AST or ALT >/= 70 U/L LDH>/= 600 U/L
3		Platelets 1 lakh -1.5 lakh/mm^3 AST or ALT >/= 40 U/L LDH >/= 600 U/L

Etiology

It is thought to arise as a consequence of endothelial and microvascular injury, increased vascular tone and platelet aggregation.

Approximately 70% of cases develop prior to delivery with a peak frequency between gestational weeks 27 and 38.10% developing before 27 weeks and remaining cases occurring postpartum, usually within 48 hours of delivery.[11]

Spectrum of Disease

Severity ranges from a mild and self-limited course to a fulminant process leading to multiple organ failure. In rare cases, occurs in normotensive pregnancy, only with epigastric pain and tenderness in right hypochondriac region as initial symptoms.[12] In most cases, resolves spontaneously within 48 hours of delivery. About 30% cases occur postpartum with majority within 48 hours. Risk of renal failure and pulmonary edema is significantly increased as compared to antenatal onset HELLP.

Differential Diagnosis

Due to many common features and laboratory parameters, following differential diagnoses has to be kept in mind.

Related to Thrombocytopenia

Immunologic thrombocytopenia (ITP).

Related to Pregnancy

- Acute fatty liver of pregnancy (AFLP)
- Gestational thrombocytopenia.

Diseases Mimicking HELLP

- Thrombotic thrombocytopenic purpura (TTP)
- Hemolytic uremic syndrome.

Other Diseases

Viral hepatitis	Appendicitis with perforation	Glomerulonephritis
Acute pancreatitis	Severe gastroenteritis	Gallbladder disease
SLE	Hyperemesis	Pyelonephritis

Maternal Mortality

The maternal mortality is reported from 1%[13,14] up to as high as 25%[15] of cases.

Cerebral hemorrhage or stroke is reported to be the primary cause of death in 26% as well as the contributing factor in another 45% of the deaths.[16] Mortality in hepatic rupture ranges from 18 to 86%.[17]

Perinatal Mortality

The perinatal mortality rate related to the HELLP syndrome is between 7.4% and 34%.[18] Prematurity, placental insufficiency, with or without intrauterine growth restriction (IUGR) and *abruptio placentae*, are the leading causes of neonatal death.[18]

Management

The initial evaluation and stabilization of patient is same as that of severe pre-eclampsia. Ideally, patient should be managed in higher center where all facilities from neonatology, anesthesia and high-risk obstetric care, intensive care, blood and blood components are easily available.

Principles of Management

- *Maintenance of oxygenation*: By nasal O_2 and monitoring by pulse oximetry.
- Initiation of magnesium sulfate regimen to control and prevent convulsions in cases of severe pre-eclampsia.
- Control of blood pressure with suitable antihypertensive.
- Corticosteroids, if <34 weeks and stable condition.
- Once stabilized, proceed to delivery (LSCS for obstetric indications only).

Investigations

- RFT (Renal function tests)
- Coagulation profile
- Urine for albumin (Dipstick)
- Depending on condition of patient other tests can be added for differential diagnosis.

Blood and blood components must be kept cross-matched, if readily available.

DELIVERY DECISION AND CONDUCT

- It is the most definite management.
- Once patient is settled one must move towards delivery of patient in women with gestational age more than 34 weeks.
- In women with gestational age less than 34 weeks, 48 hours expectant management till corticosteroids act for fetal lung maturity is recommended.
- Beyond that it is not warranted as there are profound maternal risks of abruption, pulmonary edema, ARDS, DIC, intracerebral bleeding.
- Aggressive induction for delivery with 24 hours should be aim.
- *Cesarean section*: Though the operative delivery in such situations is harmful, it may be considered in unfavorable cervices with platelet count more than $50000/mm^3$, keeping platelet infusion ready.
- Platelet consumption rate is very high in these women and minimum of 6–8 units must be kept ready initially.
- The role of steroids for improvement of platelet count is controversial and recent evidence is not favorable in antenatal as well as postnatal period.
- Sibai has mentioned some of the precautions while operating such patients.
- Drain placement (subfascial, subcutaneous or both).
- Minimal tissue trauma.
- Continuous hemodynamic monitoring.
- Serial lab evaluation for checking reversal of lab parameters which is a good sign.

REFERENCES

1. Australian and New Zealand Journal of Obstetrics and Gynaecology, 13 Feb 2008, ref to 1996 data Determinants of Maternal Mortality in Eclampsia in India. Arora R, Ganguli RP, Swain S, Oumachigui A, Rajaram P. Department of Obs & Gyn, Jawaharlal Institute of Postgraduate Medical Education and Research, Puducherry, India.
2. F Gary Cunningham, et al. William's Obstetrics, 21st edn.
3. Cochrane Database Syst Rev. 2003;(2):CD000025.
4. Belfort MA, Saade GR, Moise KJ Jr. The effect of Magnesium Sulfate on maternal retinal blood flow in preeclampsia: A randomize placebo-controlled study. Am J Obstet Gyne-col. 1992;167:1548.
5. Magpie Trial Follow-up Study Collaborative Group. The Magpie Trial: A randomized trial Comparing magnesium sulphate with placebo for pre-eclampsia. Outcome for Woman at 2 Years. BJOG. 2007;114:300-9.
6. Pritchard JA, Cunningham FG, Pritchard SA. The Parkland Memorial Hospital Protocol for treatment of eclampsia: Evaluation of 245 cases. Am J Obstet Gynecol. 1984;148:951.
7. Sibai BM, Graham JM, McCubbin JH. A Comparison of Intra-venous and intramuscular magnesium sulfate regimens in preeclampsia. Am J Obstet Gynecol. 1984;150:728.
8. Sibai BM, Mabin BC, Harvey CJ, Gonzalez AR. Pulmonary edema in severe preeclampsia–eclampsia: Analysis of thirty-seven consecutive cases. Am J Obstet Gynecol. 1987b;156:1174.
9. Haram K, Svendsen E, Abildgaard U. The HELLP syndrome: Clinical issues and management: A review, 2009, Licensee BioMed Central Ltd.
10. Weinstein L. Syndrome of hemolysis, elevated liver enzymes, and low platelet count: A severe consequence of hypertension in pregnancy. 1982. Am J Obstet Gynecol. 2005;193:859.
11. Thrombosis Research. 2010;126:e238–e240.
12. Esan K, Moneim T, Page IJ. Postpartum HELLP syndrome after a normotensive pregnancy. Br J Gen Pract. 1997;47:441-2.
13. Martin JN Jr, Thigpen BD, Rose CH, Cushman J, Moore A, May WL. Maternal benefit of high-dose intravenous corticosteroid therapy for HELLP syndrome. Am J Obstet Gynecol. 2003; 189:830-34.
14. Yücesoy, Ozkan S, Bodur H, Tan T, Caliskan E, Vural B, Corakci A. Maternal and perinatal outcome in pregnancies complicated with hypertensive disorder of pregnancy: a seven year experience of a tertiary care center. Arch Gynecol Obstet. 2005;273:43-9.
15. Matsuda M, Mitsuhashi S, Watarai M, Yamamoto K, Hashimoto T, Ikeda S. Hemolysis, elevated liver enzymes and low platelet (HELLP) syndrome associated with systemic lupus erythematosus. Intern Med. 2003;42:1052-3.
16. Isler CM, Rinehart BK, Terrone DA, Martin RW, Magann EF, Martin JN Jr. Maternal mortality associated with HELLP (hemolysis, elevated liver enzymes, and low platelets) syndrome. Am J Obstet Gynecol. 1999;181:924-8.
17. Mihu D, Costin N, Mihu CM, Seicean A, Ciortea R. HELLP syndrome: a multisystemic disorder. J Gastrointestin Liver Dis. 2007;16:419-24.
18. Gul A, Cebeci A, Aslan H, Polat I, Ozdemir A, Ceylan Y. Perinatal outcomes in severe preeclampsia-eclampsia with and without HELLP syndrome. Gynecol Obstet Invest. 2005;59:113-8.

Chapter 29

Eye in Pregnancy

Anamika Dwivedi, Richa Baharani

INTRODUCTION

Pregnancy has an important effect on eyes as on the all other systems of the body. Ocular changes appearing during pregnancy can be physiological or pathological. Overall ocular manifestations during pregnancy can be categorized as:
- Physiologic changes
- Pregnancy-specific eye disease, and
- Modifications of pre-existing eye disease.

Although mostly mild, some of the pregnancy related ocular complication can be serious and require a prompt referral to ophthalmologist.

OCULAR ADNEXAL CHANGES

Hormonally mediated increased pigmentation around the eyes known as *chloasma* is common during pregnancy. *Spider angioma* is often seen in eyelids during pregnancy perhaps related to raised estrogen level. Both of these adnexal changes often fades away postpartum. Unilateral ptosis is reported during and after pregnancy. *Ptosis* is most likely caused by an aponeurosis defect, possibly related to increased fluid retention, hormonal effects, or the effects of labor and delivery.[1]

CORNEAL CHANGES

During later part of pregnancy, there is water retention in the cornea leading to decrease in corneal sensitivity, increased corneal curvature and thickness.[2,3] These changes in cornea can give rise to temporary alteration in refraction. There can be contact lens intolerance in few. It is advisable that pregnant women wait until at least several weeks postpartum before obtaining a new spectacle prescription or new contact lens fitting. Pregnancy-induced changes in cornea make pregnancy a contraindication for refractive eye surgeries such as LASIK.

Disruption of lacrimal acinar gland during pregnancy can lead to dry eye syndrome. Krukenberg spindles on the back of cornea is noted in few during early pregnancy. These are not associated with any other sign of pigment dispersion, and usually decrease and disappear in late pregnancy and postpartum.

INTRAOCULAR PRESSURE

Studies have shown a statistically significant decrease in intraocular pressure (IOP) in all trimester of pregnancy compared to nonpregnant females.[4] This reduction in IOP increases as pregnancy advances and more in multigravida than primigravida.[5]

PREGNANCY SPECIFIC EYE DISEASES

Pre-eclampsia and Eclampsia

Pre-eclampsia typically develops in the second half of pregnancy and is characterized by hypertension, edema, and proteinuria. Eclampsia is pre-eclampsia with convulsions and usually occurs late in pregnancy. Pre-eclampsia and eclampsia place the fetus at risk because of placental vascular insufficiency. In past, severe changes in retinal arteriolar caliber were believed to reflect placental vascular insufficiency and constitute an indication for pregnancy termination. With improved medical and obstetric management of hypertension and other aspects of pre-eclampsia, retinal findings are now less frequent and less important.

Pre-eclampsia and eclampsia have been associated with a retinopathy similar to hypertensive retinopathy; serous retinal detachments; yellow, opaque retinal pigment epithelium (RPE) lesions; and cortical blindness. Focal or generalized retinal arteriolar narrowing is the most common ocular change seen in pre-eclampsia. If the constriction is severe, changes associated with hypertensive retinopathy may occur, including diffuse retinal edema, hemorrhages, exudates, and cotton-wool spots.[6]

Choroidal dysfunction is a common ocular complication of pre-eclampsia and eclampsia that manifests clinically as serous retinal detachments or yellow RPE lesions. The serous retinal detachments usually are bilateral and bullous.[7] The choroidal dysfunction is thought to be secondary to choroidal ischemia from intense arteriolar vasospasm. Primary choriocapillaris ischemia leads to RPE ischemia manifest as fluid pump dysfunction allowing subretinal fluid accumulation. Women with HELLP syndrome (*hemolysis/elevated liver enzymes/low platelet* count) may be approximately seven times more likely to develop a retinal detachment than those who do not have the syndrome.[8] These changes can cause profound decrease in vision but are usually reversible postpartum. One study suggested that serous detachments are more specific to pre-eclampsia and eclampsia, whereas retinopathy is seen more often in pre-eclampsia superimposed on pre-existing hypertension.[9]

Central Serous Chorioretinopathy

Central serous chorioretinopathy (CSCR) results in an accumulation of subretinal fluid that leads to a circumscribed neurosensory retinal detachment in the macula at the level of the RPE. Although CSCR is 10 times more common in men, in women it has a strong association with pregnancy. Elevated levels of endogenous cortisol are thought to lead to increased permeability in the blood-retinal barrier, choriocapillaris, and RPE. White fibrous subretinal exudates are found in 90% of pregnancy-associated cases of CSCR, compared with 20% of general cases.[10]

Occlusive Vascular Disorder

An increase in the level of clotting factors and clotting activity occurs during pregnancy leading to increased risk of vaso-occlusive disease. This increased risk of vaso-occlusive disease may manifest as retinal or choroidal vascular occlusions. Purtscher-like retinopathy, most likely from arteriolar obstruction by complement-induced leukocyte aggregation, has been documented in the immediate postpartum period.[11] Branch and central retinal artery occlusions, as well as retinal vein occlusions (although these are less common), have been reported in pregnancy.

PRE-EXISTING EYE DISEASES

Diabetic Retinopathy

Gestational diabetes in the absence of pre-existing diabetes does not increase the risk for diabetic retinopathy (DR). For patients with pre-existing diabetes, pregnancy is associated with an increased risk of development and progression of DR.[12] Diabetic women who may become pregnant should establish excellent glucose control before conception, since major period of fetal organogenesis may take place before the mother even aware that she is pregnant. Diabetic retinopathy status should be evaluated and stabilized prior to conception.

Risk factors that may accelerate DR in pregnant women include coexisting hypertension or pre-eclampsia, greater severity diabetes prior to pregnancy, poor prepregnancy glycemic control, rapid normalization of blood glucose levels, etc. but the major determinants remains the duration of diabetes and the degree of retinopathy at the onset of pregnancy. Macular edema may worsen by coexisting hypertension, nephropathy, and proteinuria. Both diabetic retinopathy and diabetic macular edema may spontaneously regress postpartum. Exact pathogenesis of worsening of DR in pregnancy is controversial, it is probably due to increase in retinal blood flow in diabetic patients during pregnancy, this hyperperfusion causes an added stress to an already compromised retinal circulation leading to the progression of DR.[13]

Women with diabetes who plan to become pregnant should have a prepregnancy dilated fundus examination. During pregnancy, an examination should be performed in the first trimester. Those with no retinopathy to moderate non-proliferative DR should be re-examined every three to 12 months. Patients with findings of severe nonproliferative DR (NPDR) or worse should be re-examined every one to three months. Those diagnosed with gestational diabetes do not require retinopathy screening.[14] Treatment of complications of diabetic retinopathy such as diabetic macular edema and proliferative diabetic retinopathy is same as in non-pregnant patients, i.e. laser photocoagulation with a good metabolic control.

Uveitis

For chronic noninfectious uveitis, pregnancy seems to confer a beneficial effect, with a lower incidence of flare-ups. This is possibly due to hormonal and immunomodulatory effects.

In conclusion, visual disturbances are very common during pregnancy. Physicians should have a firm understanding of the various ocular conditions that might appear pregnancy or get modified by pregnancy.

REFERENCES

1. Sanke RF. Blepharoptosis as a complication of pregnancy. Ann Ophthalmol. 1984;16:720.
2. Weinreb RN, Lu A, Beeson C. Maternal corneal thickness during pregnancy. Am J Ophthalmol. 1988;105:258-60.
3. Park SB, Lindahl KJ, Temnycky GO, Aquavella JV. The effect of pregnancy on corneal curvature. CLAO J. 1992;18:256-9.
4. Akar Y, Yucel I, Akar ME, Zorlu G, Ari ES. Effect of pregnancy on intraobserver and intertechnique agreement in intraocular pressure measurements. Ophthalmologica. 2005;219:36-42.
5. Qureshi IA, Xi XR, Yaqob T. The ocular hypotensive effect of late pregnancy is higher in multigravidae than

in primigravidae. Graefes Arch Clin Exp Ophthalmol. 2000;238:64-7.
6. Jaffe G, Schatz H. Ocular manifestations of pre-eclampsia. Am J Ophthalmol. 1987;103:309.
7. Folk JC, Weingeist TA. Fundus changes in toxemia. Ophthalmology. 1981;88:1173.
8. Vigil-De Gracia P, Ortega-Paz L. Retinal detachment in association with pre-eclampsia, eclampsia, and HELLP syndrome. Int J Gyn Obstet. 2011;114(3):223-5.
9. Saito Y, Omoto T, Kidoguchi K, et al. The relationship between ophthalmoscopic changes and classification of toxemia in toxemia of pregnancy. Acta Soc Ophthalmol Jpn. 1990;94:870.
10. Sunness JS, Haller JA, Fine SL. Central serous chorioretinopathy and pregnancy. Arch Ophthalmol. 1993;111(3):360-4.
11. Ayaki M, Yokoyama N, Furtukawa Y. Postpartum central retinal artery occlusion simulating Purtscher's retinopathy. Ophthalmologica. 1995;209:37.
12. Sheth BP. Does pregnancy accelerate the rate of progression of diabetic retinopathy? An update. Curr Diab Rep. 2008;8:270-3.
13. The Diabetic Retinopathy Study Research Group. Four risk factors for severe visual loss in diabetic retinopathy. The third report from the Diabetic Retinopathy Study. Arch Ophthalmol. 1979;97:654-5 [PubMed: 426679].
14. Preferred Practice Pattern Guidelines: Diabetic Retinopathy. American Academy of Ophthalmology; 2008. Available at *www.aao.org/ppp*.

Chapter 30

Placenta Previa: An Obstetrical Resurgence

Shashi Khare, Anupama B Solanki

INTRODUCTION

Any bleeding from or into the genital tract after 28 weeks but before the birth of the baby is termed as antepartum hemorrhage. Antepartum hemorrhage complicates 2–5% of pregnancies, in which approximately one third are due to placenta previa. Placenta previa is a condition due to an abnormal implantation of the embryo wholly or partially in the lower uterine segment.[1] Placenta accreta is a rare but important complication of placenta previa.

EPIDEMIOLOGY

The global incidence of placenta previa ranges from 0.5 to 1% in hospital deliveries. The incidence of placenta previa is rising with the increasing cesarean section rate.[2] The highest prevalence is in Asian Women, in whom the overall prevalence is 12.2 per 1000 pregnancies.

ETIOPATHOGENESIS

For reasons yet unknown, the presence of scarring or endometrial disruption in the lower uterine segment predispose to placental implantation in that area. Fortunately as pregnancy advances, the placenta follow a process of growth called trophotropisis in which the trophoblastic cells seek area of high vascularity towards fundus. As a result, in 90% of cases placenta migrate to upper uterine segment. It is only a late-gestation ultrasound which can definitively establish persistence or resolution of placenta previa. Hence, it is advisable not to create panic situation for the patient when diagnosed early and patient is asymptomatic.

Risk Factors[3]

- Previous history of placenta previa
- *Previous cesarean section (CS):*
  - Risk ratio after one CS increased by 2.2%
  - Risk ratio after two CS increased by 9.1%
  - Risk ratio after three CS increased by 22.04%
- *Advancing maternal age:* 2–3 times higher in >35 years
- Increased parity
- Smoking
- Cocaine use during pregnancy
- Previous spontaneous or induced abortion
- Deficient endometrium due to past history of manual removal of placenta, curettage and endometritis
- Twin pregnancy
- *Placental pathology:* Succenturiate lobe, battledore placenta, velamentous insertion of the cord.

CLINICAL FEATURES

Symptoms

The only symptom of placenta previa is painless and causeless bleeding (not related to activity). The first bleeding is sentinel bleed, which is often minor. Usually it ceases, only to recur.[2]

Signs

Pallor, proportionate to visible blood loss. Tachycardia and hypotension depending upon amount of blood loss. In excessive blood loss, symptoms and sign of shock (faintness, tachycardia, hypotension, sweating, cold and clammy extremities, oliguria, syncope) may be noticed. Earlier in pregnancy, the first bleeding occurs, the worse is the outcome of pregnancy.

Abdominal Palpation

- Uterus relaxed and nontender
- *Abnormal lie and fetal presentation:* Women with placenta previa have a higher risk of fetal malpresentation such as breech or transverse lie than women with normal placental sites. Mechanism of malpresentation in placenta previa is assumed to be due to the bulk of the placenta in the lower segment preventing engagement of fetal head. It is likely that malpresentation indicates situations with a significant degree of placenta previa in whom safe vaginal delivery would be unlikely.[4,5]

- High presenting part (deeply engaged presenting part) usually rules out placenta previa.[6]
- Fetal heart sound usually well auscultated, unless there is major degree of placental separation (fetal bradycardia on pressing the head down into the pelvis and prompt recovery on release of pressure is suggestive of low lying placenta especially of posterior type—Stallworthy's sign).

CLASSIFICATION

- *According to FJ Brown:*
  - *I degree:* Type I— where placenta dips into lower uterine segment by its lower margin, the greater part of it being in the upper segment.
  - *II degree:* Type II—when edge of the placenta reaches the internal os
  - *III degree:* Type III—when placenta overlaps/covers the internal os when it is closed but does not cover it entirely when fully dilated.
  - *IV degree:* Type IV—placenta covers the whole internal os when it fully dilated (**Figs 30.1 and 30.2**).
- *Ultrasound (TVS):* Classification by Oppenheimer within 28 days of term:[7]
  - \>20 mm away from internal os—cesarean section not indicated
  - 11-20 mm from os—low risk of bleeding and cesarean delivery
  - 0-10 mm from os high risk of bleeding and cesarean section
  - Overlapping of internal os by any distance—cesarean section indicated
- *Workshop sponsored by National Institute of Health:* The following classification is recommended (Dashe 2013):[2]
  - *Placenta previa*—The internal os is covered partially or completely by placenta. (In the past, these were further classified as either total or partial previa).
  - *Low lying placenta*—Implantation in the lower uterine segment is such that the placental edge does not reach the internal os and remains outside a 2 cm perimeter around the os, previously it was termed as marginal.

Clinically, placenta previa is classified as:
- **Minor**: Encompassing type I and type II anterior
- **Major**: Encompassing type II posterior, type III and type IV

Type II posterior placenta previa is also known as dangerous placenta previa.

DIAGNOSIS

Clinical

Suspicion should be high in any women with vaginal bleeding after 20 weeks of gestation. A high presenting part, an abnormal lie, and painless and causeless bleeding are highly suggestive of low-lying placenta.

Ultrasound has become the standard means of diagnosing placenta previa. Due to placental trophotropism, the diagnosis is usually not made before 20 weeks. During anomaly scan, if placenta previa is suspected and patient is asymptomatic, again scan at 36 weeks. If major placenta previa is suspected ultrasound should be repeated at 32 weeks.

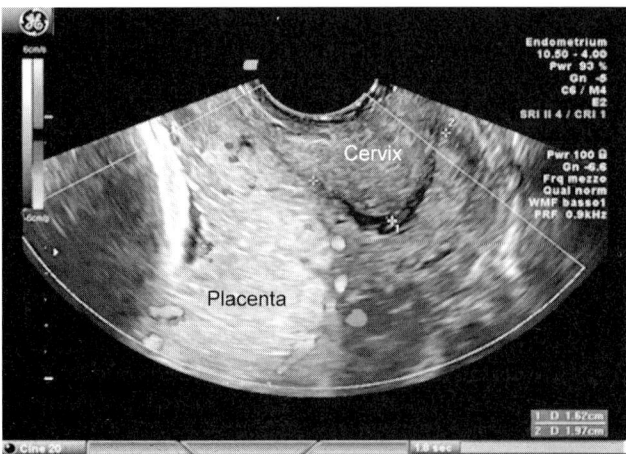

Fig. 30.1: Transvaginal sonography showing complete placenta previa *(For color version, see Plate 2)*

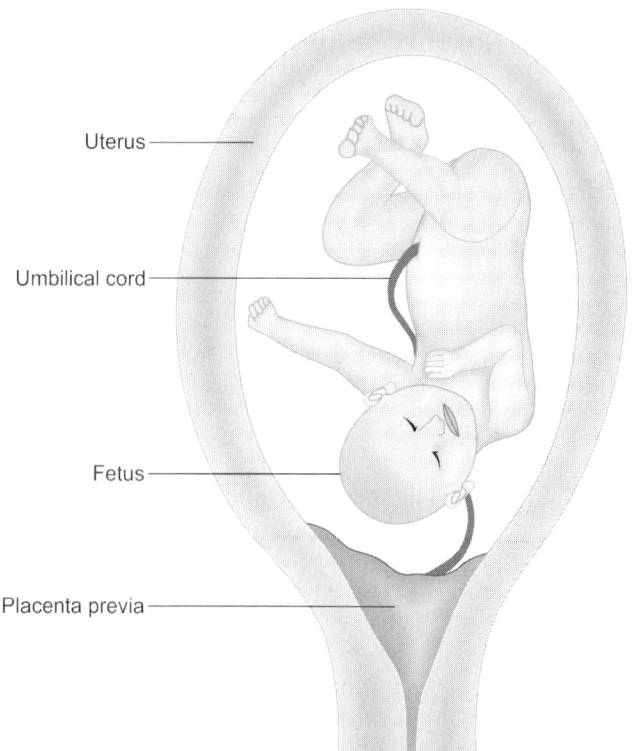

Fig. 30.2: Diagram showing complete placenta previa

Transabdominal ultrasound: It is the first test performed. An average accuracy of 96% has been reported.[2] False positive reports are due to:
- Overfilled bladder compressing lower uterine segment.
- Myometrial contraction simulating placental tissue in abnormally low position.

Transvaginal sonography: At any time in pregnancy is more accurate than transabdominal sonography because of following reason:
- Vaginal probes are closer to the region of interest and typically of high frequency, obtaining higher resolution images.
- The internal cervical os and the lower placental edge cannot be imaged adequately by the transabdominal approach as internal os is assumed rather than actually seen.
- The fetal head may obscure views of the lower placental edge when using transabdominal approach and a posterior placenta previa may not be adequately imaged.
- Safety of transvaginal ultrasound (TVS) is well established in recent studies, as the vaginal probe is under direct visualization, and hence direct contact with the cervix is avoided.
- Women who had history of placenta previa or underlying scar of previous cesarean color flow ultrasound should be performed as there is increased risk of placenta accreta.

Magnetic Resonance Imaging

Magnetic resonance imaging (MRI) is the gold standard to imaging placenta and its relationship to cervix. It may be superior to ultrasound in some setting, particularly when placenta accreta is suspected because of improved soft tissue contract and wide field of view. However, it is limited by cost, availability and concern about fetal effect.[8]

DIFFERENTIAL DIAGNOSIS

- Most common differential diagnosis is abruptio placenta
- Vasa previa
- Local cervical and vaginal lesions.

COMPLICATIONS OF PLACENTA PREVIA

Maternal

- *Antenatal period*: Antepartum hemorrhage, malpresentation, preterm labor spontaneous or induced, anemia, rhesus sensitization in Rh-negative women.
- *Intrapartum period*: Premature rupture of membranes, cord prolapse, intrapartum hemorrhage prolonged labor, increased operative interference, increased incidence of postpartum hemorrhage, retained placenta when morbidly adherent.
- *Puerperium*: Secondary postpartum hemorrhage, sepsis due to anemia, operative interference and placental site close to vagina, subinvolution, venous thromboembolism.

Fetal Complications

Intrauterine death, prematurity, asphyxia due to placental separation or cord compression, low birth weight, birth injuries, congenital malformations such as spina bifida are three times more common in placenta previa.

MANAGEMENT

Asymptomatic patients: Some women progress to the late third trimester without any bleeding and diagnosis is usually by ultrasound. These women should abstain from intercourse and avoid digital examination. There is no place for routine tocolysis to prevent bleeding. Due attention should be given to the maternal blood cell reserve. Iron and folic acid should be administered to prevent and treat anemia. The os–placental edge distance on TVS after 35 weeks' gestation is valuable in planning route of delivery. When the placental edge lies >20 mm away from the internal cervical os, women can be offered a trial of labor with a high expectation of success.

A distance of 11-20 mm away from the os is associated with a higher CS rate, although vaginal delivery is still possible depending on the clinical circumstances. In general, any degree of overlap (> 0 mm) after 35 weeks is an indication for cesarean section as the route of delivery.[6,9] Women with placenta previa and prior cesarean section are at high risk of placenta accreta. Delivery should be planned in a tertiary center with adequate resources.

McAfee and Johnson regimen may be appropriate for mild preterm bleeding with:[10]
- Good general condition of mother
- Gestational age less than 37 weeks
- Absence of active vaginal bleeding
- Patient not in labor
- Fetus in good condition.

CONDUCT OF EXPECTANT MANAGEMENT (McAfee AND JOHNSON REGIMEN)

- Bed rest
- Routine investigations and send blood for cross match
- Regular inspection of vaginal pads
- Iron, folate and calcium supplementation
- No role of tocolysis
- Inj anti-D is given to Rh-negative women
- Steroid therapy is indicated, if duration of pregnancy is less than 34 weeks.

Inpatient versus outpatient management: Patient may remain stable for 2-3 weeks requiring hospitalization between the initial warning hemorrhage & delivery of fetus. Outpatient management of placenta previa may be appropriate for stable women with home support, close proximity to a hospital and readily available transportation and telephonic communication.[2,11]

Indications for Active Management[12]

- Persistent hemorrhage
- If hemorrhage is massive and life threatening
- Gestational age more than 37 weeks
- Fetal distress in viable pregnancy
- Patient in labor
- Fetus is dead or major malformation present.

CESAREAN SECTION IN PLACENTA PREVIA

Cesarean section should be done by an experienced team of obstetrician, pediatrician and anesthesia department. Keeping adequate blood is life-saving, especially in cases of previous section and accreta.[12] This will reduce maternal and fetal morbidity and mortality. If patient is in shock and bleeding continues, cesarean section is to be performed in emergency along with resuscitation.

In major placenta previa, elective cesarean section should be performed under optimal circumstances in a tertiary center and ready availability of blood. The risk of complications for both mothers and children may be lower.[12]

Method of Anesthesia

The choice of anesthesia for cesarean section must be made by the anesthetist conducting the procedure. There is insufficient evidence to support one technique over the other.[7] Two retrospective studies conclude that regional anesthesia is safe and one small randomized trial concludes that epidural anesthesia is superior to general anesthesia with regard to maternal hemodynamic. When prolonged surgery is anticipated, general anesthesia may be preferred and regional anesthesia could be converted to general anesthesia, if undiagnosed accreta is encountered.

Skin incision: Cohen's transverse incision is preferred. Lower segment section is the choice in all varieties of placenta previa. When the placenta is anterior, large vessels are ligated and cut in between while giving the transverse incision. Avoid incision over the placenta (ward technique)—after the uterine incision, a cleavage plane is created digitally between the uterus and the placenta, until the membranes are reached and ruptured. Sometimes, incision is made through the placenta resulting in severe maternal and fetal hemorrhage. Cord should be clamped immediately to prevent fetal anemia. After the delivery of placenta, lower segment should be inspected for bleeding points which are stitched with 1.0 vicryl.[2,3] If hemostasis by sutures fails then balloon devices can be inflated to provide uterine compression and removed later through vagina.[2,3] B-Lynch and Cho's sutures can be placed over lower uterine segment,[3] bilateral uterine artery ligation (O'Leary stitch),[2,3] systemic devascularization and internal iliac artery ligation should be attempted next. Hysterectomy if all conservative measures fail.[2] Hysterectomy offer quick control of all uterine vasculature with rapid hemostasis. Decision should be taken timely before disseminated intravascular coagulation sets in.

Prognosis

Mother

Significant reduction in maternal mortality has been observed in recent years due to early diagnosis and prompt referral, availability of blood and blood products and liberal use of cesarean section. In developing countries, maternal mortality from placenta previa ranges from 1 to 5%. The causes of maternal morbidity and mortality are due to hemorrhage, shock, disseminated intravascular coagulation and operative delivery.

Fetus

Perinatal mortality is three times more than the general population in the range of 7–25%, leading cause of death being: (1) prematurity, (2) asphyxia due to placental separation, (3) cord accidents, and (4) congenital malformations. Recently, reduction in perinatal deaths has been observed due to judicious use of expectant management in preterm fetus and liberal use of cesarean section and improvement in the neonatal care unit.[6]

CONCLUSION

- Women at greatest risk of placenta previa are those who have myometrial damage caused by an earlier cesarean delivery or curettage.
- TVS is highly sensitive and specific for the diagnosis of placenta previa.
- To enhance patient safety, delivery or cesarean section (CS) be performed in tertiary care center by experienced Obstetric team. Other specialties such as urologist, general surgeon, pathologist, neonatologist and blood bank incharge should be involved. Improved maternal and neonatal outcomes have been demonstrated, when female with major degree placenta previa give birth in specialized tertiary center.
- Preoperative patient counseling should include discussion of the risk of profuse hemorrhage, blood requirement and potential need for hysterectomy.

- The timing of delivery should be individualized depending on patient circumstances. Combined maternal and neonatal outcome is optimized in stable patients with a planned delivery at 37 weeks.

REFERENCES

1. Arulkumaran, edited by Richard Warren, Sabaratnam. Best practice in labour and delivery. Cambridge: Cambridge University Press. 1st edn: 2009.pp.142-6.
2. Cunningham FG, Leveno KJ, Bloom SL, Hauth JC, Gilsstrap LC, Katharine D. Wenstrom. Obstetrical Hemorrhage. Williams Obstetrics. 24th edn. 2014.pp.799-804.
3. Ronan Bakker, Carl V Smith. Medscape. Updated; 2012.
4. Konje JC, Taylor DJ. Bleeding in late pregnancy. In: James DK, et al. High risk pregnancy management options, 3rd edn. Philadelphia: Elsevier; 2006.pp.1259-74.
5. Bhide A, Thilaganathan B. Recent advances in the management of placenta previa. Curr Opin Obstet Gynecol. 2004;16(6):447-51.
6. Brinsden, Judith Collier, Murray Longmore, Mark. Oxford Handbook of Clinical Specialties, 7th edn. Oxford: Oxford University Press. 2006.p.1970.
7. Oppenheimer LW, Farine D. A new classification of placenta previa: measuring progress in obstetrics. Am J Obstet Gynecol. 2009;201:227-9.
8. Allen BC, Leyendecker JR. Placental evaluation with magnetic resonance. Radiol Clin North Am. 2013;51(6):955-66. [Medline]
9. Vergani P, Ornaghi S, Pozzi I, Beretta P, et al. Placenta previa: distance to internal os and mode of delivery. Am J Obstet Gynecol. 2009;201(3):266.e1-5.
10. Neilson JP. Interventions for suspected placenta praevia. Cochrane Database of Systematic Reviews, 2003; Issue 2.
11. Kollmann M, Gaulhofer J, Lang U, et al. Placenta praevia: incidence, risk factors and outcome. J Matern Fetal Neonatal Med. 2015;4:1-4.
12. Placenta previa, placenta previa accreta and vasa previa: Diagnosis and management. RCOG Guidelines, Green-top 27. Retrieved 15 January 2013.

Chapter 31

Placenta Accreta

Rooplekha Chauhan

These abnormalities of placental insertion are serious as there occurs trophoblastic invasion into the myometrium to a variable extent. Bleeding from these sites can be dangerous. Placenta accreta is becoming more important to obstetricians as the number of cesarean sections is on rise.

DEVELOPMENT OF HUMAN PLACENTA

Human placenta is hemochorial, as the maternal blood directly bathes the syncytiotrophoblast.

By day 17, fetal blood vessels become functional and placental circulation is established. Villi have outer syncytium and inner Langhans cells or cytotrophoblast. Cytotrophoblast penetrates at villous tips which forms the anchoring villi which is attached to the deciduas at the basal plate.

In the early pregnancy, villi cover the entire periphery of the chorionic membrane, as the blastocyst invades the decidua, the villi facing the deciduas form chorion frondosum, which is the fetal component of placenta. The remaining villi degenerate to from chorion leave which is close contact with decidua capsularis and parietalis.

Trophoblastic Invasion

Decidual natural killer (NK) cells of deciduas in the first half of pregnancy are in direct contact with trophoblast. These cells are different from the circulating NK cells and those of endometrium before pregnancy.

Decidual NK express IL 8 and interferon-inducible protein 10 which helps trophoblastic invasion towards spiral arterioles. Decidual NK cells produce vascular endothelial growth factor (VEGF), and placental growth factor.

The extravillous trophoblast of first term of pregnancy are very invasive, they extend upto inner 1/3 of myometrium. The proteolytic enzyme secreted by trophoblast digest extracellular matrix. MMP-9 appears critical for trophoblastic invasion. Trophoblast secretes IGF which acts in autocrine manner, it promotes invasion. Decidua at the same time secretes IGF-binding protein-type 4 which blocks this autocrine loop. Thus the degree of trophoblastic invasion is controlled by regulation of matrix degradation and factors that cause trophoblastic migration. Fetal febronectin, a glycopeptide is also called trphoblast glue it promotes adhesion of trophoblast.

Invasion of Spiral Arteriole

The walls of the spiral arterioles are destroyed by cytotrophoblast which enters several centimeters along the vascular lumen. The intraluminal cytotrophoblast diminishes in number as the pregnancy advances. Cytotrophoblast does not invade decidual veins. During the process of invasion, spiral arterioles are tapped to form lacunae which are filled with maternal blood. The lacunae join to form labyrinth, which is partitioned by cytotrophoblast columns.

PLACENTA ACCRETA (FIG. 31.1)

At sites where decidua is not well formed, placental invasion may occur deeper to cause accreta, increta or percreta.

Placenta accreta is a condition in which all or part of the placenta is adherent to the uterine wall because of myometrial invasion by chorionic villi. It may occur when there is a

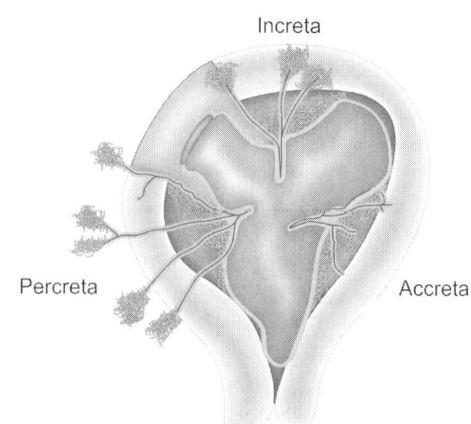

Fig. 31.1: Placenta accreta

primary deficiency or secondary damage to deciduas basalis and Nitabuch's layer. Abnormal trophoblastic invasion has been associated with upregulation of VEGF and down-regulation of VEGF receptor and Tie-2.

Three grades are described depending on the depth of invasion of myometrium **(Fig. 31.1)**.
1. *Accreta*: Chorionic villi are in contact with myometrium, rather than being contained within the decidua. This is seen in 80% cases of adherent placenta
2. *Increta*: There is the extensive villous invasion into the myometrium. Its incidence is 15%.
3. *Percreta*: Villous invasion extends up to or through serosal covering of the uterus, this form is seen in 5%.

High-risk Factors

- Multiparity
- Prior uterine surgery (myomectomy, D+C)
- Increasing maternal age
- Placenta previa
- Prior cesarean section
- Uterine irradiation
- Endometrial ablation.

Placenta accreta rarely complicates vaginal delivery, incidence being 1:22,000 in absence of placenta previa. Rare cases may have no risk factors. It is interesting to note that adhesion may be away from the site of the scar. It has also been reported in pregnancy with non-communicating rudimentary horn **(Fig. 31.2)**.

The incidence of placenta accreta has been rising from 1:2510 in 1980 to 1:533 in 2002 and 1:210 in 2006. It may be directly related to increase in number of cesarean section. Clark and coworkers showed an almost linear increase in the incidence of placenta previa with repeat cesarean sections with the rate of 10% in women with 4 prior sections. They also found high incidence of adherent placenta previa, there was a two-fold increase in adherent placenta with one section. The overall risk increases with rising number of cesarean sections, it is 3% with one section 11% with two sections 40% with three and 61% with 4 previous cesarean sections.

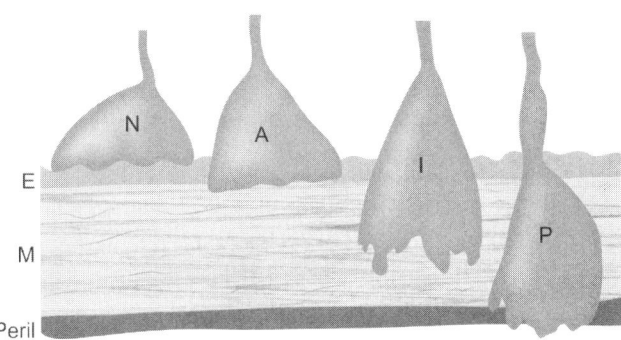

Fig. 31.2: Degree of invasion of chorionic tissue. N: Normal; A: Accreta; I: Increta; P: Percreta; E: Endometrium; M: Myometrium

In patients with placenta previa and previous cesarean section, accreta is more common when previa is anterior or central (29%) than with lateral or posterior position of placenta (6.5%). In cases of percreta intra-abdominal bleeding, bladder symptoms and hematuria may be present.

All types of adherent placenta can cause severe PPH. If the diagnosis of accreta is suspected, then ultrasound or MRI may help planning a section. Expert surgeon, skilled anesthetist, blood transfusion facilities and ICU care should be available.

Placenta percreta is associated with high mortality of up to 7%.

DIAGNOSIS

High-risk cases should be screened for this abnormality.
- *Ultrasound*: The criteria for diagnosis are-
  - Loss of hypoechoic zone especially in the third term
  - Myometrial thickness of <1 mm
  - Large intraplacental blood lakes. The last two have the sensitivity of 100%, specificity of 72%, ppv of 72% and npv of 100%.
  - Thinning or disruption of hyperechoic uterine serosa-bladder interface.
  - Blood vessels crossing this region of interface disruption.
- *MRI*: It gives conflicting results. Addition gadolinium-based contrast agent seems to improve the specificity, but gadolinium may not be safe for use in pregnancy. MRI may be done when ultrasonography diagnosis is inconclusive, especially when parametrial or posterior invasion is suspected. Abnormal placental adherence can be identified even in early pregnancy.
- *Laboratory tests*:
  - *Alpha fetoprotein*: Abnormally, high levels in II term of pregnancy are found in palcenta accreta. There is a direct relation between extent of invasion and elevation of alpha-feto-protein.
  - *Creatinine kinase*: It is also a marker of invasive variety of placenta.

MANAGEMENT

Cases can be divided into:
- *Suspected*: Where planning can be done.
- *Unsuspected*: Little time is available to make quick decisions.

Suspected Case of Placenta Accreta/Increta

Counseling

Counseling is extremely important. Patient needs to be informed about risk of bleeding, need for hysterectomy, need for blood transfusion, need for uni- or bilateral oophorectomy, risk of infection, renal or other organ damage, thrombosis, other iatrogenic complications and risk of fatality.

Multidisciplinary Approach

- *Blood bank*: About 3000–5000 mL blood may be needed for cesarean hysterectomy. Adequate amount of PRBC, FFP, platelets, cryoprecipitate should be available. Preoperative hemodilution may be done where 3 units of blood are separated preoperatively and replaced by equal amount of crystalloids.
  Cell saver: Blood recovered from abdominal cavity may need double wash to remove fetal RBC and amniotic debris before transfusion.
- *Anesthesia*: Team of expert anesthetists is required. General anesthesia is preferred, then additional epidural catheter may be placed for postoperative analgesia. Temperature control is crucial. It is important to avoid hypothermia, hypovolemia and acidosis as all of them increase the risk of coagulopathy. Timely monitoring of hematocrit, platelets and blood gas analysis should be performed every 15–30 minutes.
- *Urological preparation*: In anterior placenta previa, accrete, increate or percreta, there is hypervascularity and distortion of uterovesical junction. Preoperative cystoscopy and ureteric stenting may be necessary in some. The portion of bladder involved may be excised as there are no long-term complications.
- *Internal iliac balloon catheter*: It may have to be passed when intraoperative hemorrhage is anticipated.

Operation Room Plan

The team of surgeons must discuss the plan earlier. The role of each operation assistant must be properly assigned. The different instruments required by different surgeons may best be procured in advance.

Neonatologist: Most of the planned sections are done between 34 and 37 weeks where baby will be mature. If cesarean is planned before 34 weeks, preoperative glucocorticoids may be given.
- *Intraoperative management*:
  - Low lithotomy position will facilitate ureteric stenting, assessment of vagina after delivery and for packing the vagina.
  - Vertical skin incision is preferred
  - Intraoperative ultrasound may be needed
  - Inspect lower segment for distortion. There may be hypervascularity and dilated large vessels. LUS may appear bulbous and distended.
  - Baby is best extracted with upper segment vertical incision, sometimes even fundal or posterior classical incision may be taken for which the uterus will have to be exteriorized.
  - No attempt should be made to remove the placenta manually and the cord should be tie close to its origin
  - Oxytocin infusion or 1000 µg rectal misoprostol can be given. Uterus may be observed for some time to see, if placenta separates naturally or not. If it is accerta, uterus should be closed in single layer using locking sutures. Intramyometrial PgF2α 250 µg in 20 mL saline can be given with 22-gauge needle at multiple sites.
  - Vagina should also be packed as it places the uterus up and straightens the coils of uterine artery thus reducing its caliber.
  - If hysterectomy has to be performed, then it should be preceded by stepwise devascularization. The neovasculature at sites of placenta accreta has vessels with thin musculature therefore they are more friable. Such vessels are best tied or clipped as coagulation frequently causes more bleed. Uterine arteries may be approached from posterior, i.e. USL complex side while working from posterior to anterior.

Subtotal hysterectomy: It should be discouraged as it prolongs the operation time and causes more blood loss. Uterus in most cases is removed unnecessarily as placental encroachment is in LUS and cervix. Collateral supply to uterus must also be taken care of.

Persistent hemorrhage may continue even after surgery because of coagulation defects. Until such time that blood or blood products are available compression of aorta at infrarenal site is recommended. Sometimes cross-clamping may be required temporarily.

Internal iliac embolization: For this the patient needs to be transferred to interventional radiology suite. It may be difficult in cases who are unstable. The procedure therefore should be individualized.

Tips for hemorrhage control during surgery:
- Abandon surgery temporarily
- Aortic compression-pelvic packing
- Skin closure with towel clips
- Giving blood products
- Warming the patient
- Pelvic drain

Until such time that coagulopathy reverses and patient is out of hemodynamic shock she should be observed in OT or ICU.
- *Postoperative management*: Risks in postoperative period includes intra-abdominal bleed, venous thromboembolism, renal failure, bowel ischemia, pulmonary edema, infection and myocardial depression. Blood transfusion can lead to lung complications besides renal damage. Later in life such a case can have Sheehan syndrome and postpartum depression.
- *Conservative treatment*: When removal of placenta seems impossible or too dangerous, conservative approach must be used. Uterus should be closed with placenta *in situ* and postoperative methotrexate should be given. Some

may require uterine artery embolization. Subsequent to conservative treatment massive hemorrhage and sepsis may develop. Currently, therefore supracervical hysterectomy remains the treatment of choice for accreta.

Unsuspected Case of Placenta Accreta/Increta

Occasionally at vaginal labor, often with history of prior uterine surgery this condition is heralded by retention of placenta. If the patient is stable rule out accreta before attempting MRP by USG. If USG is not available, then it is wiser to delay attempt at MRP until arrangements have been made to deal with massive hemorrhage.

More often accreta and percreta are discovered during a repeat section. If the lower segment appears ballooned and distorted with huge dilated vessels, then uterine incision should be delayed until necessary arrangements for blood transfusions have been made.

In case of partial accreta which may sometimes be found, hemostasis must be achieved by deep myometrial sutures using a 3 cm square pattern to cover maximal bleeding area.

Alternatively, inversion of cervix into the uterine cavity and suturing the inverted cervical tissue over the area of bleeding bed may be all that should be done. Two parallel vertical sutures Lynch type may be placed in LUS to compress the placental bed.

POINTS TO REMEMBER

- High index of suspicion
- Counseling regarding treatment plan and outcome
- Keen observation in high-risk cases
- Operate the case quick enough before coagulopathy develops.
- Quick decision making appropriate for each case
- Aggressive resuscitation
- Use of blood products.

Chapter 32

Placental Abruption

Sadhana Gupta, Hema J Shobhane

GENERAL CONSIDERATION

Abruptio placentae (i.e placental abruption) refers to separation of the normally located placenta after the 20th week of gestation and prior to birth, and clinically is presented as bleeding from or in to the genital tract or both **(Fig. 32.1)**. Severe obstetric hemorrhage is the most feared obstetric emergency that can occur to any woman at childbirth. If unattended, then hemorrhage can kill even a healthy woman. The hemorrhage accounts for nearly one-quarter of all maternal deaths and for almost half of all postpartum deaths in low-income countries. The most common type of antepartum obstetric hemorrhage is placental abruption, as well as most common type of postpartum hemorrhage (PPH), mainly primary PPH occurring within 24 hours postpartum. Placental abruption occurs on average in 0.5%, or 1 in 200, deliveries[1] Placental abruption is a significant contributor to maternal mortality worldwide; early and skilled medical intervention is needed to ensure a good outcome, and this is not available in many parts of the world.[2] Treatment depends on how serious the abruption is and how far along the woman is in her pregnancy. On the other hand, the management of abruptio placentae remains a problem, despite advances in medical science due to ambiguous clinical presentation. Placental abruption has effects on both mother and fetus. The effects on the mother depend primarily on the severity of the abruption, while the effects on the fetus depend on both its severity and the gestational age at which it occurs.

CLINICAL FEATURES

Being an obstetrician, must suspect abruption placentae in any patient, who is presented with the following symptoms:
- Vaginal bleeding—80%
- Abdominal or back pain and uterine tenderness—70%
- Fetal distress—60%
- Abnormal uterine contractions (e.g. hypertonic, high frequency)—35%
- Idiopathic premature labor—25%
- Fetal death—15%.

EXAMINATION

Placental abruption is mainly a clinical diagnosis based on findings of vaginal bleeding, abdominal pain, uterine tenderness, uterine contractions, and fetal distress.

Classification of placental abruption is based on extent of separation (i.e. partial versus complete) and the location of separation (i.e. marginal versus central). Clinical characteristics are divided into the following classes:
- *Class 0:* Asymptomatic
- *Class 1:* Mild (represents approximately 48% of all cases)
- *Class 2:* > Moderate (represents approximately 27% of all cases)
- *Class 3:* Severe (represents approximately 24% of all cases).

Class 0

The diagnosis in these patients is made retrospectively by finding an organized blood clot or a depressed area on a delivered placenta.

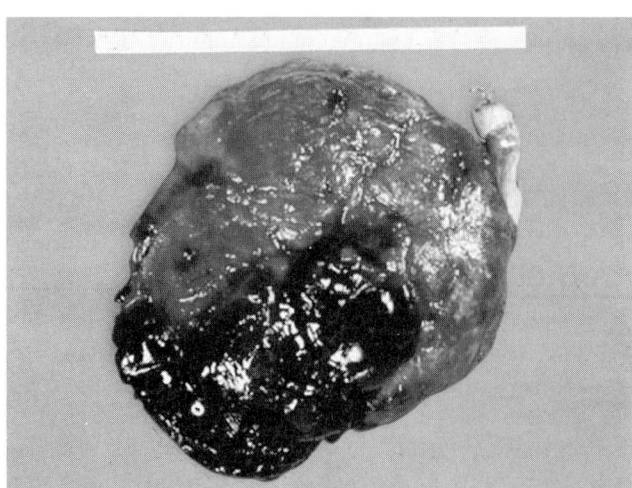

Fig. 32.1: Placenta with retroplacental hemorrhage
(For color version, see Plate 2)

Class 1

Characteristics include the following:
- No vaginal bleeding to mild vaginal bleeding
- Slightly tender uterus
- Normal maternal BP and heart rate
- No coagulopathy
- No fetal distress.

Class 2

Characteristics include the following:
- No vaginal bleeding to moderate vaginal bleeding
- Moderate-to-severe uterine tenderness, with possible tetanic contractions
- Maternal tachycardia, with orthostatic changes in BP and heart rate
- Fetal distress
- Hypofibrinogenemia (i.e. 50–250 mg/dL).

Class 3

Characteristics include the following:
- No vaginal bleeding to heavy vaginal bleeding
- Very painful tetanic uterus
- Maternal shock
- Hypofibrinogenemia (i.e. < 150 mg/dL)
- Coagulopathy
- Fetal death.

ETIOLOGY

The primary cause of placental abruption is usually unknown, but multiple risk factors have been identified.[3,4] Risk factors in abruptio placentae include the following:
- Maternal hypertension—most common cause of abruption (44%)
- Maternal trauma (e.g. motor vehicle collision [MVC], assaults, falls)—causes (1.5–9.49%)
- Prolonged rupture of membranes (24 hours or longer)
- Multiple pregnancy
- Maternal age 35 years or older
- Maternal age younger than 20 years
- Cigarette smoking
- Alcohol consumption
- Cocaine use
- Previous placental abruption
- Low socioeconomic status
- Elevated second trimester maternal serum alpha-fetoprotein (associated with up to a 10-fold increased risk of abruption)
- Subchorionic hematoma.[5]

INVESTIGATIONS

Laboratory investigations are used in the diagnosis of placental abruption include the following: Hemoglobin, Blood type, hematocrit, platelets prothrombin time/activated partial thromboplastin time, fibrinogen fibrin/fibrinogen degradation products, and D-dimer

Ultrasonography helps to determine the location of the placenta in order to exclude placenta previa. Ultrasonography is not very useful in diagnosing placental abruption (and normal ultrasonographic findings do not exclude the condition).[6]

Retroplacental hematoma may be recognized in 2–25% of all abruptions **(Figs 32.2A and B)**. This recognition depends on the degree of hematoma and on the operator's skill level.

MRI is diagnostically effective and can accurately depict placental abruption. Consider using MRI in cases where ultrasonography findings in the presence of late pregnancy bleeding are negative, but positive diagnosis of abruption would change patient management.

Some patients may not have the classic presentation of abruption, especially with posterior implantation.

Consider a diagnosis of placental abruption for every patient in premature labor. Carefully monitor patients to exclude or establish this diagnosis. Absence of vaginal bleeding does not exclude placental abruption.

PREVENTION

Treat maternal hypertension.[7] Note that although hypertensive conditions increase the risk of placental abruption, they do not appear to increase the rate of recurrence of placental abruption in subsequent pregnancies.[8]

Prevent maternal trauma/domestic violence. Prevent smoking and substance abuse.

Data from a Netherlands longitudinal-linked national cohort study of all singleton pregnancies that ended (1999–2007) revealed an increased risk of recurrence of placental abruption in women who had placental abruption in their first pregnancy.[8] The investigators suggested an elective induction from 37 weeks' gestation for women with such a history.[8]

MANAGEMENT

Management depends on the gestational age and on the condition of the mother and fetus. When there is fetal demise, the goal is to minimize morbidity to the mother. In cases of a live fetus at term, prompt delivery is indicated. When there is evidence of fetal compromise, delivery by cesarean section is usually indicated. In gestations at 34 weeks or less, conservative management may be attempted, if both the mother and the fetus are stable.

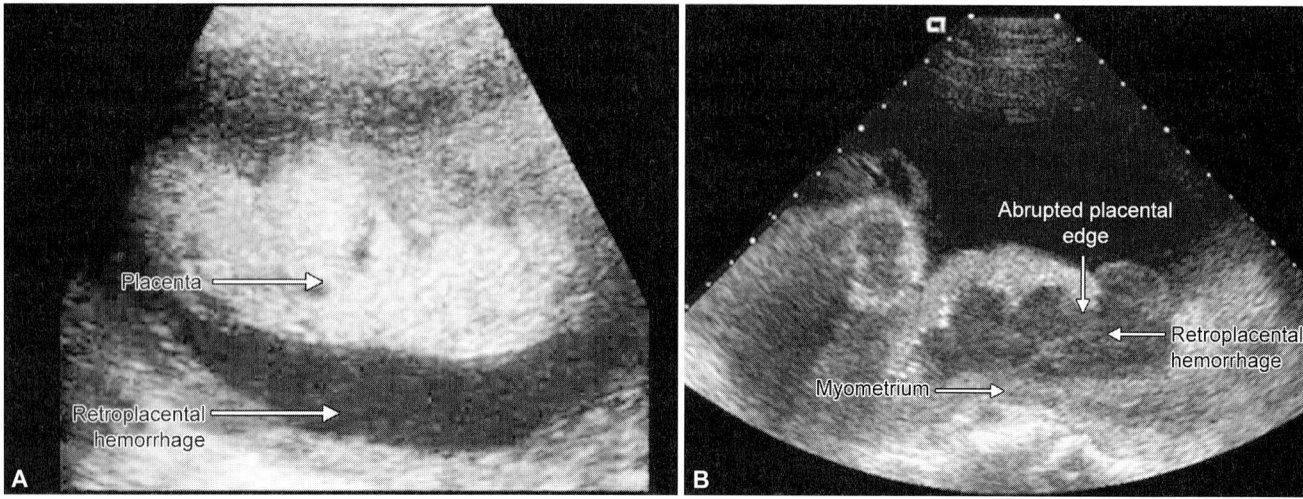

Figs 32.2A and B: Retroplacental hematoma in USG images

Initial Management

For all women with placental abruption, initial treatment should consist of stabilization and monitoring of the fetus and the mother. This includes:
- Intravenous access with wide-bore cannulas.
- FBC for evidence of anemia. Hct and Hb levels may be low.
- Coagulation profile looking for evidence of impaired coagulation. Low fibrinogen levels and a prolonged PT are suggestive of impaired coagulation due to DIC.
- Monitoring of the patient's hemodynamic status by monitoring BP, pulse, volume intake, and urine output.
- Continuous fetal monitoring.
- Anti-D immunoglobulin in Rh-negative women.
- Fluid, blood, or blood-product replacement, as indicated.
- Sonographic examination for placental location and for evidence of abruption. Placenta previa found on sonography makes placental abruption unlikely.

The goals are to prevent hypovolemia, anemia, and DIC. Blood and fluid replacement needs can be determined by estimated blood loss, and by vital signs (BP, pulse, and urine output). The goal should be to keep the Hb level above 100 g/L (10 g/dL) and Hct above 30%. Urine output should be at least 30 mL/hour.

Live Fetus: Gestational Age more than 34 Weeks (Flow chart 32.1)

The aim in these circumstances is expeditious delivery. If the mother is in a stable condition and the fetal heart tracing is reassuring, then vaginal delivery can be attempted. Often the mother is having vigorous contractions, but if the mother is not in active labor, amniotomy and oxytocin induction usually results in delivery. Blood coagulation products should be readily available and replaced aggressively, if needed.

If the maternal condition is worsening with severe hemorrhage, then the urgent cesarean delivery may be indicated (although rarely). Unnecessary delay should be avoided. A study demonstrated that neonates born to women with placental abruption and bradycardia had better perinatal outcomes, if the decision-delivery interval for cesarean delivery was <20 minutes. It is important that both blood and blood products are replaced before and during the surgery.

In cases of placental abruption, the uterus may not contract adequately, and therefore hemorrhage may be difficult to control. Uterotonic agents such as oxytocin, methylergometrine, and prostaglandin analogues may be given. In severe cases, where bleeding is unresponsive to delivery and to administration of uterotonic agents, surgical ligation of the uterine arteries or the hypogastric arteries may be life-saving. In centers with an adequately skilled interventional radiologist, selective embolisation of these vessels may lead to cessation of this life-threatening hemorrhage. In cases that fail to respond to these conservative methods, hysterectomy may be necessary. Coagulation derangement should be actively corrected while these procedures are taking place.

Live Fetus less than 34 Weeks Gestation (Flow chart 32.2)

In cases where the fetus and mother are both stable and there is no evidence of maternal coagulopathy, hypotension, or severe ongoing blood loss, conservative management with the aim of delivering a more mature fetus is the main goal of therapy. Corticosteroids should be given to promote fetal lung maturation in pregnancies between 24 and 34 weeks. Tocolytics may be used with extreme caution in

Flow chart 32.1: Algorithm for the management of placental abruption in women who are term/near term (>34 weeks' gestation)

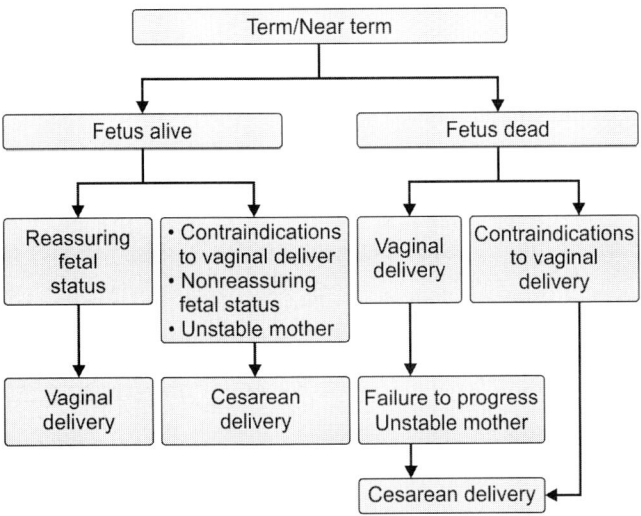

Source: Oyelese Y, Ananth CV. Placental abruption. Obstet Gynecol. 2006;108:1005-16. Used with permission

Flow chart 32.2: Algorithm for the management of placental abruption in women who are preterm (≤34 weeks' gestation)

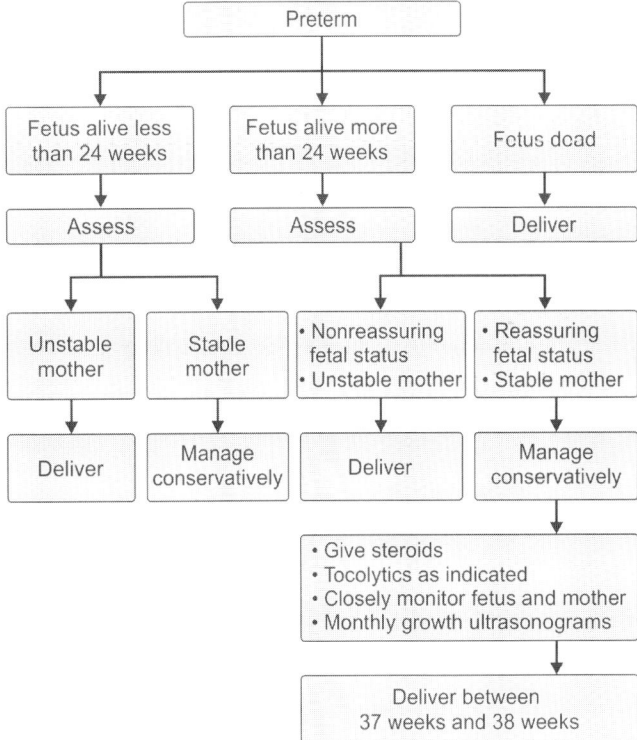

Source: Oyelese Y, Ananth CV. Placental abruption. Obstet Gynecol. 2006;108:1005-16. Used with permission

cases where there are uterine contractions in pregnancies >24 weeks. This is controversial, but small studies have confirmed that careful use of tocolytics may be safe in these circumstances. Recently, the FDA has warned against the off label use of injectable terbutaline for the long-term (i.e. >72 hours) treatment or prevention of preterm labor, due to an increased risk of maternal cardiovascular adverse effects. Oral terbutaline is now contraindicated for this indication. Therefore, terbutaline should not be used for this indication in patients with suspected abruption.

There is an increased risk of stillbirth, so it is recommended that delivery by 37–38 weeks is considered.

Fetal Demise

The approach to management is similar to when the fetus is alive (i.e. expeditious delivery, preferably by the vaginal route). If the mother is not in active labor, she can be induced by amniotomy and oxytocin. Women who have had an abruption sufficient to cause fetal demise are highly likely to have DIC. If the maternal condition is worsening with severe hemorrhage, then cesarean delivery may be indicated (although rarely). It is important that both blood and blood products are replaced before and during the surgery.

RECURRENCE

The risk of recurrence of abruptio placentae is reportedly 4–12%. If the patient has abruptio placentae in 2 consecutive pregnancies, then risk of recurrence rises to 25%.

If the abruption is severe and results in the death of the fetus, then risk of a recurrent abruption and fetal demise is 7%.

LONG-TERM MATERNAL CARDIOVASCULAR MORTALITY

A study by Pariente et al. indicated that women who have placental abruption are at increased long-term risk for cardiovascular mortality. The study examined the cardiovascular mortality rate after 653 deliveries in patients with placental abruption, with follow-up occurring over more than 10 years. Although the investigators did not find a significant connection between placental abruption and later, long-term hospitalization for cardiovascular disease, they found a 13% cardiovascular mortality rate in the women who had suffered placental abruption, compared with a 2.5% rate in women who had not.

COUNSELING

Educate patients about reversible avoidable risk factors, especially domestic violence, smoking, cocaine abuse, and these factors should be avoided before further pregnancies. Placental abruption may be due to thrombophilia, thus possibilities of thrombophilia should be rule out and is treated.

REFERENCES

1. Sheffield [edited by] Cunningham FG, Leveno KJ, Bloom SL, Spong CY, Dashe JS, Hoffman BL, Casey BM, Jeanne S. William's Obstetrics, 24th edn; 2014.
2. Placental abruption | Pregnancy | Pregnancy complications | March of Dimes. marchofdimes.org. Retrieved. 2012-10-23.
3. Ananth CV, Oyelese Y, Yeo L, Pradhan A, Vintzileos AM. Placental abruption in the United States, 1979 through 2001: temporal trends and potential determinants. Am J Obstet Gynecol. 2005;192(1):1911.
4. Rana A, Sawhney H, Gopalan S. Abruptio placentae and chorioamnionitis-microbiological and histologic correlation. Acta Obstet Gynecol Scand. 1999;78(5):363-6.
5. Tuuli MG, Norman SM, Odibo AO, Macones GA, Cahill AG. Perinatal outcomes in women with subchorionic hematoma: a systematic review and meta-analysis. Obstet Gynecol. 2011; 117(5):1205-12.
6. Ananth CV, Savitz DA, Bowes WA Jr, Luther ER. Influence of hypertensive disorders and cigarette smoking on placental abruption and uterine bleeding during pregnancy. Br J Obstet Gynaecol. 1997;104(5):572-8.
7. Hoskins IA, Friedman DM, Frieden FJ. Relationship between antepartum cocaine abuse, abnormal umbilical artery Doppler velocimetry, and placental abruption. Obstet Gynecol. 1991;78(2):279-82.
8. Tikkanen M, Luukkaala T, Gissler M, et al. Decreasing perinatal mortality in placental abruption. Acta Obstet Gynecol Scand. 2013;92(3):298-305.

Chapter 33

Preterm Labor: Diagnosis and Treatment

Anuradha Dang, Pushpa Pandey, Sneh Chaube

INTRODUCTION

Approximately, 15 million babies are born preterm each year accounting to about 1 in 10 in all babies. Almost one million children die each year due to complications preterm birth. Many survivors may face a lifetime of disability, compounded by learning disabilities and visual and hearing problems.

17th November is observed as 'World Prematurity Day' since 2011.[1]

DEFINITION

American College of Obstetricians and Gynecologists (ACOG) has defined preterm labor as the onset of labor (regular painful uterine contractions associated with effacement and dilatation of the cervix) prior to the completion of 37 weeks (259 days) of gestation counting from the first day of the last menstruation period and after completing the age of viability which is different in different countries being 20–24 weeks in developed countries (22 weeks and 500 g by WHO, 24 weeks in the United Kingdom and 28 weeks in developing countries including India.

Subcategories of preterm birth: Based on gestational age, preterm birth is subcategorized as:
- Extremely preterm (< 28 weeks)
- Very preterm (28 to < 32 weeks)
- Moderate-to-late preterm (32 to <37 weeks).

Introduction of labor or cesarean section should not be planned electively before 39 completed weeks unless medically indicated.

PATHOPHYSIOLOGY OF PRETERM LABOR

Four pathways are involved in pathophysiology of preterm labor.
1. *Inflammation*: Infection from periodontal disease, pneumonia, sepsis, pancreatitis, acute cholecystitis, pyelonephritis, asymptomatic bacteriuria, chorioamnionitis can cause preterm labor.
   Genital tract inflammations are the most common cause of very early preterm deliveries. Bacterial vaginosis facilitate overgrowth of bacteria, *Mycoplasma* species, *Gardnerella vaginalis* and gram-negative bacteria, such as *Escherichia coli* and gram-positive cocci. Asymptomatic bacteriuria and vaginal *E. coli* account for two-fold increase in risk of preterm delivery (PTD).
2. *Decidual hemorrhage*: Vaginal bleeding occurring in more than one trimester is associated with 50% risk PPROM (Preterm, premature rupture of membranes).[2] Decidual hemorrhage may be associated with inherited and acquired thrombophilias, hypertension as well as environmental stimuli including heavy cigarette smoking, cocaine, trauma, etc. It may present with vaginal bleeding or retroplacental or retrochorionic hematoma on ultrasound.
3. *Uterine distension*: Mechanical stretching of uterus from polyhydramnios and multiple gestation induces preterm delivery. Stretching increases Cox-2 expression and related prostaglandin production. It also induces oxytocin receptor, Cox-2, IL-8 connexin expressions.
4. *Premature activation of normal physiological initiation of normal labor:* Generation of prostaglandin (PG) and proteases reflects the common pathway in preterm and term delivery. Level of prostaglandins increases in genital tract tissues, maternal plasma and amniotic fluid immediately prior to or during labor. Simultaneously, prior to onset of labor due to upregulation of myometrial prostaglandin receptors, prostaglandin increases. Prostaglandin induces withdrawal of functional progesterone, enhance sensitivity to estrogens and increase MMP and IL-8 expression which leads to cervical changes and fetal membrane rupture.

RISK FACTORS

- *Prior preterm birth*: According to ACOG, prior PTB is one of the strongest risk factors for subsequent PTB. Guzman and coworkers, Andrews and coworkers stated that women with history of preterm labor had increased risk of recurrence in subsequent pregnancies.[3,4]
- *Short cervical length*: Short cervical length is most commonly defined as less than 25 mm, usually before

24 weeks gestation, as measured by transvaginal ultrasonography.
- *A history of cervical surgery*: Surgeries such as conization and loop electrosurgical procedures were thought to be risk factors but no definite link is established. Studies show that cone biopsy and LLETZ increased the risk of preterm delivery.[5] The risk was greater if the depth of excision was more than 10 mm.[6] Laser vaporization, cryotherapy and punch biopsy have not been shown to increase the risk.
- *Uterine instrumentation*: Intrauterine microbial colonization injury to the endometrium or both has been associated with an increased risk of preterm birth. Two or more prior dilatation and evacuation especially for late termination of pregnancy is associated with cervical insufficiency.[7]
- *Other factors*: Myoma, uterine septum, bicornuate uterus. Pregnancy associated with vaginal bleeding, urinary tract infections (UTIs), genital tract infections, malaria, typhoid fever, pneumonia and periodontal disease are considered potential risk factors for PTB.
- *Behavioral risk factors*: Low maternal pregnancy weight, smoking, substance abuse, short interpregnancy interval, pregnancy induced hypertension and antepartum hemorrhage can also cause preterm labor.
- *Multiple pregnancies*: Rate of preterm delivery is about 10% for single pregnancy but more for twins and to the extent of 80–90% for multiple pregnancies.
- *Alteration in fetal membrane*: Tensile strength of chorion and amnion are responsible for integrity of pregnancy, which forms the physical and functional boundary of the fetus. Preterm rupture of membrane is responsible for 30% of spontaneous birth.

Screening Methods During Pregnancy

The goal of screening is the early identification of pregnant women at an elevated risk of going into labor prematurely, so that these women can be helped to carry their pregnancies to term.

Cervical Length Screening

Short cervix was most important single predictor of preterm birth.[3]

Cervical length is also good negative predictor. Length equal or greater than 30 mm is highly reassuring. As cervical effacement occurs slowly, so cervical length less than 20 mm does not always indicate preterm labor but cervical length more than 30 mm excludes preterm labor.[8]

It most accurately measured by transvaginal sonography with empty bladder and probe in anterior fornix. Length should be measured in a straight line from internal to

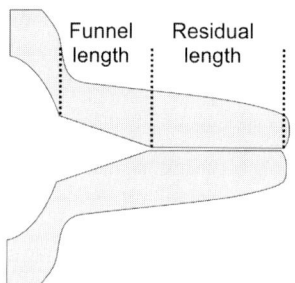

Fig. 33.1: Residual cervical length

external cervical os. As cervix is dynamic 3 measurements are made over 5 mins period.

Cervical funneling does not always increase the risk of PTL associated with a shortened cervical length. Residual length is the real cervical length and should be less than 25 mm to increase the risk of PTL **(Fig. 33.1)**.[9] A false or pseudofunnel may occur when the lower uterine segment contracts to form a funnel above a cervix of normal length.

Other Specific Tests and Monitoring Modalities

- *Salivary estriol*: Salivary estriol has very poor sensitivity and specificity and is also expensive test.
- *Home uterine activity monitoring (HUAM)*: An external tocodynamometer belted around the abdomen and connected to electronic waist recorder allows a woman to ambulate while uterine activity is recorded. It is no longer used in practice. Earlier studies showed that HUAM was effective but recently, it has showed no benefit in predicting PTL.[4]
- *Bacterial vaginosis (BV)*: In earlier studies BV was shown to increase preterm labor by two fold. However, results have been largely inconclusive.

Fibronectin Measurement

Fibronectin is present before 16–18 weeks of pregnancy and at the onset of labor. It is a marker of disruption of decidual-chorionic interface. Levels more than 50 ng/mL[10] increases the risk of preterm labor. Presence of fibronectin glycoprotein produced by fetal amnion in cervicovaginal discharge between 24 and 34 weeks is a predictor of preterm labor. When the test is negative, it reassures delivery will not occur within 7 days.

Relative Contraindication to this Test

- Cervical cerclage
- Use of lubricants or disinfectants
- Recent coitus.

INTERVENTIONS

The two main interventions for preventing PTL are progesterone supplementation and cervical cerclage.

Role of Progesterone Supplement[13]

In the 2011, the US food and drug administration approved, the use of hydroxyprogesterone caproate during pregnancy to reduce the risk of recurrent preterm birth in women with a history of at least one prior spontaneous preterm delivery[11]

- *Progesterone supplementation in women with a history of spontaneous preterm birth*: A woman with a singleton gestation and a prior spontaneous preterm singleton birth should be offered progesterone supplementation starting at 16–24 weeks of gestation, regardless of transvaginal ultrasound cervical length, to reduce the risk of recurrent spontaneous birth.
- *Progesterone in women with cervical shortening*: Cervical shortening is a known risk factor for preterm birth in both low- and high-risk populations. Progesterone administration significantly reduced the rate of spontaneous preterm birth before 34 weeks. Vaginal progesterone is recommended as a management risk of preterm birth in asymptomatic woman with a singleton gestation without a prior preterm birth with an incidentally identified very short cervical length less than or equal to 20 mm before or at 24 weeks of gestation.
- *Women with a cerclage*: It is not clear whether progesterone provides additional benefit to women with a cervical cerclage in place.
- *Multiple gestation*: Progesterone treatment does not reduce the incident of preterm birth in women with twin or triplet gestation and therefore, is not recommended as an intervention to prevent preterm birth in women with multiple gestation.

Dose of Progestogens

Use of 17-hydroxy progesterone caproate 500 mg intramuscularly weekly or oral hydrogesterone 10–20 mg daily or vaginal progesterone 200 mg daily is recommended.

Cervical Cerclage[14]

Cervical cerclage provides physical support for structurally weak cervix and improves cervical immunological barrier by improving retention of the mucus plug.[12] History indicated cerclage may be offered between 13 week and 14 week. Cervical length screening strategy for women with a history suspicious for insufficiency initiate TV ultrasound at 14 week.
- If Cl > 30 mm, repeat every 2 week until 23
- If Cl 25–29 mm, repeat every one week until 23
- If Cl less than 25 mm prior to 24 weeks, offer cerclage placement.

Vaginal cerclage is most common (Macdonald or shirodekar) and can be placed during pregnancy between 12 and 24 weeks of gestation. Abdominal cerclage is usually reserved for women with prior failed vaginal cerclage.

Other Interventions

Other interventions, such as pharmacotherapy with indomethacin or antibiotic, activity restriction, or supplementation with omega-3 fatty acids are not recommended for women with an incidentally diagnosed short cervical length.[13]

Diagnosis of Preterm Labor

Diagnosis of preterm labor should be made, if patient is between 20 and 37 weeks, if contraction occurs at a frequency of 4 per 20 mins or 8 in 60 mins accompanied by one of the following.
- Premature rupture of membranes (PROM)
- Cervical dilatation > 2 cm
- Cervical effacement of 50%
- Change in dilatation or effacement on serial examination.

Routine Physical Examination in Preterm Labor

- Pulse, temperature, blood pressure measurement and dipstick urine analysis.
- Abdominal examination for fetal presentation, fetal heart and uterine activity.
- Vaginal speculum examination to assess cervix, membrane status and for taking swabs.
- Digital assessment of the cervix may be used but is not always necessary.

Routine Investigations for Preterm Labor

- Urine for glucose, proteins, ketones, microscopy and culture.
- *Swabs*: One or more of the following should be taken.
  - High vaginal swab for gram staining and culture, pH and Fern test.
  - Endocervical swab for *Neisseria gonorrhoeae* and *Chlamydia trachomatis* culture.
  - Urethral swab in indicated cases.
- Cardiotocography (CTG) for uterine contraction and fetal heart.
- Ultrasound for fetal maturity, fetal anomalies, presentation liquor assessment, estimated fetal weight. Transvaginal

ultrasound assessment for cervical length and funneling internal os.
- Swab from cervicovaginal area for fetal fibronectin, if available.

Management of preterm labor

- Corticosteroids should be given to the mother to reduce the risk of neonatal respiratory distress syndrome and other neonatal complications.
- *In utero* transfer of the mother for delivery in a unit where appropriate neonatal care can be provided.
- Tocolytic drugs can be used for a short period to prolong gestation for 2–7 days, unless contraindicated.
- Antibiotics is reserved for cases with infection (hemolytic *Streptococcus*) in whom delivery is imminent.
- Careful intrapartum monitoring, minimal trauma and involvement of the neonatologist during delivery are essential.
- Vaginal delivery is preferred, unless cesarean section is indicated for obstetric reasons.

Administration of Corticosteroids

For prophylaxis against neonatal respiratory distress syndrome (RDS) betamethasone 2 doses of 12 mg intramuscularly 24 hours apart or dexamethasone 6 mg bid for 4 doses.

Repeat dose is not required as many may have side effects:
- Maternal sepsis
- Neonatal sepsis
- Reduced birth weight
- Reduced fetal head circumference

However, a few author suggest a single rescue dose, if delivery does not occur in next seven days.

Contraindication to Corticosteroids

Chorioamnionitis, maternal tuberculosis, porphyria, pregnancy >34 weeks, maternal or fetal infections. Maternal diabetes is a relative contraindication. Additional dose of insulin may be required to tide over hyperglycemic periods.

Antibiotics

The ORACLE trial has confirmed that antibiotic are not of any benefit in reducing neonatal mortality or serious neonatal morbidity in preterm labor with intact membranes. However, antibiotic for group B *Streptococcus* prophylaxis may be started at least 4 hours before delivery with Ampicillin, Clindamycin or Erythromycin with ruptured membranes.

Tocolysis (Table 33.1)

It is indicated:
- Gestation<34 weeks
- No fetal or maternal compromise
- *In utero* transfer

They may be classified as first line tocolytic and second line tocolytic.

It prolongs pregnancy by at least 48 hours, allowing administration of betamethasone and shifting the patient to a center equipped with better neonatal facilities (*in utero* transfer).

Contraindications to tocolysis for treatment of preterm labor include fetal distress, eclampsia, fetal demise, etc.

First-line Tocolytics[15-17]

- *Nifedipine*: Unless contraindicated, it should considered as first-line agent in developing countries
- Side effects
- Hypotension, headache, nausea, flushing and increase in liver enzymes.
- It should not be combined with other betamimetics or magnesium sulfate.
- It enhances neuromuscular blocking effect of magnesium which can interfere with pulmonary and cardiac functions.

Dosage
- Initial dose of 20 mg of nifedipine orally should be started with a normal blood pressure (BP) (Not slow release nifedipine and not sublingual which usually causes sudden fall of BP).
- After 30 mins, it contractions persist, another 20 mg oral dose can be repeated.
- After a further 30 mins, it still contracting, follow-up with a further 20 mg orally.
- If BP is stable, a maintenance dose of 20 mg three times a day for 48–72 hours may be given where indicated. Maximum doses 120 mg per day.

Precautions
- IV line started.
- Baseline electrolytes, urea creatinine, liver function test measured.
- Half-hourly pulse, BP, respiratory rate measured.
- Continuous electronic fetal heart rate monitoring.
- Auscultation of lung bases every 8 hourly.

Second-line Tocolysis[18-20]

- Salbutamol may be used as the second-line tocolytic, in the absence of contraindications or when nifedipine cannot be given.
- It must not be added to nifedipine.

It is contraindicated
- Presence of maternal or fetal cardiac disease.
- Insulin-dependent diabetes.
- Thyroid disorder.

Table 33.1: Tocolytic therapy in preterm labor

Drug	Mechanism of action	Contraindication	Maternal side effects	Fetal side effects
Terbutaline	B₂ agonist	• Cardiac • Arrhythmias • Diabetes	• Cardiac and pulmonary arrhythmias • Pulmonary edema • Myocardial infarction • HT • Tachycardia	• Tachycardia • Hyperinsulinemia • Hypoglycemia • Myocardial and septal hypertrophy
Ritodrine	B-mimetic	• Diabetes mellitus • Poorly controlled thyroid disorder	• Hyperinsulinemia • Hypocalcemia • Altered thyroid functions	• Neonatal Hyperinsulinemia • Hypocalcemia • Intraventricular hemorrhage
Salbutamol	B₂ agonist	Diabetes mellitus	• Hyperinsulinemia • Hypocalcemia • Altered thyroid functions	• Neonatal Hyperinsulinemia • Hypokalemia • Intraventricular hemorrhage
Nifedipine	Calcium-channel blocker	Cardiac diseases	• Hypotension dizziness • Nausea	None
Atosiban	Oxytocin receptor antagonist	Gest. age <24 >30 weeks	Nausea	
Indomethacin	Nonsteroidal anti-inflammatory drug	• Late pregnancy • Renal or hepatic insufficiency	• Heart burn • Nausea	• Constriction of ductus arteriosus • Pulmonary HT • Reversible • Decrease in renal function • Intraventricular hemorrhage • Hyperbilirubinemia • Necrotizing enterocolitis
Magnesium sulphate	Myosin light chain inhibitor	Myasthenia gravis	• Flushing • Lethargy • Muscle weakness • Diplopia • Pulmonary edema	• Lethargy • Hypotension • Respiratory depression

Dosage: Infusion is commenced at 12 mL/hour (10 µg/min) and increased by 4 mL/hour (3.3 µg/min) every 30 mins. The end point is as follows:
- Till contractions cease
- Maternal pulse rate reaches 120 beats/minute or
- The infusing rate reaches a maximum of 36 mL/hour (30 µg/min).

Glyceryl Trinitrate

Glyceryl trinitrate (GTN) is a nitric oxide donor and causes smooth muscle relaxation. Peak action occurs 1–2 hours after application of the patch form.

Dosage: About 5–10 mg transdermal GTN patch is applied the contractions persist (maximum does 20 mg in 24 hours).

Side effects: Headache, facial flushing, hypotension and tachycardia.

Indomethacin

It is well-tolerated, especially if pregnancy is less than 32 weeks and other drugs are contraindicated.

Dosage: 100 mg rectal suppositories followed by 24 mg oral every four hours till 48 hours.

Side effects: Prolong use of indomethacin, especially in the presence of a relatively mature fetus, may lead to narrowing or occlusion of the fetal ductus and/or reduction In fetal rental function.

Magnesium sulfate: It can be used in diabetic mother. Loading dose 4-6 g over 20-30 mins followed by 1-2 g per hours infusion is given. It is used between 24 and 32 weeks for atleast 12 hours. It has tocolytic and neuroprotective role by decreasing incidence of cerebral palsy (Beneficial effects of antenatal magnesium sulfate, BEAM Study 2008).[21,22]

Ritodrine, isoxsuprine and terbutaline: Are not much advocated due to complications, especially pulmonary edema. However, ritodrine may be started with 0.05 mg/minute (5 drops/minute) till contractions cease usually at a dose of 0.15 mg/minute (30 drops/minute). But maximum of 3.0 mg/minute (30 drops/minute) and continued for 48 hours. Effective dose is 0.05-0.15 mg/minute. Than oral ritodrine table (10 mg) every 4-6 hours can be given until 37th week of pregnancy or at least up to one week after stoppage of contractions but its role is doubtful.

Isoxsuprine regimen: It can also be given by intravenous infusion at a rate of 60 µg (8 drops) per minute (60 mg in 500 mL 5% dextrose) increasing or reducing it depending on efficacy and effect on blood pressure and heart rate. Isoxsuprine 10 mg IM every 4-6 hours may also be used initially, followed by maintenance dosage of 60-80 mg daily orally.

Terbutaline: It is given as IV bolus of 250 µg followed by 10-50 µg/minute until the labor stops. Then administer subcutaneously 0.25-0.5 mg every 2-4 hours for 12 hours. A maintenance dose of 2.5-5 mg orally may be given 4-6 times a day.

Atosiban: It is a oxytocin antagonist. It is used as an intravenous medication as a tocolytic to halt premature labor. It is given as initial bolus dose of 6.75 mg over 1 minute, followed by an infusion of 18 mg/hour for 3 hours, then 6 mg/hour for up to 45 hours (maximum 330 mg). It is safest choice in multiple pregnancy, in cases of expanded blood volume and anemia where use of other tocolytics predisposed to pulmonary edema.

Management of Labor

- Various factors such as presentations of baby, severe IUGR or pre-eclampsia and fetal status on admission is considered
- Vaginal delivery is preferred in low socioeconomic set-ups. Earlier cesarean section was considered as the choice of delivery but in low socioeconomic set-ups with no good nursery care, neonatal mortality was high. Chances of repeat surgery in next pregnancy is more and it also increased economic burden of family.
- Operative vaginal deliveries are relatively contraindication in labor less than 34 weeks. Use of vacuum causes increased incidence of intra- and extracranial hemorrhage, brachial plexus injury, etc.

Delayed Cord Clamping

- Early cord clamping (within 60 sec of birth) was initially thought to improve management of preterm baby.
- Currently, WHO recommends delayed cord clamping 1-3 min after birth with infant held at or below level of placenta.

Contraindications to Delayed Cord Clamping[23,24]

- Infants requiring urgent resuscitation
- Presence of placental abnormalities such as placenta previa, vasa previa or placental abruption
- Thick meconium-stained liquor
- Multiple pregnancy
- Severe IUGR with absent or reversed and diastolic flow in umbilical artery on Doppler study
- Alloimmunization.

New strategy is proposed to milk the cord (3 times over duration of less than 30 sec) achieves significant improvement in hemodynamic stability.

IMPORTANT POINTS

Fruitful outcome of preterm labor accomplishes:
- Prevention and early diagnosis of preterm labor
- Cervical ultrasound examination and fetal fibronectin testing have good negative value thus either approach or combined may be helpful in determining which patients do not need tocolysis.
- Use of tocolytic agents to delay labor for short period.
- Calcium-channel blockers are preferable to other agents..
- Use of corticosteroids for better neonatal outcome.
- *In utero* transfer to a center with appropriate maternal and neonatal facilities.

REFERENCES

1. World Prematurity Day. EHO/PMNCH. Retrieved; 2014;29.
2. Harger JH, Hsing AW, Tumala RE, et al. Risk factors for preterm premature rupture of membrane, a multicentric-case control study. American of Obstet Gyn. 1990;163:13.
3. Guzman ER, Mellon R, Vintzileos AM, Ananth CV, Walters C, Gipson K. Relationship between endocervical canal length between 15-24 weeks gestation and obstetric history. J Matern Fetal Med. 1998;7(6):269-72.
4. Andrews WW, Copper R, Hauth JC, Goldenberg RL, Neely C, Dubard M. Second-trimester cervical ultrasound: associations with increased risk for recurrent early spontaneous delivery. Obstet Gyne. 2000;95(2):222-6.
5. Kyrgiou MKG, Martin-Hirsch P, Arbyn M, Prendiville W, Paraskevaidis E. Obstetric outcomes after conservative treatment for intraepithelial or early invasive cervical lesions: systematic review and meta-analysis. Lancet. 2006;367(9509):489-98.
6. Berghella VTJ, Kuhlman K, Weiner S, Bolognese RJ. Cervical ultrasonography compared with manual examination as a

predictor of preterm delivery. Am J Obstet Gynecol. 1997;177(4):723-30.
7. Visintine J, Berghella V, Henning D, Baxter J. Cervical length for prediction of preterm birth in women with multiple prior induced abortions. Ultrasound Obstet Gynecol. 2008;31(2):198-200.
8. Murakawa H, Utumi T, Hasagawa I, Tanaka K, Fuzimori R. Evaluation of threatened preterm delivery by transvaginal ultrasonographic measurement of cervical length. Obstet Gynecol. 1993;82:829-32.
9. Zilianti M, Azuaga A, Calderon F, Pages G, Mendoza G. Monitoring the effacement of the uterine cervix by transperineal sonography: A new perspective. J Ultrasound Med. 1995;14:719-24.
10. Lockwood CJ, Senyei AE, Dische MR, et al. Fetal fibronectin in cervical and vaginal secretions as a predictor of preterm delivery. N Engl J Med. 1991;325(10):669-74.
11. Norwitz ER. Progesterone supplementation and the prevention of preterm birth. Rev Obstet Gynecol. 2011;4(2):60-72. PMCID PMC3218546.
12. Alabi-Isam L, Chandiramani M, et al. Time interval from elective removal of cervical cerclage to onset of spontaneous labour. Eur Jobst Gynecol Reprodu Biol. 2012;165(2):235-8.
13. Committee on Practice Buletins-Obstetrics American College of Obstetricians and Gynecologists. Practice bulletin no.130: prediction and prevention of preterm birth. Obstet Gynecol. 2012;120(4):946-73.
14. Defranco E, Atkins KL. Spontaneous preterm Birth, Evans AT, Defranco E (Eds). Manual of Obstetrics, 8th edn. Published by Wolter Kluwr (India) Pvt Ltd, New Delhi. 2014.pp.146.
15. Gyetvai K, Hannah ME, Hodnett ED, Ohlsson A. Tocolysis for preterm labour: a systematic review. Obsetet Gynecol. 1999;94(5pt2):869-77.
16. Flenady V, Wojcieszek AM, Papatsonis DN, Ayock OM, Murray L, Jardine LA, el al. Calcium-channel blockers for inhibiting preterm labour and birth. Cochrane Database Syst Rev. 2014;6:CD002255.
17. King JF, Flenady V, Papatsonis D, Dekker G, Carbonne B. Calcium channel blockers for inhibiting preterm labour. a systematic review of the evidence and a protocol for administration of nifedipine. Aust NZJ Obstet Gynaccol. 2003;43(3):192-8.
18. Duckitt K, Thornton S. Nitric oxide donors for the treatment of preterm labour (Cochrane review). The Cochrane Library. Oxford: Update Software; 2003(1).
19. Souter D, Harding J, McCowen L, O'Donnell C, McLeay E, Baxendale H. Antenatal Indomethacin: adverse fetal effect confirmed. Aust NXJ Obstetrics and Gynaecol. 1998;38(1):11-6.
20. Morales WJ, Smith SG, Angel JL, O'Brien WF, Knuppel RA. Efficacy and safety of indomethacin versus ritsuodrine in the management of preterm labour: a randomized study. Obsetet Gynaecol. 1989;74(4):567-72.
21. Nelson KB, Grether JK. Can magnesium sulfate reduce the risk of cerebral palsy in very low birthweight infants? Pediatrics. 1995;95(2):263-9.
22. Kinney HC. The near-term (late preterm) human brain and risk for periventricular leukomalacia: a review. Semin perinatal. 2006;30(2):81-8.
23. Hutton EK, Hassan ES. Late versus early clamping of the umbilical cord in fill-term neonates: systematic review and meta-analysis of controlled trials. JAMA. 2007;23(297):1241-52.
24. Backs CH, Rivera BK, Haque U, et al. Placental transfusion strategies in very preterm neonates: a systematic review and meta-analysis. Obstet Gynecol. 2014;124:47-56.

Chapter 34

Premature Rupture of Membranes

Jyoti Bindal

Premature rupture of membranes is a significant obstetric problem. It complicates only 2% of pregnancies but is responsible for approximately 30% of all preterm deliveries[1] and causes important perinatal morbidity and mortality, because it is associated with brief latency from membrane rupture till delivery, perinatal infection, and umbilical cord compression caused by oligohydramnios.

The three causes of neonatal death associated with preterm premature rupture of membranes (PPROM) are prematurity, sepsis and pulmonary hypoplasia. Women with intrauterine infection deliver earlier than noninfected women and infants born with sepsis have a mortality four times higher than those without sepsis.[2] In addition, there are maternal risks associated with chorioamnionitis.

DEFINITION

Premature rupture of membranes (PROM) is defined as spontaneous membrane rupture or rupture of chorioamnion that occurs before the onset of labor.

When spontaneous membrane rupture occurs before 37 weeks of gestation, it is referred to as PPROM.

Previable PROM occurs before the limit of viability, i.e. less than 23 weeks of gestation. Preterm PROM remote from term is from viability to 32 weeks of gestation and preterm PROM near term is between 31 and 36 weeks of gestation.

INCIDENCE

Preterm premature rupture of membranes occurs in 3% of pregnancies.[2] Incidence of PROM has been quoted as 2.6–14%.[3]

Amnionitis (13–60%) and clinical abruption placentae (4–12%) occur in PPROM.

PATHOPHYSIOLOGY

PROM is multifactorial in nature. Each of the following factors may cause PPROM through membrane stretch or degradation, local inflammation, or a weakening of maternal resistance to ascending bacterial colonization. This is believed to be related to progressive weakening of the membranes seen with advancing gestation, largely resulting from collagen remodeling and cellular apoptosis. However, in most cases, ultimate cause is unknown.

- Choriodecidual infection or inflammation
- Decreased membrane collagen content
- Increase in amniotic fluid matrix metalloproteases
- Decrease in tissue inhibitors of matrix metalloproteases
- Potential genetic link through polymorphisms for inflammatory cytokines
- Lower socioeconomic status
- Cigarette smoking
- Sexually transmitted infections
- Prior cervical conization
- Prior preterm delivery
- Prior preterm labor in current pregnancy
- Uterine distention (e.g. twins, hydramnios)
- Cervical cerclage
- Amniocentesis
- Vaginal bleeding in pregnancy
- Short cervix
- Positive cervicovaginal fetal fibronectin screen.

Pathologic changes in structure of prematurely ruptured membranes have been documented. There is thinning of the epithelium at the site of rupture with a decrease in its tensile strength. Collagen sheets and fibril bundles are dissolved and replaced by amorphous material signifying disorientation of the extra-cellular matrix.[4]

The amnion is five times stronger than the chorion despite being only one-third as thick. Decidual prolactin may induce osmolality changes in the amniotic fluid. These may effect the viscous component of the membranes.

ETIOLOGY

There are three etiologic subtypes of preterm rupture of membranes. These are:
- Placental (50%)
- Silent infections (38%)
- Immunologic (30%)

Table 34.1: Risk factor for PPROM

- Socioeconomic factors
- Lower socioeconomic class
- Previous PPROM
- Short cervix
- Presence of fetal fibronectin
- Multiple pregnancy
- Intrauterine death
- Genital tract infection or colonization with
  - *Chlamydia trachomatis*
  - *Neisseria gonorrhoeae*
  - Bacterial vaginosis
  - *Trichomonas vaginalis*
  - Group B *Streptococcus*
- *Gardnerella vaginalis*
- Cervical incompetence
- Polyhydramnios
- Fetal abnormalities
- Latrogenic
  Invasive procedures, e.g. amniocentesis, fetal blood sampling

Table 34.2: Clinical risk factors for PROM

Risk factor	Odds ratio
Previous preterm PROM	3.3–6.3
Previous preterm delivery	1.9–2.8
Cigarette smoking	2.1
Bleeding during pregnancy	
During first trimester	2.4
During second trimester	4.4
During third trimester	6.4
More than one trimester	7.4
Acute pulmonary disease	1.8
Bacterial vaginosis	1.5

- Uterine/cervical (14%)
- Miscellaneous (24%)
- True idiopathic (4%).

Causes can be listed **(Tables 34.1 and 34.2)**:
- Idiopathic—40–50%
- Infections—Group B streptococcal infections, bacterial vaginosis
- Cervical incompetence
- Polyhydramnios
- Multiple pregnancy
- *Malpresentations*: Because the presenting part is not fitting against the lower uterine segment
- Low tensile strength of the membranes
- Collagen degradation

- Nutritional deficiency of vitamin C, zinc and copper deficiencies
- Increased intrauterine pressure
- Prenatal diagnostic procedures. Cervical cerclage
- Diet and habits
- Coitus
- Placental pathology
- Genetic disorders
- Maternal smoking
- External cephalic version
- Trauma
- Second and third trimester bleeding.
- Maternal connective tissue disorders (e.g. Ehlers-Danlos syndrome).

PPROM is associated with 40% of cases of preterm labor. As can be seen in table listed below, most of the risk factors for PROM and Preterm labor are common.

DIAGNOSIS

Diagnosis of PROM may be difficult either due to the presence of other fluids in vagina or because there is no fluid.

History (Table 34.3)

- Gush of fluid from vagina (noted in 90% of women with PROM) or moistening is noted in perineum
- Duration of leakage
- Quantity of the discharge
- Type of discharge (clear/blood stained/cream colored/green colored)
- Consistency of the fluid
- Presence of vernix
- Presence and duration of pain
- LMP for period of gestation
- Assessment of fetal movements
- Any history of infections like repeated vaginal examinations elsewhere, *Dais* interference, fever/symptoms of lower genital tract infection/urinary tract infection
- Detailed present and past-obstetric, medical and surgical history.

Physical Examination (Table 34.4)

- *General physical examination*: Hydration of the patient and monitoring of vitals (temperature, pulse, blood pressure and respiratory rate).
- Abdominal examination
  - Confirm the period of gestation by measuring fundal height, which may be small for dates due to drainage of fluid.
  - Look for uterine tenderness to see if chorioamnionitis has set in.
  - Determine fetal lie.
  - Fetal heart sounds to be auscultated.

Table 34.3: Symptoms of PROM

- Uterine activity, e.g. contractions or frequent tightening
- Passage of a show
- Lower abdominal pain or cramping sensation of vaginal discharge
- Vaginal bleeding

Table 34.4: Routine physical examination in PROM

- Routine pulse, temperature, blood pressure measurement and dipstick urinalysis
- Abdominal examination
- Vaginal speculum assessment to assess cervix, membranes status, for swabs taking
- Digital assessment of the cervix may be useful but is not always necessary
- Assess uterine activity and fetal viability—a cardiotocograph (CTG) is ideal for the purpose

Table 34.5: Investigation for PPROM

- Urine for microscopy and culture
- Swabs
  - High vaginal for gram staining and culture
  - Endocervical for *Neisseria gonorrhoeae*
  - Endocervical for *Chlamydia*
  (if genital infection is suspected, urethral and anorectal swabs are indicated)
- Ultrasound examination for fetal assessment and amniotic fluid measurement
- Collected vaginal fluid for
  - Microbiological culture
  - Demonstrate ferning to confirm amniotic fluid
  - Fetal lung maturity studies, e.g. lecithin/sphingomyelin ratio

Other tests
- Amniocentesis to provide uncontaminated amniotic fluid for:
- Microbiological culture (this is the best indicator of chorioamnionitis)
- Fetal lung maturity studies, e.g. lecithin/sphingomyelin ration

- *Local examination*
  - Speculum examination reveals pooling of fluid in vagina.
  - Leaking from the cervical canal may be seen.
  - Leak may be visualized by asking the woman to cough, applying pressure on uterine fundus.
  - After application of vulval pad, patient is asked to ambulate for an hour, soakage on pad is noted.
- *Examination of the collected amniotic fluid* **(Table 34.5)**:
  - *Litmus paper test*: Amniotic fluid is more alkaline than vaginal pH 9 normal vaginal pH is 4.5 and pH of liquor is 7.8. Vaginal secretions containing amniotic fluid turns the litmus paper blue.
  - *Nitrazine paper test*: Nitrazine paper is orange and turns blue when in contact with alkaline amniotic fluid. False positive reactions occur due to alkalization of vagina by blood, semen, soap, antiseptic, infected urine and infection with trichomonas or bacterial vaginosis.
  - *Ferning or arborization test*: A drop of amniotic fluid when placed on a clean slide and allowed to dry demonstrates ferning (microscopic crystallization) on microscopic examination due to the interaction of amniotic fluid proteins and salt. This test has a sensitivity of 96–99%, a specificity of 96–98% and a negative predictive value of 90–99%.
  - *Microscopy of fluid*: The gross presence of specks of vernix caseosa and the microscopic detection of lanugo hair in the fluid from the vagina will confirm the presence of amniotic fluid.
  - *Cytological methods for detection of fetal cells*: Fluorescent microscopy, Papanicolaou smear, staining for lipids in cells: Sudan III, Nile blue sulfate, etc. When amniotic fluid is treated with Nile blue sulfate, fetal cells with a higher fat content take an orange color stain against a blue background. This test is not very reliable in preterm PROM.
- *Special investigations*
  - *Amniocentesis*: In doubtful cases, a dilute solution of 1 ampule of indigo carmine dye is injected into the amniotic fluid and a pad is kept at vulva. A leak of blue fluid in vagina confirms the diagnosis of PROM.
  - *High vaginal swab*: For culture and sensitivity and fetal fibronectin.
  - *Ultrasound*
    - Estimation of gestational age
    - Amount of liquor
    - Fetal presentation, number
    - Estimated fetal weight
    - Placental localization and maturity
- *Complete blood count*: Including hemoglobin, TLC, DLC and if possible, C reactive proteins.
- *Urine examination*: Routine, microscopy and culture.

Signs of Chorioamnionitis

- Fever ≥ 100°F/37.8°C
- Maternal tachycardia (PR > 100 bpm or > 20 bpm above the base line
- Fetal tachycardia
- Uterine tenderness
- Foul odor of amniotic fluid

- Maternal leukocytosis (≥12000–15000/cc and shift to left)
- CRP (if possible)
- Gram stain of amniotic fluid (if possible)
- Biophysical profile (BPP) (if possible)
  - Decreased fetal breathing movements
  - Decreased gross fetal body movement
  - Nonreactive NST.

MANAGEMENT (FLOW CHARTS 34.1, 34.3 TO 34.8)

- Management of chorioamnionitis (**Flow chart 34.2**)
- Routine monitoring of expectant management (**Table 34.6**).

RCOG Guidelines

There is evidence demonstrating an association between ascending infection from the lower genital tract and PPROM. In patients with PPROM, about one-third of pregnancies have positive amniotic fluid cultures[4] and studies have shown that bacteria have the ability to cross intact membranes.

Table 34.6: Routine monitoring in expectant management of PPROM

Maternal markers of infection
- Temperature measurements 4 times a day
- Maternal pulse 4 times a day
- 3 x weekly white cell count
- 3 x weekly C-reactive protein (CRP)
- Daily note of vaginal loss (for detection of purulent discharge)

Fetal well-being
- 2–3 weekly growth scan
- Up to weekly amniotic fluid assessment depending gestation
- Fetal biophysical profile (including CTG) is of limited value in detecting fetal infection.

- Guidelines to achieve the diagnosis of PPROM:
  - The diagnosis of spontaneous rupture of the membranes is best achieved by maternal history followed by a sterile speculum examination.
  - Ultrasound examination is useful in some cases to help confirm the diagnosis.

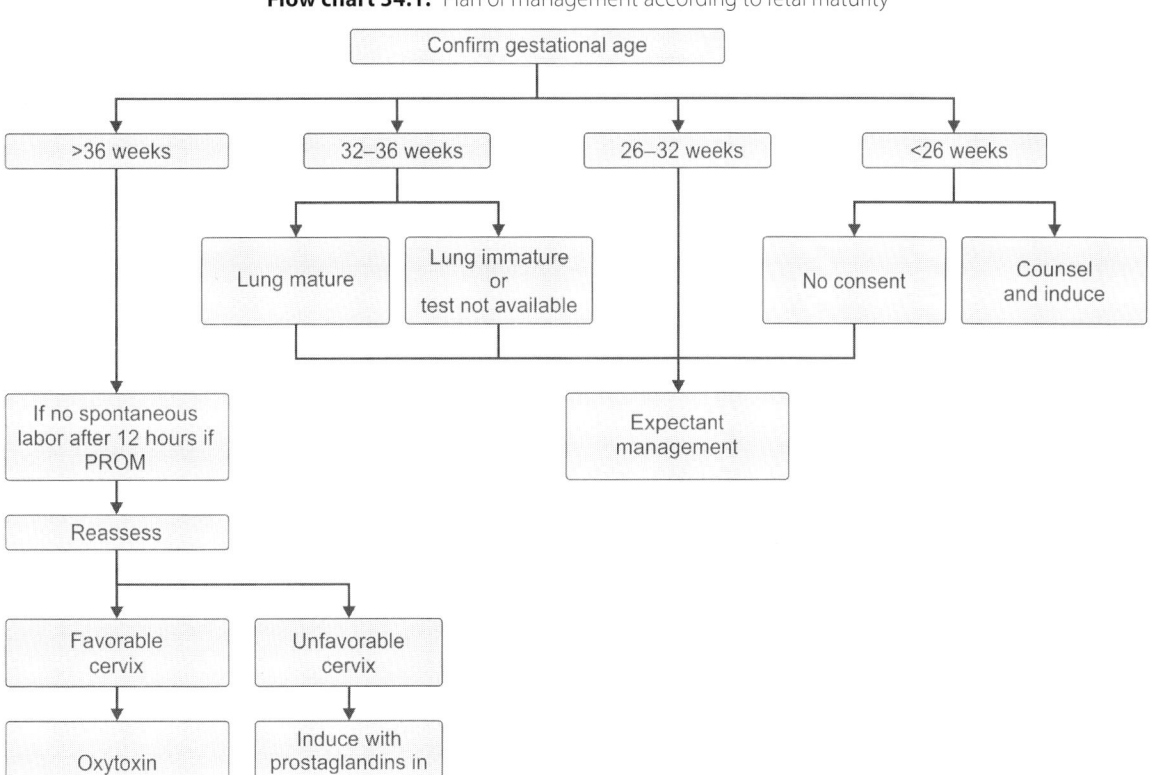

Flow chart 34.1: Plan of management according to fetal maturity

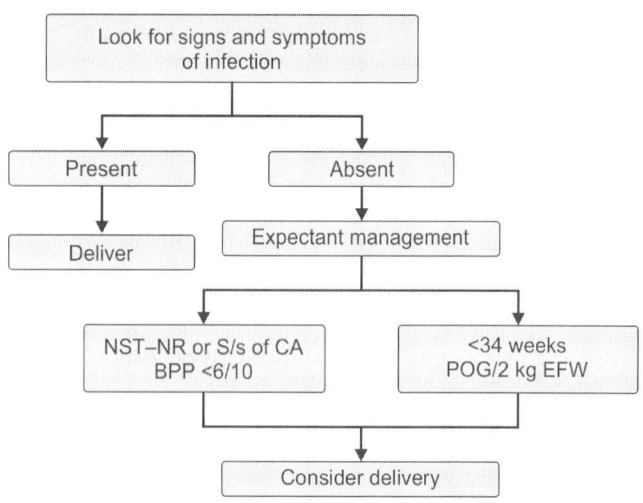

Flow chart 34.2: Management of chorioamnionitis

Abbreviation: POG, poor outcome group

- The presence of a pool of fluid in the vagina at sterile speculum examination is highly suggestive of amniorrhexis.
- A range of tests have been used to confirm membrane rupture; the most widely used has been the Nitrazine test, which detects pH change.
- Other tests which have been used include microscopic examination of the vaginal fluid for the characteristic ferning of the crystalline pattern of dried amniotic fluid owing to its sodium chloride and protein content, examination for lanugo hair, and fetal epithelial cells stained with Nile blue.
- The diagnosis is made by a history suggestive of spontaneous rupture of membranes followed by a sterile speculum examination demonstrating pooling of fluid in the posterior vaginal fornix; a Nitrazine test is not necessary. Digital vaginal examination is best avoided unless there is a strong suspicion that the woman may be in labor. This is because micro-organisms may be transported from the vagina into the cervix leading to intrauterine infection, prostaglandin release and preterm labor. Indeed, a retrospective study reported that the latency interval between spontaneous rupture of membranes and delivery in those who had a digital vaginal examination was significantly shorter than if a sterile speculum examination only was performed.
- Guidelines for antenatal tests to be performed:
  - Women should be observed for signs of clinical chorioamnionitis.
  - Weekly high vaginal swab need not be performed.
  - It is not necessary to carry out weekly maternal full blood count or C-reactive protein because the sensitivity of these tests in the detection of intrauterine infection is low.
  - Cardiotopography is useful and indeed fetal tachycardia is used in the definition of clinical chorioamnionitis. Biophysical profile score and Doppler velocimetry can be carried out, but women should be informed that these tests are of limited value in predicting fetal infection.
- The criteria for the diagnosis of clinical chorioamnionitis include maternal pyrexia, tachycardia, leukocytosis, uterine tenderness, offensive vaginal discharge and fetal tachycardia. During observation, the woman should be regularly examined for such signs of intrauterine infection and an abnormal parameter or a combination of them may indicate intrauterine infection. The frequency of maternal temperature, pulse and fetal heart rate auscultation should be between every 4 and 8 hours.
- Guidelines for the role of amniocentesis:
  - Although there are data documenting an association between subclinical intrauterine infection and adverse neonatal outcome, the role of amniocentesis in improving outcome remains to be determined. There is insufficient evidence to recommend the use of amniocentesis in the diagnosis of intrauterine infection.
  - Intrauterine infection, as defined by positive amniotic fluid cultures, is found in 36% of women with PPROM. Most infections are subclinical without obvious signs of chorioamnionitis.[5] Positive amniotic fluid cultures increase the risks of preterm delivery, neonatal sepsis, respiratory distress syndrome, chronic lung disease, periventricular leukomalacia, intraventricular hemorrhage and cerebral palsy.
- Current evidence suggests that infection is a cause rather than a consequence of amniorrhexis. Amniocentesis has the potential to detect subclinical infection before the onset of maternal signs of chorioamnionitis and before the onset of fetal sepsis, allowing appropriate intervention such as administration of antibiotics in infected cases and/or delivery depending on the gestation, and expectant management for patients with negative amniotic fluid cultures. Rapid tests on amniotic fluid such as Gram stain and assay of cytokines such as interleukins 6 and 18, which indicate intrauterine infection, may be performed.
- Guidelines for prophylactic antibiotics (**Flow chart 34.9**): Erythromycin should be given for 10 days following the diagnosis of PPROM.
- This review shows that routine antibiotic administration reduces maternal and neonatal morbidity. Antibiotic therapy also delays delivery, thereby allowing sufficient time for prophylactic prenatal corticosteroids to take effect. The data also showed that prenatal co-amoxiclav increased the risk of neonatal necrotizing enterocolitis and this antibiotic is best avoided. Erythromycin or penicillin appears the antibiotic of choice. Erythromycin may be used in women who are allergic to penicillin.

Flow chart 34.3: Evaluation and protocol of management of PPROM

```
┌─────────────────────────────────────────────┐
│ Diagnosis confirmed fluid per cervical os   │
│ or vaginal pool with positive Nitrazine or  │
│ ferning test result or Indigo–carmine       │
│ amnioinfusion                               │
└─────────────────────────────────────────────┘
                      │
                      ▼
┌─────────────────────────────────────────────┐
│ Ultrasonography for gestational age,        │
│ growth, anomalies as appropriate            │
│ Cervical cultures; Chlamydia, gonorrhea     │
│ Ano-vaginal cultures; Group B Streptococcus │
│ Urine cultures                              │
│ Initial continuous monitoring for labor,    │
│ fetal distress                              │
└─────────────────────────────────────────────┘
                      │
                      ▼
┌──────────────────────────────┐   Yes   ┌─────────┐   ┌──────────────────────────────┐
│ Amnionitis, abruption        │ ──────▶ │ Deliver │──▶│ Intrapartum group B           │
│ placentae, fetal death,      │         └─────────┘   │ Streptococcus prophylaxis if  │
│ nonreassuring testing, or    │                       │ no recent negative ano-       │
│ advance labor                │                       │ vaginal culture results       │
└──────────────────────────────┘                       │ Broad-spectrum antibiotics    │
              │ No                                     │ if amnionitis                 │
              ▼                                        └──────────────────────────────┘
```

Branches:

- *Previable PPROM:* Less than 23 weeks of gestation
- *PPROM remote from term:* 23–31 weeks of gestation
- *PPROM near term:* 32–33 weeks of gestation
- *PPROM near term:* 34–36 weeks of gestation

Previable PPROM (<23 weeks):
- Initial monitoring for infection, labor, abruption placentae initial bed rest to encourage resealing
- Recounsel
- Induction with oxytocin, PgE2 or misoprostol or Dilatation and evacuation
- Evaluate for persistent oligohydramnios and pulmonary hypoplasia with serial ultrasonograpy
- Recounsel
- If discharged before viability and remains pregnant, readmit at fetal viability for conservative management

PPROM remote from term (23–31 weeks):
- Conservative management
- Serial evaluation for amnionitis, labor, abruption, fetal well-being, growth
- Modified bed rest and pelvic rest to encourage resealing, reduce infection
- Administer corticosteroids and antibiotics (NH protocol), increased or decreased short-term tocolysis
- Deliver for amnionitis, nonreassuring fetal testing, abruption, advanced labor
- Deliver at 34 weeks of gestation if stable until then

PPROM near term (32–33 weeks):
- Documented fetal pulmonary maturity
  - Immature testing or fluid unavailable → No → Consider conservative management for corticosteroid benefit with concurrent antibiotic therapy followed by delivery after 24–48 hours or at 34 weeks of gestation or Expeditious delivery
  - Yes → Expeditious deliver
- Intrapartum group B Streptococcus prophylaxis if no recent negative ano-vaginal culture results
- Broad-spectrum antibiotics if amnionitis

PPROM near term (34–36 weeks):
- Expeditious deliver

- Guidelines for role of antenatal corticosteroids: Antenatal corticosteroids should be administered in women with PPROM.
- Guidelines for using tocolytic agents:
  - Tocolysis in women with PPROM is not recommended because this treatment does not significantly improve perinatal outcome.
    - Prophylactic tocolysis

Flow chart 34.4: Plan of management of PROM

Flow chart 34.6: Management of PROM at term

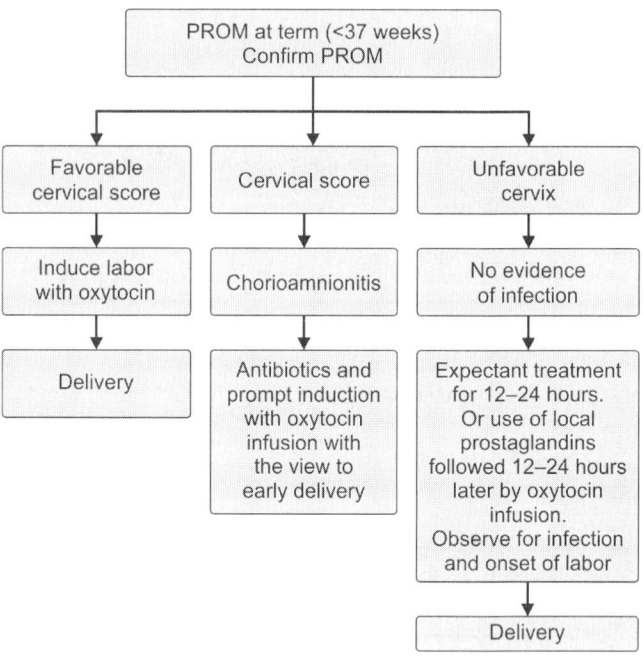

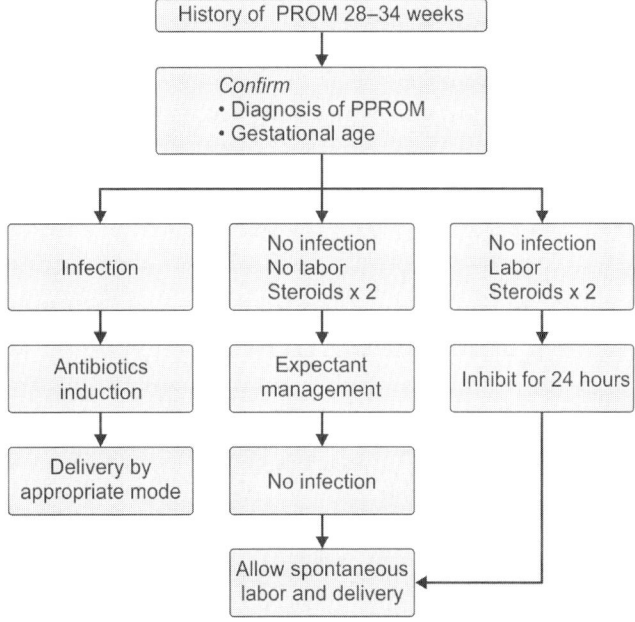

Flow chart 34.5: Management of PROM at 28–34 weeks

- A retrospective case—control study showed that tocolysis after PPROM did not increase the interval between membrane rupture and delivery or reduce neonatal morbidity.
  - Therapeutic tocolysis
- In the absence of clear evidence that tocolysis improves neonatal outcome following PPROM, it is reasonable not to use it. Additionally, with PPROM in the presence of uterine contractions, it is possible that tocolysis could have adverse effects, such as delaying delivery from an infected environment, since there is an association between intrauterine infection, prostaglandin and cytokine release and delivery.
- Guidelines for the appropriate time to deliver the baby:
  - Delivery should be considered at 34 weeks of gestation. Where expectant management is considered beyond this gestation, women should be informed of the increased risk of chorioamnionitis and the decreased risk of respiratory problems in the neonate.
  - The decision to deliver or manage expectantly in cases of PPROM requires an assessment of the risks related to the development of intrauterine infection in those pregnancies managed expectantly compared with the gestational age-related risks of prematurity in pregnancies delivered earlier.
  - Until the results of these trials become available, published data question the benefit of continued expectant management beyond 34 weeks of gestation. There is little evidence that intentional delivery after 34 weeks adversely affects neonatal outcome. There

CHAPTER 34: Premature Rupture of Membranes

Flow chart 34.7: Algorithm for the management of PPROM

```
                        Symptomatic women
                                │
                                │ Clinical assessment
                                ▼
  Expedite delivery by labor    Yes    Is there any indication
  induction, cesarean section ◄──────  for immediate delivery?
                                        │
                                        │ No
                                        ▼
                                   Is PPROM confirmed?  ──No──►  Observe
                                        │                          │
                                        │ Yes              ┌───────┴───────┐
                                        ▼            PPROM confirmed   Symptoms resolved
  • Arrange in utero transfer           
    unless in advance labor    Yes     Are there appropriate        PPROM           Discharge
  • Give corticosteroids,      ◄────── facilities available for    confirmed
  • Tocolyse as if contracting         the preterm infant?
                                        │
                                        │ Yes
                                        ▼                      Cervix >3 cm
  Uncomplicated PPROM    No     Are uterine contractions     ──────────►   In established labor
  what is the gestation? ◄──── present?                                     How advanced is labor?
       │                                                                      │
       │                                                              ┌───────┴───────┐
       ▼                                                             Yes              No
```

16–23 weeks
- Expectant management
- Give a single of corticosteroids at 24 weeks
- Prophylactic erythromycin at 24 weeks (in singletons)
- Limited role for amniotic fluid infusion if severe oligohydramnios
- Deliver electively at 34–36 weeks

24–23 weeks
- Expectant management
- Give corticosteroids
- Prophylactic erythromycin (in singletons)
- Limited role for further course of corticosteroids on a "rescue" basis
- Delivery electively at 34–36 weeks

35–36 weeks
- Give corticosteroids
- Expedite delivery after 24–48 hours of corticosteroids

Established labor
- Give corticosteroids
- No role for tocolysis
- Antibiotic prophylaxis againts of Group B *Streptoccous*

Suspected of early labor
- Give corticosteroids
- Tocolysis
- Prophylactic erythromycin

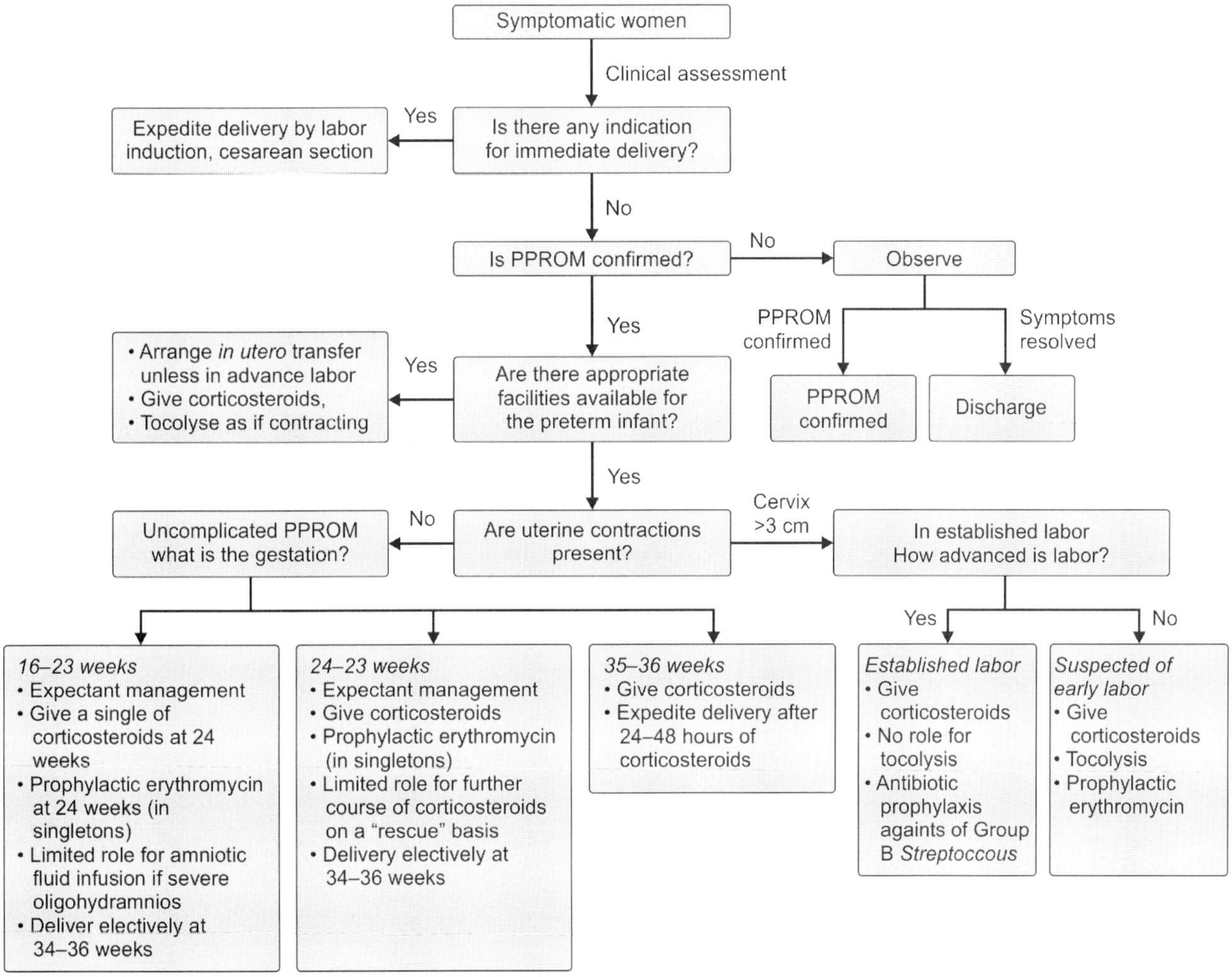

Flow chart 34.8: ACOG vs RCOG protocol for the management of PPROM

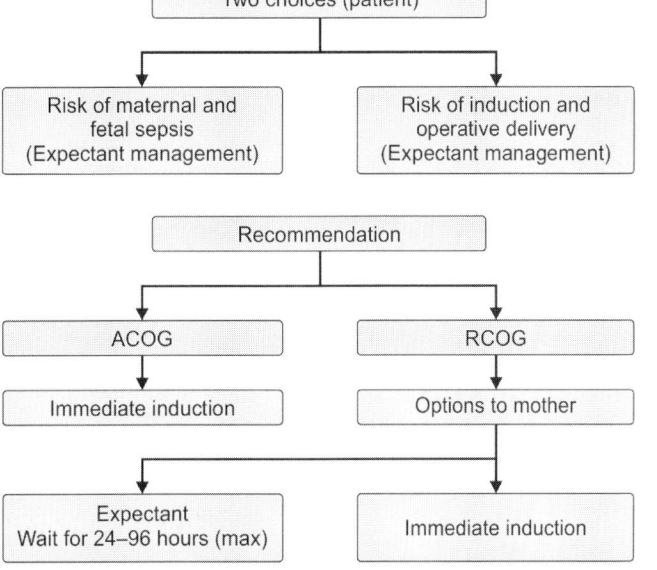

Flow chart 34.9: Antibiotic protocol for the management

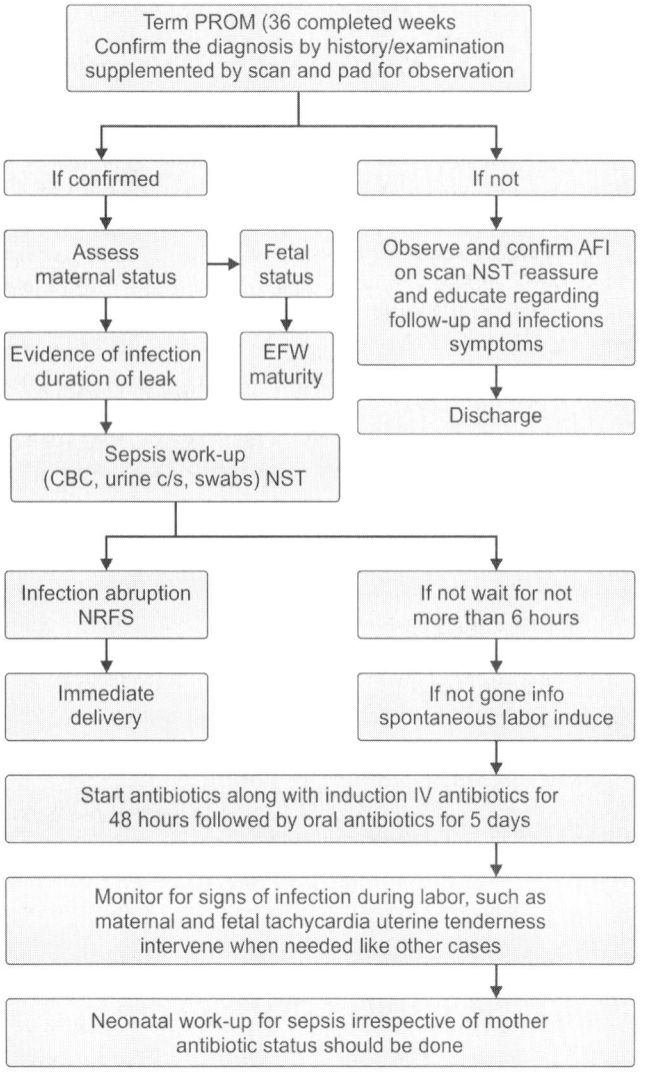

is a suggestion from these studies that expectant management beyond 34 weeks is associated with an increased risk of chorioamnionitis. A longer latency interval with expectant management may allow time for clinical chorioamnionitis, which either is subclinical at the time of membrane rupture or develops with ascending bacterial infection subsequent to membrane rupture.

- A Cochrane review of planned early birth versus expectant management for women with PPROM before 37 weeks of gestation was published in 2010. The conclusion were that there is insufficient evidence to guide clinical practice on the benefits and harms of immediate delivery compared with expectant management.

- Guidelines on women to be monitored at home:
  - There are insufficient data to make recommendations for home and outpatient monitoring rather than continued hospital admission in women with PPROM. The decision to allow the woman home should incorporate the finding that women presenting with PPROM and subclinical intrauterine infection deliver earlier than noninfected patients. It would be considered reasonable to keep the woman in hospital for at least 48 hours before a decision is made to allow her to go home. This method of management should be individualized and restricted to certain women. Women should be instructed to take regular temperature recordings at home every 4–8 hours.

- Guidelines for amnioinfusion in labor:
  - Amnioinfusion during labor is not recommended in women with preterm rupture of membranes.
  - PPROM places the fetus at risk of umbilical cord compression. Amnioinfusion has been described as a method of preventing this complication. Amnioinfusion during labor has been the subject of a Cochrane review, which examined one randomized controlled trial involving 66 women with spontaneous rupture of membranes between 26 and 35 weeks of gestation who received amnioinfusion during labor. The results showed no significant differences between amnioinfusion and no amnioinfusion for cesarean section, low Apgar scores and neonatal death. The implication is that there is insufficient evidence to guide clinical practice concerning the use of amnioinfusion.

- Guidelines for role of transabdominal amnioinfusion in the prevention of pulmonary hypoplasia
  - There is insufficient evidence to recommend amnioinfusion in very preterm PPROM as a method to prevent pulmonary hypoplasia.

- Guidelines for role of fibrin glue in the sealing of chorioamniotic membranes to prevent pulmonary hypoplasia:
  - There is insufficient evidence to recommend fibrin sealants as routine treatment for second-trimester oligohydramnios caused by PPROM.
  - There are publications involving small numbers of women with midtrimester PPROM describing transvaginal or transabdominal injection of fibrin

into the amniotic fluid with the aim of sealing the membranes. The 'amniopatch' resulted in an increase in amniotic fluid volume in some cases. Larger studies are needed examining neonatal outcome before this treatment can be recommended as routine practice.

REFERENCES

1. Arias F, Tomich P. Etiology and outcome of low birth weight and preterm infants. Obstet Gynecol. 1982;60:277.
2. Meis PJ, Ernest JM, Moore ML. Causes of low birth weight births in public and private patients. Am J Obstet Gynecol. 1987;156:1165-8.
3. Lebherz TB, Austin JA. Controversies in Obstetrics and Gynecology Reid DE, Baron TC (Eds). Philadelphia: WB Saunders Company; 1969.
4. Akhter MS, Deacon J, Akhter IA, Wren F, Cumming D, Sharma B. Premature rupture of the fetal membrane. J Obst Gynaecol. India. 1980;30:81-7.
5. Artal R, Sokol RJ, Nessman RJ, et al. The mechanical properties of prematurely and nonprematurely ruptured membranes. Am J Obst Gynecol. 1976;125:655-9.

Chapter 35
Management of Multiple Pregnancy: The Recent Evidence

Sushma Dikhit, Shalini Agrawal

INTRODUCTION

Increasing incidence of multiple gestation seen during recent times[1] has been attributed to due to various factors, such as advanced maternal age, use of ovulation inducing drugs and Assisted Reproductive Techniques.[2] Perinatal morbidity and mortality rates along with preterm delivery rates are, however, higher for twins and triplets than for singletons.[3] The careful management of these pregnancies can, however, help in decreasing the risk of complications.

CLASSIFICATION OF TWIN PREGNANCIES

Dizygotic: These fetuses are from two different ova and have different genetic material. All are dichorionic and diamniotic (DCDA) **(Figs 35.1A and B)**.

- *Monozygotic*: These form from the same ova, however, placentation is more complex and depends upon the time at which the zygotic division occurs after fertilization. This can be:
  - *Dichorionic and diamniotic (DCDA)*: When the zygotic division occurs within 72 hours of fertilization **(Figs 35.1A and B)**.
  - *Monochorionic and diamniotic (MCDA)*: When the zygotic division occurs within 4–8 days of fertilization **(Fig. 35.2)**.
  - *Monochorionic and monoamniotic (MCMA)*: When the zygotic division occurs more than 8 days after fertilization **(Fig. 35.3)**.
  - *Conjoined or siamese twins*: When the zygotic division occurs after 13 days of fertilization **(Fig. 35.4)**.

Complications Associated with Multiple Gestation

- *Maternal antenatal postnatal*
  - Anemia
  - PIH
  - Gestational diabetes
  - Venous thromboembolism
  - Postpartum hemorrhage
  - Failing lactation
  - Postpartum blues and depression
- *Fetal*:
  - Prematurity
  - Intrauterine growth restriction
  - Congenital anomalies
  - Chromosomal disorders
  - Increased neonatal morbidity and mortality.

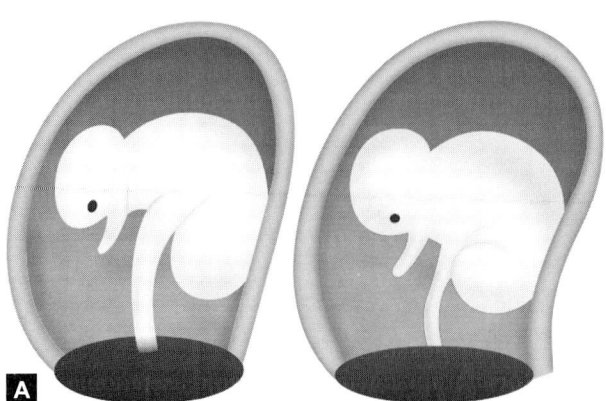 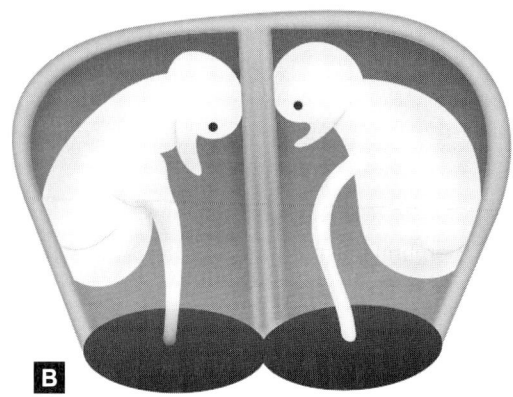

Figs 35.1A and B: (A) Dichorionic and diamniotic placenta; and (B) Fused dichorionic and diamniotic placenta four separating membranes—2 amnion and 2 chorion

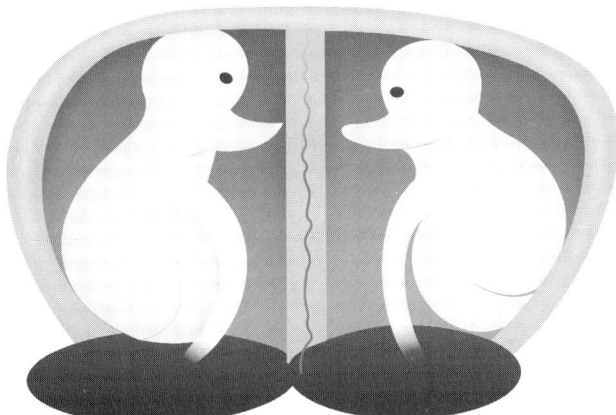

Fig. 35.2: Monochorionic diamniotic placenta—two amnion and one chorion (Dividing membrane)

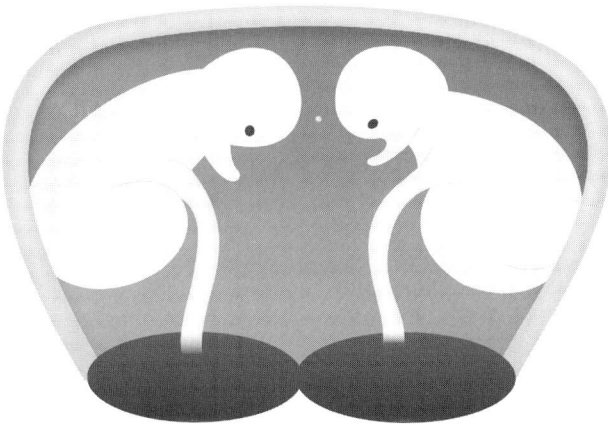

Fig. 35.3: Monochorionic monoamniotic placenta

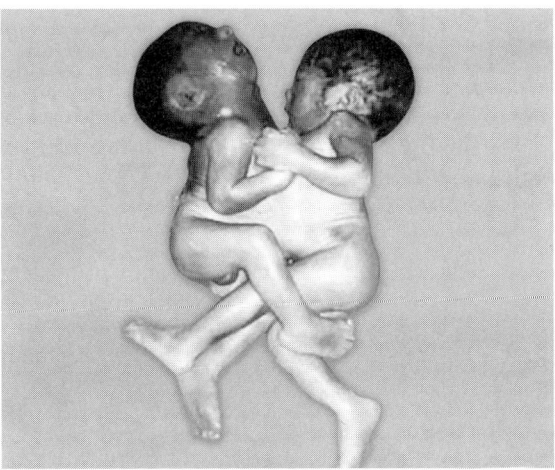

Fig. 35.4: Conjoined twins (monozygotic) *(For color version, see Plate 3)*

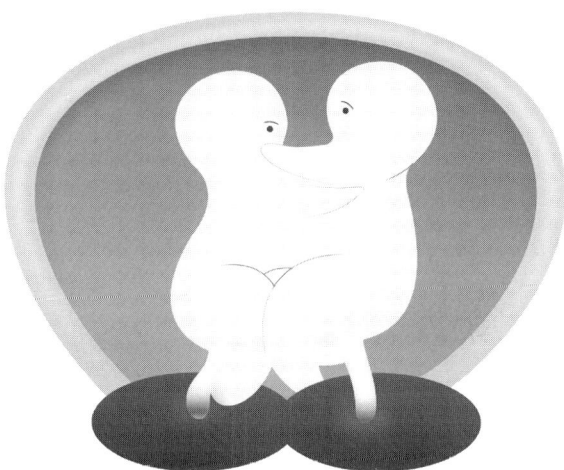

- *Specific complications*: Associated with monochorionic pregnancies—vascular placental anastomoses that connect the umbilical circulations of both twins result in unique complications.
  - Twin–twin transfusion syndrome (TTTS), including twin reversed arterial perfusion (TRAP)
  - The consequences of fetal death to the co-twin
  - Cord entanglement in MCMA pregnancies (1% of twin pregnancies)
- *Long-term consequences*:
  - Cerebral palsy
  - Learning disabilities.

Principles of Management

- Early identification of multifetal gestation, determine accurate gestational age and chorionicity.
- Screening for potential complications, prevention and management
- Growth assessment and regular growth scans
- Counseling of pregnant woman and her family regarding need for additional care, antenatal visits and check-ups.

Determining Gestational Age and Chorionicity

Gestational Age

All pregnant women must be offered an early scan at 6–7 weeks to identify multiple gestation, confirm the gestational age and determine chorionicity. If the pregnant woman reports after this period, ultrasound should be offered when crown–rump length measures from 45 mm to 84 mm (at approximately 11 weeks 0 days to 13 weeks 6 days) to estimate gestational age, determine chorionicity and screen for Down's syndrome. Use the largest baby to estimate gestational age in twin and triplet pregnancies to avoid the risk of estimating it from a baby with early growth pathology.

Chorionicity

- Because of the increased rate of complications associated with monochorionicity, determination of chorionicity by late first trimester or early second trimester in pregnancy is important for counseling and management of women with multifetal gestations.[4]
- Chorionicity is better assessed by ultrasound before 14 weeks than after 14 weeks.
- Determine chorionicity at the time of detecting twin and triplet pregnancies by ultrasound using the number of placental masses, the lambda or twin peak sign in Dichorionic and or T-sign in monochorionic pregnancies and membrane thickness. If it is not possible to determine chorionicity by ultrasound at the time of detecting the twin or triplet pregnancy, seek a second opinion from a healthcare professional who is competent in determining chorionicity by ultrasound scan as soon as possible.
- If it is difficult to determine chorionicity, even after referral (i.e. because the woman has booked late in pregnancy), manage the pregnancy as monochorionic until proved otherwise.
- If transabdominal ultrasound scan views are poor because of a retroverted uterus or a high body mass index (BMI), use a transvaginal ultrasound scan to determine chorionicity.
- Do not use three-dimensional ultrasound scans to determine chorionicity.

Maternal Complications

Anemia

- Check the complete blood count at first antenatal visit and repeat at 20 weeks and further at 28 weeks.[4]
- Educate the woman about the need for additional diet and care in preventing deficiencies.
- Start iron and folic acid supplementation early in second trimester. For those with anemia, investigate to find the cause and treat on priority basis.

Hypertension

Blood pressure and urine for proteinuria should be checked at every antenatal visit to screen for hypertensive disorders. About 75 mg of aspirin should be given daily from 12 weeks until the birth of the babies, if they have one or more of the one or more risk factors for hypertension.[4] These risk factors are; Primigravida, age 40 years or older, pregnancy interval of more than 10 years, BMI of 35 kg/m^2 or more at first visit and family history of pre-eclampsia.

Women with high-order multiple gestations should be queried about nausea, epigastric pain, and other unusual third-trimester symptoms because they are at increased risk to develop HELLP syndrome, in many cases before symptoms of pre-eclampsia have appeared.[5]

Gestational Diabetes

The higher incidence of gestational diabetes in high-order multiple gestations warrants screening and monitoring for this complication.[5]

Fetal Complications

Screening for Chromosomal Anomalies Especially Down's Syndrome

Women should be informed about the increased chance of Down's syndrome in multiple gestations, the various options of screening available, higher false positives, possible need for invasive testing.

Use the combined screening test (nuchal translucency, beta-hCG, PAPP-A) for Down's syndrome between 11 week 0 day to 13 week 6 days. Calculate the risk of Down's syndrome per pregnancy in monochorionic twin and triplet pregnancies. Calculate the risk of Down's syndrome for each baby in dichorionic twin and triplet and trichorionic triplet pregnancies.

Screening for Structural Abnormalities

Offer screening for structural abnormalities in twin and triplet pregnancies as in routine antenatal care by doing a level II USG at 18–20 weeks and fetal echo between 22 and 24 weeks.

Consider scheduling ultrasound scans in twin and triplet pregnancies at a slightly later gestational age than in singleton pregnancies.

Preterm Birth

Predicting the Risk of Preterm Birth

Women with twin pregnancies have a higher risk of spontaneous preterm birth, if they have had a spontaneous preterm birth in a previous singleton pregnancy.[4] However, as per the current evidence, the use of fetal fibronectin testing alone, cervical length (with or without fetal fibronectin) or home uterine activity monitoring should not be used to predict the risk of spontaneous preterm birth in twin or triplet pregnancies.[4,6]

Preventing Preterm Birth

Neither the National Institute for Health and Care Excellence (NICE) nor the American Congress of Obstetricians and Gynecologists (ACOG) recommend the use of bed rest at home or in hospital, intramuscular or vaginal progesterone, cervical cerclage, oral tocolytics (alone or in combination) routinely to prevent spontaneous preterm birth in twin or triplet pregnancies as these have not been proved to decrease neonatal morbidity or mortality.[4,5] In fact, studies demonstrate that cerclage may increase the risk of preterm birth in women with a twin pregnancy and an ultrasonographically detected cervical length less than 25 mm and is not recommended even in these patients.

Use of Tocolytics

Tocolytic agents should be used judiciously in multiple gestations.[5] Beta-mimetics such as Terbutaline, Ritodrine can result in pulmonary edema when used in multiple gestation.

Use of Corticosteroids

Unless a contraindication exists, one course of antenatal corticosteroids should be administered to all patients who are between 24 weeks and 34 weeks of gestation and at risk of delivery within 7 days, irrespective of the fetal number.[4,5]

Do not use single or multiple untargeted (routine) courses of corticosteroids in twin or triplet pregnancies as there is no benefit in using untargeted administration of corticosteroids.[4]

Use of Magnesium Sulphate

Magnesium sulfate reduces the severity and risk of cerebral palsy in surviving infants, if administered when birth is anticipated before 32 weeks of gestation, regardless of fetal number.[6]

Monitoring for Intrauterine Growth Restriction

- Do not use abdominal palpation or symphysis–fundal height measurements to predict intrauterine growth restriction in twin or triplet pregnancies.[4]
- Estimate fetal weight discordance using two or more biometric parameters at each ultrasound scan from 20 weeks. Aim to undertake scans at intervals of less than 28 days and every 2–3 weeks in uncomplicated monochorionic pregnancies from 16 weeks. Consider a 25% or greater difference in size between twins or triplets as a clinically important indicator of intrauterine growth restriction and offer referral to a tertiary level fetal medicine centre.[4]
- Do not use umbilical artery Doppler ultrasound to screen for intrauterine growth restriction or birth weight differences in twin or triplet pregnancies.

Specific Monochorionic Complications

Clinicians and women should be aware that MC twin pregnancies have higher fetal loss rates than DC twin pregnancies, mainly due to second trimester loss and, overall, may have a propensity to excess neurodevelopmental morbidity.[7]

Monitoring for Fetofetal or Twin-to-twin Transfusion Syndrome

Twin-to-twin transfusion syndrome (TTTS) affects identical twins (or higher multiple gestations), who share a common monochorionic placenta. The shared placenta contains abnormal blood vessels, which connect the umbilical cords and circulations of the twins. Depending on the number, type and direction of the connecting vessels, blood can be transfused disproportionately from one twin (the donor) to the other twin (the recipient). The transfusion causes the donor twin to have decreased blood volume, slower than normal growth than its co-twin and poor urinary output causing little to no amniotic fluid or oligohydramnios. The recipient twin becomes overloaded with blood which puts a strain on this baby's heart to the point that it may develop heart failure, and also causes polyhydramnios and hydrops fetalis.

The diagnosis of TTTS is based on ultrasound criteria of the presence of a single placental mass, concordant gender, oligohydramnios with maximum vertical pocket (MVP) less than 2 cm in one sac and polyhydramnios in other sac (MVP>8 cm). Discordant bladder appearances, hemodynamic and cardiac compromise are indicative of severe TTTS.

Start diagnostic monitoring with ultrasound for fetofetal transfusion syndrome from 16 weeks.[7] Repeat monitoring every two weeks until 24 weeks. Carry out weekly monitoring of twin and triplet pregnancies with membrane folding or other possible early signs of fetofetal transfusion syndrome (specifically, pregnancies with intertwin membrane infolding and amniotic fluid discordance) to allow time to intervene, if needed.[7]

The Quintero system of staging TTTS (**Table 35.1**) has some prognostic value but the course of the condition is unpredictable and may involve improvement or rapid deterioration.

There has been controversy about the Quintero staging of TTTS, since stage 1 disease may not necessarily be associated with the best outcomes.[9]

Fetal echocardiography of MC pregnancies at risk of or with TTTS may be more useful in defining the risk of severe TTTS.

Twin–twin transfusion syndrome should be managed in conjunction with regional fetal medicine centers with recourse to specialist expertise. Severe twin–twin transfusion

Table 35.1: The Quintero classification system[8]

Stage	Amniotic volume	Bladder	Doppler studies	Other features
I	MVP<2 cm in one sac and >8 cm in other	Bladder of donor twin visible	Normal	None
II	MVP<2 cm in one sac and >8 cm in other	Bladder of donor twin not visible over the length of examination over 1 hour	Not critically abnormal	None
III	MVP<2 cm in one sac and >8 cm in other	Bladder of donor twin not visible over the length of examination over 1 hour	Critically abnormal in either twin and are characterized as abnormal or reversed end-diastolic velocities in the umbilical artery, reverse flow in the Ductus venosus or pulsatile umbilical venous flow	None
IV	MVP<2 cm in one sac and >8 cm in other	Bladder of donor twin not visible over the length of examination over 1 hour	Critically abnormal in either twin and are characterized as abnormal or reversed end-diastolic velocities in the umbilical artery, reverse flow in the Ductus venosus or pulsatile umbilical venous flow	Ascites, pericardial or pleural effusion, scalp edema or overt hydrops present
V	MVP<2 cm in one sac and >8 cm in other	Bladder of donor twin not visible over the length of examination over 1 hour	Critically abnormal in either twin and are characterized as abnormal or reversed end-diastolic velocities in the umbilical artery, reverse flow in the Ductus venosus or pulsatile umbilical venous flow	One or both babies are dead

syndrome presenting before 26 weeks of gestation should be treated by laser ablation rather than by amnioreduction or septostomy (the deliberate creation of a hole in the dividing septum with the intention of improving amniotic fluid volume in the donor sac).[7]

Some women request termination of pregnancy when severe TTTS is diagnosed and this should be discussed as an option. Another option is to offer selective termination of pregnancy using bipolar diathermy of one of the umbilical cords; with inevitable sacrifice of that baby.[10] There are few data to inform how frequently ultrasound surveillance is required after fetoscopic laser ablation (or amnioreduction). However, some experts advocate that ultrasound examination (with brain imaging, fetal measurement and Doppler assessment) should be performed at least weekly, with consideration given to delivery of the surviving twin(s) at 34 weeks.[11] Often, the mode of delivery at this gestation is by ccsarean section.

Death of a Single Twin

After the single fetal death in a monochorionic pregnancy, the risk to the surviving twin of death or neurological abnormality is of the order of 12 and 18%, respectively. Clinicians should be aware that the risks are much higher than in dichorionic pregnancies and that management of such pregnancies iscomplex.[7] Single fetal death in a monochorionic pregnancy should be referred and assessed in a regional fetal medicine center.

Damage to MC twins after the death of a co-twin is now thought to be caused by acute hemodynamic changes around the time of death, with the survivor essentially hemorrhaging part of its circulating volume into the circulation of the dying twin. This may cause transient or persistent hypotension and low perfusion, leading to the risk of ischemic organ damage, notably but not exclusively, to the brain.

Fetal anemia may be assessed in the surviving twin by measurement of the fetal middle cerebral artery peak systolic velocity using Doppler sonography.

Clinical management is complex and is best overseen by fetal medicine experts. Rapid delivery is usually unwise, unless there are significant cardiotocographic abnormalities or evidence of anemia in the survivor twin. Brain imaging by 4 weeks and earlier by fetal MRI, help in deciding the future course of action including termination of pregnancy.

Management of Conjoined Twins

Conjoined twins are very rare, occurring in around one in 90000–100000 pregnancies worldwide. Antenatal use of ultrasound in all pregnant women helps in diagnosing these cases earlier.

Elective termination of pregnancy, intrauterine death are the common outcomes. B-mode ultrasound, Doppler, color

Doppler and three-dimensional imaging techniques, with detailed assessment of cardiovascular anatomy important for determining prognosis and planning management. The overall individual survival rate to discharge of those attempting pregnancy continuation in a series was about 25%.[12] Most cases are now antenatally diagnosed and delivered by elective cesarean section but vaginal deliveries of conjoined twins are reported. Risk of dystocia and uterine rupture has been reported in association with antenatally undiagnosed cases.

Timing of Delivery

Numerous population-based studies indicate that the nadir of perinatal complications occurs at earlier gestational ages in multiple pregnancies compared with singletons.[13] Twins at 37-38 weeks had stillbirth rates equivalent to post-term singletons.[14]

A rational delivery approach, supported by the 2011 NICHD and SMFM workshop, is to plan elective delivery at 38 weeks in dichorionic pregnancies. In these, prolongation of the pregnancy past 39 weeks is not advisable because of clear risk without any known benefit.

Monochorionic, diamniotic twins: They are at a greater risk for variety of pregnancy complications. Based on these concerns, some experts recommend offering elective delivery at 36-37 weeks in uncomplicated cases.[7]

Most monochorionic, monoamniotic twins have cord entanglement and are best delivered at 32 weeks (RCOG) and 32-34 weeks (ACOG), by cesarean section, after corticosteroids.[7]

If uncomplicated triplets remain undelivered at 36 weeks, elective delivery should be undertaken. Triplet pregnancies that include a monochorionic pair have higher fetal loss rates than dichorionic triplet pregnancies along with higher risk of TTTS and individualized management is required in these cases.

Multiple gestations complicated by maternal or fetal abnormalities will require individualized assessment and decision making.

Mode of Delivery

Twin gestation represents a high-risk intrapartum situation that requires expert management. The variables which decide the mode of delivery include gestational age, chorionicity, fetal weight, fetal position relative to each other, availability of USG machine in the delivery room and capability of monitoring each twin independently during the entire intrapartum period.

Combinations of twin presentation (for DCDA and MCDA) can be classified into three groups:

1. *Twin A vertex and twin B vertex*: A trial of labor is appropriate regardless of age and weight of fetuses. Presentation of 2nd twin may change in 10-20% of cases. For this reason, patient should be counseled and a clear plan for management of an non-vertex 2nd twin must be in place prior to delivery.
2. *Twin A non-vertex and twin B non-vertex*: Nearly, all singleton breech fetuses are delivered by cesarean section nowadays and cesarean delivery is optimal mode of delivery when presenting twin fetus is non-vertex.
3. *Twin A vertex and twin B non-vertex*: In this situation, the route of delivery is subject to significant debate. For 2nd twin, there are three options for vaginal delivery: breech extraction, external cephalic version or internal podalic version. Breech extraction is a preferable option, if fetal weight is >1500 gm. Attending obstetrician should have the skills needed to safely perform vaginal breech delivery. External cephalic version is associated with more fetal distress and higher rate of cesarean section for second twin than breech extraction.

For monochorionic (MCDA) twins, it is appropriate to aim for vaginal birth unless there are specific indications of cesarean.[7] Discussion with mother should take place at 32-34 weeks of pregnancy about mode of delivery and intrapartum management.

Most monochorionic, monoamniotic twins have cord entanglement and are best delivered at 32 weeks (RCOG) and 32-34 weeks (ACOG), by cesarean section, after corticosteroids.[6,7]

Women with one previous low transverse cesarean delivery, who are otherwise appropriate candidates for twin vaginal delivery, may be considered candidates for trial of labor after cesarean delivery (VBAC).[6]

Triplets: Monitoring of three fetuses throughout labor is challenging. As a result, elective cesarean delivery of patient with 3 or more live fetuses of viable gestational age is a reasonable management strategy.

Intrapartum Management of Twin Vaginal Delivery

Safe vaginal delivery of multiples requires multidisciplinary co-operation between obstetrics, anesthesia, nursing and neonatology. On admission for delivery, fetal presentation, weight of the fetuses should be confirmed by USG. Both fetuses should be monitored throughout the labor. The delivery is best performed in OT, as anesthesia or cesarean may be urgently needed.

The administration of neuraxial analgesia in women with multifetal gestations facilitates operative vaginal delivery, external or internal cephalic version, and total breech extraction and is recommended.[6]

Time Interval Between Deliveries

After delivery of first twin, uterine inertia may develop, umbilical cord of 2nd twin can get prolapsed, non-reassuring CTG may develop, cervix can close and placental abruption may render the 2nd twin hypoxic. Some 2nd twins may require rapid delivery, others can be safely followed with FHR surveillance and remain undelivered for substantial period of time. Many reports have suggested that the interval between deliveries should ideally be 15 minutes or less and not more than 30 minutes.

Postpartum Care

Prevention and Management of PPH

Careful watch for postpartum hemorrhage (PPH), active management of third stage, prophylactic use of Misoprost 600 µg, especially in low resource settings are a must, as overdistended uterus is more prone for postpartum hemorrhage. Availability of blood must be ensured prior to taking up these patients for delivery.

Problems with Lactation

Inadequate milk production, difficulty in breastfeeding two babies together are some of the issues affecting mothers of multiple pregnancy. Counseling the mothers, constant encouragement, teaching correct feeding techniques such as the double football and double cradle position along with judicious use of galactagogues such as domperidone and metoclopramide will help in overcoming these problems.[15]

Postpartum Mental Health Issues

Caring for twins and triplets can be challenging for a young mother. Most investigations that compared mental health outcomes in parents of multiples versus parents of singletons found that parents of multiples experience heightened symptoms of depression, anxiety, and parenting stress.[16] Mothers of multiple births have been found to have 43% greater odds of having moderate/severe, 9-month postpartum, depressive symptoms, compared with mothers of singletons.[17] Awareness of mental health issues, counseling the mother with her family and early recognition of the signs and symptoms such as excessive crying, difficulty in sleeping, feeling anxious, guilty, panic attacks, etc. are important in managing these problems.

Venous Thromboembolism

Multiple pregnancy is a risk factor for venous thromboembolism (VTE). Presence of one more risk factor such as elective cesarean, age more than 35, pre-eclampsia, preterm delivery warrants postpartum prophylaxis for 10 days with low molecular weight heparin.[18] Early ambulation and avoidance of dehydration is a must to lower the risk of VTE.

Primary Prevention

Multiple gestation pregnancy rates are high in assisted reproductive treatment cycles because of the perceived need to stimulate excess follicles and transfer excess embryos in order to achieve reasonable pregnancy rates. Since the goal of infertility therapy is a healthy child, and multiple gestation puts that goal at risk, multiple pregnancy must be regarded as a serious complication of assisted reproductive treatment cycles. If there are more than three mature follicles, the cycle should be converted to an IVF cycle, or it should be cancelled and intercourse should be avoided. In IVF cycles two embryos can be transferred without reducing birth rates in most circumstances. In the United States, physicians and patients jointly decide how many embryos to transfer. However, in England, no more than two embryos may be transferred in most cases. In Canada, a maximum of three embryos are recommended for transfer.

Embryo reduction involves extremely difficult decisions for infertile couples and should be used only as a last resort. Women who underwent pregnancy reduction from triplets to twins, as compared with those who continued with triplets, were observed to have lower frequencies of pregnancy loss, antenatal complications, preterm birth, low-birth-weight infants, cesarean delivery, and neonatal deaths, with rates similar to those observed in women with spontaneously conceived twin gestations.[6]

Indications for Referral to a Tertiary Level Fetal Medicine Center

Seek a consultant opinion from a tertiary level fetal medicine centre for:
- Monochorionic monoamniotic twin pregnancies
- All triplet pregnancies
- Pregnancies complicated by any of the following: Discordant fetal growth, fetal anomaly, discordant fetal death, fetofetal transfusion syndrome.

REFERENCES

1. Martin JA, Park MM. Trends in twin and triplet births: 1980-97. Natl Vital Stat Rep. 1999;47(24).
2. http://sogc.org/publications/multiple-birth/
3. Blondel B, et al. Am J Public Health. 2002;92(8):1323-30.
4. National Collaborating Centre for Women's and Children's Health. Multiple pregnancy: The management of twin and triplet pregnancies in the antenatal period. London (UK): National Institute for Health and Clinical Excellence (NICE). 2011;38.p. (Clinical guideline; no. 129).
5. Multiple gestation: complicated twin, triplet, and high-order multifetal pregnancy. American College of Obstetricians and

Gynecologists (ACOG). Multiple gestation: complicated twin, triplet, and high-order multifetal pregnancy. ACOG; 2004;15. p. (ACOG practice bulletin; no. 56).

6. Multifetal gestations: twin, triplet, and higher-order multifetal pregnancies. American College of Obstetricians and Gynecologists (ACOG). Multiple gestation: twin, triplet, and high-order multifetal pregnancy. ACOG; 2004;15.p. (ACOG practice bulletin; no. 144).

7. Management of monochorionic twin pregnancy. RCOG green-top guideline no. 51 December 2008

8. Quintero RA, Morales WJ, Allen MH, Bornick PW, Johnson PK, Kruger M. Staging of twin-twin transfusion syndrome. J Perinatol. 1999;19:550-5.

9. Ville Y. Twin-to-twin transfusion syndrome: time to forget the Quintero staging system? Ultrasound Obstet Gynecol 2007;30:924-7.

10. Taylor MJ, Shalev E, Tanawattanacharoen S, Jolly M, Kumar S, Weiner E, et al. Ultrasound-guided umbilical cord occlusion using bipolar diathermy for Stage III/IV twin-twin transfusion syndrome. Prenat Diagn. 2002;22:70-6.

11. Consensus views arising from the 50th Study Group: Multiple Pregnancy. In: Kilby M, Baker P, Critchley H, Field D (Eds). Multiple pregnancy. London: RCOG Press; 2006. p. 283-6.

12. Agarwal U, Dahiya P, Khosla A. Vaginal birth of conjoined thoracopagus: a rare event. Arch Gynecol Obstet. 2003;269:66-7.

13. Steven G Gabbe, et al. Obstetrics: Normal and Problem Pregnancies, 6th edn.

14. Sairam S, et al. Prospective risk of still birth in multiple gestation pregnancies: a population-based analysis. Obstet Gynecol. 2002;100:638.

15. O Flidel-Rimon, et al. Breast feeding twins and high multiples. Arch Dis Child Fetal Neonatal Ed. 2006;91(5):F377-80.

16. Wenze SJ1, Battle CL, Tezanos KM. Raising multiples: mental health of mothers and fathers in early parenthood. Arch Womens Ment Health. 2015;18(2):163-76. doi: 10.1007/s00737-014-0484-x. Epub 2014 Dec 18.

17. Choi Y, Bishai D, Minkovitz CS.Pediatrics. 2009;123(4):1147-54. doi: 10.1542/peds.2008-1619.

18. Reducing the risk of venous thromboembolism during pregnancy and the puerperium. RCOG Green-Top Guideline 37a.

Chapter 36

Teenage Pregnancy: A Global Issue

Shruti Agrawal, Nisha Sahu

Teenage pregnancy is a global issue. Interestingly, teenage pregnancy is one of the few issues that connect the east with the west, albeit in shades of negativity. Even developed nations such as the United States are facing the same big problem of teenage pregnancy. But, there is a sharp difference in terms of the reason, why teenagers get pregnant in more modernized societies such as the United States and in developing nations such as India. While in developing nations such as India, early marriages are to be blamed primarily for early pregnancies; while in the United States, maximum teenage pregnancies occur out of unplanned sexual activity—an issue which is gradually gripping the Indian urban teenagers as well.

A RISING ISSUE

Pregnancies that occur below the age of 20 years are called as teenage pregnancies.[1,2] It is notable that the age of women, at the time of giving birth, is taken into consideration and not at the time of conception. Adolescent childbearing has a negative impact on three major dimensions: health of the adolescent and their infants, individual social and economic effects, and societal-level impacts.

About 16 million adolescent girls aged 15–19 give birth each year,[3] roughly 11% of all births worldwide and 4.4 million have abortions. Almost, 95% of these births occur in developing countries.

Evidence in developing world indicates that one-third to one-half of women become others within 19 years of age, making pregnancy-related causes as leading cause of death.[4] Relatively, the situation in South Asian countries is severe as there are higher proportion of teenage pregnancies in this region due to the common practice of early marriage and social expectations to have a child soon after marriage.[5,6]

Evidence further indicates that nearly 60% of all girls are married by the age of 18 years and one-fourth are married by the age of 15 years in South Asia,[7] whereas within South Asia, the recorded teenage pregnancy rate is highest in Bangladesh (35%), followed by Nepal (21%) and India (21%).[8]

Data show that globally 5,29,000 women die every year due to pregnancy- and childbirth-related complications,[3] and this risk increases greatly as maternal age decreases with adolescents under 16 years facing four times the risk of maternal death as women over 20 years.[9] The outcomes are influenced by biological immaturity, unintended pregnancy, inadequate perinatal care, poor maternal nutrition and stress. Long-term follow-up studies have shown that the children born to teenage mothers are at higher risk and are usually plagued by intellectual, language and social economic delays.

FACTORS INFLUENCING ADOLESCENT PREGNANCY AND CHILDBIRTH

- *Declining age of menarche:* The age of menarche has declined, especially in urban areas.
- Duration of education and societal demands—in rural areas, marriages still occur very early for young girls. They are then pushed into early motherhood because of societal demands and pressure. Women with little or no education also have lack of access to information and contraceptive services, and hence may soon become pregnant.
- *Early initiation of sexual activity is on the increase:* Possibly because of influence of media, cross-cultural influences, decreased supervision by adults (nuclear families, migration) more opportunities, etc. This coupled together with ignorance, further increases the magnitude of the problem.
- *Socioeconomic factors:* Risky sexual behaviors are more likely to occur in poor families and among those with single parents. Teens who focus on academic activities and are more involved religiously are less likely to experience teen pregnancy. Involvement in religious activities is one of the strongest factors related to delayed sexual activity.
- Lack of access to information and to contraceptive services has a significant bearing on early pregnancy and childbirth. Adolescent pregnancy tends to be highest in areas with the lowest contraceptives prevalence. Contraceptive prevalence has increased mostly among older, married women and not adolescents.

Potential Behavioral Patterns for a Teenage Girl Becoming Pregnant

- Early dating behavior
- High-risk behavior (smoking, alcohol and substance abuse)
- Peer pressure
- Lack of support group or few friends
- Unhealthy environment at home
- Stress and depression
- Delinquency/criminal behavior
- Exposure to domestic and sexual violence
- And most important, financial constraints

COMPLICATIONS

Complications of pregnancy and childbirth that occur more commonly in adolescents than in adults

- Pregnancy-induced hypertension
- Anemia during antenatal period
- HIV—higher incidence of mother to child transmission.
- Higher severity of malaria
- Preterm birth
- Obstructed labor
- Anemia during postpartum period
- Pre-eclampsia
- Postpartum depression
- Too early repeat pregnancies
- Low birth weight
- Parenteral and neonatal mortality
- Inadequate child care and breastfeeding practices

Problems in Antenatal Period

- Pregnancy-induced hypertension (PIH)—studies report an increased incidence of the condition in young adolescents, compared to older women.
- *Anemia:* There is an increased risk of anemia in adolescents, because of nutritional deficiencies, especially of iron and folic acid and by malaria and intestinal parasites. Being in the growing age herself, her body has special nutritional need and when pregnancy occurs, it is a strain on already depleted reserves, especially if she belongs to a low socioeconomic background.
- *STIs/HIV:* Sexually active adolescents are at an increased risk of contacting STIs, including HIV infection, owing to their biological and social vulnerability. The presence of other STDs (syphilis, gonorrhea and *Chlamydia*) with local inflammation may increase viral shedding and recently contracted HIV (with high viral load), may increase the risk of mother to child transmission during labor.
- Higher severity of malaria is a common cause of anemia in this group.
- Vitamin deficiencies are more common.

Problems during Labor and Delivery

- Preterm birth is common in women under twenty years of age because of immaturity of the reproductive organs, social factors such as poverty at play. Biologically, an adolescent's body is still developing and not yet ready to take on an added strain.
- *Obstructed labor in young girls (below 15 years of age):* Pelvic bones do not reach their maximum size until about the age of 18, therefore, the pelvis of the teenage mother may not have grown enough to allow vaginal delivery of a normal-size baby. For this reason, the incidence of cesarean section is higher in teenage mothers.
- Lack of access to medical and surgical care—can result in complications like vesicovaginal and rectovaginal fistulae and other birth injuries like cervical, vaginal and perineal tears and lacerations.

Problems in the Postpartum Period

Anemia is common and further aggravated by blood loss during delivery, thereby also increasing the risk of infection.

Eclampsia—studies report an increased incidence among young adolescents.

Postpartum depression and mental health problems are common as the young girl may not be mentally prepared for motherhood with all its responsibilities.

Too early repeat pregnancies because of difficulty in accessing reliable contraception.

Problems Affecting the Baby and Impact of Teenage Pregnancy on the Child

- Since the teenage mother is herself in the growing phase and since she is less likely to eat correctly during pregnancy her baby often has a low birth weight, making it more likely that the baby will become ill.
- Babies born to teenage mothers are more likely to die in the first year of life, compared to babies born to mothers older than 20 years of age. Hence, the high perinatal and neonatal mortality in developing countries.
- Early motherhood can affect the psychosocial development of the infant. Children born to teenage mothers are less likely to receive proper nutrition, healthcare and cognitive and social stimulation. As a result, they are at risk for lower academic achievement. Also, they are at increased risk for abuse and neglect. In short, developmental disabilities

and behavioral issues are increased in children born to teenage mothers.

Consequences of Pregnancy and Childbirth in Adolescent Girls

- Married
  - More likely to seek and receive ANC
  - May access safe MTP services
  - Chronic ill health and depression due to complications during pregnancy labor and childbirth.
- Unmarried
  - Less likely to seek and receive ANC
  - May resort to illegal and unsafe abortion practices.
  - Guilt and depression due to social stigma.
  - Chronic ill health and infertility due to complications during abortion.

CARE OF THE ADOLESCENTS DURING PREGNANCY, CHILDBIRTH AND THE POSTNATAL PERIOD

Adolescent pregnancies and deliveries require much more care than adult pregnancies and all efforts must be made to reduce the occurrence of problems. This includes early diagnosis of pregnancy, effective antenatal care, effective care during labor and delivery and during the postpartum period (**Flow chart 36.1**).

Early Diagnosis of Pregnancy

Healthcare worker and family members should create a conducive environment for the adults in which she feels able to share information about her pregnant situation, especially if she is unmarried. By ensuring early diagnosis of pregnancy, care is started early and complications are avoided.

Antenatal Care

At least four antenatal checkups are recommended for all pregnant women under the RCH programme. The antenatal period provides us with a valuable opportunity for the provision of information and counseling. It also provides us with a golden opportunity for the prevention, early diagnosis and treatment of complications.

Anemia, malaria and pregnancy-induced hypertension can be timely detected and treated early. In case of more serious complications (such as pre-eclampsia, eclampsia and abruption placentae) referral to a hospital is essential.

Since adolescents are more at risk of STIs, including HIV/AIDS, voluntary counseling and testing services should be made available to them and timely treatment should be delivered.

Iron and folic acid supplementation and tetanus toxoid immunization should always be taken care of.

Counseling should also include care of the newborn, including exclusive breastfeeding and prevention of an early repeat pregnancy, by accessing reliable and timely contraceptive services.

Management of Labor and Delivery

- Hospital delivery should always be encouraged and timely arrangement for transportation to an equipped center should be made.
- If the pregnancy in an adolescent is normal and with no complications and anemia treated adequately, labor starts at term, and the infant is in cephalic presentation, then the labor is not at increased risk, but as such, the teenage pregnancy is always a high-risk pregnancy.
- Besides observing and monitoring, continuous empathetic support by a technically qualified nurse or midwife is essential.

Postpartum Care

- This includes prevention, early diagnosis and treatment of postnatal complication in the mother and her baby.

Flow chart 36.1: Role of the health sector regarding pregnancy in adolescents girls

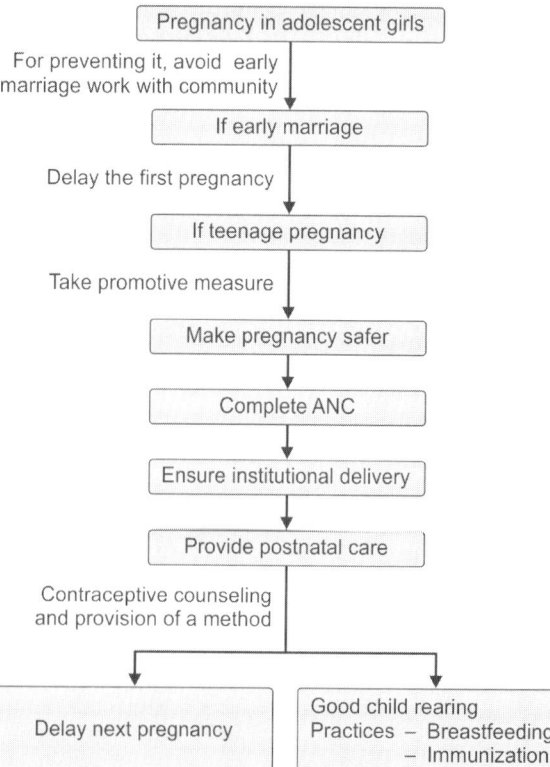

- Information and counseling on breastfeeding, nutrition, contraception and care of the baby is essential.
- Family counseling is vital and provides a lifeline to the adolescent mother and her baby.

PREVENTION

As healthcare professional: The most important role of physicians is to be proactive and ask all teenaged patients about sexual activity, sexual health issues and also inquire about the contraceptive used. Also abortion counseling and referral should be provided when needed.

Parents, schools and healthcare professionals can have open, honest and educational talks with teenagers and pre-teenagers. The teenagers should be advised to prevent unwanted pregnancies and also contraceptive counseling.

INITIATIVES BY FOGSI

In this context, it is apt to mention the "Growing-up" program. Initiated through the FOGSI in partnership with Johnson & Johnson (J&J), the program educated school girls on menstruation, its myths hygiene and sexual issues.

'Let's talk'—is another program initiated by the FOGSI for the college-going students, and it educates women about the various forms of contraception.

The need of the hour is that we should all join our hands together for a fight against "Motherhood in Childhood."

REFERENCES

1. Chedraui P, Hidalgo L, Chavez M, Glenda SM. Determinant factors in Ecuador related to pregnancy among adolescent aged 15 or less. Journal of Perinantal Medicine. 2004;32:337-41.
2. Lawlor DA, Shaw M. Teenage pregnancy rates: high compared with where and when? Journal of the Royal Society of Medicine. 2004;97:121-3.
3. WHO. Facts and figures form the World Health Report. 2005. Geneva: World Health Organization 2005 [*http://www.who.jnt/whr/2005/media_ centre/facts_en.pdf*] Accessed 15/12/2008.
4. Viegas OA, Wiknsosastro G, Sahagun GH, Chaturachinda K, Ratnam SS. Safe childbirth needs more than medical services, World Health Forum. 19921;13:59-65.
5. Adhikari R. Early marriage and childbearing: risk and consequences. Geneva: World Health Organization, 2003 [*http://apps.who.int/reproductive-health/pulications/towards_adulthood/7.pdf*], accessed on 02/02/2011.
6. Stone N, Ingham R, Simkhada P. Knowledge of sexual health issue among unmarried young people in Nepal. Asia Pacific Population Journal. 2003;18:33-54.
7. Mehra S, Agrawal D. Adolescent health determinants for pregnancy and child health outcomes among the urban poor. Indian Pediatrics. 2004;41:137-45.
8. Acharya DR, Bhattarai R, Poobalan A, Van TE, Chapman G. Factors associated with teenage pregnancy in South Asia: a systematic review. Health Science Journal. 2010;4:1-13.
9. Population References Bureau. The world's youth. Washington DC: Population References Bureau: 2000 [*http://www.prb.org/pdf/WorldsYouth_Eng.pdf*].

Chapter 37

Obesity and Pregnancy

Bharati Dhorepatil

Globally, approximately 2.3 billion adults are overweight and more than 700 million adults are obese, as projected by the World Health Organization (WHO).[1] Many low-income countries are affected by rising levels of obesity. India has the world's second-largest population and its economy is growing rapidly with urbanization, industrialization, and changes in lifestyle—all of which predispose to obesity and other health-related conditions associated with it. Despite this, the overall prevalence of overweight adults in India is low and that of undernutrition is high, with obesity most common among women in urban and high-socioeconomic status groups.[2] National Family Health Surveys in India indicated an increase in obesity from 10.6% in 1998–1999 to 14.8% in 2005–2006.[3] Obese women are at increased risk of pregnancy-related complications, including subfertility, early spontaneous abortion, pre-eclampsia, and gestational diabetes mellitus (GDM), and are more likely to require instrumental and/or cesarean delivery than women of a normal weight.[4] Although there are several published reports from India on obesity in both adolescents and the general population, none exists on the prevalence of maternal obesity and risk of adverse perinatal outcome in the country. But as obesity becomes more common in the general population, it is not surprising that the prevalence of obese pregnant women is on the rise globally.

Obesity during pregnancy is not without consequences, and obesity-related complications are an important burden for obstetrical care providers.

DEFINITION OF OBESITY

The most common and objective way to classify obesity is by body mass index (BMI) (defined as kg/m^2) with the following definitive zones:

> *Currently recommended cut-offs of BMI by WHO[1]*
> *Normal:* 18.5–24.9 kg/m^2
> *Overweight:* 25.0–29.9 kg/m^2
> *Obesity:* 30 kg/m^2

> *Consensus meeting statement based on various studies all over India[5]*
> Normal BMI: 18.5–22.9 kg/m^2
> Overweight: 23.0–24.9 kg/m^2
> Obesity in Indians: 25 kg/m^2

Although calculating BMI may be the best method for measuring adiposity, it is not without limitations. Body fat distribution, an independent predictor of health risk, is not accounted for when calculating BMI, nor is body composition. Therefore, some muscular individuals, such as athletes, may be misclassified as obese using BMI alone.

The goal of recommendations for weight gain in pregnancy based on BMI **(Table 37.1)** is the full-term delivery of a live infant with birth weight between 3000 g and 4000 g.[6]

EFFECTS OF OBESITY ON FERTILITY AND EARLY PREGNANCY

Fertility

Obesity is associated with several reproductive disturbances.[8] Body weight influences the timing of menarche and the capacity to achieve pregnancy.[9] Early reproductive dysfunction among obese women includes precocious menarche, irregular menstrual cycles, oligomenorrhea and amenorrhea, and chronic anovulation. A U-shaped relationship between body weight and fertility has been described.[9] Excess body mass has an independent and deleterious effect on fertility, even after controlling for confounding factors such as maternal age.[10] Among obese women, subfertility is often related to ovulatory dysfunction,[11] likely because of the effect of obesity on many neuroendocrine and ovarian functions.[12] Moreover, obesity creates a state of sex hormone imbalance that is not favorable for reproduction. The negative effect of obesity on fertility in general also influences the success of assisted reproductive technology. Although some studies report that clinical pregnancy and

Table 37.1: Optimal weight gain in pregnancy

Maternal pre-pregnancy weight (BMI)	Weight gain			
	Total (lbs)	Rate (lbs/wk)*	Total (kg)	Rate (kg/wk)*
Underweight (<19.8 kg/m²)	24–40	1.25	12.7–18.2	0.575
Normal weight (19.8–26.0 kg/m²)	25–35	1.00	11.4–15.9	0.45
Overweight (26.1–29.0 kg/m²)	15–25	0.70	8.8–11.4	0.3
Obese (>29.0 kg/m²)	15	0.50	6.8	0.225
Twin gestation	35–45	1.50	15.9–20.4	0.675

*In second and third trimester
Adapted from: American College of Obstetricians and Gynecologists.[129]

delivery rates after IVF or ICSI are not affected by obesity,[13-15] the evidence in support of a negative effect on IVF and ICSI success rates is stronger.[16-20] Obese women undergoing IVF require higher doses of exogenous gonadotropins to achieve superovulation[21-23] and have fewer oocytes retrieved.[24,25] There is also a direct relationship between BMI and the risk of miscarriage[26] with a progressively increasing risk in overweight, obese, and very obese groups (adjusted OR 1.29, 1.71, and 2.19, respectively).[26] One of the largest cohort studies examining the success rate of IVF determined that women with a BMI > 27 kg/m² had significantly lower delivery rates (OR 0.67) than women with a BMI 20 kg/m² to 27 kg/m², and that a BMI > 27 kg/m² reduced the chance of a live birth in the first IVF cycle by 33%.[27]

Early Pregnancy

Obesity has been identified as an independent risk factor for miscarriage in women receiving fertility treatments.[28] However, reports on the risk of miscarriage in obese women who conceive naturally are scarce and contradictory.[29-31] In a recent case-control study, the risks of early miscarriage (at 6–12 weeks of gestational age) and recurrent early miscarriage were significantly higher among obese women (OR 1.2 and 3.5, respectively).[29] Further research is needed regarding the association between obesity and miscarriage in naturally conceived pregnancies.

ANTEPARTUM COMPLICATIONS

Gestational Diabetes Mellitus

In the general population, obesity is strongly related to the risk of T2DM,[6] and obese women are more likely to have pre-existing T2DM at the time of conception.[32-34] A similar trend is described in the literature for obesity and the risk of developing GDM; after excluding pre-existing T2DM, numerous studies have shown a significantly increased risk of GDM in overweight and obese women.[7,30,35-42]

A retrospective cohort study of 2,87,213 completed singleton pregnancies in the United Kingdom found that overweight and obese women were significantly more at risk of GDM (OR 1.68 and 3.6, respectively).[34] In Canada, a retrospective cohort study of 603 First Nations women showed even greater risks of GDM among overweight and obese women (OR 3.86 and 8.32, respectively).[43]

The pathophysiologic mechanisms underlying the development of GDM include an inadequate insulin response coupled with maternal pre-pregnancy insulin resistance.[44] In an attempt to prove causality, Villamor et al.[45] examined the association between change in prepregnancy BMI from the first to the second pregnancy and the risk of adverse outcomes during the second pregnancy in a nationwide Swedish study of 1,51,025 women. Women whose BMI increased by more than 3 kg/m² between pregnancies had twice the risk of GDM regardless of their initial weight.[45] Even a weight gain of 10 lbs between pregnancies has been shown to increase the risk of GDM in obese women (OR 1.47).[46]

Hypertensive Disorders

Hypertensive disorders are more prevalent among pregnant women who are obese,[36-38,47-54] and excessive maternal BMI has been identified as an independent risk factor for developing hypertensive disorders of pregnancy.[33,55-58] Pregnant women who are obese are more likely to have pre-existing hypertension at the time of conception.[32,34] Moreover, they are at significantly greater risk of developing hypertension during pregnancy, with odds ratios that vary from 2.01 to 7.93 in women with a BMI > 30 kg/m².[31,35]

Obesity is also strongly associated with the development of pre-eclampsia.[39,42,59] In their meta-analysis of 13 cohort studies, O'Brien et al. demonstrated that the risk of pre-eclampsia typically doubled if BMI increased by 5 kg/m² to

7 kg/m^2; this increased risk persisted after adjustment for confounders and exclusion of chronic hypertension and diabetes.[60] In a prospective cohort study of 3480 women with morbid obesity (BMI > 40 kg/m^2), 12,698 women with a BMI of 35 kg/m^2 to 40 kg/m^2, and 5,35,900 women of normal weight (BMI 19.8–26 kg/m^2), the risk of pre-eclampsia was found to be four times greater in obese women and almost five times greater in the morbidly obese.[61] A similar risk of pre-eclampsia was found in overweight and obese First Nations women in Canada.[43] The risk of pre-eclampsia is not related to the current maternal weight. Indeed, regardless of their pre-pregnancy weight, women whose BMI increased by more than 3 kg/m^2 between pregnancies have a two-fold risk of developing pre-eclampsia in the subsequent pregnancy.[45]

The mechanism behind this increased risk of pre-eclampsia in obese women is unknown. Other than mediation through syndromes of metabolic derangement associated with obesity,[62] current theories involve C-reactive protein, which may share a common pathway to pre-eclampsia with high BMI.[62] Important mediators of the association between increased BMI and pre-eclampsia may include inflammation and increased serum triglyceride levels before 20 weeks' gestation.[63]

Thromboembolism

A significant association between the risk of venous thromboembolism and body weight in pregnant women weighing 90 to 120 kg (OR 2.17) and women weighing more than 120 kg (OR 4.13) has been reported in a large Canadian population-based cohort study.[39]

Antepartum Infections

Women who are overweight or obese have an increased risk of various infections, especially urinary and genital tract infections, during the antepartum period.[34] These women are also at increased risk of pyrexia of unknown origin.[34] Chorioamnionitis is also more likely in overweight and obese women.[48,50]

Preterm Delivery

Publications regarding the risk of preterm birth in overweight and obese women show conflicting data. Several retrospective cohort studies have described an increased risk of delivery at less than 32 weeks' gestation in obese women,[38,50,61] but others have found no difference [32,35,39,47] or even a decreased risk.[33,34] A population-based Cohort Study in the United States found that, compared with lean women, women with a BMI of greater than 30 kg/m^2, had 1.6 times the risk of delivering prematurely; this risk remained significant after adjusting for antenatal complications.[36] Contrasting results were found in a population-based cohort analysis in the United Kingdom, which showed that women with an increased BMI were less likely than women of normal weight to deliver at less than 32 weeks' gestation.[34]

Multiple Pregnancy

An increased incidence of twin pregnancy in women with increased BMI has recently been reported in two large studies.[64,65] In one of these studies, a significantly greater risk of twinning (OR 1.44) was noted in[43,48] obese women not reporting fertility treatment.[65] In the Collaborative Perinatal Project, which studied 51,783 pregnancies (of which 561 were twins) pre-dating the use of fertility drugs, a significantly greater incidence of dizygotic but not monozygotic twins was found among obese women.[64] The relationship between increased BMI and the incidence of twinning may be related to increased levels of FSH in obese women.

INTRAPARTUM COMPLICATIONS

Labor

In a Canadian cohort study, 35 women with a BMI > 25 kg/m^2 were found to have a shorter duration of labor than those with a BMI < 25 kg/m^2. Conversely, in a study of nulliparous women, the rate of cervical dilatation was inversely associated with maternal weight: for each 10 kg increment in weight, the rate of dilatation decreased by 0.04 cm/hour.[66] Similarly, the duration of labor was positively associated with maternal weight.[66] In this study, neither lower rates of oxytocin administration to heavier women nor diminished uterine responsiveness accounted for the slower progress of labor. Buhimschi et al. studied intrauterine pressure during the second stage of labor and found that although women with a BMI >30 kg/m^2 had a longer active phase, the duration of the second stage was similar among all BMI groups.[67] More specifically, they found no significant differences in uterine contractility between obese women, overweight women, and women of normal weight.[67] Thus, the poor progress of labor that seems to be associated with obesity is more likely due to disturbance of active phase function rather than poor progression in the second stage. In a large retrospective population-based study, obese women were found to be more likely to present with failure to progress in the first stage of labor than their normal weight counterparts, but there was no difference in the duration of the second stage.[30]

Reports describing the augmentation of labor with oxytocin in obese gravidas are limited and conflicting. In a study of 1,42,404 pregnancies in Nova Scotia, no association between obesity and augmentation of labor was noted.[39] However, in a prospective study focusing on the second stage of labor in obese women, Buhimschi et al. determined that gravidas with a BMI >25 kg/m^2 were more likely to need augmentation using oxytocin.[67]

Induction of Labor

Several studies have shown that obesity is associated with the need for induction of labor.[30,31,34,61] This association appears to remain significant after adjustment for complications of pregnancy such as hypertension and diabetes.[39] Furthermore, obese gravidas have been found to be at greater risk of having a failed induction.[18] For each 10 kg increase in body weight, an increase of 0.3 hours in the interval from oxytocin administration to delivery was observed in nulliparous women.[68]

Vaginal Birth after Cesarean Section

Obesity decreases the odds of women succeeding at VBAC,[69-76] and it is an independent risk factor for failed trial of labor after a primary CS.[77,78] In a study involving over 28,000 women, the rate of failed trial of labor increased from 15% in women of normal weight to 22% in overweight women, 30% in obese women, and 39% in morbidly obese women.[74] Moreover, morbidly obese women were at significantly greater risk of uterine dehiscence and rupture, composite morbidity, and neonatal injury.[74]

Operative Vaginal Delivery

An increased BMI does not appear to increase the risk of requiring an operative vaginal delivery.[35,37,39,50,67,79] In the North West Thames study in the UK, the odds ratios for operative vaginal delivery among overweight and obese women were 1.04 and 0.95, respectively.[34] In another UK population-based cohort analysis, obese parturients had a greater risk of failure during an instrumental delivery, although they were not at increased risk of requiring an assisted vaginal delivery.[80] It seems, however, that the risk of operative vaginal deliveries increases in women who are severely obese (BMI > 35 kg/m^2) or morbidly obese (BMI > 40 kg/m^2).[42,61]

Rate of Cesarean Section

Delivery by CS has been shown to occur more frequently in obese women.[30,40-42,51,61,79-81] The association between excessive BMI and the need for CS is independent of other factors such as maternal height and age, primiparity, macrosomia, and maternal diabetes.[82,83]

The indication for CS in obese women is most often cephalopelvic disproportion[35,84] and failure to progress in labor.[83,85] It has been speculated that obese women may have suboptimal uterine contractility or increased fat deposition in pelvic soft tissues.[34]

Obese women not only undergo CS more frequently than women of normal weight but also are at greater risk for intrapartum and postoperative complications such as longer operating time, increased blood loss, and endometritis.[34,69,86] Wound infections are also more common in obese women.[87-89] This association remains significant even when the procedure is elective and prophylactic antibiotics are administered.[87] It remains unclear whether the reapproximation of subcutaneous tissue and/or the use of subcutaneous drains is useful in preventing postoperative infection. Two recent studies found that subcutaneous drains were not effective in preventing infection in obese women[90,91]; however, one small study found that the use of a drain in women with more than 2 cm of subcutaneous fat may help in reducing wound infection.[92] In a meta-analysis of the value of suture closure of the subcutaneous dead space in preventing wound complications after CS, suture closure resulted in a 34% decrease in the risk of wound disruption in women with a fat thickness greater than 2 cm.[93]

Another area of concern in obese women undergoing CS is anesthesia management. A Canadian Study of over 1,40,000 pregnancies identified a significant increase in anesthesia complications in women weighing more than 120 kg.[39] Airway management and the insertion of regional nerve blocks are technically difficult in these women, and the incidence of failed intubation is greater than in women of normal weight.[86] Although the failure rate of initial insertion of an epidural catheter is high and multiple attempts are often necessary, these challenges should not prevent the use of epidural anesthesia in obese parturients. Other practical factors to be considered include the weight-bearing capacity of operating tables, the availability of suitable equipment, and the availability of sufficient personnel for safe transfer. Because of these issues, evaluation of obese pregnant women by an anesthesiologist before labor is recommended.

FETAL COMPLICATIONS

Stillbirth and Intrauterine Fetal Death

Maternal obesity is associated with a greater risk of both intrauterine fetal death and stillbirth. In their review of the etiology and prevention of stillbirth, Fretts et al. identified obesity as one of 15 independent risk factors for stillbirth.[94]

The risk of fetal death, particularly late and unexplained fetal demise, increases with rising BMI.[95-97] A maternal BMI of greater than 29 kg/m^2 or a weight greater than 68 kg has been associated with unexplained fetal death.[98,99] The magnitude of the risk is difficult to determine, but the risk may be as much as tripled.[100]

No single cause of death seems to predominate in the higher mortality of the infants of obese women, although more stillbirths are caused by unexplained intrauterine death and fetoplacental dysfunction in obese women than in women of normal weight.[100,101]

Large-for-gestational-age Babies and Macrosomia

Pre-pregnancy obesity and excessive weight gain during pregnancy have been identified as key factors in determining infant birth weight.[102] Infants born to obese women are significantly more likely to weigh more than 4000 g[32,33,40,41,103] or more than 4500 g.[35,42] Moreover, obesity has been identified as an independent risk factor for macrosomia, even with adjustment for diabetes.[104,105] This association has also been observed among First Nations Women in Canada.[43]

In a Swedish cohort, the prevalence of macrosomia increased by 23% between 1991 and 2001.[106] Contributing factors likely include increased insulin resistance (even in non-diabetic women) and higher plasma triglyceride levels.[34,107] Triglycerides can be cleaved by placental lipases, thereby transferring free fatty acids to the fetus.[34,107] The combination of increased energy-rich fatty acid delivery and fetal hyperinsulinemia caused by amino acid stimuli can account for increased birth weight.[34,107]

After adjusting for fetal macrosomia, maternal obesity is not an independent risk factor for shoulder dystocia.[108,109] Nonetheless, in a recent retrospective cohort study, deliveries complicated by shoulder dystocia were more likely to be associated with neonatal injury in obese women than in women of normal weight.[110] Despite the fact that obesity may not be directly causative, shoulder dystocia remains an important complication of deliveries in obese women, and obstetrician should be prepared to manage such a complication.

Fetal Distress and Resuscitation

The evidence suggesting that maternal obesity is a risk factor both for fetal distress and for requiring resuscitation at birth is controversial. Many studies describe a lack of association between maternal obesity and low Apgar scores or low umbilical cord pH.[40,47,52,80] Others have shown an increased risk of cord pH < 7.15 and Apgar score <7 at 5 minutes.[50,61] Respiratory distress and a need for resuscitation including mechanical ventilation appear more likely to occur in infants of obese parturients.[31,37]

Admission to NICU

While two prospective Cohort studies have indicated that infants born to obese mothers are not at increased risk of requiring NICU admission,[40,52] more recent evidence suggests the opposite. Indeed, several large retrospective cohort analyses, including the North West Thames Study,[34] found children of obese parturients to be at greater risk of requiring NICU admission than those born to women of normal weight.[33,41,103] This risk increased as BMI rose.[37,50] A Canadian cohort study of over 18,000 pregnancies revealed that women with BMI >3 25 kg/m^2 were more likely to have their newborn admitted to the NICU (OR 1.21 for BMI 25–29.9 kg/m^2; OR 1.60 for BMI 31–39.9 kg/m^2; and OR 2.89 for BMI >40 kg/m^2).[35] Requirements for an incubator and tube feeding have also been reported to be increased in infants born to mothers with a BMI > 30 kg/m^2.[80] Unfortunately, most studies do not specify the reasons for NICU admission; therefore, it is difficult to explain how maternal obesity influences the infant's need for admission to NICU. In fact, many confounding factors, such as the presence of maternal diabetes, could explain this observation.

Neonatal Death

Several cohort analyses show an increased risk of death in the neonatal period in infants born to obese mothers.[36,50,61] Strikingly, a pre-pregnancy BMI >30 kg/m^2 has been associated with a risk of neonatal death more than double that of infants born to women of normal weight, even after adjusting for confounding factors such as smoking and alcohol intake.[100] However, this finding was not confirmed in two independent retrospective studies.[35] More research is needed to clarify this relationship and the mechanism behind it; until then, obese parturients and their newborns should be followed closely.

Congenital Anomalies

There is increasing evidence to support an association between maternal obesity and congenital malformations, particularly neural tube defect (NTD) and cardiac malformations. The risk of spina bifida in the offspring of obese gravidas has been found to be 2 to 3 times greater than in the infants of women of normal weight.[111-113] In a retrospective Canadian cohort trial, there was a significant increase in the rate of NTD according to weight increments.[114] For each 10 kg increase in maternal weight, the odds ratio of NTD increased by 1.2. Obese women appear to have a substantially increased risk of delivering a baby with anencephaly.[115] Odds ratios for NTD become greater when the joint effects of maternal obesity and gestational diabetes are present, which provide evidence for interaction on a multiplicative scale.[115] Hyperinsulinemia has been identified as a strong risk factor for NTD and may account for most of the observed risk in obese women, but even after adjustment for hyperinsulinemia, obesity continues to be a modest risk factor.[111] It has been suggested that obesity and diabetes mellitus may act synergistically in the pathogenesis of such anomalies.[116] Measures to prevent NTD (i.e., folic acid supplementation) may also lack efficacy. It is possible that folic acid supplementation in obese women does not reduce the risk of NTD to the same extent as in women of normal weight because of poor absorption and higher metabolic demand.[107] Fetal cardiac anomalies, especially septal defects, also appear to occur more frequently when the mother is obese.[117-119] The Atlanta Birth Defects Risk Factor Surveillance Study found that obese women were at greater risk of having offspring with heart defects, omphalocele, and multiple anomalies.[113]

Finally, while some studies found an increased risk of oralfacial clefting in the babies of obese women,[120] others have not confirmed this finding.[121] The mechanism behind the relationship between maternal obesity and congenital anomalies is unknown, but is likely related to an alteration of the nutritional environment provided for the developing fetus.[102] Possible alterations include increased serum insulin, triglycerides, uric acid, and endogenous estrogens;[113] other theories suggest increased insulin resistance, chronic hypoxia, and hypercapnia as possible mechanisms.[107] Another possible explanation is that women who are obese have a higher incidence of diabetes, which is a known risk factor for birth defects.[116] Nevertheless, the relationship between obesity and congenital anomalies persists even when women with known diabetes are excluded[117] or after adjustment is made for diabetes.[111] Women who are obese may be more likely than women of normal weight to have poor quality diets, which could lead to nutritional deficits that increase the risk for congenital anomalies.[113]

It is imperative to counsel obese mothers regarding these risks, especially given the difficulties encountered with sonographic visualization of the fetus in obese women. Obese women overall are at greater risk than women of normal weight to have poor fetal visualization, and this risk increases with greater degrees of obesity.[122] For example, women with a BMI of 30 kg/m² to 35 kg/m² have 2.4 times the risk of suboptimal ultrasound scans of fetal cardiac structures compared with women of normal weight; women with a BMI 35 kg/m² to 40 kg/m² have 5 times the risk and women with a BMI >40 kg/m² have 8 times the risk. The risk of suboptimal visualization of craniospinal structures is also greater in obese women.[122]

POSTPARTUM COMPLICATIONS

Maternal Mortality

There is little available information on the risk of maternal mortality in obese women. Both Sheiner et al.[30] and Raatikainen et al.[50] found in retrospective cohort analyses that pregnant women with a BMI > 30 kg/m² were at increased risk of mortality. The findings of these authors are supported by the report of the Confidential Enquiry on Maternal and Fetal Death, conducted in the United Kingdom between 2000 and 2002. This report identified obesity as one of eight risk factors for maternal death.[123] Thirty-five percent of all women who died were obese, which is a significantly greater proportion than in the general population. Thirty-five percent of all women who died were obese, whereas only 23% of women of reproductive age in the general population were obese at the time of the study.

Postpartum Hemorrhage

Several recent large cohort studies have reported that as a woman's BMI rises, there is an increased risk of postpartum hemorrhage (PPH).[31,35,39,80] In the North West Thames study, the incidence of PPH was 30% higher in overweight women and 70% higher in obese women.[34] Similarly, Cedergren et al. reported that morbidly obese women were almost twice as likely as women of normal weight to have a PPH.[61] Proposed reasons for the association between obesity and PPH include increased bleeding from a larger area of placental attachment because of macrosomia[34] and reduced bioavailability of uterotonic agents arising from the relative increase in volume of distribution associated with obesity.[102]

Breastfeeding

The association between obesity and excessive weight gain during pregnancy and the likelihood of initiation and duration of breastfeeding has been recently examined in retrospective cohort studies. These found that women with a BMI > 30 kg/m² were significantly less likely to initiate breastfeeding and more likely to discontinue sooner than their normal weight counterparts.[124-126] Although the exact reason for the association between poor breastfeeding and obesity is unclear, it has been suggested that it may be endocrine in nature. Indeed, overweight and obese women appear to have a decreased prolactin response to suckling; in turn, this would reduce the ability to produce milk and would ultimately lead to failure of lactation.[127] A delay in lactogenesis may be another reason for failure to initiate breastfeeding in obese women.[128] It has also been postulated that breast morphology might be a barrier to breastfeeding: obese women tend to have larger breasts and areolas, as well as flat nipples, and this may make it difficult for the baby to latch on.[128]

Overweight and obese women should be referred to a lactation consultant in order to optimize breastfeeding techniques.

CONCLUSION

Obesity causes significant complications during pregnancy for the mother and fetus. Interventions promoting pre-pregnancy weight loss and the prevention of excessive weight gain during pregnancy must begin in the preconception period. Obstetrical care providers need to counsel their obese patients about the risks and complications conferred by obesity and the importance of weight loss before pregnancy. Surveillance may need to be heightened during pregnancy, and a multidisciplinary approach to the management of obese women during pregnancy is useful. Women need to be informed about both maternal and fetal complications and about the measures that are necessary to optimize outcome. However, no measure has greater consequences than addressing the weight issue before pregnancy.

REFERENCES

1. World Health Organization. Obesity and overweight. Factsheet 311. *www.who.int. www.who.int/mediacentre/factsheets/fs311/en/index.html*. Published. 2006. Updated 2011.
2. Wang Y, Chen HJ, Shaikh S, Mathur P. Is obesity becoming a public health problem in India? Examine the shift from under- to overnutrition problems over time. Obes Rev. 2009;10(4):456-74.
3. International Institute for Population Sciences. Key Indicators for India from NFHS-3. *www.nfhsindia.org. http://www.nfhsindia.org/pdf/India.pdf*. Published. 2006. Accessed 2011.
4. Cedergren MI. Maternal morbid obesity and the risk of adverse pregnancy outcome. Obstet Gynecol. 2004;103(2):219-24.
5. National Task Force on the Prevention and Treatment of Obesity. Overweight, obesity, and health risk. Arch Intern Med. 2000;160:898-904.
6. Subcommittee on Nutritional Status and Weight Gain during Pregnancy. Nutrition during pregnancy. Washington: Institute of Medicine, 1990.
7. Lu GC, Rouse DJ, DuBard M, Cliver S, Kimberlin D, Hauth JC. The effect of the increasing prevalence of maternal obesity on perinatal morbidity. Am J Obstet Gynecol. 2001;185:845-9.
8. Pasquali R, Pelusi C, Genghini S, Cacciari M, Gambineri A. Obesity and reproductive disorders in women. Hum Reprod Update. 2003;9:359-72.
9. Davies MJ. Evidence for effects of weight on reproduction in women. Reprod Biomed Online. 2006;12:552-61.
10. Wang JX, Davies M, Norman RJ. Body mass and probability of pregnancy during assisted reproduction treatment: retrospective study. BMJ. 2000;321:1320-1.
11. Rich-Edwards JW, Spiegelman D, Garland M, Hertzmark E, Hunter DJ, Colditz GA, et al. Physical activity, body mass index, and ovulatory disorder infertility. Epidemiology. 2002;13:184-90.
12. Pasquali R, Gambineri A. Metabolic effects of obesity on reproduction. Reprod Biomed Online. 2006;12:542-51.
13. Dechaud H, Anahory T, Reyftmann L, Loup V, Hamamah S, Hedon B. Obesity does not adversely affect results in patients who are undergoing in vitro fertilization and embryo transfer. Eur J Obstet Gynecol Reprod Biol. 2006;127:88-93.
14. Dokras A, Baredziak L, Blaine J, Syrop C, VanVoorhis BJ, Sparks A. Obstetric outcomes after in vitro fertilization in obese and morbidly obese women. Obstet Gynecol. 2006;108:61-9.
15. Spandorfer SD, Kump L, Goldschlag D, Brodkin T, Davis OK, Rosenwaks Z. Obesity and in vitro fertilization: negative influences on outcome. J Reprod Med. 2004;49:973-7.
16. Cano F, Landeras J, Mollá M, Gomez E, Ballesteros A, Remohí J. The effect of extreme of body mass on embryo implantation at oocytes donation program. Fertil Steril. 2001;76:S160-S161.
17. Loveland JB, McClamrock HD, Malinow AM, Sharara FI. Increased body mass index has a deleterious effect on in vitro fertilization outcome. J Assist Reprod Genet. 2001;18:382-6.
18. Nichols JE, Crane MM, Higdon HL, Miller PB, Boone WR. Extremes of body mass index reduce in vitro fertilization pregnancy rates. Fertil Steril. 2003;79:645-7.
19. vanSwieten EC, van der Leeuw-Harmsen L, Badings EA, van der Linden PJ. Obesity and clomiphene challenge test as predictors of outcome of in vitro fertilization and intracytoplasmic sperm injection. Gynecol Obstet Invest. 2005;59:220-4.
20. Carrell DT, Jones KP, Peterson CM, Aoki V, Emery BR, Campbell BR. Body mass index is inversely related to intrafollicular hCG concentrations, embryo quality and IVF outcome. Reprod Biomed Online. 2001;3:109-11.
21. Dodson WC, Kunselman AR, Legro RS. Association of obesity with treatment outcomes in ovulatory infertile women undergoing superovulation and intrauterine insemination. Fertil Steril. 2006;86:642-6.
22. Fedorcsak P, Dale PO, Storeng R, Ertzeid G, Bjercke S, Oldereid N, et al. Impact of overweight and underweight on assisted reproduction treatment. Hum Reprod. 2004;19:2523-8.
23. Frattarelli JL, Kodama CL. Impact of body mass index on in vitro fertilization outcomes. J Assist Reprod Genet. 2004;21:211-5.
24. Fedorcsak P, Storeng R, Dale PO, Tanbo T, Abyholm T. Obesity is a risk factor for early pregnancy loss after IVF or ICSI. Acta Obstet Gynecol Scand. 2000;79:43-8.
25. Wittemer C, Ohl J, Bailly M, Bettahar-Lebugle K, Nisand I. Does body mass index of infertile women have an impact on IVF procedure and outcome? J Assist Reprod Genet. 2000;17:547-52.
26. Wang JX, Davies MJ, Norman RJ. Obesity increases the risk of spontaneous abortion during infertility treatment. Obes Res. 2002;10:551-4.
27. Lintsen AM, Pasker-de Jong PC, de Boer EJ, Burger CW, Jansen CA, Braat DD, et al. Effects of subfertility cause, smoking and body weight on the success rate of IVF. Hum Reprod. 2005;20:1867-75.
28. Bellver J, Rossal LP, Bosch E, Zuniga A, Corona JT, Melendez F, et al. Obesity and the risk of spontaneous abortion after oocyte donation. Fertil Steril. 2003;79:1136-40.
29. Lashen H, Fear K, Sturdee DW. Obesity is associated with increased risk of first trimester and recurrent miscarriage: Matched case-control study. Hum Reprod. 2004;19:1644-6.
30. Sheiner E, Levy A, Menes TS, Silverberg D, Katz M, Mazor M. Maternal obesity as an independent risk factor for caesarean delivery. Paediatr Perinat Epidemiol. 2004;18:196-201.
31. Doherty DA, Magann EF, Francis J, Morrison JC, Newnham JP. Pre-pregnancy body mass index and pregnancy outcomes. Int J Gynaecol Obstet. 2006;95:242-7.
32. LaCoursiere DY, Bloebaum L, Duncan JD, Varner MW. Population-based trends and correlates of maternal overweight and obesity. Utah 1991-2001. Am J Obstet Gynecol. 2005;192:832-9.
33. Kumari AS. Pregnancy outcome in women with morbid obesity. Int J Gynaecol Obstet. 2001;73:101-7.
34. Sebire NJ, Jolly M, Harris JP, Wadsworth J, Joffe M, Beard RW, et al. Maternal obesity and pregnancy outcome: a study of 287,213 pregnancies in London. Int J Obes Relat Metab Disord. 2001;25:1175-82.
35. Abenhaim HA, Kinch RA, Morin L, Benjamin A, Usher R. Effect of prepregnancy body mass index categories on obstetrical and neonatal outcomes. Arch Gynecol Obstet. 2007;275:39-43.
36. Baeten JM, Bukusi EA, Lambe M. Pregnancy complications and outcomes among overweight and obese nulliparous women. Am J Public Health. 2001;91:436-40.
37. Callaway LK, Prins JB, Chang AM, McIntyre HD. The prevalence and impact of overweight and obesity in an Australian obstetric population. Med J Aust. 2006;184:56-9.
38. Cnattingius S, Lambe M. Trends in smoking and overweight during pregnancy: prevalence, risks of pregnancy

complications, and adverse pregnancy outcomes. Semin Perinatol. 2002;26:286-95.
39. Robinson HE, O'Connell CM, Joseph KS, McLeod NL. Maternal outcomes in pregnancies complicated by obesity. Obstet Gynecol. 2005;106:1357-64.
40. Rode L, Nilas L, Wojdemann K, Tabor A. Obesity-related complications in Danish single cephalic term pregnancies. Obstet Gynecol. 2005;105:537-42.
41. Rosenberg TJ, Garbers S, Chavkin W, Chiasson MA. Prepregnancy weight and adverse perinatal outcomes in an ethnically diverse population. Obstet Gynecol. 2003;102:1022-7.
42. Weiss JL, Malone FD, Emig D, Ball RH, Nyberg DA, Comstock CH, et al. Obesity, obstetric complications and cesarean delivery rate—a population-based screening study. Am J Obstet Gynecol. 2004;190:1091-7.
43. Brennand EA, Dannenbaum D, Willows ND. Pregnancy outcomes of First Nations women in relation to pregravid weight and pregnancy weight gain. J Obstet Gynaecol Can. 2005;27:936-44.
44. Catalano PM, Kirwan JP, Haugel-de Mouzon S, King J. Gestational diabetes and insulin resistance: Role in short- and long-term implications for mother and fetus. J Nutr. 2003;133:1674S-83S.
45. Villamor E, Cnattingius S. Interpregnancy weight change and risk of adverse pregnancy outcomes: a population-based study. Lancet. 2006;368:1164-70.
46. Glazer NL, Hendrickson AF, Schellenbaum GD, Mueller BA. Weight change and the risk of gestational diabetes in obese women. Epidemiology. 2004;15:733-7.
47. Jensen DM, Damm P, Sorensen B, Molsted-Pedersen L, Westergaard JG, Ovesen P, et al. Pregnancy outcome and prepregnancy body mass index in 2459 glucose-tolerant Danish women. Am J Obstet Gynecol. 2003;189:239-44.
48. Kabiru W, Raynor BD. Obstetric outcomes associated with increase in BMI category during pregnancy. Am J Obstet Gynecol. 2004;191:928-32.
49. Power ML, Cogswell ME, Schulkin J. Obesity prevention and treatment practices of U.S. obstetrician-gynecologists. Obstet Gynecol. 2006;108:961-8.
50. Raatikainen K, Heiskanen N, Heinonen S. Transition from overweight to obesity worsens pregnancy outcome in a BMI-dependent manner. Obesity (Silver Spring). 2006;14:165-71.
51. Steinfeld JD, Valentine S, Lerer T, Ingardia CJ, Wax JR, Curry SL. Obesity-related complications of pregnancy vary by race. J Matern Fetal Med. 2000;9:238-41.
52. Yogev Y, Langer O, Xenakis EM, Rosenn B. The association between glucose challenge test, obesity and pregnancy outcome in 6390 non-diabetic women. J Matern Fetal Neonatal Med. 2005;17:29-34.
53. Frederick IO, Rudra CB, Miller RS, Foster JC, Williams MA. Adult weight change, weight cycling, and prepregnancy obesity in relation to risk of preeclampsia. Epidemiology. 2006;17:428-34.
54. Leeners B, Rath W, Kuse S, Irawan C, Imthurn B, Neumaier-Wagner P. BMI: new aspects of a classical risk factor for hypertensive disorders in pregnancy. ClinSci (Lond). 2006;111:81-6.
55. Bodnar LM, Siega-Riz AM, Cogswell ME. High prepregnancy BMI increases the risk of postpartum anemia. Obes Res. 2004;12:941-8.

56. Conde-Agudelo A, Belizan JM. Risk factors for preeclampsia in a large cohort of Latin American and Caribbean women. BJOG. 2000;107:75-83.
57. Ray JG, Vermeulen MJ, Shapiro JL, Kenshole AB. Maternal and neonatal outcomes in pregestational and gestational diabetes mellitus, and the influence of maternal obesity and weight gain: the DEPOSIT study. diabetes endocrine pregnancy outcome study in Toronto. QJM. 2001;94:347-56.
58. Grossetti E, Beucher G, Regeasse A, Lamendour N, Herlicoviez M, Dreyfus M. Obstetrical complications of morbid obesity. J Gynecol Obstet Biol Reprod (Paris). 2004;33:739-44.
59. Murakami M, Ohmichi M, Takahashi T, Shibata A, Fukao A, Morisaki N, et al. Prepregnancy body mass index as an important predictor of perinatal outcomes in Japanese. Arch Gynecol Obstet. 2005;271:311-5.
60. O'Brien TE, Ray JG, Chan WS. Maternal body mass index and the risk of preeclampsia: a systematic overview. Epidemiology. 2003;14:368-74.
61. Cedergren MI. Maternal morbid obesity and the risk of adverse pregnancy outcome. Obstet Gynecol. 2004;103:219-24.
62. Wolf M, Kettyle E, Sandler L, Ecker JL, Roberts J, Thadhani R. Obesity and preeclampsia: The potential role of inflammation. Obstet Gynecol. 2001;98:757-62.
63. Bodnar LM, Ness RB, Harger GF, Roberts JM. Inflammation and triglycerides partially mediate the effect of prepregnancy body mass index on the risk of preeclampsia. Am J Epidemiol. 2005;162:1198-206.
64. Reddy UM, Branum AM, Klebanoff MA. Relationship of maternal body mass index and height to twinning. Obstet Gynecol. 2005;105:593-7.
65. Basso O, Nohr EA, Christensen K, Olsen J. Risk of twinning as a function of maternal height and body mass index. JAMA. 2004;291:1564-6.
66. Nuthalapaty FS, Rouse DJ, Owen J. The association of maternal weight with cesarean risk, labor duration, and cervical dilation rate during labor induction. Obstet Gynecol. 2004;103:452-6.
67. Buhimschi CS, Buhimschi IA, Malinow AM, Weiner CP. Intrauterine pressure during the second stage of labor in obese women. Obstet Gynecol. 2004; 103:225-30.
68. Maasilta P, Bachour A, Teramo K, Polo O, Laitinen LA. Sleep-related disordered breathing during pregnancy in obese women. Chest. 2001;120:1448-54.
69. Chauhan SP, Magann EF, Carroll CS, Barrilleaux PS, Scardo JA, Martin JN Jr. Mode of delivery for the morbidly obese with prior cesarean delivery: vaginal versus repeat cesarean section. Am J Obstet Gynecol. 2001;185:349-54.
70. Brill Y, Windrim R. Vaginal birth after caesarean section: Review of antenatal predictors of success. J Obstet Gynaecol can. 2003; 25:275-86.
71. Carroll CS S, Magann EF, Chauhan SP, Klauser CK, Morrison JC. Vaginal birth after cesarean section versus elective repeat cesarean delivery: weight-based outcomes. Am J Obstet Gynecol. 2003;188:1516-20; discussion 1520-2.
72. Durnwald CP, Ehrenberg HM, Mercer BM. The impact of maternal obesity and weight gain on vaginal birth after cesarean section success. Am J Obstet Gynecol. 2004;191:954-7.
73. Edwards RK, Harnsberger DS, Johnson IM, Treloar RW, Cruz AC. Deciding on route of delivery for obese women with a prior cesarean delivery. Am J Obstet Gynecol. 2003;189:385-9;discussion 389-90.

74. Hibbard JU, Gilbert S, Landon MB, Hauth JC, Leveno KJ, Spong CY, et al. Trial of labor or repeat cesarean delivery in women with morbid obesity and previous cesarean delivery. Obstet Gynecol. 2006;108:125-33.
75. Juhasz G, Gyamfi C, Gyamfi P, Tocce K, Stone JL. Effect of body mass index and excessive weight gain on success of vaginal birth after cesarean delivery. Obstet Gynecol. 2005;106:741-6.
76. Landon MB, Leindecker S, Spong CY, Hauth JC, Bloom S, Varner MW, et al. The MFMU cesarean registry: factors affecting the success of trial of labor after previous cesarean delivery. Am J Obstet Gynecol. 2005;193:1016-23.
77. Bujold E, Hammoud A, Schild C, Krapp M, Baumann P. The role of maternal body mass index in outcomes of vaginal births after cesarean. Am J Obstet Gynecol. 2005; 193:1517-21.
78. Goodall PT, Ahn JT, Chapa JB, Hibbard JU. Obesity as a risk factor for failed trial of labor in patients with previous cesarean delivery. Am J Obstet Gynecol. 2005;192:1423-6.
79. Ramos GA, Caughey AB. The interrelationship between ethnicity and obesity on obstetric outcomes. Am J Obstet Gynecol. 2005;193:1089-93.
80. Usha Kiran TS, Hemmadi S, Bethel J, Evans J. Outcome of pregnancy in a woman with an increased body mass index. BJOG. 2005;112:768-72.
81. Rhodes JC, Schoendorf KC, Parker JD. Contribution of excess weight gain during pregnancy and macrosomia to the cesarean delivery rate, 1990-2000. Pediatrics. 2003;111:1181-5.
82. Ehrenberg HM, Durnwald CP, Catalano P, Mercer BM. The influence of obesity and diabetes on the risk of cesarean delivery. Am J Obstet Gynecol. 2004;191:969-74.
83. Kaiser PS, Kirby RS. Obesity as a risk factor for cesarean in a low-risk population. Obstet Gynecol. 2001;97:39-43.
84. Young TK, Woodmansee B. Factors that are associated with cesarean delivery in a large private practice: the importance of prepregnancy body mass index and weight gain. Am J Obstet Gynecol. 2002;187:312-8; discussion 318-20.
85. Vahratian A, Siega-Riz AM, Savitz DA, Zhang J. Maternal pre-pregnancy overweight and obesity and the risk of cesarean delivery in nulliparous women. Ann Epidemiol. 2005;15:467-74.
86. Saravanakumar K, Rao SG, Cooper GM. Obesity and obstetric anaesthesia. Anaesthesia. 2006;61:36-48.
87. Myles TD, Gooch J, Santolaya J. Obesity as an independent risk factor for infectious morbidity in patients who undergo cesarean delivery. Obstet Gynecol. 2002;100:959-64.
88. Schneid-Kofman N, Sheiner E, Levy A, Holcberg G. Risk factors for wound infection following cesarean deliveries. Int J Gynaecol Obstet. 2005;90:10-5.
89. Tran TS, Jamulitrat S, Chongsuvivatwong V, Geater A. Risk factors for postcesarean surgical site infection. Obstet Gynecol. 2000;95:367-71.
90. Magann EF, Chauhan SP, Rodts-Palenik S, Bufkin L, Martin JN Jr, Morrison JC. Subcutaneous stitch closure versus subcutaneous drain to prevent wound disruption after cesarean delivery: a randomized clinical trial. Am J Obstet Gynecol. 2002;186:1119-23.
91. Ramsey PS, White AM, Guinn DA, Lu GC, Ramin SM, Davies JK, et al. Subcutaneous tissue reapproximation, alone or in combination with drain, in obese women undergoing cesarean delivery. Obstet Gynecol. 2005;105:967-73.
92. Allaire AD, Fisch J, McMahon MJ. Subcutaneous drain vs. suture in obese women undergoing cesarean delivery. A prospective, randomized trial. J Reprod Med. 2000;45:327-31.
93. Chelmow D, Rodriguez EJ, Sabatini MM. Suture closure of subcutaneous fat and wound disruption after cesarean delivery: a meta-analysis. Obstet Gynecol. 2004;103:974-80.
94. Fretts RC. Etiology and prevention of stillbirth. Am J Obstet Gynecol. 2005;193:1923-35.
95. Froen JF, Arnestad M, Frey K, Vege A, Saugstad OD, Stray-Pedersen B. Risk factors for sudden intrauterine unexplained death: epidemiologic characteristics of singleton cases in Oslo, Norway, 1986-1995. Am J Obstet Gynecol. 2001;184:694-702.
96. Chibber R. Unexplained antepartum fetal deaths: what are the determinants? Arch Gynecol Obstet. 2005;271:286-91.
97. Stephansson O, Dickman PW, Johansson A, Cnattingius S. Maternal weight, pregnancy weight gain, and the risk of antepartum stillbirth. Am J Obstet Gynecol. 2001;184:463-9.
98. Conde-Agudelo A, Belizan JM, Diaz-Rossello JL. Epidemiology of fetal death in Latin America. Acta Obstet Gynecol Scand. 2000;79:371-8.
99. Huang DY, Usher RH, Kramer MS, Yang H, Morin L, Fretts RC. Determinants of unexplained antepartum fetal deaths. Obstet Gynecol. 2000;95:215-21.
100. Kristensen J, Vestergaard M, Wisborg K, Kesmodel U, Secher NJ. Pre-pregnancy weight and the risk of stillbirth and neonatal death. BJOG. 2005;112:403-8.
101. Nohr EA, Bech BH, Davies MJ, Frydenberg M, Henriksen TB, Olsen J. Prepregnancy obesity and fetal death: a study within the Danish national birth cohort. Obstet Gynecol. 2005;106:250-9.
102. Nuthalapaty FS, Rouse DJ. The impact of obesity on obstetrical practice and outcome. Clin Obstet Gynecol. 2004; 47:898,913;discussion 980-1.
103. Michlin R, Oettinger M, Odeh M, Khoury S, Ophir E, Barak M, et al. Maternal obesity and pregnancy outcome. Isr Med Assoc J. 2000;2:10-3.
104. Ehrenberg HM, Mercer BM, Catalano PM. The influence of obesity and diabetes on the prevalence of macrosomia. Am J Obstet Gynecol. 2004;191:964-8.
105. Jolly MC, Sebire NJ, Harris JP, Regan L, Robinson S. Risk factors for macrosomia and its clinical consequences: a study of 350,311 pregnancies. Eur J Obstet Gynecol Reprod Biol. 2003;111:9-14.
106. Surkan PJ, Hsieh CC, Johansson AL, Dickman PW, Cnattingius S. Reasons for increasing trends in large for gestational age births. Obstet Gynecol. 2004;104:720-6.
107. Yu CK, Teoh TG, Robinson S. Obesity in pregnancy. BJOG. 2006;113:1117-25.
108. Robinson H, Tkatch S, Mayes DC, Bott N, Okun N. Is maternal obesity a predictor of shoulder dystocia? Obstet Gynecol. 2003;101:24-7.
109. Poggi SH, Stallings SP, Ghidini A, Spong CY, Deering SH, Allen RH. Intrapartum risk factors for permanent brachial plexus injury. Am J Obstet Gynecol. 2003;189:725-9.
110. Mehta SH, Blackwell SC, Bujold E, Sokol RJ. What factors are associated with neonatal injury following shoulder dystocia? J Perinatol. 2006;26:85-8.
111. Hendricks KA, Nuno OM, Suarez L, Larsen R. Effects of hyperinsulinemia and obesity on risk of neural tube defects among Mexican Americans. Epidemiology. 2001;12:630-5.
112. Shaw GM, Todoroff K, Finnell RH, Lammer EJ. Spina bifida phenotypes in infants or fetuses of obese mothers. Teratology. 2000;61:376-81.

113. Watkins ML, Rasmussen SA, Honein MA, Botto LD, Moore CA. Maternal obesity and risk for birth defects. Pediatrics. 2003;111:1152-8.
114. Ray JG, Wyatt PR, Vermeulen MJ, Meier C, Cole DE. Greater maternal weight and the ongoing risk of neural tube defects after folic acid flour fortification. Obstet Gynecol. 2005;105:261-5.
115. Anderson JL, Waller DK, Canfield MA, Shaw GM, Watkins ML, Werler MM. Maternal obesity, gestational diabetes, and central nervous system birth defects. Epidemiology. 2005;16:87-92.
116. Moore LL, Singer MR, Bradlee ML, Rothman KJ, Milunsky A. A prospective study of the risk of congenital defects associated with maternal obesity and diabetes mellitus. Epidemiology. 2000;11:689-94.
117. Mikhail LN, Walker CK, Mittendorf R. Association between maternal obesity and fetal cardiac malformations in African Americans. J Natl Med Assoc. 2002;94:695-700.
118. Cedergren MI, Kallen BA. Maternal obesity and infant heart defects. Obes Res. 2003;11:1065-71.
119. Watkins ML, Botto LD. Maternal prepregnancy weight and congenital heart defects in offspring. Epidemiology. 2001;12:439-46.
120. Cedergren M, Kallen B. Maternal obesity and the risk for orofacial clefts in the offspring. Cleft Palate Craniofac J. 2005;42:367-71.
121. Shaw GM, Todoroff K, Schaffer DM, Selvin S. Maternal height and prepregnancy body mass index as risk factors for selected congenital anomalies. Paediatr Perinat Epidemiol. 2000;14:234-9.
122. Hendler I, Blackwell SC, Bujold E, Treadwell MC, Wolfe HM, Sokol RJ, et al. The impact of maternal obesity on midtrimester sonographic visualization of fetal cardiac and craniospinal structures. Int J Obes Relat Metab Disord. 2004;28:1607-11.
123. Confidential Enquiry into Maternal and Child Health. The National Institute for Clinical Excellence, Scottish Executive Health Department; Department of Health, Social Services and Public Safety, Northern Ireland. In: Lewis G (Ed). Why Mothers Die. 2000-2002. The Sixth Report of the Confidential Enquires into Maternal Deaths in the United Kingdom. 2000-2002. London: RCOG Press; 2004:291.
124. Donath SM, Amir LH. Does maternal obesity adversely affect breastfeeding initiation and duration? Breastfeed Rev. 2000;8:29-33.
125. Hilson JA, Rasmussen KM, Kjolhede CL. Excessive weight gain during pregnancy is associated with earlier termination of breast-feeding among white women. J Nutr. 2006;136:140-6.
126. Li R, Jewell S, Grummer-Strawn L. Maternal obesity and breast-feeding practices. Am J Clin Nutr. 2003;77:931-6.
127. Rasmussen KM, Kjolhede CL. Prepregnant overweight and obesity diminish the prolactin response to suckling in the first week postpartum. Pediatrics. 2004;113:e465-71.
128. Hilson JA, Rasmussen KM, Kjolhede CL. High prepregnant body mass index is associated with poor lactation outcomes among white, rural women independent of psychosocial and demographic correlates. J Hum Lact. 2004;20:18-29.
129. American College of Obstetricians and Gynecologists. Nutrition during pregnancy. ACOG technical bulletin No. 179. Int J Gynaecol Obstet. 1993;43:67-74.

Chapter 38

Cesarean Scar Pregnancy

Mahesh Gupta, Richa Baharani

INTRODUCTION

Ectopic pregnancy accounts for 1–2% of all pregnancies.[1,2] Those occurring within a previous cesarean section scar are rare with potential fatal consequences and account for 0.05–0.04% of all pregnancies.[1] Implantation of a pregnancy within a cesarean fibrous tissue scar is considered to be the rarest form of ectopic pregnancy and a life-threatening condition.[3] This is because of the very high risk for uterine rupture and all the maternal complications related to it.[4] The diagnosis and treatment of cesarean scar pregnancy (CSP) is challenging. Hence, in these women issues concerning early detection is of utmost importance, and it is the cornerstone to reduce heavy complications related to the CSP.[5]

EPIDEMIOLOGY

It has an estimated incidence of 1 in 1800 to 1 in 2500 of all cesarean deliveries performed.[6,7] It is estimated that 0.15% of all pregnancies with a history of a previous cesarean delivery will be followed by a CSP in the woman's next pregnancy. The overall incidence is, however, thought to be increasing,[8] representing up to 6% of ectopic pregnancies in patients with a history of a cesarean section.[9] There may be two different types of cesarean scar pregnancies. The first type involves implantation of the gestational sac on the scar with progression towards either the cervix or the uterine cavity. In this type, the fetus may grow to viability but there is a risk of life-threatening hemorrhage from the implantation site. The second type involves a deep implantation in a cesarean scar defect with possible rupture and bleeding during the first trimester of pregnancy.[10]

Risk Factors

Previous dilatation and curettage, previous placental pathology, previous manual removal of placenta, previous ectopic pregnancy, *in vitro* fertilization (IVF), two or more previous cesarean sections, and other uterine surgery such as myomectomy, metroplasty, or hysteroscopy.[11]

DIAGNOSIS

An easy and clinically practical diagnosis of CSP[12] is based upon having a history of previous cesarean delivery, a positive pregnancy test, and the following sonographic criteria (**Fig. 38.1**):

- Empty uterine cavity and closed, empty endocervical canal.
- Chorionic/gestational sac and/or placenta located in low and in the anterior wall of the uterus, below the bladder, in close proximity and at the level of the internal os, at the site of the previous hysterotomy scar/niche, with or without fetal or embryonic pole and/or yolk sac, with or without heartbeats (depending on gestational age).
- Absent or thin myometrial layer between the chorionic/gestational sac and unusually close proximity to the bladder wall.
- Abundant blood flow around the chorionic/gestational sac concentrated on the anterior side of the chorionic sac

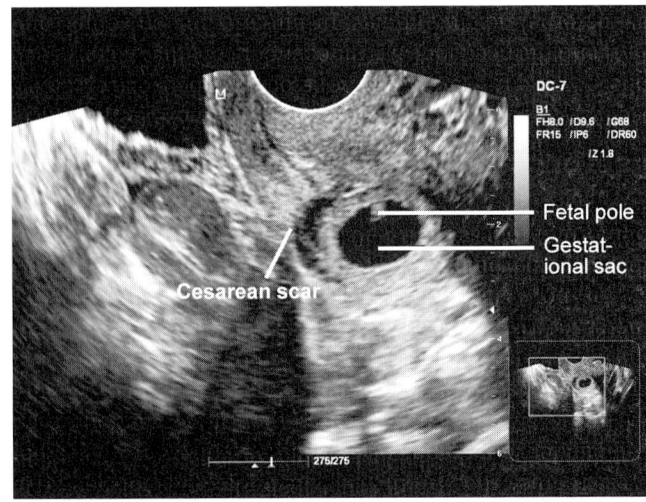

Fig. 38.1: Transvaginal sonography showing cesarean scar pregnancy *(For color version, see Plate 3)*

"marking" the site of the placental implantation. Rarely, the typical sonographic appearance of an arteriovenous malformation (AVM) can be seen.
- Before 7 weeks, the gestational sac may assume the shape of the niche. At or after 7 weeks, the sac is "forced" to extend toward the uterine cavity, elongate, and mold to finally assume an intracavitary position. Importantly, the placenta stays anchored in the area of the scar/niche, in its initial site of implantation.

The specificity of three-dimensional (3D) ultrasound imaging has been reported to be better than two-dimensional (2D) scans as the 3D image incorporates an additional coronal section that is not possible with 2D imaging.[13]

MAGNETIC RESONANCE IMAGING

Although transvaginal sonography is the first-line tool in diagnosis, magnetic resonance imaging is useful as a troubleshooting tool when sonography is equivocal or inconclusive before intervention or therapy. Sagittal, coronal, and transverse sections of T1- and T2-weighted magnetic resonance imaging sequences can be used to show the gestational sac embedded in the anterior lower uterine segment, better evaluate pelvic anatomy, improve intraoperative orientation, and assess the possibility of myometrial invasion and bladder involvement. Magnetic resonance imaging can also be used to measure the lesion volume to help assess the indication for and success of local methotrexate treatment.[14]

MANAGEMENT

The cause of this condition and the best management of CSP are unclear but early diagnosis and appropriate treatment is crucially important to prevent serious complications. The options are medical, surgical or a combination of both methods.

Aim of the treatment would be avoidance of uterine rupture, hemorrhage, hysterectomy and preserve fertility.

Once a diagnosis of CSP has been established, the patient should be counseled about her options. The presence of a live CSP requires immediate and decisive action to prevent further growth of the embryo or fetus.

In general, treatment should be individualized, based on the patient's age, number of previous cesarean deliveries, number of children, and the expertise of the clinicians managing her care. Options include:
- Termination of the pregnancy
- Continuation of the pregnancy with the possibility of delivering a live offspring, provided the patient understands that a morbidly adherent placenta may occur, often necessitating emergency hysterectomy.

Medical Treatment

It is preferred for asymptomatic women with <8 weeks gestation and myometrial thickness <2 mm between gestation sac and bladder.[15] Different techniques have been described and these include:

Systemic Administration

Systemic administration of Methotrexate (MTX), CSPs have been shown to respond well to Methotrexate (dose of 50 mg/m^2), especially in those with β-hCG levels < 5000 miu/mL.[16,17] Conservative medical treatment is appropriate for a woman who is pain free and hemodynamically stable. Before MTX treatment women should have prior baseline full blood count and liver and renal function tests performed. They must be agreeable to surgery if medical treatment fails or if the CSP ruptures.[18] The disadvantage with the former is need for repeated doses of MTX since its half life is short, women should also be prepared for a long follow-up since it can take 4–16 weeks for β-hCG level normalization. This is due to the placental implantation on mainly fibrous tissue and hence absorption of the gestation sac is extremely slow.[17] Mifepristone may be used prior to methotrexate. The anti-progesterone activity of mifepristone helps to destroy and detach the chorionic villi, thus making MTX more effective.

Local Injection of Embryocides

This has been successfully reported with local injection of MTX,[19,20] potassium chloride.[21] under ultrasound guidance these drugs can be injected locally to the gestation sac via transabdominal or transvaginal route. Ultrasound-guided methotrexate injection emerges as the treatment of choice to terminate cesarean scar pregnancy.[22]

Combined Medical Treatment

Combined medical treatment in varying regimens has been described by many authors, e.g. local injection of 8 mEq potassium chloride (2 mEq/mL) followed by 60 mg of MTX injected into the gestation sac,[23] multi-dose systemic MTX (1 mg/kg) with alternate day folinic acid rescue,[24] failed systemic MTX followed by successful local MTX.[25]

Medical Treatment Combined with Surgical Sac Aspiration

Various sequences of combination have been described:
- Local potassium chloride/TVS-guided sac aspiration/local MTX injection/intramuscular MTX injection
- Systemic MTX/TVS-guided sac aspiration

- Sac aspiration (transvaginal or transabdominal)/local MTX injection
- Sac aspiration under ultrasound guidance/systemic MTX
- Systemic MTX/sac aspiration by vaginal route/local MTX.[24]

Serial transvaginal color flow Doppler is useful for monitoring the response to medical treatment and appears to correlate well with β-hCG levels.[26]

Surgical Treatment

If treatment with MTX fails, open or endoscopic surgery is the treatment of choice. Wedge resection and repair of the implantation site via laparotomy or laparoscopic or hysteroscopic excision can be done.[27] Hysteroscopy is a minimally invasive operative technique that offers direct visualization, low morbidity, and high primary success rates.[28] Surgical or invasive techniques, including dilatation and curettage are not recommended for cesarean scar pregnancy due to high morbidity and poor prognosis. Bilateral uterine artery embolization to minimize bleeding has been used as an adjunct to medical therapy.[29]

DIFFERENTIAL DIAGNOSIS

The diagnosis and treatment of cesarean scar pregnancy (CSP) is challenging.

Transvaginal sonography and color Doppler ultrasound are the best diagnostic tools for its detection , and if needed, for treatment as well. A low, anteriorly displaced gestational sac in a pregnancy with a history of previous cesarean delivery is almost certainly a CSP. Location of the placenta and its vessels by color Doppler determines the implantation site.Its differential diagnoses include cervical pregnancy and miscarriage in progress.[30]

COMPLICATIONS

Catastrophic hemorrhage (secondary to placental invasion and vascularity) and rupture at the site of implantation as in any ectopic pregnancy. It is likely that if a developing pregnancy in a cesarean section scar continue to the second or third trimesters, there would be a substantial risk of uterine rupture with catastrophic hemorrhage, with a high risk of hysterectomy causing serious maternal morbidity and loss of future fertility.

Bladder invasion is a possible sequel, if the myometrium is breached completely and there is also a danger of invasion of the bladder by the growing placenta or a secondary abdominal pregnancy.

However, if the pregnancy continues within the uterus, the risk of placenta accreta is significantly increased, up to three- to five-fold .

REFERENCES

1. Rotas M, Haberman S, Levgur M. Cesarean scar ectopic pregnancies: etiology, diagnosis, and management. Obstet Gynecol. 2006;107:1373-81.
2. Santos-Ribeiro S, Tournaye H, Polyzos NP. Trends in ectopic pregnancy rates following assisted reproductive technologies in the UK: a 12-year nationwide analysis including 160000 pregnancies. Hum Reprod. 2016;31:393-402.
3. Fylstra DL. Ectopic pregnancy within a Caesarean scar: a review. Obstet Gynecol Surv. 2002;57:537-43. Cross Ref Medline Web of Science
4. Herman A, Weinraub Z, Avrech O, Maymon R, Ron-El R, Bukovsky Y. Follow up and outcome of isthmic pregnancy located in a previous caesarean section scar. Br J Obstet Gynecol. 1995;102,839-41.
5. Maymon R, Halperin R, Mendlovic S, Schneider D, Vaknin Z, Herman A, et al. Ectopic pregnancies in caesarean section scars: the 8 year experience of one medical centre. Hum Reprod. 2004;19(2):278-84. [PubMed].
6. Jauniaux E, Jurkovic D. Placenta accreta: pathogenesis of a 20th century iatrogenic uterine disease. Placenta. 2012;33:244-251.
7. Jurkovic D, Hillaby K, Woelfer B, Lawrence A, Salim R, Elson CJ. Cesarean scar pregnancy. Ultrasound Obstet Gynecol. 2003;21:310.
8. Levine D. Ectopic pregnancy. Radiology. 2007;245(2):385-97. doi:10.1148/radiol.2452061031. Pubmed citation
9. Dibble EH, Lourenco AP. Imaging Unusual Pregnancy Implantations: Rare Ectopic Pregnancies and More. Am J Roentgenol. 2016; 1-13. doi:10.2214/AJR.15.15290. Pubmed citation
10. Vial Y, Petignat P, Hohlfeld P. Pregnancy in a cesarean scar. Ultrasound Obstet GynecoI. 2000;16:592-3.
11. Larsen V, Solomon MH. Pregnancy in a uterine scar sacculus: an unusual cause of postabortal haemorrhage: a case report. S Afr Med. 1978;53:142-3.
12. Timor-Tritsch IE, Monteagudo A, Santos R, Tsymbal T, Pineda G, Arslan AA. The diagnosis, treatment, and follow-up of cesarean scar pregnancy. Am J Obstet Gynecol. 2012;207:44.e1-e13.
13. Ruano R, Reya F, Picone O, Chopin N, Pereira PP, Benachi A, et al. Three-dimensional ultrasonographic diagnosis of a cervical pregnancy. Clinics (Sao Paulo). 2006;61:355-8.[PubMed]
14. Osborn DA, Williams TR, Craig BM. Cesarean scar pregnancy: Sonographic and magnetic resonance imaging findings, complications, and treatment. J Ultrasound Med. 2012;31(9):1449-56.
15. Weimin W, Wenqing L. Effect of early pregnancy on a previous lower segment cesarean section scar. Int J Gynaecol Obstet. 2002;77: 201-7.
16. Shufaro Y, Nadjari M. Implantation of a gestational sac in a cesarean section scar. Fertil Steril. 2001;75:1217.
17. Ravhon A, Ben-Chetrit A, Rabinowitz R, Neuman M, Beller U. Successful methotrexate treatment of a viable pregnancy within a thin uterine scar. Br J ObstetGynaecol. 1997;104:628-9.
18. Lam PM, Lo KWK, Lau TK. Unsuccessful medical treatment of cesarean scar ectopic pregnancy with systemic methotrexate: a report of two cases. Acta Obstet Gynecol Scand. 2004;83:108-16.

19. Godin P-A, Bassil S, Donnez J. An ectopic pregnancy developing in a previous caesarean section scar. Fertil Steril. 1997;67:398-400.
20. Lai YM, Lee JD, Lee CL, Chen TC, Soong YK. An ectopic pregnancy embedded in the myometrium of a previous cesarean section scar. Acta Obstet Gynecol Scand. 1995;74:573-6
21. Hartung J, Meckies J. Management of a case of uterine scar pregnancy by transabdominal potassium chloride injection. Ultrasound Obstet Gynecol. 2003;21:94-5.
22. Seow KM, Huang LW, Lin YH, Lin MY, Tsai YL, Hwang JL. Cesarean scar pregnancy: issues in management. Ultrasound Obstet Gynecol. 2004;23(3):247-53.
23. Donnez J, Godin P-A, Bassil S. Successful methotrexate treatment of a viable pregnancy within a thin uterine scar. Br J Obstet Gynaecol. 1997;104:1216-7.
24. Hwu YM, Hsu CY, Yang HY. Conservative treatment of caesarean scar pregnancy with transvaginal needle aspiration of the embryo. BJOG. 2005;112:841-2.
25. Persadie RJ, Fortier A, Stopps RG. Ectopic pregnancy in a caesarean scar: a case report. J Obstet Gynaecol Can. 2005;27:1102-6.
26. Seow KM, Huang LW, Lin YH, Yan-Sheng Lin M, Tsai YL, Hwang JL. Caesarean scar pregnancy: issues in management. Ultrasound Obstet Gynecol. 2004;23:247-53.
27. Local metothrexate treatment of cesarean scar ectopic pregnancy .Open Journal of Obstetrics and Gynecology. 2012; 2:329-30 OJOG http://dx.doi.org/10.4236/ojog.2012.24069 Published Online November 2012 (http://www.SciRP.org/journal/ojog/)
28. Open Journal of Obstetrics and Gynecology. 2012;2:329-30 OJOG http://dx.doi.org/10.4236/ojog.2012.24069 Published Online November 2012 (http://www.SciRP.org/journal/ojog/) Local metothrexate treatment of cesarean scar ectopic pregnancy DavutGüven, KadirBakay*, A. SertaçBatıoğlu Department of Obstetrics and Gynecology, Faculty of Medicine, OndokuzMayis University, Samsun, Turkey Email: *drkadirbakay@gmail.com
29. Yang MJ, Jeng MH. Combination of transarterial embolization of uterine arteries and conservative surgical treatment for pregnancy in a cesarean section scar. Reprod Med. 2003;48:213-6
30. Contemporary OB/GYN Obstetrics-Gynecology and Women's Health Cesarean delivery Cesarean scar pregnancy diagnosis and management November 24, 2015 By Ilan E Timor-Tritsch MD, Ana Monteagudo MD, Andrea Kaelin Agten MD.

SECTION 7: INFECTIONS DURING PREGNANCY

Chapter 39

Malaria During Pregnancy

Richa Baharani, Pushpa Pandey, Anand Baharani

INTRODUCTION AND MAGNITUDE OF PROBLEM

Malaria remains a formidable challenge to everyone including physicians, gynecologists and health administrators. Globally, Malaria is reported to cause 250-300 million infections and more than a million deaths every year. Actual number of cases may be as high as 300-660 million.[1]

Two-to-three fold increase in the incidence of malaria over the last 35 years has been attributed to a coincidence of several factors such as population movements into malarious regions, changing agricultural practices, building of dams, deforestation, drug-resistant parasites, insecticides resistant mosquitoes, global climate change, continuing poverty, and political instability.[2]

Malaria has been ever present in India since ancient times. It causes immense suffering to millions of Indians. Even ruthless conquerors, who always won in the battle fields, lost their lives to malaria. At present in India, 1.5-2 million confirmed malaria cases and 1000 deaths are reported annually. Of the total malaria burden in India rural malaria accounts for more than 90-95% cases and urban malaria less than 5-10% cases.[3,4]

EPIDEMIOLOGY

There are five identified species that cause human malaria: P. Falciparum, P. Vivax, P. Ovale, P. Malariae and *P. Knowlesi.* About 85% of cases and most of the deaths are caused by Falciparum. Infection is transmitted by female anopheles mosquito.

Malaria has made a come back in India causing an estimated 15 million cases and 20000 deaths annually with Odisha and Maharashtra (particularly tribal belts) being worst affected. In a study from undivided MP estimated annual incidence of malaria in pregnancy has been reported to be in excess of 2,20,000 infections contributing to 76,000 abortions, 19,800 still births and 1000 maternal deaths.

PATHOPHYSIOLOGY

Malaria is transmitted when an infected mosquito takes a human blood meal and the *Plasmodium* sporozoites are transferred from the saliva of the host. Within hours parasite will migrate to the liver, where it undergoes further cycling and replication before being released in to host's bloodstream.

Incubation period: 7-30 days

CLINICAL MANIFESTATIONS OF MALARIA

Today malaria is known as plasmodial infection of RBCs. That can present not just as a case of fever with chills but as a multisystem disease with myriad manifestations ranging from an asymptomatic infection to a rapidly progressive fatal disease.

The clinical manifestations of malaria depend on several factors :

Parasite species, genotype, age of host, geographical origin of parasite, premorbidity, pregnancy, prior chemoprophylaxis, immune status with respect to malaria, severity of infection, duration and status of infection.

In *P. falciparum* infection sequence of chills, fever, followed by sweating can occur. Headache, vomiting, dry cough are most common symptoms of malaria. Most studies have reported presence of headache in 50-85% of cases, vomiting in 25-35% of patients, diarrhea in 5-38% of patients, occurrence of cough in 63% of cases and Jaundice in 2.5-62% of cases. Generalized weakness and prostration and anemia are fairly common in malaria. Edema and hypoglycemia are particularly more common in pregnant women.

MALARIA IN PREGNANCY

Malaria has a devastating impact on pregnancy largely due to immunological and hormonal changes that occur in pregnancy and the availability of placental tissue with chondroitin sulfate, disease tends to be more severe in pregnant women with adverse impact on mother as well as the growing fetus: Clinical manifestations of malaria during pregnancy vary greatly according to the level of immunity of the host. Nonimmune pregnant women with *P. falciparum* infection are more susceptible to all its complications such as cerebral malaria, acute renal failure, hyperpyrexia, etc. and have 2-10 times higher mortality compared with non pregnant population.

Effects of Malaria on Pregnant Women

- Anemia megaloblastic (due to folic acid deficiency and haemolysis). Malaria causes upto 15% of anemia in pregnancy. It can cause severe anemia.
- Hypoglycemia due to increased glucose consumption.
- Metabolic acidosis
- Jaundice due to hepatic dysfunction, hepatic failure, hypotension
- Renal failure due to block of renal microcirculation
- Pulmonary edema and respiratory distress
- Convulsions and coma, cerebral malaria
- Disseminated intravascular coagulation
- High fever, placental infection, puerperal sepsis and high MMR

(Pregnant women are 3 times more likely to suffer from severe disease as a result of malarial infection compared with their non pregnant counterparts and have a mortality rate from severe disease that approaches 50%, second trimester appears to bring highest rate of infection).

Effects of Malaria on Mother

- Anemia tends to occur between 16-29 weeks due to hemolysis of parasitized cells and increased demands of pregnancy +/-folate and iron deficiency.
- An Indian study reported that pregnant women with malaria are at increased risk of hypoglycemia, cerebral malaria, renal failure, hepatic failure and hypotension. Acute pulmonary edema occurs much more commonly in pregnant women and carries high mortality.
- Disseminated intravascular coagulation can occur and carries a high mortality risk.

Effects of Malaria on Fetus

- Spontaneous abortion
- Missed abortion
- Preterm labor
- Intrauterine growth retardation
- Intrauterine fetal death
- Low birth weight
- Congenital infection
- Perinatal death
- Still birth

Pathogenesis of Severe Malaria

Red blood cells undergo progressive and dramatic structural biochemical and mechanical modifications after invasion by malaria parasites. Infected erythrocytes become rigid, sticky, irregular. Increased cytoadherence causes microvascular obstruction placental dysfunction more hypoxia. Rosetting is the adhesion phenomenon by which parasitized RBCs bind to unparasitized RBCs to form clumps of cells causes microvascular obstruction and impaired tissue perfusion.

Diagnosis of Malaria

Clinical Diagnosis

Based entirely on symptoms of malaria.

WHO has recommended the following for a clinical diagnosis of malaria.[5,6]

- In settings where the risk of malaria is low, clinical diagnosis of uncomplicated malaria should be based on the degree of exposure to malaria and a history of fever in the previous 3 days with no features of other severe disease.
- In settings where risk of malaria is high clinical diagnosis, especially in young children and pregnant women should be based on a history of fever in the previous 24 hours and the presence of anemia (for which pallor of the palms appears to be the most reliable sign).
- In malaria epidemics, all patients with a history of fever should normally be treated for the disease.

Parasitological Diagnosis

- Confirmation of malaria infection is based on identification of either malaria parasites or antigens in the patient's blood. Thick blood smear technique used as a "gold standard" technique even today. Presence of malaria pigment in the circulating phagocytic leukocytes is a pathognomonic sign of recent malaria infection and may be useful in the diagnosis of malaria, when parasites cannot be found on the blood film.
- Rapid diagnostic tests
- Serological tests for detection of antibodies against asexual blood stage malaria parasites.
- Molecular tools (PCR assays)
- *Placental blood smear:* Negative test does not rule out malaria, a positive test may not confirm malarial infection as the cause for patient's illness.

If the test is negative in the presence of high clinical suspicion, then test must be repeated 2-3 times at intervals of 6-12 hours to firmly rule out malaria.

In following conditions, parasites sometimes may not be detected in peripheral smear:

- Sequestration deep vascular bed
- Partially treated patients

- Prophylactic antimalarial treatment
- Inexperienced microscopist
- Poor quality staining

Prevention of Malaria

Pregnant women are more prone to complications of malaria infection than nongravid women. Prevention involves chemoprophylaxis and mosquito avoidance. Because of changes in women's immune system during pregnancy and the presence of a new organ (the placenta with new places for parasites to bind), pregnant women lose some of their immunity to malaria infection. In malaria-infected human placenta examined under microscope intervillous spaces are filled with red blood cells, most of which are infected with *Plasmodium falciparum* malaria parasite. Parasites appear as black dots under microscope. Placenta which is infected by malaria unable to carry its normal function to provide nutrient to fetus.

Prevention involves chemoprophylaxis and mosquito prevention.

Currently recommended interventions for pregnant women are:
- Use of insectiside treated bed nets.
- Intermittent preventive treatment (IPT) for women in high transmission areas.
- Diagnosis and treatment of illness women should also receive iron/folate supplementation to protect them against anemia, a common occurrence against all pregnant women.
- Application of repellants use of 20% diethyltoluamide (DEET) is considered to be safe in pregnancy.[7]
- Wearing clothing with long sleeves, pants and footwear.

Chemoprophylaxis During Pregnancy

WHO recommends that all pregnant women in area of stable malaria transmission should receive atleast 2 doses of IPT after quickening.[8]

1st Choice Chloroquine

300 mg base weekly starting 1 week before arrival in endemic area, continuing weekly during travel and 4 weeks after leaving endemic area.

In areas resistant to Chloroquine
or
Sulphadoxine (500 mg) + Pyrimethamine (25 mg) one tablet once weekly
SP should be avoided during 1st 16 weeks of antenatal period.

Intermittent Presumptive Treatment

Drug of choice sulfadoxine/pyrimethamine dose 3 tablets twice during pregnancy
1st dose between 20–24 weeks pregnancy
Second dose between 28–32 weeks

WHO recommends that in areas of moderate-to-high malaria transmission of Africa, IPTp-SP be given to all pregnant women at each scheduled ANC visit, starting as early as possible in the second trimester, provided that the doses of SP are given at least 1 month apart. WHO recommends a package of interventions for preventing malaria during pregnancy, which includes promotion and use of insecticide-treated nets, as well as IPTp-SP. To ensure that pregnant women in endemic areas start IPTp-SP as early as possible in the second trimester, policy-makers should ensure health system contact with women at 13 weeks of gestation.[9,10]

Recurrence of Malaria During Pregnancy

- Recurrence is very common in pregnancy
- WHO recommended
- Artesunate 2 mg/kg/day or 100 mg daily for seven days and clindamycin 450 mg three times daily for seven days.

Management of Malaria in Pregnancy

It involves:
- Treatment of malaria
- Management of complications
- Management of labor

Treatment of Malaria in Pregnancy

- Energetic
- Anticipatory
- Careful

Energetic

- One should not waste time
- Admit all cases of *P. falciparum*
- *Assess severity:*
  - Pulse, BP, pallor, jaundice, temperature, hemoglobin, parasite count, SGPT, S. bilirubin, blood sugar, S. Creatinine

Anticipatory

- Look for complications by regular monitoring
- Monitor maternal and fetal vital parameters
  - RBS 4–6 hourly
  - Hemoglobin and parasite count 12 hourly

- S. creatinine
- S. bilirubin
- Intake output chart

Careful

- Drugs which are contraindicated should be avoided
- Over/under dosing of drugs should not be done
- Fluid overload and dehydration should be avoided
- Adequate intake of calories should be maintained
Treatment depends on whether *P. vivax* or *P. falciparum*

Treatment of Vivax Malaria

If patient is *P. vivax* positive, then she should be treated with chloroquine.
Drug schedule for treatment of *P. vivax* malaria:
10 mg/kg body weight on day 1
10 mg/kg body weight on day 2
5 mg/kg body weight on day 3
Or
Chloroquin 600 mg base
4 tablet (each 150 mg) stat 0000
2 tablet (each 150 mg) after 6 hours 00
2 tablet (each 150 mg) after 24 hours 00
2 tablet (each 150 mg) after 48 hours 00

Note: Chloroquine 250 mg tablet is having 150 mg base
Primaquine is contraindicated in pregnancy

Treatment of vivax malaria in chloroquine-resistant cases:
Quinine salt 10 mg/kg twice a day × 7 days
Or
Artesunate 4 mg/kg body weight in divided loading dose followed by 2 mg/kg body weight daily × 6 days.

Treatment of Pregnant Women with Uncomplicated *P. falciparum* Malaria[11]

Treatment During First Trimester

Quinine salt 10 mg/kg three times daily × 7 days.
Quinine may induce hypoglycemia. Pregnant women should not take quinine on an empty stomach and should eat regularly while on quinine treatment.

Treatment during 2nd and 3rd Trimester

In north-eastern states ACT–AL: Coformulated tablet of artemether (20 mg) – Lumefantrine (120 mg)
- Dose twice daily for 3 days
- In other states, ACT-SP

Dose

- Artesunate 4 mg/kg BW × 3 days
- Plus Sulfadoxine (25 mg/kg BW)
- Pyrimethamine 1.25 mg/kg BW on first day

Chemotherapy in Severe and Complicated Malaria

Initial parental treatment for atleast 48 hours.

Quinine

20 mg Quinine salt/kg body weight on admission (IV Infusion in Dex 5% over 4 hours followed by 10 mg/kg over 4 hours 8 hourly. Infusion rate should not exceed 5 mg/kg/hour. Loading dose of 20 mg/kg should not be given if patient has already received quinine.
Or
Artesunate 2.4 mg/kg IV or IM given on admission (time = 0) then at 12 hour and 24 hour then once a day.

Follow-up treatment when patient take oral medicine following parentral treatment.
Those who received injectable quinine are given quinine 10 mg/kg 3 times a day × 7 days.
With clindamycin 10 mg/kg bodyweight 10 hourly × 7 days.
Those who received injectable artesunate are given fully oral course of area specific ACT.
In north-eastern state, age specific ACT-AL × 3 days.
In other states, treat with ACT-SP for 3 days.

Note: Pregnant women with severe malaria in any trimester can be treated with artemisinin derivatives which in contrast to quinine do not risk aggravating hypoglycemia.

Supportive Treatment

- Patients with severe anemia may need blood transfusion
- Folic acid 10 mg should be given daily to prevent megaloblastic anemia.
- Fluid replacement needs to be very carefully monitored to prevent pulmonary edema.
- If anemia requires transfusion Hb <7–8 g/dL, then packed cells are preferred to avoid fluid overload.
- Complications of malaria should be managed aggressively and carefully.

Drugs which should not be used during malaria management in pregnancy
- Tetracyclin
- Doxycyclin
- Primaquin

Management of Labor

All efforts should be made to rapidly control body temperature by cold sponging, antipyretics. Careful fluid management is also very important. If situation demands induction of labor may have to be considered. Fetal or maternal distress may indicate the need to shorten the second stage of labour. If need even cesarean section must be considered.

Radical Cure

For prevention of relapse of *P. vivax* Tab. Chloroquine 300 mg/week is given until stoppage of lactation. Complete therapeutic treatment is given after stoppage of lactation chloroquine and primaquin for 14 days.

REFERENCES

1. Kakkilaya Srinivas, The problem of malaria, malaria modern day management, Macmillan medical communications, 1st edn 2012 Pg.
2. Tren R. Malaria and climate change. working Gpaper series: Julian Simoncentre for Policy Research. 2002.
3. Kumar A, Valecha N, Jain T, Dash AP, Burden of malaria in India, retrospective and prospective view. MJ Trop Med. Hyg. 2007;(6 suppl):69-78.
4. Malaria situation National vector born disease control programme. Available in *http://nvbdcp.gov.in/Doc/malaria %20situationpdf.*
5. WHO expert committee on malaria. Twentieth report. Geneva, World Health Organisation, 2000 (WHO Technical report series, No.892).
6. Guidelines for the treatment of malaria, 2nd edition. WHO, Geneva, 2010
7. World Health Organisation. A strategic framework for malaria prevention and control during pregnancy in the African region. Brazzaville; WHO Regional Office for Africa, 2004. AFR/AML 04/01. Available at http://whqlid who.int/afro/2004/AFR MAL 04.01 pdf
8. Chen LH, Wilson ME, Schlagenhauf P. Prevention of malaria in long term travelers. JAMA. 2006;296(18):2234-44.
9. WHO recommendations on antenatal care for appositive pregnancy experience2016 [Internet][cited on28nov2016] Available from *www.Who.int/reproductive health/publications/maternal_perinatal_health/ anc-positive-pregnancy-experience/en/.*
10. Guidelines for the treatment of malaria, 3rd edn. Geneva: World Health Organization; 2015 (*http://apps.who.int/iris/ bitstream/10665/162441/1/9789241549127_*).
11. National Drug Policy on Malaria 2013. Directorate of National Vector Borne Disease Control Programme (Directorate General of Health Services) Ministry of Health and Family Welfare. Delhi.

Chapter 40

Management of Influenza, Swine Flu and Dengue During Pregnancy

Priti Kumar, Phagun Shah

INFLUENZA AND SWINE FLU IN PREGNANCY

Introduction

Influenza is an acute, viral respiratory infection that causes significant morbidity and mortality among high-risk groups like pregnant women and infants. Physiological and immunological changes during pregnancy including decreased tidal volume and lung capacity, increased oxygen consumption and cardiac output, and selective suppression of T-helper-type 1 cell-mediated immunity that impairs maternal response to infection and poses pregnant women at high risk of complications and hospitalizations.[1-3]

The symptoms of influenza are fever, headache, chills, muscle aches, coughing, congestion, runny nose, and sore throat. Influenza sometimes causes vomiting and diarrhea. Influenza is contagious. The virus spreads through contact with respiratory droplets from the nose and mouth of infected individuals. When people cough or sneeze, droplets containing the virus are spread through the air. The incubation period (the time between exposure and the development of symptoms) is about 1 to 4 days. A person with the flu is contagious for upto a week after he or she first develops symptoms.

Influenza viruses are a group of RNA viruses belonging to the family *Orthomyxoviridae*. They are classified into 3 distinct genera: influenza A, B, and C.

Influenza A can be divided further into a number of subtypes according to the expression pattern of two viral antigens: hemagglutinin (which mediates viral attachment) and neuraminidase (which mediates viral release). There are 16 hemagglutinin and 9 neuraminidase variants. Thus, H1N1 (*H*emagglutinin-*1*, *N*euraminidase-*1*) designates a specific subtype of influenza A. Influenza B and C are not divided into subtypes. Both influenza A and B strains cause seasonal infections of viral influenza (flu) and the dominant strains are included in each year's influenza vaccination. Influenza C typically causes only a mild respiratory illness.[4]

Human infection with the novel H1N1 strain of the influenza A virus (formerly called *swine flu*) was first identified in April 2009. The outbreak has since reached pandemic status. Pregnant women are at especially high risk for the development of complications of H1N1 influenza A.[5,6] During pregnancy, healthy women have a 4- to 5-fold increased rate of serious illness and hospitalization with influenza.[6] For this reason, it is critical that all obstetric care providers be familiar with the symptoms, treatment, and prevention of H1N1 infection in pregnant women.

Clinical Manifestation of H1N1 Infection

Patients with novel H1N1 typically present with symptoms of an acute respiratory illness, including cough, sore throat, rhinorrhea, and fever. Other complaints may include headache, fatigue, body aches, vomiting, and diarrhea. Their clinical presentation can be complicated by development of a secondary bacterial infection (such as pneumonia). Symptoms commonly develop within 1 week of exposure, and patients are contagious for approximately 8 days thereafter. Most pregnant women will have an uncomplicated course, but there have been reports of adverse pregnancy outcome, including maternal death.[7]

The risk of morbidity from seasonal influenza is higher among pregnant women.[6,8-10] Pregnancy-related complications of novel H1N1 infection include nonreassuring fetal testing (most commonly fetal tachycardia) and febrile morbidity. Hyperthermia in early pregnancy has been associated with neural tube defects and other congenital anomalies, and fever during labor and birth is a risk factor for neonatal seizures, newborn encephalopathy, cerebral palsy, and death.

If influenza is suspected in a pregnant patient, she should undergo immediate testing for novel H1N1. A rapid influenza antigen test is commonly used in patients suspected of having influenza, which should be confirmed by reverse transcription polymerase chain reaction (RT-PCR), the recommended test.

Treatment

Pregnant women and women up to 4 weeks postpartum are also at high risk for influenza-related complications.[12] Increased severity of illness, increased hospitalizations, and increased mortality have been observed, particularly in women with influenza in their third trimester. Influenza in pregnancy has also been associated with effects on the fetus, including congenital abnormalities, low birth weight, preterm delivery, and fetal death.[12,13]

Oseltamivir is considered the antiviral medication of choice for pregnant women for the treatment of influenza.[11,13] Results from studies of pregnant women during the H1N1 pandemic in 2009 suggest that early treatment with oseltamivir may reduce ICU admissions and mortality. Current data do not suggest any increased risk to the developing fetus, if oseltamivir is taken during pregnancy. Treatment guidelines from the Association of Medical Microbiology and Infectious Disease, Canada, Centers for Disease Control and Prevention, and the Infectious Diseases Society of America all recommend oseltamivir use for the treatment of suspected and confirmed influenza in the pregnant population.

The CDC recommendation for pregnant women is oseltamivir (75 mg twice daily for 5 days) or zanamivir (25 mg inhalations twice daily for 5 days). Oseltamivir and zanamivir are both pregnancy category C drugs, but no adverse events have been reported to date among women who received these agents during pregnancy. Treatment should ideally be started as soon as possible after the onset of symptoms because the benefit of antiviral medications is greatest, if started within 48 hours of symptom onset. However, studies on antiviral use in seasonal flu have shown some benefit for hospitalized patients, even if started after 48 hours. In addition to specific antiviral medications, acetaminophen should be given, if the patient is febrile.[14-16]

Isolation

Patients with suspected pandemic H1N1 should wear a facemask and be placed in an isolated room away from providers and other hospitalized patients. If pandemic H1N1 infection is confirmed, contact precautions (gown and gloves) should be added. If aerosolization of droplets is possible (e.g. while the patient is receiving a nebulizer treatment or being intubated), goggles should be worn. Symptomatic patients should be placed on droplet precautions (including gowns, gloves, and N95 respirators), although most hospitals will only require droplet precautions for confirmed cases of novel H1N1. Due to the pandemic nature of the disease, patients do not need to be placed in negative-pressure rooms.[2,4]

If a pregnant patient delivers while infected with H1N1, she should be separated from her infant immediately after delivery. She should avoid close contact with her infant until she has been on antiviral medications for at least 48 hours, her fevers have resolved, and she can control her coughing and secretions. After this initial period of isolation, she should continue to practice good hand hygiene and cough etiquette, and wear a facemask for the next 7 days.

Prophylaxis

Postexposure prophylaxis should be considered for pregnant women with close contacts who have suspected or confirmed H1N1. Two regimens are recommended: zanamivir (10 mg inhaled daily) or oseltamivir (75 mg daily by mouth). Although zanamivir may be the drug of choice due to its limited systemic absorption, an inhaled route of administration may not be tolerated, especially in women with underlying respiratory disease such as asthma or chronic obstructive pulmonary disease. In this setting, oseltamivir is a reasonable alternative. Chemoprophylaxis should probably be continued for 10 days after the last known exposure, but may need to be extended at the discretion of the obstetric care provider in settings where multiple exposures are likely to occur (such as within households). Close monitoring for symptoms of influenza is recommended.[2]

Breastfeeding

The risk of transmission of novel H1N1 through breast milk is unknown. However, since reports of viremia with seasonal flu are rare, it seems highly unlikely that the H1N1 virus will cross into breast milk. On the other hand, breastfeeding is known to strengthen the neonatal immune response, and infants who are not breastfed may actually be more vulnerable to viral infection.

Use of antiviral medication for H1N1 treatment or chemoprophylaxis is not a contraindication to breastfeeding. The concentration of both oseltamivir and zanamivir in breast milk has been estimated to be less than the pediatric dose of each. If the infant needs to be isolated from its infected mother, healthy adults should provide bottle feedings of expressed breast milk until the mother and child can be reunited. If no assistance is available, the mother should be allowed to breastfeed her child, but she should use a facemask and practice strict hand hygiene and cough etiquette.

Prevention

Recommendations for the prevention of pandemic H1N1 infection in pregnant women are similar to those for seasonal flu.[2,4] Patients should be advised to cover their cough, practice good hand hygiene, and minimize sick contacts. They should be encouraged to stay home, if sick. In the office or hospital setting, sick or potentially infected patients should be separated from the healthy pregnant population.

Vaccination

A seasonal trivalent influenza vaccine is available which is surface antigen inactivated vaccine and should be offered to all pregnant women during flu season (November–March). Such vaccinations are low-cost interventions that have been shown to have substantial benefits for both mother and baby. There are recommendations of many member bodies to promote influenza vaccination in pregnancy, such as WHO, ACOG and FOGSI. The vaccination is recommended in second and third trimester of pregnancy and in case of epidemic, it can be given in the first trimester as well.[17,18]

Conclusion

Pregnant women and their fetuses are at high risk of infection with the novel H1N1 influenza A virus. Obstetric providers need to be prepared to provide the care necessary to address the increased morbidity, mortality, and pregnancy-related complications (including spontaneous miscarriage and preterm birth) faced by pregnant women during such an influenza pandemic.

PREGNANCY AND DENGUE FEVER

Dengue fever is a viral disease caused by any of 4 closely related serotypes of Flavivirus (RNA virus). *Aedes* mosquitoes, particularly *A. aegypti* is a vector transmitting it to human. Most of the states in India are dengue endemic. *Early detection and access to proper medical care reduces fatality from 20% to below 1%.* When this viral infection is not asymptomatic, it is diagnosed as dengue fever (DF), dengue hemorrhagic fever (DHF), and dengue shock syndrome. The effect of dengue infection on pregnant women and their fetuses is unclear, although several cases and case series have been reported.[19-21]

The clinical manifestations, treatment and outcome of dengue in pregnant women are similar to those of nonpregnant women. The clinical presentation of dengue may overlap with some of the complications of pregnancy, e.g. HELLP syndrome, pneumonia, pulmonary embolism, various obstetric causes of pervaginal bleeding and other infectious diseases. It is still uncertain whether dengue is a significant factor for adverse pregnancy outcomes such as preterm birth, low-birth weight and cesarean deliveries. The risk of vertical transmission is well established among women with dengue during the perinatal period. Severe bleeding may complicate delivery and/or surgical procedures performed on pregnant patients with dengue *during the critical phase*, i.e. the period coinciding with marked thrombocytopenia with or without plasma leak. Dengue fever does not warrant termination of pregnancy. There is insufficient data of probable embryopathy to mothers who had DF in first trimester.[22]

Challenges in Recognition of Dengue Disease and Plasma Leakage in Pregnancy

Vomiting which is one of the warning sign may be taken as hyperemesis of pregnancy. Baseline tachycardia, lower baseline BP and lower baseline hematocrit attributed to physiological rise in blood volume. Failure to recognize plasma leakage and shock early will lead to decompensated shock and multiorgan failure.

Clinical Presentation (Flow chart 40.1)

Dengue fever happens in three stages: Febrile phase, critical phase and recovery phase.

Acute Febrile Phase

- There is a high grade fever, (Day 1-7) with facial flushing, skin erythema, congested pharynx and conjunctiva. Body ache, myalgia, arthralgia, retroorbital eye pain, headache sore throat, anorexia, nausea and vomiting.
- Rash looks like flushed skin on Day 1/2, later looks like measles. General and systemic examination may be normal petechial and mucosal membrane bleeding. Liver may been larged and tender after few days off ever.
- Tourniquet test is positive

(Inflate BP cuff to midpoint between SBP and DBP for 5 minutes. Test is positive when >10 petechial spots appear/1sq inch area).

The earliest abnormality in the progressive decrease in WBC, which should alert the physician to a high probability of dengue.

Critical Phase (Phase of Capillary Leak)

When fever starts subsiding (Day 3-8) critical phase starts. One or all of following complications may develop, and if not intervened in time results in fatality.
- Significant plasma leak from intravascular compartment to extravascular compartment leading to shock and death.
- Hemorrhagic manifestations
- Severe organ involvement may develop (Hepatitis, encephalitis, myocarditis, bleeding)

Warning Signs of Plasma Leak

- Persistent vomiting and severe abdominal pain, increasing lethargic but usually remains mentally alert, increasing liver size and a tender liver
- Progressive signs of shock and death
- Fall in WBC, Platelets fall and rise in hematocrit (PCV)
- Cold extremities capillary refill time of > 2 seconds
- Rapid breathing cold and cyanosed extremities
- Mottled skin, BP unstable/not recordable
- Pulse pressure of ≤20 mm Hg, systolic BP may be normal.
- Tachycardia, weak pulse, very feeble pulse. Pulse oxymetry may be normal. Confused, restless
- Lethargic

Flow chart 40.1: Classification (WHO Classification 1997)

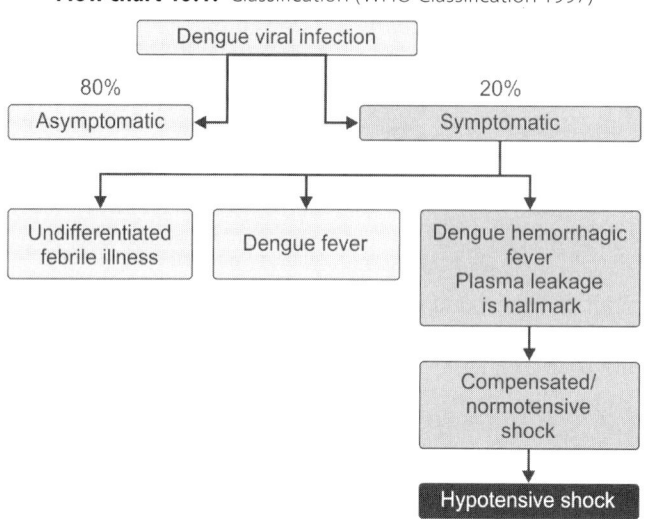

	Febrile phase	Critical phase	Recovery phase
Symptoms	Fever with	Fever starts subsiding	Afebrile
	Headache/arthalgia/myalgia		
	Tourniquet test +	Warning signs appear	
Potential complication	Dehydration	Shock	Volume overload
		Bleeding	
		Multiorgan involvement	
Lab change	WBC low	Platelet Low	Hct: Stable/normal
		Hct rise	WBC increase
			Platelet increase
	1–4 days	3rd to 6th day	7th to 10th day

Recovery Phase

As the patient survives the 24–48 hour of critical phase, a gradual reabsorption of extravascular compartment fluid takes place in the following 48–72 hours. General well-being improves, appetite returns, gastrointestinal symptoms abate, hemodynamics status stabilizes, and diuresis ensues.

Management of Dengue Fever in Pregnancy

All pregnant patients with suspected dengue fever are advised admission for close monitoring. The management of pregnant female with dengue depends on the severity of the illness **(Flow charts 40.2 and 40.3)**:

Monitor (Pregnant Female with Group A)

- Do baseline CBC on D1/D2 of fever.
- If WBC count normal/lower side, suspect dengue fever.
- Repeat CBC after 24 hours and compare further fall in platelets/rise in PCV (10% rise is considered as significant).
- Temperature charting, pulse, BP and pulse pressure every four hours
- Ensure urine output at least 4-6 hours (minimum 100 cc every 4 hours)
  - Intake output record.
  - *Labs:* Daily CBC, other investigations, if necessary.

Treatment

- Paracetamol 500-650 6 hourly. *Not* to exceed 4 g paracetamol in 24 hours.
- NSAID such as ibuprofen and diclofenac sodium. Should not be taken. Tepid sponging for fever.
  - Aspirin should be avoided.
  - Oral Intake encouraged. ORS, coconut water, Kanji, juice, all are encouraged apart from routine food. Aim of at least 2.5 L of fluid intake. If nausea/vomiting of

Flow chart 40.2: Inpatient management for dengue patients with warning signs

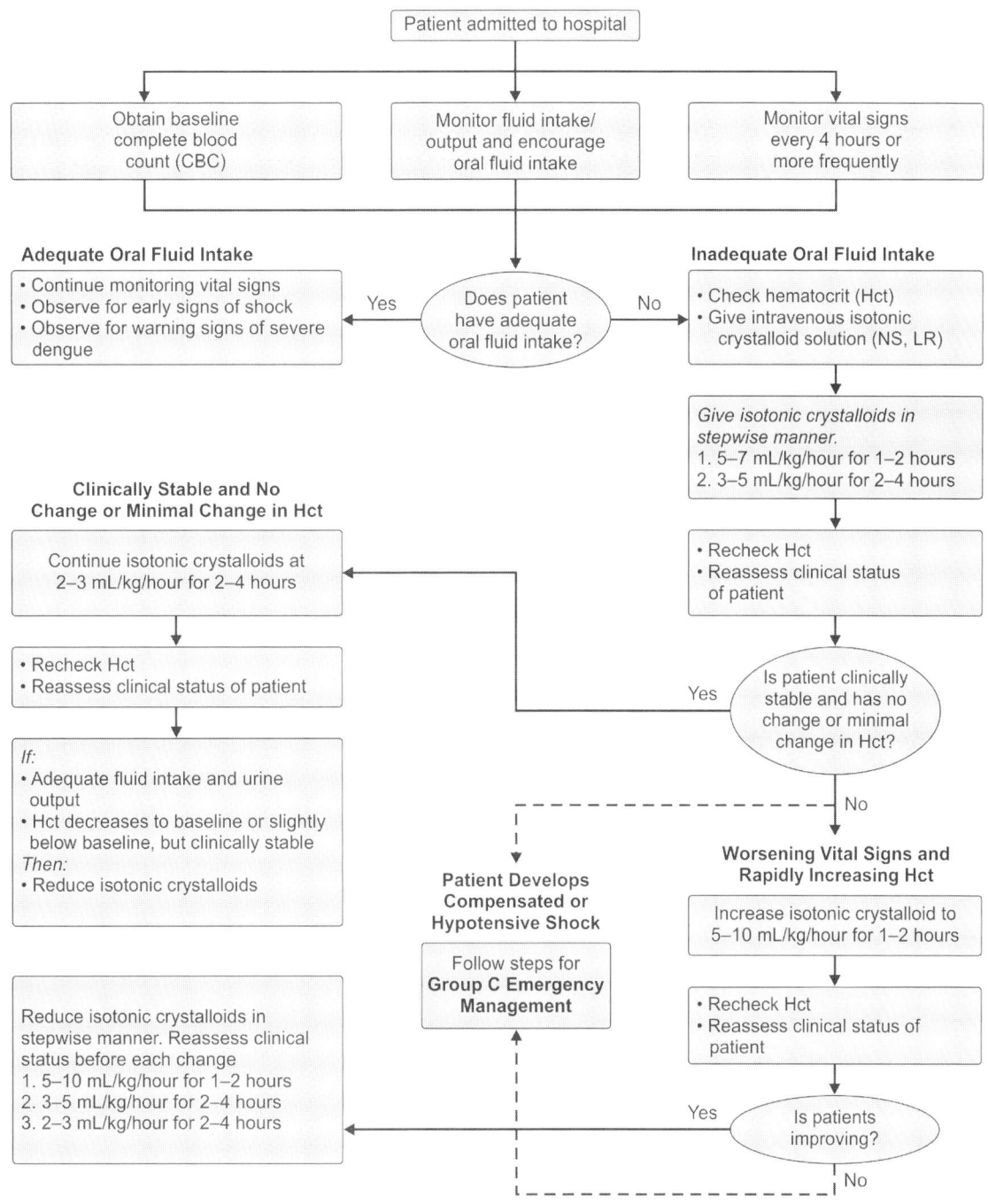

Abbreviations: NS, normal saline; LR, Ringer's lactate

pregnancy restrict oral intake, give IV fluid (NS) 100 cc/hour. One should be cautious, if urine output is less, vomiting, lethargy, narrowing of pulse pressure (<20) is noticed.
- Warning symptoms and signs for capillary leak are to be looked for vigilantly especially so when fever starts subsiding. As warning signs hallmarks capillary leak and she can progress to severe dengue. These are patients for IV fluid therapy.
- Warning symptoms are abdominal pain and tenderness, persistent vomiting, lethargy, restlessness, liver enlargement >2 cm, urine output is less, mucosal bleed: epistaxis, gum bleed and petechial.

Flow chart 40.3: Dengue case management

Assessment

Presumptive diagnosis
Live in/travel to endemic area plus fever and two of the following:
- Nausea and vomiting
- Rash
- Acnes and pains (headache, eye pain, muscle ache or joint pain)
- Warning signs
- Tourniquet test positive
- Leukopenia

↓

Warning signs
- Severe abdominal pain or tenderness
- Porsistent vomiting
- Mucosal bleed
- Liver enlargement >2 cm
- Clinical fluid accumulation
- Lethargy; restiesness
- Increase in Hct concurrent with rapid decrease in platelet count

↓

No warning signs	For patients with warning signs of severe dengue or co-existing conditions: • Pregnancy • Infancy • Diabetes mellitus • Poor social situation • Old age • Renal failure	For patients with any of: • Severe plasma leakage with shock and/or fluid accumulation with respiratory distress • Severe bleeding • Severe organ impairment
Group A Outpatient management	**Group B** Inpatient management	**Group C** Inpatient management

– Rise in Hct (20% of baseline) (If baseline is not known consider 36 as baseline)

Dengue Fever with Warning Sign (Group B)

- Monitor vitals (BP, pulse and pulse pressure hourly)
- Catheterize to know precise UOP hourly (Aim 0.5 mL/kg/hour).
- Intense fluid resuscitation. (Normal saline). Bolus of 5–10 mL/kg/hour × 2 hours given followed by 3–5 mL/kg/hour as a maintenance. This is monitored by UOP and Pulse pressure.
- Avoid induction of labor/-planned surgery in this phase.

Dengue Fever with Shock on Admission (Group C)

These patients need institutional management in ICCU setup. Timely fluid management with appearance of any warning symptom practically prevents further complication. Before transferring this patient

- Draw blood for CBC, to know Hct.
- ABO/Rh, SGOT, SGPT, electrolytes, blood sugar, blood urea and serum creatinine.
- Fluids bolus given as (NS) 10 cc/kg over 15 minutes. Before transfer NS is preferred to Ringer lactate and DNS. *Plain Dextrose solution NOT to be used. Colloids can be given only after 2 fluid boluses in patients of shock.* And second bolus as 10 mL/kg for next 1 hour during transfer.

  Hand over all reports, fluid bolus details for reference for further treatment
- *Transfusion trigger:* Trigger is low for dengue than in any other blood tranfusion indication.
- *Fresh blood transfusion (BT):* If there is overt blood loss nearing 500 cc.

Convalescent Phase

Rise of WBC count followed by rise of platelet count, stabilization of Hct marks convalescent phase. Now watch for signs of fluid overload—cough, wheez, tachypnea, rise of both SBP and DBP.

Discharge from Hospital

- If afebrile for 24 hours without antipyretics
- If the appetite is normal
- Hct at baseline value and rising trends of WBC and platelets.

WORD OF CAUTION

- No Other NSAID (Ibuprofen/Diclofenac) for fever. Only Paracetamol to be given. Daily dose should not exceed 4 g. Normal saline 0.9% should be used for initial resuscitation.
- No overt bleeding but *drop in Hct without clinical improvement* despite adequate fluid replacement, the patient should be referred to higher center.
- Prophylactic platelet transfusion is *not* recommended unless delivery is inevitable (in coming 6 hours) platelet count > 50000/cc, and 75000/cc for operative delivery. Clinically stable dengue with low or very low platelet count in critical/recovery phase—no platelet transfusion. Platelet transfusion may be given in presence of overt bleeding with low platelet counts.
- There is no role of steroid/IV immunoglobulin/prophylactic antibiotics.
- Operative delivery for obstetric indications only. Avoid Planned *induction*/surgery. The presence of wounds or trauma during the critical phase of dengue with marked thrombocytopenia, and plasma leak creates a substantial risk of severe hemorrhage.

- Delivery should take place in a hospital where blood/blood components and a team of skilled obstetricians and a neonatologist are available.
- Tocolytic agents and measures to postpone labor to a suitable time may be considered during the critical phase of dengue illness. However, there is currently a lack of evidence on this practice.
- Intramuscular injections, Hypotonic, Steroids and antibiotics are avoided

Inevitable Delivery During Critical Phase

If delivery is inevitable, then bleeding should be anticipated and closely monitored. Blood and blood products should be cross-matched and saved in preparation for delivery. Trauma or injury should be kept to the minimum, if possible. It is essential to check for complete removal of the placenta after delivery.

- Transfusion of platelet concentrates should be initiated during or at delivery but not too far ahead of delivery, as the platelet count is sustained by platelet transfusion for only a few hours during the critical phase.

Fresh whole blood/fresh packed red cells transfusion should be administered as soon as possible, if significant bleeding occurs. If blood loss can be quantified, it should be replaced immediately. Do not wait for blood loss to exceed 500 mL before replacement, as in postpartum hemorrhage. Do not wait for the hematocrit to decrease to low levels.

Oxytocin infusion should be commenced to contract the uterus after delivery to prevent postpartum hemorrhage. Misoprostol may be given for PPH—prophylaxis/treatment.

- Intramuscular injections are to be avoided.

Post-delivery

Newborns with mothers who had dengue just before or at delivery, should be closely monitored in hospital after birth in view of the risk of vertical transmission. At or near-term/delivery, severe fetal or neonatal dengue illness and death may occur when there is insufficient time for the production of protective maternal antibodies. Baby to be evaluated for congenital dengue.

REFERENCES

1. Jamieson DJ, Theiler RN, Rasmussen SA. Emerging infections and pregnancy. Emerging Infectious Diseases. 2006;12(11):1638-43.
2. Gaunt G, Ramin K. Immunological tolerance of the human fetus. The American Journal of Perinatology. 2001;18(6) 299-312.
3. Laibl VR, Sheffield JS. Influenza and pneumonia in pregnancy. Clinics in Perinatology. 2005;32(3):727-38.
4. Neumann G, Noda T, Kawaoka Y. Emergence and pandemic potential of swine-origin H1N1 influenza virus. Nature. 2009;459:931-9. [PMC free article] [PubMed]
5. Centers for Disease Control and Prevention Web site, authors. Pregnant women and novel influenza A (H1N1): considerations for clinicians. [Accessed August 24, 2009]. http://www.cdc.gov/h1n1flu/clinician_pregnant.htm. Updated June 30, 2009.
6. Jamieson DJ, Honein MA, Rasmussen SA, et al. Novel Influenza A (H1N1) Pregnancy Working Group, authors. H1N1 2009 influenza virus infection during pregnancy in the USA. Lancet. 2009;374:451-8. [PubMed]
7. Dawood FS, Jain S, Finelli L, et al. Novel Swine-Origin Influenza A (H1N1) Virus Investigation Team, authors. Emergence of a novel swine-origin influenza A (H1N1) virus in humans. N Engl J Med. 2009;360:2605-15. [PubMed]
8. Shinde V, Bridges CB, Uyeki TM, et al. Triple-reassortant swine influenza A (H1) in humans in the United States, 2005-2009. N Engl J Med. 2009;360:2616-25. [PubMed]
9. Neuzil KM, Reed GW, Mitchel EF, et al. Impact of influenza on acute cardiopulmonary hospitalizations in pregnant women. Am J Epidemiol. 1998;148:1094-102. [PubMed]
10. Dodds L, McNeil SA, Fell DB, et al. Impact of influenza exposure on rates of hospital admissions and physician visits because of respiratory illness among pregnant women. CMAJ.
11. Mertz D, Kim KH, Johnstone J, et al. Populations at risk for severe or complicated influenza illness: Systematic review and meta-analysis. BMJ. 2013;347:f5061.
12. Luteijn JM, Brown MJ, Dolk H. Influenza and congenital anomalies: a systematic review and meta-analysis. Hum Reprod. 2014;29:809-23.
13. Haberg SE, Trogstad L, Gunnes N, et al. Risk of fetal death after pandemic influenza virus infection or vaccination. N Engl J Med. 2013;368:333-40.
14. Ward P, Small I, Smith J, et al. Oseltamivir (Tamiflu®) and its potential for use in the event of an influenza pandemic. J Antimicrob Chemother. 2005;55(suppl 1):i5-i21. [PubMed]
15. Hayashi M, Yamane R, Tanaka M, et al. Pregnancy outcome after maternal exposure to oseltamivir phosphate during the first trimester: a case series survey [in Japanese]. Nihon Byoin Yakuzaishi Gakkai Zasshi. 2009;45:547-50.
16. Freund B, Gravenstein S, Elliott M, Miller I. Zanamivir: a review of clinical safety. Drug Saf. 1999;21:267-81. [PubMed]
17. World Health Organization Website, authors. Vaccines for the new influenza A (H1N1) [Accessed August 24, 2009]. http://www.who.int/csr/disease/swineflu/frequently_asked_questions/vaccine_preparedness/en/index.html. Updated July 12, 2009.
18. Macdonald NE, Riley LE, Steinhoff MC. Influenza immunization in pregnancy. Obstet Gynecol. 2009;114:365-8. [PubMed]
19. Carles G, Talarmin A, Peneau C, Bertsch M. Dengue fever and pregnancy: a study of 38 cases in French Guiana. J Gynecol Obstet Biol Reprod. 2000;29(8):758-62.
20. Janjindamai W, Pruekprasert P. Perinatal dengue infection: a case report and review of literature. Southeast Asian J Trop Med Public Health. 2003;34(4):793-6.
21. Sirinavin S, Nuntnarumit P, Supapannachart S, Boonkasidecha S, Techasaensisi C, Yoksarn S. Vertical dengue infection: case reports and review. Pediatr Infect Dis J. 2004;23(11):1042-7.
22. FOGSI Guidelines for the Management of Dengue, 2014.

Chapter 41

Tuberculosis in Pregnancy: Update on an Archenemy

Alka Pandey, Ajay Sinha

INTRODUCTION

Tuberculosis is an archenemy of humankind from time immemorial. Almost one-third of the world population is infected with tuberculosis. TB is bacterial disease caused by *Mycobacterium tuberculosis* and spreads through air droplets. In 2014, an estimated 3.2 million women suffered from TB; and, out of that, 4,80,000 women died including 1,40,000 deaths among HIV-positive women. Most of the victims are from South-East Asia and Africa. This disease is the greatest cause of death in people living with HIV.

Tuberculosis in pregnancy is very common in India and is among the three leading causes of death among women aged 15–45 years. The exact incidence of TB in pregnancy is not available in India, however, it is expected that the incidence among pregnant women would be as high as in general population in India. TB in pregnancy is associated with six-fold increase in perinatal deaths and two-fold risks of premature birth and low birth weight. Genital TB, which is challenging to diagnose, has been identified as an important cause of infertility. TB among mothers living with HIV, is associated with 300% increased risk of infant and perinatal mortality and is associated with more than double the risk of vertical transmission of HIV to the unborn child.

Tuberculosis in pregnancy is described as a double-edged sword, one blade being the effect of tuberculosis on pregnancy and growth of the newborn, while the other is the effect of pregnancy on the progression of tuberculosis. The factors which have got effects of TB on pregnancy include the severity of the disease, how advanced the pregnancy has gone at the time of diagnosis, the presence of extrapulmonary spread, HIV co infection and nutritional status of the patient.

DIAGNOSIS OF TUBERCULOSIS IN PREGNANT WOMEN

Diagnosis of TB in pregnancy can be difficult because of the vague, non-specific nature of the symptoms. Fatigue, sweating and tiredness, shortness of breath, all characteristics of TB can also be due to pregnancy. Between 20% and 67% of pregnant patients presenting with pulmonary TB, are unaware of their disease and have no significant symptoms. Therefore, high suspicion is important for treating gynecologist and physician. Many physicians are reluctant to order a chest X-ray for diagnosis, for fear of harming fetus particularly in first trimester. If the chest X-ray is necessary, suitable lead apron shielding will limit fetal radiation exposure to less than 0.3 mrads and should not harm the fetus. MRI scan chest and abdomen is an option in selected group of patient. There are no reported harmful effects from MRI on the pregnant women or fetus.

Diagnostic work-up includes:
- *History and clinical examination in suspected patient*
- Lab investigation, including complete blood count, PCR, Interferon-gamma-release assay (IGRA) (TB gold). IGRA is usually obsolete in diagnosing HIV-negative active tuberculosis, but it has got a role in diagnostic work-up of extrapulmonary tuberculosis.
- Tuberculin skin test (Mantoux test)—mostly in latent TB infection (LTBI) and HIV patient, sometimes, it can be of help in diagnosing extrapulmonary TB. Likewise, IGRA (TB gold) has usually no role in diagnosing active TB but, sometimes, it may help like Mantoux test (superior to Mantoux test in India due to high BCG vaccination)
- X-ray chest PA view
- Sputum for AFB and culture (Cornerstone), 3 specimen early morning sample
- Gene codons for multidrug resistant tuberculosis (MDR-TB)
- Fine-needle aspiration cytology (FNAC) and biopsy of lymph node and tissue (definitive diagnosis)
- USG in extrapulmonary tuberculosis
- MRI chest and abdomen.

Latent TB Infection

Latent TB infection (LTBI) is a condition in patients who have no clinical or radiological evidence of active disease. In these cases, TB bacteria lie dormant in body, but have produced antibodies against them, which is detected by most of our screening test, including Mantoux test. The prevalence rate of latent tuberculosis in India is very high and ranges from 40% to 50% (in west only 0.5%). This means that India has 500 million population suffering from LTBI; out of which, 5–10% of these cases may convert into active TB disease. The goal of testing for LTBI is to identify individuals who are at increased risk for the development of TB and, therefore, who would benefit from treatment of LTBI. Contrary to Western countries, treatment LTBI is usually not recommended in India except in HIV-positive and immune compromised patient.

TREATMENT

After diagnosis, treatment is planned as per recommendation of the WHO, British Thoracic Society, International Union against Tuberculosis. For patients with drug susceptible TB and good adherence, first-line drugs will cure more than 90% TB in pregnancy in India. Treatment is mostly done on outdoor basis except aggressive vigilance of early drug-induced side effects. The preferred initial treatment regimen is INH, Rifampicin, and Ethambutol daily for 2 months, followed by INH and Rifampicin for 7 months. Streptomycin should not be used because it has been shown to have harmful effects in the fetus. Pyrazinamide is not recommended in the USA because its effects on fetus are unknown. However, in some countries, it has been used because of its peculiar effect on TB bacteria without having bad effect on fetus.

INH: ADEC category A, 5 mg/kg, max 300 mg, side effects—hepatotoxicity 2%, others—nausea, peripheral neuropathy, rash, arthralgia, psychosis.

Rifampicin: ADEC category C, 10 mg/kg, max 450 (<50 kg), 600 (>50 kg), side effects—hepatotoxicity, bone marrow suppression, nausea, rash and polyarthralgia and finally hemorrhagic tendency in newborn, if used late in pregnancy (administer postpartum vitamin K to the newborn baby).

Ethambutol: ADEC category A, 20 mg/kg max 1000 mg, side effects—optic neuritis, headache, confusion, nausea, vomiting and malaise.

Pyrazinamide: Limited pregnancy data available, but no reports of fetal malformations or significant adverse events reported, 25 mg/kg max 1500 mg. Side effects—hepatotoxicity, rash, arthralgia.

Detailed guidelines can be downloaded from *website// www.health.qld.gov.au.*

BREASTFEEDING

Antituberculosis drugs are compatible with breastfeeding. The amounts of drugs excreted in breast milk are very small without any harmful effect to the baby, and insufficient to kill BCG vaccine. If the mother is still sputum positive just before delivery, then infant needs preventive chemotherapy ideally with Isoniazid for 6 months. Breastfeeding is continued. BCG vaccination is done in all newborns (only in HIV-infected infant where extraprecaution for immunity development is taken).

MULTIDRUG RESISTANT TUBERCULOSIS IN PREGNANCY

There is no conclusive evidence to aid clinicians for managing MDR TB. Only case reports provide guidance for management of MDR TB in pregnancy. The best way to deal with MDR TB and pregnancy is to prevent it. Patient and their relatives should be involved in management decisions. Individualized approach is selected based on risks and benefit to the patient and pregnancy, use of injections should be avoided (exception-high mortality risk).

Streptomycin/Amikacin/Kanamycin: Safety uncertain but evidence of risk class *D* usually avoided.

Capreomycin category C, but to be avoided usually because of 8th nerve damage and renal toxicity in fetus.

Fluoroquinolones/ethionamide/cycloserine/PAS/Linezolid: Safety uncertain but no human or animal studies reveal an adverse effect *C* can be used.

HIV COINFECTION AND PREGNANT WOMEN WITH TUBERCULOSIS

HIV infection in pregnancy increases the chance of tuberculosis. Early recognition of TB is important to prevent neonatal TB among these women. This can be done primarily on the basis of maternal history and relevant investigations of the mother and newborn. There are WHO guidelines for maternal therapy and prophylaxis and also prophylaxis to the newborn on the stage of maternal disease. When the CD4 count is less than 200, mother should be treated with combination of antiretroviral. The combination of antiretroviral and antituberculous therapy poses difficulties which can be resolved by combination of different drugs. In both the conditions, exclusive breastfeeding is recommended.

Pregnancy does not appear to influence the progression of HIV disease and it does not seem to affect survival of women infected with HIV. Concern was raised that anti-HIV (anti-retroviral) therapy may increase the incidence of adverse pregnancy outcome. But studies have shown that most of anti-retroviral, except protease inhibitors, had no negative effect on pregnancy. Antiretroviral therapy has led to marked decrease of HIV transmission in mother to child (from 25% to 2%). Pregnancy alters the pharmacokinetics of a number of antiretroviral drugs, therefore, selection of both anti-tuberculous and antiretroviral drugs should be optimized.

CONCLUSION

Due to high prevalence of tuberculosis in pregnancy and diagnostic dilemma, increased awareness for early diagnosis is important for treating clinician. Skin testing on suspected pregnant patient and strategic efforts to identify active disease are key steps to successful management. Pregnancies complicated by MDR-TB and/or AIDS require special consideration.

BIBLIOGRAPHY

1. 2010/2011 tuberculosis global fact; World Health Organization, http://www.who.int/tb/country/en/index.html, Nov. 2010.
2. Facts about health in African Subregion, Factsheet N-314 World Health Organization, 2011.
3. Friedman LN, Tanoue LT. Tuberculosis in pregnancy. Up to date [online] 2014 Mar [cited 2014 Apr 28]; [9 screens]. Available from URL: http://www.uptodate.com/contents/search.
4. Global tuberculosis control 2010, Tech. Rep. World Health Organization, Geneva, Switzerland (WHO/HTM/TB/2010), 2010.
5. National Health and Medical Research Council (NHMRC). The Australian Immunisation Handbook, http://www.health.gov.au/internet/immunise/publishing.nsf/Content/Handbook-home Ed. Canberra: Australian Government Publishing Service; 2013.
6. National TB Advisory Committee. Position Statement on interferon-γ release assays in the detection of latent TB infection. CDI. 2012;36:125-31. Available from URL: http://www.health.gov.au/internet/main/publishing.nsf/content/cda-cdi3601-pdf-cnt.htm/$FILE/cdi3601i.pdf.
7. Palasanthiran P, Starr M, Jones C. Management of perinatal infections. Sydney: Australasian Society for Infectious Diseases (ASID); 2002. recommendations, 2006.
8. Pathways to Better Diagnostics for Tuberculosis. A Blueprint for Development of TB Diagnostics. World Health Organization, Geneva, Switzerland, 2009.
9. Therapeutic Guidelines, Antibiotic-Mycobacterial infections (Tuberculosis) [revised June 2010] In: eTG complete [internet]. Melbourne: Therapeutic Guidelines Limited; 2014 March.
10. WHO guideline for intensified tuberculosis case finding and isoniazid preventive therapy for people living with HIV, WHO, Geneva, Switzerland, 2011.

Chapter 42

Viral Infections in Pregnancy and Labor

Madhuri Chandra

INTRODUCTION

Viral infections during pregnancy not only contribute to maternal morbidity and mortality but also carry the risk of adverse pregnancy outcome, including spontaneous abortions, stillbirths, premature birth and intrauterine growth restriction. Physiological adaptions in pregnancy alter the maternal immune system and its response to bacterial and viral infections. Infections like influenza may have a more virulent course in pregnancy while other infections carry risk of vertical transmission and spread from the woman to her fetus or newborn. Common viral infections with risk of mother-to-child transmission are discussed.

Infections with risk of mother-to-child transmission:
- *Intrauterine*: Transplacental
  - *Viruses*: Varicella zoster, coxsackie, parvovirus B19, rubella, CMV, HIV
  - *Bacteria*: Treponema pallidum, Listeria monocytogenes, Borrelia
  - *Protozoa*: Toxoplasmosis, *Plasmodium falciparum*.
- *Intrauterine*: Ascending infection
  - Group B streptococcus, coliforms, HSV
- Ascending maternal infection and chorioamnionitis causing fetal infection, usually subsequent to prolonged rupture of membranes (PROM), prolonged labor, obstetric manipulations.
- Perinatal infection (during birth)—hematogenous or genital route—gonorrhea, chlamydia, tuberculosis, Group B streptococcus, HIV, herpes (HSV), HPV, hepatitis B and C, varicella.
- Postnatal infection—*Staphylococcus*, HSV, HIV, coliforms. Childbirth involves an abrupt transition from a highly protected environment to exposure to a vast array of new pathogens ex utero. It places the baby with an immature immune system in direct contact with maternal blood or genital secretions and infections may result, especially in PROM. Some protection is provided by maternal antibodies (IgG) crossing the placenta.

Antenatal screening is advised for:
- Rubella susceptibility
- Syphilis
- Hepatitis B
- HIV I and II
- Pap's smear, gonococcal, chlamydia, tuberculosis screening and Group B streptococcus culture.

Preconception counseling and vaccination for protection against influenza, rubella, tetanus and varicella is advocated.

RUBELLA (GERMAN MEASLES)

Introduction

Rubella or German measles is an acute contagious viral infection, which occurs most often in children and young adults.

Epidemiology

Rubella occurs worldwide. Rubella has a seasonal pattern, with epidemics in spring. Widespread use of MMR vaccination in childhood has eliminated rubella and congenital rubella syndrome from developed countries.

Etiopathogenesis

Rubella is an RNA virus of Togavirus family, its infection causes a mild disease, with fever, coryza and a maculopapular rash, it is often asymptomatic. Posterior auricular, cervical and suboccipital lymphadenopathy may be present. However, if the infection occurs during pregnancy, it can cross the placenta and cause fetal death or Congenital Rubella Syndrome (RS). Incidence of CRS in developing countries is 0.4–4.3/1000 live births. Birth defects are most likely (85%) in infants infected during the first eight weeks of pregnancy. Infants with CRS suffer retarded growth, classic triad of sensorineural deafness, eye defects—retinopathy, cataract, microphthalmia and congenital heart disease. Other manifestations include microcephaly, blood disorders, thrombocytopenia, purpuric skin rash, intellectual disability or pneumonia. They may also develop problems later in childhood, including autism, hearing loss, brain syndromes, insulin-dependent diabetes mellitus, immune system disorders, or thyroid disease. Infections after 20 weeks gestation usually cause no fetal problems. Thus an accurate knowledge of gestational age at exposure is most important factor to predict fetal manifestation **(Table 42.1)**.

Diagnosis

Rubella is usually asymptomatic, or causes mild fever, cold and rash. Posterior auricular and cervical lymph nodes may be enlarged. Diagnosis depends on history of contact, symptoms and serology for rubella specific antibodies. Rubella can also be diagnosed by viral RNA detection with PCR usually in oral, nasal, throat samples. IgG avidity differentiates between primary infection and reinfection, however, test facilities not universally available **(Table 42.2)**.

Management

- Routine screening of all antenatal for rubella susceptibility is not advised.[1] In India, most women are exposed to rubella during childhood and have high immunity. Childhood MMR vaccine provides good immunity, a history of vaccination should be taken from all pregnant women.
- Serological tests should be offered to any pregnant woman with fever and rash or in woman with history of exposure or contact. If within a week of exposure, IgG is positive and IgM negative, there is previous immunity and no evidence of recent infection. If both IgG and IgM are not detected, the person is susceptible to rubella and retest after 4 weeks is advised. If rubella IgM detected irrespective of IgG result, further reference testing is advised.[3]
- There is no specific treatment for rubella, symptomatic relief with antipyretics and analgesics may be provided. If maternal infection occurs prior to 10 weeks of gestation, the patient is counseled about fetal risks and offered medical termination of pregnancy.
- USG markers of CRS/fetal rubella infection—IUGR, microcephaly, ventriculomegaly, hydrocephalus, cardiac abnormality. Amniocentesis for viral PCR may be offered after 6 weeks of exposure, however, positive viral PCR does not guarantee fetal or neonatal effects.

Prophylaxis

All woman susceptible to rubella and planning pregnancy, should be offered 2 doses of MMR vaccine, 4 weeks apart or rubella vaccine single dose and advised to avoid pregnancy for one month post-vaccination. Vaccination can be done in postpartum period also.[2]

CYTOMEGALOVIRUS

Introduction

Cytomegalovirus (CMV) is a double-stranded DNA virus of herpes family. CMV is a common virus and most women have had an episode in their lifetime. The prevalence of CMV antibody increases with age, the age of acquisition of CMV being influenced by socioeconomic status, ethnic background, social and sexual practices and childcare settings.

Table 42.1: Risk of congenital rubella syndrome[2]

Period of gestation	Risk of congenital rubella syndrome (CRS)
<10 weeks	80–90%—consider medical termination of pregnancy
11–16 weeks	10–20%
16–20 weeks	20% deafness
>20 weeks	<1%

Table 42.2: Serologic evaluation of pregnant woman exposed to Rubella

Sera at 1st visit

IgG	IgM	Interpretation
Positive	Negative	Immune
Negative	Negative	Susceptible, repeat IgG and IgM, 3 to 4 weeks from suspected exposure: If IgM and IgG positive—acute infection; If negative—repeat test after 6 weeks.
Negative	Positive	Acute infection, collect 2nd sera 5–10 days later for IgG, IgM, IgG avidity testing.
Positive	Positive	Low avidity, rise in IgG titer—acute infection. High avidity, no rise in IgG titer—false positive. False positive seen in parvovirus B19, Epstein Barr virus infection and rheumatoid arthritis.

Epidemiology

CMV is not highly contagious, its spread requires close contact with infected secretions. The infection passes unnoticed or there may be mild flulike symptoms. Primary CMV infection involves about 1% of all pregnancies, with a 40% risk of transmission to fetus, risk being greatest in third trimester, though most adverse fetal outcomes occur with first trimester infection.[2] Once infection has taken place, the virus remains dormant within the body and recurrences of the virus in body fluids may occur at intervals. It is the primary infection that is more likely to result in severe fetal infection though CMV reactivation or reinfection has a <1% risk of transmission from mother to fetus **(Table 42.3)**.

Etiopathogenesis

Cytomegalovirus is the most common congenital infection, occurring in 0.2–2.2% of newborns. Transplacental CMV transmission represents the most significant risk of developing clinical sequelae. Over 90% of infected babies are asymptomatic at birth. Only 10% will have measurable symptoms at birth. The mortality rate for these symptomatic newborns is 20–30%. Surviving infants with CMV may suffer from hearing problems (15%) or mental retardation (30%). Sensorineural deafness may develop later in life in apparently normal infants. Risk of neurological damage is more likely in CMV infection in first-half of pregnancy, while infection late in pregnancy, during or shortly after birth may present with acute visceral disease, i.e. Pneumonia, hepatitis, hepatosplenomegaly, purpura or thrombocytopenia.

Diagnosis and Management in Primary CMV

Routine antenatal screening for CMV by serology is not recommended.[4] Serologic testing for CMV may be considered for women who develop influenza-like illness during pregnancy or following detection of sonographic findings suggestive of CMV infection or in seronegative healthcare and childcare workers. CMV is readily inactivated by soaps, detergents and alcohol **(Table 42.4)**.

Prevention

Proper hygiene, frequent handwashing and wearing gloves while handling infective secretions.

HERPES SIMPLEX

Introduction

Genital herpes simplex virus (HSV) infection is the most common viral sexually transmitted infections. HSV can cause cold sores on face (HSV-1) or genital (HSV-2). Cold sores are extremely common by the age of twelve years, one quarter of children have contracted the virus, mostly without having any symptoms. Genital HSV-2 is more common in women, initial infection of the female genital tract can present with clinical disease or can be subclinical (asymptomatic).

Table 42.3: Risk of fetal transmission with cytomegalovirus[3,5]

Gestation	Primary CMV	Recurrent CMV
	90% mothers asymptomatic 10% fever, malaise, fatigue, sore throat. Risk of preterm labor, PROM.	Mothers usually asymptomatic
<20 weeks	40% fetus infected. Of which, 10% symptomatic at birth. Tetrad of mental retardation, cerebral calcifications, microcephaly and chorioretinitis. 90% asymptomatic at birth. *Risks in symptomatic at birth* 25% neonatal death 75% of symptomatic will have late complications (at age 2–3 years)—bilateral sensorineural hearing loss, mental retardation, seizures, spastic diplegia, learning disabilities and visual motor dysfunction. *Risks in asymptomatic at birth* Infants do well. 5–15% develop late complications—hearing loss, learning disabilities, microcephaly, behavioral difficulties and motor defects	Pre-existing maternal antibodies do not prevent reactivation or recurrence of infection, nor do they prevent fetal transmission. However, infants are usually asymptomatic at birth and are less likely to develop long-term consequences, <5% chance of hearing loss.
>20 weeks	Usually asymptomatic at birth.	
Intrapartum	Usually no permanent sequelae. Infants excrete virus (in urine) for up to 2 years.	
Breast feeding	40–60% infants of seropositive mothers will be infected.	

Table 42.4: Diagnosis and management in primary CMV[4-6]

Test result	Interpretation
IgG positive	Does not differentiate between current and previous infection. Four-fold rise in titer in 3–4 weeks supports recent infection.
IgM positive	Takes 4 weeks after infection for titer to rise. May persist for 18 months after infection. May be positive in recurrent infection also. Sensitivity, specificity 75%.
IgG avidity	Low avidity—primary CMV. High avidity—reactivation or reinfection.
Antenatal serial USG (every 2–4 weeks after exposure)	CMV infection—IUGR, poly- or oligohydramnios, microcephaly, hydrocephaly, ascites, nonimmune hydrops, intracranial calcifications, hyperechogenic bowel, intrahepatic calcifications.
Amniocentesis—amniotic fluid PCR for CMV DNA	Advised if clinical or serologic evidence of maternal infection or suspicious USG findings. Should be done after 20 weeks gestation or 5–6 weeks after acute maternal infection. Positive DNA PCR cannot predict which fetus will be symptomatic or have permanent sequelae.
Fetal MRI	Sensitivity optimal at 32–34 weeks, a gestation at which pregnancy termination not an option in most countries.

Etiopathogenesis

In primary infection, lesions occur through perineum and cervix, with an incubation period of 2–14 days. There are multiple vesicular eruptions with an erythematous base, these are painful, may ulcerate and cause difficulty in urination, vaginal discharge and local lymphadenopathy. Once infected, the virus like herpes virus remains dormant within body for life, and the person is prone to recurrences. In recurrent herpes, lesions are usually one to three in number and recur at the same anatomical site as the primary lesion. Asymptomatic reactivation and shedding of HSV virus occurs in subclinical infections also and virus may be transmitted to sexual partner or newborn.

Risk to fetus with primary maternal HSV-2 infection in first half of pregnancy is controversial **(Table 42.5)**. An increased risk of abortion, prematurity, IUGR and rare cases of congenital herpes has been reported. Congenital infection is very rare phenomenon of fetal acquisition of HSV in utero (transplacental). The fetal manifestations include microcephaly, hepatosplenomegaly, IUGR, and IUFD. Fulminant hepatitis is rare but associated with a maternal mortality rate of 43%.

Risk for neonatal infection seems to be greatest when maternal primary infection occurs in the third trimester.[3] Here the mother acquires infection but is unable to complete seroconversion to IgG prior to delivery, and the infant is delivered in the absence of protective passive IgG from the mother. Neonatal herpes occurs in 5–8% of infants born to mothers with active herpetic lesions in genital tract. About 1 in 1,000 and 1 in 5,000 infants are born with HSV infections. About 80% of these infections are acquired during birth (intranatal), the virus enters the infant through its eyes, skin, mouth, and upper respiratory tract. Of the infants born with HSV infection, about 20% will have localized infections of the eyes, mouth, or skin and about 50% will develop disseminated infection, producing meningoencephalitis with jaundice and hepatosplenomegaly, and, sometimes, bleeding within 9–11 days after birth. Disseminated herpes infections attack the liver and adrenal glands, as well as other body organs. Without treatment, the mortality rate is 80%. Even with antiviral medication, the mortality rate is still 15–20%, and 40–55% of the survivors having long-term damage to the central nervous system.

Table 42.5: Risks of transmission of HSV[2-4]

HSV-2 infection	Risk of transmission
Primary genital herpes in 3rd trimester	30–50%
Active recurrent genital herpes	4–8%
Subclinical shedding	0.3–3%

Diagnosis

Diagnosis depends on clinical symptoms and signs, serology and virus detection in tissue culture. PCR assays for HSV-DNA are helpful in confirming diagnosis.

Management

- Routine screening of pregnant women for HSV is also not recommended.[7] Routine antepartum genital HSV cultures in asymptomatic patients with recurrent disease are not recommended.

- Women with primary HSV infection during pregnancy should be treated with antiviral therapy. (Valacyclovir 1,000 mg twice a day for 7-14 days. Acyclovir 200 mg five times a day or 400 mg three times a day for 7-14 days. Famciclovir 250 mg three times a day for 7-14 days).[2,7]
- Women with active recurrent genital herpes should be offered suppressive viral therapy (acyclovir, famciclovir and valacyclovir) at or beyond 36 weeks of gestation. Acyclovir therapy decreases viral shedding, prevents neonatal herpes, reduces the need for cesarean delivery, and decreases clinical recurrences of herpes simplex virus infection. Because of their increased bioavailability, valacyclovir and famciclovir require less frequent dosing to achieve the same therapeutic benefits as acyclovir.[2,3,7]
- Cesarean delivery is indicated in women with first episode genital herpes, active genital lesions or prodromal symptoms, such as vulvar pain or burning at delivery, unless the membranes have been ruptured more than 4 hours.[2,7] Cesarean delivery is not recommended for women with a history of HSV infection but no active genital disease during labor.[7] Elective cesarean section can reduce the risk of infant exposure to infected secretions during birth and has become the standard of care for women with symptomatic lesions. However, most neonatal infections occur with asymptomatic mothers, who are subclinically shedding virus.
- In women with PROM, there is no consensus on the gestational age at which the risks of prematurity outweigh the risks of herpes simplex virus (HSV). Expectant management in patients with preterm labor or preterm premature rupture of membranes and active HSV.
- A pregnant woman who does not have a history of HSV but who has a partner with genital HSV, should have type-specific serology testing to determine her risk of acquiring genital HSV in pregnancy. Testing should be repeated at 32-34 weeks' gestation. Practice abstinence or use condoms in 3rd trimester.
- Neonatal cultures for HSV should be performed following delivery, and the neonate should be observed carefully for signs of HSV infection.
- If a woman with herpes simplex virus has an obvious lesion on the breast, breastfeeding is contraindicated.[7]

VARICELLA ZOSTER (CHICKENPOX)

Introduction

Varicella zoster is a highly contagious DNA virus of herpes family, responsible for chickenpox and herpes zoster. It is transmitted by respiratory droplets and by direct personal contact with vesicular fluid. The primary infection (chickenpox) is characterized by fever, malaise, and a pruritic rash that develops into crops of maculopapules, which become vesicular and crust over before healing. Incubation period lasts 10-21 days. Patient is infectious 48 hours before the rash appears and continues to be infectious until the vesicles crust over. Reactivation of virus in nervous tissue results in herpes zoster.

Epidemiology

Varicella affects 1/2,000 pregnancies. There is a 10-15% risk of fetal infection (majority transient and asymptomatic). Chickenpox is a common childhood disease. It usually causes mild infection. It is estimated that >90% of the antenatal population are seropositive for VZV IgG antibody and therefore, almost invariably immune to infection. Following primary infection, the virus may remain dormant in sensory nerve root ganglia but can be reactivated to cause a vesicular erythematous skin rash in a dermatome distribution known as herpes zoster or shingles. As shingles in pregnancy is not associated with viremia, it does not appear to cause fetal sequelae.

Etiopathogenesis

Primary varicella in adults, especially in nonimmune pregnant women, is more serious. About 5-10% of pregnant women with varicella infection develop pneumonitis. Risk factors for the development of varicella pneumonitis in pregnancy include cigarette smoking, more than 100 skin lesions and onset of disease in the third trimester. Mortality rates (1-2%) increase with age, they are higher in pregnant women than in nonpregnant adults, and death usually results from respiratory complications.[3]

When chickenpox occurs at <20 weeks gestation, 2-3% infants develop congenital varicella syndrome, which involves:
- Damage to brain—encephalitis, microcephaly, hydrocephaly, aplasia of brain.
- Damage to eye—optic stalk, optic atrophy, microphthalmia, cataract, chorioretinitis.
- Damage to cervical and lumbosacral spinal cord, motor and sensory deficits, anisocoria/Horner's syndrome.
- Damage to body—ipsilateral limb hypoplasia, anal and bladder sphincter dysfunction.
- Skin disorders—cicatricial skin lesion, hypopigmentation.

Risk of Congenital Varicella Syndrome (CVS) is low, being 0.7% in 1st trimester, 2% in 2nd and 0% in 3rd trimester.[8] Highest risk between 13-20 weeks **(Table 42.6)**. Detailed ultrasound and appropriate follow-up is recommended to all women who develop varicella in pregnancy to screen for fetal consequences for infection. Diagnosis of fetal infection may require amniocentesis with VZR PCR of amniotic fluid.

Infection with chickenpox in the later stages (>20w) of pregnancy can cause premature delivery or neonatal

Table 42.6: Risks of transmission of varicella	
Gestation at infection	Risk of transmission
1st trimester	0.7%
2nd trimester	2.0% (highest at 13–20 weeks) causes CVS
3rd trimester	0.0%
Peripartum	Neonatal chickenpox

chickenpox infection. Neonatal chickenpox (severe pneumonia and fulminant hepatitis) can occur if the mother is infected 5 days before to 2 days after the delivery. It is associated with up to 30% of neonatal mortality.[2]

Diagnosis

History, symptoms of fever with vesicular rash in different stages and in clusters, tending to be central in distribution. Serology for varicella specific antibodies. Confirmation by scraping of a lesion and Tzanck smear, tissue culture, direct fluorescent antibody testing or NAAT test.

Management

Pregnant women must avoid exposure to people with chickenpox or herpes zoster. If they develop chickenpox; avoid scratching, maintain hydration, have lukewarm baths, use calamine lotion and antihistamines to prevent scratching. Use paracetamol and avoid aspirin.

Women with significant varicella infection (pneumonitis) in pregnancy should be treated with oral acyclovir 800 mg 5 times daily. Hospitalization and IV acyclovir is recommended for severe complications (pneumonia, encephalitis, disseminated disease) in pregnancy as oral forms have poor bioavailability.[5] The dose is usually 10–15 mg/kg of BW or 500 mg/m^2 IV every 8 h for 5–10 days for varicella pneumonitis, and it should be started within 24–72 h of the onset of rash. VZIG has been shown to lower varicella infection rates if administered within 72–96 hours after exposure.[2,5] VZIG leads to reduction of the maternal risks of varicella infection-related complications associated with adult disease and some effect in decreasing the risk of fetal infection even in those women who develop varicella.

If varicella occurs around the time of delivery, there is risk of neonatal varicella. Prescribe oral acyclovir 800 mg five times daily X 5–7 days.[8] Babies of mothers with perinatal chickenpox should receive varicella-zoster immune globulin (VZIG).[5,8] If the baby has developed the varicella rash, VZIG is not helpful and treatment for neonatal chickenpox should be started with acyclovir. If at least a week passes between the rash and delivery, then maternal IgG should give adequate protection. The initial antibody response is IgM but this does not cross the placenta.

Intrauterine infection after 20 weeks of gestation can result in neonatal herpes zoster. This usually presents in the first year of life and most commonly involves a thoracic dermatome.

Prophylaxis

India: Varicella-zoster vaccine is not currently recommended for susceptible women of child-bearing age or for routine use in children. (High incidence in childhood ensures 85% adults are seropositive for VZ IgG antibody).

UK, USA, Canada: The antenatal varicella immunity status of all pregnant women should be documented by history of previous infection, varicella vaccination, or varicella zoster IgG serology. Varicella immunization by Varivax (attenuated live virus vaccine) 2 doses, 4–8 weeks apart is recommended for all nonimmune women as part of prepregnancy and postpartum care.

Vaccine-induced immunity diminishes overtime. 5% breakthrough infection rate after 10 years. Varicella vaccination should not be administered in pregnancy. However, termination of pregnancy should not be advised because of inadvertent vaccination during pregnancy.

HEPATITIS B

Introduction

Hepatitis B is an infectious disease caused by hepatitis B virus (HBV). Hepatitis B is a DNA virus transmitted through infected blood and body fluids. Transmission can occur, through sexual contact, contaminated blood exposure or perinatal transmission from mother to baby. Many of those infected with the virus remain asymptomatic and, therefore do not suspect a diagnosis.

Epidemiology

The WHO estimates that over 350 million people worldwide are chronically infected with HBV. In many high-prevalence countries, 10% or more of the population have chronic hepatitis B infection. Maternal transmission of HBV is the most common and efficient way in which HBV is spread, fortunately, this has been reduced to 5% in countries with postpartum neonatal HBV vaccination and immunoprophylaxis program.

Etiopathogenesis

Acute infections with hepatitis B may be subclinical or cause flu-like illness. The incubation period is on an average 60–90 days. Jaundice only occurs in about 10% of children and in 30–50% of adults. However, acute infection may occasionally lead to fulminant hepatic necrosis, which is often fatal. The illness usually starts insidiously, with malaise, anorexia, nausea, mild fever and right upper abdomen pain. Jaundice persists for 4–6 weeks. About 10–20% may develop hepatomegaly and splenomegaly.

Chronic hepatitis B is the presence of detectable hepatitis B surface antigen (HBsAg) in the blood or serum for longer than six months. Chronic hepatitis B may be inactive and cause no significant health problems, but may progress to liver fibrosis, cirrhosis and hepatocellular carcinoma. Chronic hepatitis B can be divided into e-antigen (HBeAg)-positive or HBeAg-negative disease based on the presence or absence of e-antigen. The presence of HBeAg is associated with higher rates of viral replication and higher infectivity, including perinatal (vertical) transmission.

Risk of fetal transmission depends on gestational period, viral load and viral markers (antigens):
- 1st trimester—Minimal risk of neonatal transmission
- 2nd trimester—10% risk of neonatal transmission.
- 3rd trimester—90% risk of neonatal transmission (95% intrapartum, 5% transplacental).

Chronic HBV depends on age of acquisition of infection. Infants who are infected during birth are at a high risk (>90%) of becoming chronic carriers. This significantly increases their risks of developing chronic liver disease which can cause premature death. If HBV infection is acquired at 7–12 months, 40% progress to chronic infection, at age 1–3 years, 10–20% progress to chronic infection, while acquisition in adulthood, 15–20% progress to chronic infection.

Vertical transmission of infection can occur in 65–90% of pregnancies where the mother is HBeAg positive and in about 10% of HBsAg positive but HBeAg negative mothers.

Diagnosis

HBsAg is the only serological marker detected during the first 3–5 weeks after being infected. The persistence of HBsAg for more than 6 months defines carrier status.

Among those who are HBsAg-positive, those in whom HBeAg is also detected in the serum, are the most infectious. The presence of HBeAg implies high infectivity. HBeAg is usually present for 1½–3 months after the acute illness.

Antibodies to hepatitis B core antigen (HBcAg), i.e. anti-HBc—imply past-infection.

Antibodies to HBsAg, i.e. anti-HBs—alone imply vaccination.

Patients with acute infection have raised levels of IgM to HBcAg (anti-HBc).

Management

Screen all pregnant women for HBV infection. HBsAg-positive women should be tested for HBeAg and anti-HBe, HBV DNA level, and have a Liver Function Test. They should also be offered HCV and HIV testing.[9]

Patients who have high viral loads, should be considered for therapy with a potent antiviral agent from 32nd week of pregnancy. Treating mother in the last month of pregnancy with lamivudine/tenofovir may reduce the transmission rate.[9]

All co-infected patients (HBV, HCV, HIV) should be treated with combination antiretroviral therapy. Patients co-infected with hepatitis C should be offered elective cesarean section.

Infants born to HBsAg-positive mothers should be given HBIG[2] (within 12 hours of birth) and a dose of monovalent hepatitis B vaccine on the day of birth, concurrently but in separate thighs. This therapy is 85–95% effective in preventing HBV chronic carrier state in newborn.[3] Vaccination should not be delayed beyond 7 days after birth, as vaccination alone has been shown to be reasonably effective in preventing infection. Hepatitis B vaccination should be repeated at 2, 4 and 6 months of age, so that the infant receives a total of 4 doses of hepatitis B vaccines. Anti-HBs antibody and HBsAg levels should be measured in infants born to mothers with chronic hepatitis B infection 3–12 months after completing the primary vaccine course.

Prevention

All pregnant women should be routinely screened for HBsAg and HBsAb.

All HBsAg-positive women should have partner and children screened. Those non-immune or not already infected should be vaccinated.

HBV vaccine (3 doses) to be included in childhood universal immunization.

All healthcare workers should be vaccinated and standard precautions against exposure to blood and bodily fluids should be used.

HIV AIDS

Introduction

Human immunodeficiency virus (HIV) belongs to a group of retroviruses known as lentivirinae. HIV enters through wet mucus membranes like rectum, female genital tract, glans penis and urethra. Blood, bloody fluids, genital secretions and breast milk are infectious fluids. Like all viruses, to survive, the HIV virus requires a host cell, it mainly infects the CD4 lymphocytes (T cells) but also to a lesser degree monocytes, macrophages and dendritic cells. Once infected, the cell turns into an HIV replicating cell and loses its function in human immune system. HIV gradually disrupts the immune system, kills CD4 lymphocytes and throws the immune system out of balance. HIV also destroys the immune system memory and CD4 cells which have been programmed to recognize infections become depleted. For this reason, opportunistic infections like *Pneumocystis carinii* pneumonia, tuberculosis, candidiasis develop as CD4 count falls.

Epidemiology

The first HIV-positive person was identified in India in 1986, and since then, there has been a rapid spread of the epidemic in some parts of the country. India has about 20.9 lakh HIV-positive adult population. Of which, women form 39% and children 7% of HIV positive cases.[10] By virtue of its 1.2 billion population, India has the third highest number of people living with HIV AIDS. The prevalence of HIV is high in the 15–49 age group and accounts for majority of infections.

The spread of HIV in India has been uneven. Although much of India have a low rate of infection, certain places have been more affected than others. HIV epidemics are more severe in the southern half of the country and the far north-east, high prevalence states being Manipur, Andhra Pradesh, Maharashtra, Karnataka, Tamil Nadu and Nagaland. Across India, HIV prevalence appears to be low among the general population, but disproportionately high among high-risk groups, such as IDUs, female sex workers, men who have sex with men (MSM) and STD clinic attendees. The mode of transmission of STI and HIV are same; presence of STIs, especially syphilis, enhances the HIV acquisition and transmission risk by 4–10 times.

Etiopathogenesis

Though largely sexually transmitted, what is alarming is the risk of vertical transmission, i.e. from mother to child (MTCT). Transmission from HIV infected mother to baby is the key mode of HIV infection in children. About 0.13% women tested at antenatal clinic are HIV positive. Annually, about 14,000 new HIV infections occur among children in India and HIV infection causes about 10,000 deaths annually among children in India.[10] Pediatric HIV is amenable to prevention as well as effective management. Currently available anti-retroviral drug regimen, if given to HIV-infected pregnant women, can eliminate risk of HIV transmission.

Estimated risk of MTCT in absence of any intervention is about 25–40%. MTCT may occur during pregnancy (transplacental 5–10%), during labor and delivery (10–15%) and during breastfeeding (5–20%). Risk of MTCT depends on the viral load. If viral load >1,00,000 HIV RNA copies/mL, the transmission risk is about 40%, if viral load <50 HIV RNA copies/mL (undetectable range), there is <1% transmission risk **(Table 42.7)**.

Management

The management of an HIV-positive pregnant woman is based on current NACO guidelines.[10] The National Technical

Table 42.7: Risk factors for perinatal transmission of HIV

HIV-related factors	High viral load (HIV-RNA level) Viral load >1,00,000 HIV RNA copies/mL = 40% transmission risk. Viral load <50 HIV RNA copies/mL (undetectable range) ≤1% transmission risk. Genital tract viral load CD4 cell count
Maternal factors increasing risk	• Clinical stage of HIV, acute infection with HIV during pregnancy and late stages (AIDS) are associated with increased vertical transmission. • Maternal malnutrition • Unprotected sex with multiple partners • Smoking cigarettes, injectable drugs, substance abuse, vitamin A deficiency • STDs (ulcerative) and other coinfections • Viral or parasitic placental infection (especially malaria) • Antiretroviral agents
Labor and delivery factors increasing risk	• Preterm labor • Mode of delivery, vaginal birth associated with more admixture of maternal and fetal body fluids and trauma. CS before onset of labor and PROM, is advised if maternal HIV RNA >1000 copies/mL with or without ART. • Placental Abruption • Prolonged rupture of membranes (>4 hours) • Injury to birth canal during child birth, Instrumental delivery/ episiotomy • Antepartum procedures, amniocentesis, CVS. • Acute chorioamnionitis • Invasive fetal monitoring • Delayed infant cleaning and eye care
Fetal Conditions increasing risk	• Premature delivery • Low birth weight, immature immune status • First infant in a multiple birth • Oral diseases • Breastfeeding • Routine infant airway suctioning

Guidelines have been revised to meet the global target of "elimination of new HIV infections among children". Department of AIDS control has decided to provide life-long

ART (triple drug regimen) for all pregnant and breastfeeding women living with HIV. All pregnant women living with HIV (including 1st trimester) receive a triple drug ART regimen (TDF + 3TC + EFV) regardless of CD4 count or WHO clinical stage, both for their own health and to prevent vertical HIV transmission from mother-to-child.

Triple drug ART to all pregnant and lactating women will help in maximum coverage for those needing treatment for keeping them alive and for their own health, avoiding stopping and starting drugs with repeat pregnancies, providing early protection against mother-to-child transmission in future pregnancies, increasing adherence and avoiding drug resistance. This will also reduce sexual transmission of HIV AIDS. These guidelines were implemented across the country from 1st January 2014.[10]

The objectives of EMTCT are:
- To detect more than 80% HIV-infected pregnant women in India. (As of now, HIV test is offered to all pregnant women as early as possible after counseling with "opt out" option).
- To provide access to comprehensive PPTCT services to more than 90% of the detected pregnant women.
- To provide access to early infant diagnosis to more than 90% HIV-exposed infants.
- To ensure access to anti-retroviral drug (ARV) prophylaxis or anti-retroviral therapy (ART) to 100% HIV-exposed infants.
- To ensure more than 95% compliance with ARV/ART in HIV-infected pregnant women and exposed children.

Essential Package of PPTCT Services[10]

- Routine offer of HIV counseling and testing with "opt-out" option
- Ensuring involvement of spouse and family members
- Providing ART to HIV positive pregnant women
- Promoting institutional deliveries of positive pregnant women
- Provision of care for STI/RTI, TB and OI
- Nutritional counseling and psychosocial support to positive pregnant women
- Antiretroviral prophylaxis to infants
- Follow-up of HIV-exposed infants
- Co-trimoxazole prophylactic therapy and early infant diagnosis

Four Prongs of PPTCT[10]

- Primary prevention of HIV, especially among adolescents and child-bearing ages.
- Prevent unintended pregnancy among women living with HIV through meeting family planning needs of HIV-positive women.
- Prevention of MTCT/vertical transmission, through a complete cascade of PPTCT services to HIV-positive pregnant women.
- Care, support and treatment of HIV-positive women by linkage to ART services.

Antenatal Care

- All women must receive minimum 3 antenatal visits with high-risk identification.
- Routine antenatal investigations to include: Complete blood picture, urine routine and microscopic, blood group and type, screen for diabetes, thyroid disease, blood VDRL, HBsAg, HBC and HIV. A screening USG at 18–22 weeks gestation.
- In addition to advocated lab tests in pregnancy, women on ART would require monitoring of blood sugar, renal function test, liver function test, CD4 count at baseline and 6 month intervals.
- Tetanus immunization.
- Iron and folic acid supplementation.
- Adherence counseling to 1st line triple drug ART.
- Cotrimoxazole prophylaxis prevents opportunistic infections (OIs) such as *Pneumocystis jiroveci* pneumonia (PCP), toxoplasmosis, diarrhea as well as bacterial infections. Cotrimoxazole should be started if CD4 count is <250 cells/mm^3 and continued through pregnancy, delivery and breastfeeding as per the national guidelines.
- Motivate for institutional delivery and exclusive breastfeeding.

All HIV-positive pregnant women including those presenting in labor and breastfeeding women with HIV should be initiated on a triple ART irrespective of CD4, for preventing mother-to-child transmission risk and should continue lifelong ART.[10]

The recommended first-line ART regimen for HIV-positive pregnant women, is:

Tenofovir (TDF 300 mg) + Lamivudine (3TC 300 mg) + Efavirenz (EFV 600 mg).

Certain Situations

- *Pregnant women identified as HIV positive during ANC checkup (new initiation):* Start ART (TDF + 3TC + EFV) as soon as possible, after proper preparedness counseling and continue ART throughout pregnancy, delivery, and thereafter lifelong.
- *Pregnant women already receiving ART:* Continue same ART regime (even if taking EFV) during pregnancy, labor, delivery and lifelong. Change only if intolerable side effects or toxicity.
- *ART regimen for pregnant women having prior exposure to NNRTI (like Nevirapine) for PPTCT:* A small number

of HIV-positive pregnant women have had previous exposure to single-dose NVP for PPTCT prophylaxis in prior pregnancies. Because of the risk of resistance to NNRTI drugs in this population, an NNRTI-based ART regimen such as TDF/3TC/EFV may not be effective. Thus, these women will require a protease inhibitor-based ART regimen (Lopinavir/Ritonavir).

- *Women presenting directly-in-labor (unbooked, uninvestigated women):* Labor room nurse will offer bedside counseling and HIV-screening test. If women consents, screen using the *Whole Blood Finger Prick test* in delivery room or labor ward. If detected positive, *initiate TDF + 3TC + EFV immediately*. Collect blood sample and send next morning to ICTC for confirmation and ART center for CD 4 count. ICTC counselor to ensure immediate linkage to ART center.
- *Women found HIV positive after delivery:* Woman delivered at home or found HIV positive after delivery, should be counseled and linked to ART center for initiation of lifelong ART. If breastfeeding the infant must be provided extended NVP prophylaxis for 12 weeks, if on replacement feeds, provide NVP for 6 weeks to baby.
- *Breastfeeding mother interrupts ART:* Breastfeeding mother may miss dose, refuse ART or interrupt due to toxicity or out of stock drugs, such mothers should have adherence counseling, offered alternative ART and infant provided NVP prophylaxis for 6 weeks after maternal ART is restarted or till 1 week after breastfeeding has ended.

Labor

The route of delivery depends on viral load, ART status and obstetric indications.

If viral load is high (HIV RNA levels >1000 copies/mL) then schedule cesarean delivery at 38 weeks' gestation in HIV +ve women irrespective of administration of antepartum antiretroviral drugs to prevent mother-to-child transmission.

In women with HIV RNA levels ≤1000 copies/mL, cesarean delivery is performed for standard obstetrical indications at 39 weeks' gestation. However, NACO advocates vaginal delivery for HIV-positive women, CS to be done for obstetric indication only.

Risk of mother-to-child transmission increases 2% per hour after ROM. Cesarean section before labor and/or rupture of membranes reduces risk of mother-to-child transmission by 50–80% compared with other modes of delivery in women on no antiretroviral therapy or on ZDV alone. There is no benefit with cesarean section after onset of labor or membranes have ruptured. Cesarean section, however, increases risk of morbidity and possible mortality to mother. Give antibiotic prophylaxis for cesarean section in HIV-infected women.[10]

Precautions during Labor

Do's	Don'ts
- Standard/Universal work precautions - Personal protection gear - Minimize vaginal examination and use aseptic techniques - Clean vagina with chlorhexidine 0.25% - Use oxytocic's to prevent blood loss - Monitor contractions and FHS - Give ART to the mother as prescribed - Early cord clamping - Clean all the secretion from the skin before needle puncture - Promote EBF - Initiate ARV for baby	- Avoid rupture of membranes - Avoid use of invasive procedures - Avoid prolonged difficult and traumatic delivery - Avoid instrumental delivery. If instrumental delivery is indicated, prefer forceps over ventouse - Avoid episiotomy - Avoid milking of umbilical cord, clamp and cut the cord as soon as possible - Avoid suctioning newborn with a nasogastric tube unless MSL

Infant Care

Newborn care—Dry and warm baby, clear airway, mouth and nostrils to be wiped as soon as head is delivered. Initiate breastfeeding within 1 hour, administer ARV prophylaxis to the baby as prescribed (**Table 42.8**). Nevirapine prophylaxis to infant be given for minimum 6 weeks, extend to 12 weeks if ART to mother was started in late pregnancy, during or after delivery and mother has not been on adequate period of ART as to be effective to achieve optimal viral suppression (which is at least 24 weeks). This recommendation on extended NVP duration applies to infants of breastfeeding women only and not those on exclusive replacement feeding.[10]

Cotrimoxazole prophylaxis for infant should be started at 6 weeks and continued up to 18 months (5 years if HIV positive). Syrup cotrimoxazole 5 mL = 40 mg trimethoprim + 200 mg sulphamethoxazole (**Table 42.9**).

Childhood vaccination as per the National Immunization Schedule.

Early Infant Diagnosis (EID) at 6 weeks, 6 months, 12 months using DBS (Dry Blood Spot), WBS (Whole Blood Sample) for HIV DNA PCR and confirmatory test (HIV antibody tests) at 18 months. HIV antibody tests are also useful for identifying potentially uninfected infants as early as 6–18 months of age if they are not breastfed, or if they ceased breastfeeding 6 weeks prior.

All infants and young children <24 months of age with confirmed HIV infection should be started on ART,

Table 42.8: Nevirapine prophylaxis and dosage (NVP 10 mg in 1 mL)

Birth weight	NVP in mg	NVP in mL
<2000 gms	2 mg/kg OD	0.2 mL/kg OD
2000–2500 gms	10 mg OD	1 mL OD
>2500 gms	15 mg OD	1.5 mL OD

Table 42.9: Cotrimoxazole for infants

Weight in kgs	Dose	Side effects
<5	2.5 mL	Mild: rash, nausea
5–10	5 mL	Severe: jaundice, anemia
10–15	7.5 mL	
15–22	10 mL	

irrespective of stage or CD4 count. Where virological testing is not available, infants and young children <18 months of age with clinically diagnosed presumptive severe HIV should be started on antiretroviral therapy. Presumptive diagnosis of severe HIV disease: 2 or more of the following: Oral thrush, severe pneumonia, severe sepsis.

HIV-infected children ≥24 months treat according to clinical and CD4% criteria. Initiate ART for all clinical stage 3 and 4, irrespective of CD4 count or percentage. In children with TB, LIP, OHL, thrombocytopenia (stage 3): Use CD4 to guide ART initiation.

Children ≥5 years of age: Follow CD4 count as in adult ART guidelines.

Breastfeeding

In India, the national policy is to promote breastfeeding. As per NACO guidelines, Mothers whose infants are HIV uninfected or of unknown HIV status should exclusively breastfeed their infants for the first six months of life. They should then introduce appropriate complementary foods and continue breastfeeding for the first 12 months of life. Breastfeeding should stop only after a nutritionally adequate and safe diet without breast-milk can be provided. In EID positive babies, breastfeeding can be continued up to 2 years along with early initiation of pediatric ART. Avoid mixed feeding as it increases the risk of HIV transmission. If mother does not desire to breastfeed or is not able to breastfeed, exclusive replacement feeding must be advised.[9]

REFERENCES

1. The UK NSC recommendations on Rubella susceptibility screening in pregnancy. May 2012.
2. The UK NSC recommendations on Cytomegalovirus screening in pregnancy. May 2012.
3. The UK NSC recommendations on Genital Herpes screening in pregnancy. July 2006.
4. National Guidelines Clearinghouse 7745.
5. ACOG Practice Bulletin 151 June, 2015. Cytomegalovirus, Parvovirus B19, Varicella Zoster and Toxoplasmosis in pregnancy. Obstetrics and Gynecology. 2015;125(6):1510-25.
6. Sgrinio Cyn Geni Cymru Antenatal Screening Wales – Infections in Pregnancy: A guide for Maternity Services, when requesting serology or virology tests. October 2012.
7. Hepatitis B: NICE Quality Standards. July 2014.
8. SOGC Clinical practice Guidelines No 274, Mar'12.
9. Operational Guidelines for Lifelong ART for all Pregnant Women Living with HIV for Prevention of Parent-to-Child Transmission (PPTCT) of HIV in India. NACO. Dec'2013.
10. Obstetric Medicine – Management of medical disorders in pregnancy. Editors: Wayne R Cohen, Phyllis August. 6th Edition.

Chapter 43

Toxoplasmosis During Pregnancy

Alka Pandey, Richa Baharani

INTRODUCTION

Toxoplasmosis is a protozoan disease caused by *Toxoplasma gondii*. *Toxoplasma gondii* is an obligate intracellular protozoan that can infect all mammals, who serve as intermediate hosts.[1] Human infection with *Toxoplasma gondii* occurs worldwide. The infection is usually benign and asymptomatic in children and adults but can lead to severe complications if it occurs in an immunocompromised patient or in a developing fetus.

EPIDEMIOLOGY

The prevalence of *Toxoplasma* antibodies varies according to age and geographic area. Seropositivity is highest in areas with warm, moist climates, where the survival of the oocysts is good and lower in cold regions and high altitudes.

Signs and Symptoms in Mother During Toxoplasmosis

In immunocompetent subjects 90% of *T. gondii* infections are asymptomatic. Symptomatic infections usually cause mononucleosis such as illness with low-grade fever, malaise, cervical lymphadenopathy, muscle aches and pains that last more than a month.

Other manifestations such as encephalitis, myocarditis, hepatitis and pneumonia are rare but can complicate acute toxoplasmosis.[1] In some studies, it has been found that mothers who gave birth to congenitally infected offspring could not recall, experiencing an infection relate illness during pregnancy.[2]

TOXOPLASMOSIS IN PREGNANCY

Women who are infected for the first time in their life by the parasite (primoinfection) lack protective immunity. In these cases, *Toxoplasma gondii* may cross the placental border and infect the fetus. Depending on gestational week infection may cause, to various probabilities, different afflictions of the central nervous system, such as hydrocephalous, intracranial calcifications and retinochoroiditis leading to lifelong disabilities in children. Often congenital toxoplasmosis is a symptomatic at birth and sequels may appear later in life leading to under reporting, if the outcome is only studied at delivery.[3]

Abnormalities related to congenital toxoplasmosis are: Miscarriage, stillbirth, premature birth, vision loss due to damage to retina at birth or later in life. Brain damage causing mental disability or seizures, heart defect, mental retardation can happen at birth or later in life.

Risk of maternal fetal transmission and abnormalities related to congenital toxoplasmosis infection is related to the gestation at maternal seroconversion.[4-6]
- *< 13 week's gestation:*
  - 5–15% risk of maternal fetal transmission
  - > 60–80% chance of abnormalities, if detected.
- *Second trimester:*
  - 25–40% risk of maternal fetal transmission
  - 15–25% chance of abnormalities, if detected.
- *Third trimester:*
  - 30–75% risk of maternal fetal transmission.
- *36 week's gestation:*
  - 72% risk of maternal fetal transmission
  - 2–10% chance of abnormalities, if detected.

MODE OF TRANSMISSION

Toxoplasma gondii is an obligate intracellular protozoan parasite.[7] It has a complex life cycle with asexual reproduction taking place in diverse tissues of mammals and birds (secondary hosts) and sexual reproduction taking place in digestive epithelium of cats (primary hosts). Cats mainly become contaminate by eating animal flesh (mouse, bird, encysted with *T. gondii* and rarely by ingesting oocysts directly from the feces of other cats.[8,9] Infected cats are usually asymptomatic and begin to shed unsporulated (non-infectious) oocysts (up to one million per day) in their feces 1–2 weeks are exposure.[9,10] Most cats shed oocysts only once in their lives within days to weeks, the oocysts sporulate and become infectious. Oocysts survive best in humid conditions (garden, litter, sandbox) and can remain infectious for many months. Oocysts also withstand exposure to freezing for up to 18 months, especially if they are covered and out of direct sunlight. After ingestion by a secondary host (human, bird, rodent, domestic animal) oocysts release sporozoites, which change into tachyzoites. Tachyzoites are present during acute infection and are capable of invading cells and replicating. They are disseminated widely and circulate from 3 to 10 days in the immunocompetent host before changing into bradyzoites and forming cysts in tissues. These cysts remain present during latent infection. Once infected human are believed to remain infected for life. Unless immunosuppression occur and the organism reactivates, human hosts usually remain asymptomatic.

ROUTES OF TRANSMISSION

- Ingestion of raw or undercooked meats
  Exposure to oocyst infected cat feces
- Vertical transmission
- Transfusion or organ transplantation from an infected person can also transmit the organism.

In pregnancy, most common mechanism of acquiring infection are through consuming raw or very undercooked meats or contaminated water, or exposure to soil (gardening without gloves) or cat litter.[7,8,11]

Incubation period: 5–18 days.

DIAGNOSIS

Serological testing is after the first step in diagnosis, using IgG and IgM antibodies. Presence of IgM antibodies cannot be considered reliable for making a diagnosis of acute toxoplasmosis infection. IgM antibody titers rise from 5 days to weeks following acute infection, reaching a maximum after 1–2 months and decline more rapidly than IgG.[12] Although IgM antibodies can decrease to low or undetectable levels, in many cases they may persist for years following the acute infection.[12,13] IgG antibodies appear later than IgM and are usually detectable within 1–2 weeks after the infection, with the peak reached within 12 weeks to 6 months after acute infection. They will be detectable for years after acquired infection and are usually present throughout life.

- If IgG and IgM are both negative, this indicates the absence of infection or extremely recent acute infection.[14]
- If testing reveals a positive IgG and negative IgM this indicates an old infection (infection greater than 1 year ago)
- If both IgG and IgM are positive this indicates either a recent infection or false positive test result.[13]

- If acute infection is suspected, repeat testing is recommended within 2–3 weeks.[12] A 4-fold rise in IgG antibody titers between tests indicates a recent infection.[15] Commercial serologic diagnostic test kits can be unreliable, therefore it is important that positive antibody results be confirmed by a toxoplasmosis reference laboratory.
- Knowing when infection occurred during pregnancy is important in evaluating the risk of fetal transmission, initiating antibiotic therapy and ensuring appropriate prenatal counselling.[14]
- Additional specific tests, *Toxoplasma* IgG avidity test, to assist in determining the timing of infection.[14] The IgG avidity test measures the strength of IgG binding to the organism.[15] Avidity in most cases but not all, shifts from low to high after about 5 months. If the avidity is high, this suggests infection occurred at least 5 months before testing.[15] Patients with a high IgG avidity test results in the first trimester of pregnancy can be reassuring suggesting past infection that is unlikely to harm the fetus. However a positive result in the second or third trimester of pregnancy cannot completely exclude the possibility of transmission. In this case, invasive testing should be offered to parents in order to completely rule out fetal infection.

Ultrasound Findings in Fetus

If on sonography findings (such as ventricular dilatation, numerous intracranial lesions, liver lesions, hepatosplenomegaly, pleural effusion, pericardial effusion and ascites, ocular abnormalities (cataracts), placental enlargement and hyperdensity) are seen, there is possibility for presence of toxoplasmosis. Ultrasound is recommended for women with suspected or diagnosed acute infection acquired during or shortly before gestation.

If ultrasonography findings associated with the fetus are present and there is possibility of development of toxoplasmosis in the fetus due to recent development of this disease in the mother supplementary tests will be needed.[16]

Amniocentesis and Polymerase Chain Reaction

Confirmed positive maternal serological screening should be accompanied by fetal diagnosis. Prenatal diagnosis of congenital toxoplasmosis is primarily based on ultrasonography and polymerase chain reaction (PCR) with amniotic fluid.[15,17] Polymerase chain reaction (PCR) amplification of toxoplasmosis DNA from amniotic fluid has been deemed the most reliable and safe method of prenatal diagnosis and has replaced direct sampling of fetal blood.[15,17-19] Amniocentesis for PCR is not recommended in pregnancies with maternal human immunodeficiency virus (HIV) infection due to procedural risks of fetal HIV transmission.[15] PCR can be performed as early as 18 weeks' gestation.[15,20,21]

A negative PCR at any gestation cannot completely rule out congenital infection so we should consider continued follow-up via serial ultrasounds, prophylaxis with spiramycin therapy and neonatal testing.[18]

Histologic Diagnosis

Demonstration of tachyzoites in tissue sections or smears of body fluid (e.g. CSF and amniotic fluid) establishes the diagnosis of acute infection.

Infants

Clinical signs of congenital toxoplasmosis in newborns are rare and nonspecific. The diagnosis has to rely on laboratory confirmation such as demonstration of parasites from blood or body tissues obtained within the first six months of life, positive specific IgM and or IgA which are demonstrated in approximately two-thirds of the cases or persistently positive IgG beyond the first year of life. In some infected treated infants, however the therapy has had the result that *Toxoplasma* IgG antibodies are not detectable at the end of the treatment, but antibodies may appear later.

PREVENTIVE MEASURES

Measures to Prevent Primary *Toxoplasma Gondii* Infection during Pregnancy[22]

- Cook meat to "well done" thoroughly to 67°C (153°F), meat should not be pink in the center.
- Meat that is smoked, cured in brine, dried may still be infectious.
- Avoid mucous membrane contact when handling raw meat.
- Wash hands carefully after contact with raw meat.
- Kitchen surfaces and utensils that have come in contact with raw meat should be washed wearing gloves.
- Refrain from skinning and butchering animals.
- Avoid contact with materials potentially contaminated with cat feces, when handling cat litter or gardening, wearing gloves is recommended when these activities cannot be avoided.
- Disinfect emptied cat litter box with near boiling water for 5 minutes before refilling.
- Wash peel fruits and vegetables before consuming.
- Avoid drinking water potentially contaminated with oocysts.
- Wash your hands before and after preparing food.
- Drink only pasteurized milk products.

PREVENTION

Primary Prevention

Preventive measures must be reinforced continually throughout pregnancy for seronegative women.[22,23]

Educational materials on how to prevent pregnant women from becoming infected should be distributed. Educational measures may be in the form of (books, magazines, simple handouts) available in different languages and integrated into existing prenatal programs, visits and classes.

Secondary Prevention (Serological Testing)

It is important to identify those women who acquire *T. gondii* infection during gestation, and if fetal infection is detected by prenatal testing, therapeutic options, including termination of pregnancy and antibiotic treatment of the fetus *in utero* should be discussed with the patient. Women and their partners have the right to know whether their fetus is at risk for congenital toxoplasmosis or whether their fetus has already been infected.

Universal screening program to detect acute *T. gondii* infection acquired during gestation can be done.

USG should be performed every month for pregnant women with suspected or proven *T. gondii* infection acquired during pregnancy.

Postnatal screening of newborns for *Toxoplasma gondii*.

MANAGEMENT

- Management depends on whether or not fetal infection has occurred.
- If maternal infection has occurred but the fetus is not infected, spiramycin is used for fetal prophylaxis particularly during 1st trimester of pregnancy.[24] It is given at a dose of 1 g (3 million U) orally every 8 hours for 3 weeks duration of pregnancy and to be repeated after 2 weeks interval till parturition if the amniotic fluid polymerase chain reaction is reported negative for *T. gondii*.
- If fetal infection has been confirmed by positive PCR on amniocentesis or is highly suspected, combination of pyrimethamine, sulfadiazine and folinic acid used as treatment for pregnant women who acquire infection after 18 weeks of gestation. Pyrimethamine is a folic acid antagonist that acts synergistically with sulfonamides. This drug should not be used in the first trimester because it is potentially teratogenic. It produces a reversible dose related depression of bone marrow so must be combined with folinic acid.[24]
- All patients who received pyrimethamine should have complete blood counts frequently monitored. Folinic acid (not folic acid) is used for reduction and prevention of haematological toxicities of the drug.

DOSE

Pyrimethamine 50 mg every 12 hours for 48 hours followed by 50 mg daily, sulfadiazine 75 mg/kg, followed by 50 mg/kg every 12 hours and folinic acid (leucovorin) 10–20 mg daily.[25]

INTRAPARTUM CARE[26]

- Pediatrician at delivery
- Following delivery newborn assessment should include physical examination for evidence of congenital toxoplasmosis (including ophthalmological examination and cerebral ultrasound).
- Placenta for histology/PCR
- May direct room-in with mother following initial assessment in nursery.

Babies that are asymptomatic at birth should undergo a prolonged follow up. It has been reported that some manifestations of congenital toxoplasmosis such as chorioretinitis can occur even after as long as 12 years of age. Babies that are asymptomatic at birth should undergo a prolonged follow-up.

REFERENCES

1. Jeffrey D Kravetz, Daniel G Federman. Toxoplasmosis in pregnancy: The American Journal of Medicine (internet) 2005; (cited on 2016 July 4) 118:212-6.
2. Jose G Montoya, Jack S Remington. Management of *Toxoplasma gondii* infection during pregnancy: Clinical Practice.
3. Villena l, Ancelle T, Deimas C, Garcia P, Brezin AP, et al. Congenital toxoplasmosis in France in 2007: first results from a National Surveillance System Euro Surveill. 2010.p.15.
4. Dunn, Wallon M, Peyron F, Peterson E, Peckham C, Gilbert R. Mother to child transmission of toxoplasmosis: risk estimates for clinical counseling. The Lancet. 1999;353:1829-33 (Level IV).
5. Langford KS. Infectious diseases and pregnancy. Current Obstet Gynaecol. 2002;12:125-30.
6. Palasanthiran P, Starr M, Jones C, Giles M, (Eds). Management of perinatal infections. Sydney: Australian Society for Infectious Diseases (ASID), 2014. Available from: URI: *http://www.asid.net.au/resources/clinical-guidelines*.
7. Skariah S, McIntyre MK, Mordue DG. *Toxoplasma gondii:* determinants of tachyzoite to bradyzoite conversion. Parasitol Res. 2010;107(2):253-60.
8. Elmore SA, Jones JL, Conrad PA, Patton S, Lindsay DS, Dubey JP. *Toxoplasma gondii:* epidemiology, feline clinical aspects, and prevention. Trends Parasitol. 2010;26(4):190-6.
9. Dubey JP, Lindsay DS, Lappin MR. Toxoplasmosis and other intestinal coccidial infections in cats and dogs. Vet Clin North Am Small Anim Pract 2009;39(6):1009-34, v.
10. Cook AJ, Gilbert RE, Buffolano W, Zufferey J, Petersen E, Jenum PA, et al. Sources of *Toxoplasma* infection in pregnant women: European multicentre case-control study. European Research Network on Congenital Toxoplasmosis. BMJ. 2000;321(7254):142-7.
11. Jones JL, Kruszon-Moran D, Wilson M, McQuillan G, Navin T, McAuley JB. *Toxoplasma gondii* infection in the United States: seroprevalence and risk factors. Am J Epidemiol. 2001;154(4):357-65.
12. Stray-Pedersen B. Toxoplasmosis in pregnancy. Baillieres Clin Obstet Gynaecol. 1993;7(1):107-37.
13. Liesenfeld O, Press C, Montoya JG, Gill R, Isaac-Renton JL, Hedman K, et al. False-positive results in immunoglobulin M (IgM) *Toxoplasma* antibody tests and importance of confirmatory testing: the Platelia Toxo IgM test. J Clin Microbiol. 1997;35(1):174-8.
14. Flori P, Chene G, Varlet MN, Sung RT. *Toxoplasma gondii* serology in pregnant woman: characteristics and pitfalls [article in French]. Ann Biol Clin (Paris). 2009;67(2):125-33.
15. Montoya JG. Laboratory diagnosis of *Toxoplasma gondii* infection and toxoplasmosis. J Infect Dis. 2002;185(Suppl 1):S73-82.
16. Holhfeld P, MacAleese J, Capella-Pavlovski M, Giovanqrandi Y, Thulliez P, Forestier F, et al. Fetal toxoplasmosis; ultrasonographic signs. Ultrasound Obstet Gynaecol. 1991; 1(4):241-4.
17. Lappalainen M, Koskiniemi M, Hiilesmaa V, Ammala P, Teramo K, Koskela P, et al. Outcome of children after maternal primary *Toxoplasma* infection during pregnancy with emphasis on avidity of specific IgG. The Study Group. Pediatr Infect Dis J. 1995;14(5):354-61. PubMed
18. Romand S, Wallon M, Franck J, Thulliez P, Peyron F, Dumon H. Prenatal diagnosis using polymerase chain reaction on amniotic fluid for congenital toxoplasmosis. Obstet Gynecol. 2001;97(2):296-300. | Article | PubMed.
19. Grover CM, Thulliez P, Remington JS, Boothroyd JC. Rapid prenatal diagnosis of congenital *Toxoplasma* infection by using polymerase chain reaction and amniotic fluid. J Clin Microbiol 1990;28(10):2297301. | Article | PubMed Abstract | PubMed Full Text.
20. Hedman K, Lappalainen M, Seppaia I, Makela O. Recent primary *Toxoplasma* infection indicated by a low avidity of specific IgG. J Infect Dis 1989;159(4):736-40. |Article|PubMed.
21. Sever J. Toxoplasmosis in pregnancy. Contemp Obstet Gynecol. 1998;43:21-4.
22. Foulon W, Naessens A, Lauwers S, De Meuter F, Amy JJ. Impact of primary prevention on the incidence of toxoplasmosis during pregnancy. Obstet Gynecol. 1988;72:363-6.
23. Wong S, Remington JS. Toxoplasmosis in pregnancy. Clin Infect Dis. 1994;18:853-62.
24. Montoya JG, Remington JS. Management of *Toxoplasma gondii* infection during pregnancy. Clin Infect Dis. 2008;47(4):554-66.
25. Francesco D' Antonio. Fetal infections. Amarnath Bhide, Sabaratnam Arulkumaran (Eds). Arias practical guide to high risk pregnancy and delivery. India: Elsevier; 2015.
26. Clinical guideline. Toxoplasmosis in pregnancy, 24 June 2015, Govt of South Australia.

Chapter 44

Zika Fever and Parvovirus Infection During Pregnancy

Shruti Agrawal, Pushpa Pandey

ZIKA VIRUS DISEASE

INTRODUCTION

Zika fever (also known as Zika virus disease or simply Zika) is an infectious disease caused by the Zika virus.[1]

Zika fever is probably a top of the mind concern right now, and for two good reasons; firstly, because of its scary multi-country advancement; and, secondly, because of potentially devastating consequences for pregnant women and their babies. Today, this mosquito-borne virus is dominating the headlines. The gravity of the problem can be envisaged from the fact that president Obama has earmarked approximately $1.9 billion from Congress in February 2016, an amount that will be earmarked for research to create vaccines and diagnostic tests for Zika and to aid the US territories, where cases of the virus have been confirmed. This money will also go towards mosquito control programs in at-risk US states.

VIROLOGY

The Zika virus belongs to the Flaviviridae family and the Flavivirus genus, and is thus related to the dengue, yellow fever, Japanese encephalitis and West Nile viruses like other flaviviruses. The virus is 'enveloped' and 'icosahedral' and has a 'nonsegmented' single-stranded, 10 kilobase positive sense RNA genome. The incubation period ranges from 3 to 12 days after the bite of mosquito.

EPIDEMIOLOGY

The very first known case of Zika fever was in a rhesus macaque monkey, that had been placed in a cage in the Zika forest of Uganda in 1947.[2] It was not until 1954 that the isolation of Zika from a human was published. After that, a few outbreaks have been reported in tropical Africa and in some areas in S-E Asia.[3]

The first major outbreak, with 185 confirmed cases, was reported in 2007 in the Yap islands of the Federated State of Micronesia.[4] In 2013, another large outbreak.[5] From 2007 to 2016, the virus spread eastwards, across the Pacific ocean to the Americas, leading to the 2015-16 Zika virus epidemic.[5-7]

In May 2015, the Pan American Health Organization (PAHO) issued an alert regarding the first confirmed Zika virus infection in Brazil.[8] Mosquito-borne Zika virus is suspected to be the cause of 2,400 cases of microcephaly and 29 infant deaths in Brazil in 2015.[9,10]

Indian scenario—no cases reported till date but the day is not far off, when the Zika fever will be reported in Indians, because India with its huge garbage yards provides a good breeding site for *Aedes aegypti* mosquitoes and also because the cases of Zika fever have been detected in the Indians residing in Singapore.

PATHOGENESIS

Zika is primarily spread by the female *Aedes aegypti* mosquito which is active mostly in the day time. The mosquito must feed on the blood in order to lay eggs. The virus has also been isolated from a number of Arboreal mosquito species in the Aedes genus with an extrinsic incubation period in mosquitoes of about 10 days.

Mosquitoes become infected when they feed on a person already infected by the virus. Infected mosquitoes can then spread the virus to other people through bites. Zika virus replicates in the mosquito's midgut epithelial cells and then its salivary gland cells. After 5-10 days, the virus can be found in the mosquito's saliva. If the mosquito's saliva is inoculated into human skin, the virus can infect epidermal keratinocytes, skin fibroblasts in the skin and the Largerhans cells. The pathogenesis of the virus is hypothesized to continue with a spread to lymph nodes and the blood stream.

Transmission of Zika virus is through the following four ways:
a. Through mosquito bites.
b. From mother to child.[5]
c. Through sexual contact.[11-13]
d. Occasional cases, reported through blood transfusion.[6,14]

Through Mosquito Bites

- Zika virus is transmitted to people primarily through the bite of an infected Aedes species mosquito (*A. aegypti* and *A. albopictus*).[15-17]
- These mosquitoes typically lay eggs in and near standing water, in things such as buckets, bowls, animal dishes, flower pots and vases.
- Mosquitoes that spread chikungunya, dengue and Zika are aggressive daytime biters. They can also bite at night.

From Mother to Child

- It is possible that Zika virus could be passed from a mother to her baby during pregnancy.
- A mother already infected with Zika virus near the time of delivery can pass on the virus to her newborn around the time of birth.
- Zika virus has been detected in fetal tissue, amniotic fluid, full-term infants and in the placenta, according to ACOG and trace amounts of the virus have also been found in breast milk,[18] but because the amount is tiny, it is unlikely to pose a threat. Moreover, the many benefits of breast-feeding outweigh the possible risk.

Symptoms of Zika Virus

Only about 1 in 5 people (or roughly 20%), with the virus, will exhibit symptoms.[19] A Zika infection is similar to a mild case of the flu and the signs and symptoms which are as follows, are similar to those of dengue and chikungunya.
- Low-grade fever (between 37.8°C and 38.5°C)[20]
- Arthralgia, notably of small joints of hands and feet, possibly swollen joints
- Myalgia
- Headache, retro-ocular headache.
- Conjunctivitis (pink eye).
- Cutaneous maculopapular rash.
- Post-infection asthenia, which seems to be frequent.
  More rarely observed symptoms include:
- Digestive problems
- Abdominal pain
- Diarrhea
- Mucous membrane ulcerations.

Effects of Zika Virus Infection

As discussed above, only about 20% (or approx 1 in 5 people) infected with Zika virus will actually become ill. But in pregnant women, the effects can be devastating in the form of:
- Miscarriages[21]
- Stillbirth
- Microcephaly

In adults, Zika virus may rarely result in Guillain-Barre syndrome,[22] which is a condition where the immune system of the body attacks the nerves. Also a possible link between Zika and ADEM (Acute disseminated encephalomyelitis) has been cited.

What is the Connection between Zika, Pregnancy and Microcephaly?

Zika virus causes microcephaly in babies born to infected pregnant women, the Centers for Disease Control and Prevention (CDC) confirmed this year. Microcephaly is a condition where the baby is born with an abnormally small head and brain. While the pathophysiology is not yet fully known, it is reported to involve infection of the primary neural stem cells of the fetal brain, known as radial glial cells, which reside in a stem cell layer called the ventricular zone.[23] Infection of brainstem cells can cause cell death, which reduces the production of future neurons and leads to a smaller brain. Microcephaly may be associated with:
- Developmental delays
- Vision abnormalities
- Mental retardation
- Seizures
- In some cases, may be fatal.

Infection during the earliest stage of pregnancy results in worst outcomes for the fetus. But fetus can be harmed by infection, even later in pregnancy. While the Zika virus remains in the blood of an infected person for a few days to a week, according to the CDC, there's no current evidence to suggest that it poses a risk of birth defects in future pregnancies and virus will not cause infections in a baby that's conceived after the virus has left the bloodstream.

DIAGNOSIS

According to the CDC, the FDA still has not approved a commercially available diagnostic test for Zika virus. But two institutions in Texas did develop the first rapid hospital-based ones.
- The first test detects Zika genetic material or ribonucleic acid (RNA)[24] in a pregnant woman's amniotic fluid, or anytime in blood, urine, spinal or amniotic fluid. Result is available in a matter of hours. This test is currently available to hospital patients who have traveled to an affected region and have acute symptoms of Zika virus.
- The second test detected the presence of antibodies (proteins) produced in response to the Zika virus infection. Commercial assays for Zika antibodies though now available, but have not yet been FDA approved.[25,26]
- Ig M, Ig G and PCR for Zika virus.[2]

Two samples to be taken, acute serum (taken within 5 days of symptom onset) and convalescent serum (2–3 weeks later).

The two samples are important to rule out false positive test due to cross-reactivity.

In a nutshell, the diagnosis is by testing the blood, urine or saliva for the presence of Zika RNA when the person is sick.[1,27]

SCREENING IN PREGNANCY

The CDC recommends screening of some pregnant women even if they do not have symptoms of infection. Pregnant women who have traveled to affected areas should be tested between two and twelve weeks after their return from the travel.[28] For women living in affected areas, the CDC has recommended testing at the first prenatal visit with a doctor, as well as in the mid-second trimester. Additional testing should be done if there are any signs of Zika virus disease. Women with positive test results for Zika virus infection, should have their fetus monitored by ultrasound every three to four weeks to monitor fetal anatomy and growth.

Specific Recommendations by the CDC After Exposure to Zika Virus

- *What if a woman is not planning to get pregnant?*
  - The CDC says that to reduce the risk of sexual transmission, women who have possibly been exposed to Zika, should ask their partners to use condoms in addition to their regular birth control or abstain from sex for at least 8 weeks (2 months).
  - Man with possible exposure, even if they did not have Zika symptoms, should use a condom or abstain from sex for at least 6 months,[6,11,29] because the viability of Zika in sperm still is not clear.
- *What if the patient is planning to become pregnant?*
  - Couple planning pregnancies "in the near future" should consider avoiding areas with Zika transmission. Check out the CDC's travel information site for updates, and avoid traveling to the areas mentioned in the list.
  - Couples who are trying to have a baby should wait a few months to get pregnant if either partner has traveled to an area, where Zika is spreading, even if they did not have a confirmed infection, the CDC says.
  - The agency advises women to wait for 2 months and men to wait at leat for 6 months after possible exposure, even if the man did not have symptoms.
- *What if you are pregnant and have been exposed to Zika virus?*
  - Because of the "growing evidence of a link between Zika and microcephaly", in January, 2016, the CDC issued a travel alert advising pregnant women to consider postponing travel to countries and territories with ongoing local transmission of Zika virus.[30] Later, the advice was updated to caution pregnant women to avoid these areas entirely, if possible, and if travel is unavoidable, to protect themselves from mosquito bites.[31] Male partners of pregnant women and couples contemplating pregnancy, who must travel to areas where Zika is active, are advised to use condoms or abstain from sex entirely. The agency also suggested that women pregnant should consult with their physicians before traveling.[30,32]

PRECAUTIONS AND PREVENTION

An integral response is required involving action in several areas, including health education and the environment.

The approach should be two-pronged approach:
- Eliminating and controlling *Aedes aegypti* mosquito breeding sites.
- Abstinence or use of barrier contraceptives (For the at risk period).

To eliminate and control the mosquitoes, it is recommended to:
- Avoid allowing standing water in outdoor containers (flower pots, bottles and containers that collect water), so that they do not become mosquito-breeding sites.
- Cover domestic water tanks so that mosquitoes cannot get in.
- Avoid accumulating garbage.
- Unblock drains that would accumulate standing water.
- Use screens and mosquito nets in windows and doors to reduce contact between mosquitoes and people.[33,34]
- Opt for air-conditioning.

To prevent mosquito bites, it is recommended that people who live in areas where there are cases of the disease, as well as travelers and, especially pregnant women, should:
- Wear shirts with long sleeves and pants, rather than shorts.[35]
- Using bug spray with DEET,[36] which is safe for pregnant and nursing women.
- Using environmental protection agency-registered insect repellents with DEET, picaridin, IR3535, oil of lemon eucalyptus.
- Treating clothes with permethrin, a type of insecticide.

However, simply visiting the region is not the only factor for contracting the disease. Risk also depends on a person's length of stay, how many mosquito bites he received and whether prevention measures were taken to prevent the bites.

TREATMENT

No effective vaccine or treatment is available uptill date. Treatment is mainly symptomatic and conservative.[24]
- Plenty of rest
- Drink fluids to prevent dehydration.
- Take acetaminophen for fever and pain.

(Some authorities have recommended against using aspirin and other NSAIDs as they have been associated with hemorrhagic syndrome, when used for other flaviviruses.[6,21] Additionally, aspirin use is generally avoided in children when possible due to the risk of Reye syndrome[37]).
- Aspirin and other NSAIDs not to be taken.
- Avoiding mosquito bites at least for the first week of illness.
- Admission to hospital is rarely necessary.

VACCINES

Till date, no commercial vaccine against Zika virus is available. The WHO experts have suggested that the priority should be to develop inactivated vaccines and other non-live vaccines, which are safe to use in pregnant women and in those of childbearing age. In June 2016, the FDA granted the first approval for a human clinical trial for a Zika vaccine.[38,39]

PARVOVIRUS B19 (PB 19)

INTRODUCTION

Parvovirus (PB 19) is a single-stranded DNA virus member of parvoviridae family, discovered in 1975 in asymptomatic donor during routine blood screening for hepatitis B antigen. Small virus (Parvum being Latin for small) infects only human, animal strain infect animal not human.[40] Causative agent of erythema infectiosum (Fifth disease of childhood). Parvovirus B19V infection may affects 1–5% of pregnant women, mainly with normal pregnancy outcome.[41] Acute infection in pregnancy may lead to fetal loss or hydrops fetalis. Adverse outcome is increased, if maternal infection occurs during first two trimester of pregnancy but may also happen during third trimester.

EPIDEMIOLOGY

Parvovirus B19 infection can occur at any time. The majority of outbreaks tend to occur in winter or spring time. Viremia occurs 4–14 days after exposure and last up to 20 days.[42] Fever and prodromal symptom may develop in last few days of incubation period, but many people remain asymptomatic.[43] Rash arthralgia may begin around day 15 by which time patient is usually no longer infectious. As Par B19V infection confers life-long immunity, 50–70% women of reproductive age develop immunity. All nonimmune individuals are at increased risk of infection. Women at increased risk include mother of preschool and school-age children, worker at day-care centers and school teachers. Infection spreads through respiratory droplets or from hand to mouth contact.[44] Other mode of transmission includes blood product infusion and transplacental transfer.

CLINICAL PRESENTATION

Maternal

- *Asymptomatic:* About 70% of infected pregnant women may remain asymptomatic.[45-51]
- *Erythema infectiosum (fifth disease):* Facial rash consistent with as slapped-cheek appearance and a lace-like rash on trunk and extremeties. This rash may be accompanied by fever malaria and lymphadenopathy. Onset of rash usually coincides with appearance of IgM antibodies.[43]
- *Arthropathy:* The onset of arthritis is coincident with increase in parvovirus B19 antibodies (IgM) similar to erythema infectiosum. It is most common symptom in adults.
- Myocarditis
- Anemia PB19 virus preferentially infects erythroid cells, leukocytes and megakaryocyte cell lines, through P antigen. The virus attacks the red cell lines in bone marrow, causing red blood aplasia.[41] The anemia, however, may be significant in those with underlying hematogenic disorders such as sickle cell disease and thalassemia.
- *Immunocompromised patient:* Parvovirus infections cause severe anemia in immune-deficient patients those with HIV, leukemia and on chemotherapy.

Fetal Effects

- *Spontaneous abortion*: The spontaneous loss of fetuses affects with parvovirus B19 before 20 weeks gestation is 14.8% and after 20 weeks gestation is 2.3%.[52]
- *Congenital anomalies*: There have been case report of central nervous system, craniofacial musculoskeletal and eye anomalies.[40,45]
- *Fetal hydrops*: PB19 has been associated with hydrops fetalis, possible mechanisms are fetal anemia due to virus crossing the placenta combined with the shorter half-life of fetal red cells, leading to severe anemia, hypoxia and high output cardiac failure. Other possible cases are fetal viral myocarditis leading to cardiac failure, impaired hepatic function caused by direct damage of hepatocytes and indirect damage due to hemosiderin deposits.[52-57]
- *Ultrasound features*: Increased nuchal translucency and abnormal flow in ductus venosus in first trimester.
- Middle cerebral artery peak systolic velocity (MCA-PSV) is high sensitive means for determining the degree of fetal anemia.
- If a fetus develops hydrops, ultrasound signs include ascites, skin edema, pleural, pericardial and placental edema. It is estimated that parvovirus B19 infection accounts for the 8–10% of nonimmune hydrops. Interval between maternal infection and appearance of fetal hydrops is between 2 weeks and 4 weeks.[58-59]

- *Long-term neonatal outcome:* Neonatal complications include hepatic insufficiency, myocarditis, CNS abnormality, learning disability, neurological handicaps. Most children born to mothers who develops parvovirus B19 infection in pregnancy do not appear to suffer long-term sequelae.[45]

DIAGNOSIS

- IgM antibodies are present in 90% of patients approximately 2 weeks after infection, peak around 30 days post-infection and last up to 3-4 months.
  - IgG antibodies start to appear after 3-4 weeks and persist for life.[60]
- Diagnosis of fetal infection parvovirus B19 cannot culture in regular culture media. It can be identified histologically or characteristic intranuclear inclusions or by the presence of virus particles by electron microscopy.[40]

Proposed algorithm of care for parvovirus B19 antibody status		
Result	Indication	Action
IgG +	Past infection immune or infected 6 months before	Reassure patient
IgG –, IgM –	No past infection (nonimmune)	Repeat testing, repeat IgG, IgM after 2 weeks; negative, no current infection
IgG +, IgM +	Recent infection	Ultrasound + MCA Doppler → Hydrops / Nonhydrops serial ultrasound + MCA Doppler up to 12 weeks
IgG –, IgM +	Recent infection or false positive; Repeat IgG, IgM after 2 weeks, IgG + recent infection	

- A woman is non-immune and susceptible to infection, if both parvovirus B19 IgM are negative. Counseling is needed in such cases. Frequent handwashing may be recommended as a simple measure to reduce the risk of acquiring the infection. IgG and IgM tests should be repeated 2-4 weeks later, if she has had a recent exposure to virus and may be incubating the infection.
- Fall in concentration (IgM) after 3 months from maternal infection may lead to false negative diagnosis, fetus may show sign of fetal hydrops. In this scenario, PCR analysis of maternal blood may help in the diagnosis. Virus DNA may also be identified by PCR of amniotic fluid or fetal blood by cordocentesis. The most reliable method to diagnose acute fetal infection is to detect viral DNA by PCR or viral particle by electron microscopy. The presence of viral particles, however, can only be seen during viremic stage.

B19 IgM test in fetal blood is not reliable. As fetus does not begin to make its own IgM until 22 weeks gestation.

MANAGEMENT

Expectant mother infected with PB19 does not carry a high risk of maternal morbidity except in immunocompromised patients or patient with underlying hematological disorders including sickle cell disease, hereditary spherocytosis, pyruvate kinase deficiency, thalassemia or autoimmune hemolytic anemia, with low hemoglobin levels prior to infection.

- Routine screening for parvovirus immunity in a low-risk pregnancy is not recommended.[61]
- Pregnant women presenting with rash should be tested for PB19 IgG and IgM. Investigation for B19 infection is recommended as part of standard workup for fetal hydrops of intrauterine fetal death.[61]
- IgG-positive, IgM-negative patients should be reassured that B19 virus infection is not a cause for concern during their pregnancy [61-66]
- Positive IgM antibody test or in recent infection fetus should be followed by ultrasound or MCA Doppler for fetal anemia or hydrops. If fetal anemia hydrops identified, it should be referred to fetal specialist. In case of negative ultrasound, follow-up scan every 1-2 weeks up to 12 weeks after infection, if no fetal abnormality at 30 weeks gestation, it is unlikely to be any adverse sequelae from PB19 infection.[22-27]

Every pregnancy identified with fetal hydrops should be referred to a tertiary care center with a fetal medicine specialist. The current management of hydrops fetuses due to parvovirus B19 infection is somewhat controversial, but the primary management tool is cordocentesis to assess fetal hemoglobin and reticulocyte count. Severely anemic fetus with a low reticulocyte count may benefit from intrauterine transfusion. If hydrops develops, an intrauterine blood transfusion via cordocentesis should be considered. If reticulocyte count is high, marrow is in resolution phase hydrops would resolve without therapy. The fetus is term or near term, delivery should be considered. If delivery is not imminently required, amniocentesis for lung maturity may be considered. The use of corticosteroids to accelerate lung maturity is not contraindicated.

REFERENCES

1. "Zika virus". World Health Organization. January 2016. Retrieved 3 February 2016.
2. Hayes, Edward B. "Zika Virus Outside Africa". Emerging Infectious Diseases. 2009;15(9):1347-50. doi:10.3201/eidl509.090442. PMC 2819875%. PMID 19788800.

3. Simpson DIH. "Zika virus infection in man". Transactions of the Royal Society of Tropical Medicine and Hygiene. 1964;58(4): 339-48. doi.lO.1016/0035-9203(64)90201-9. ISSN 0035-9203.
4. Duffy MR, Chen TH, Hancock WT, et al. "Zika Virus Outbreak on Yap Island. Federated States of Micronesia". New England Journal of Medicine. 2009;360(24):2536-43. doi:10.1056/NEJMoa0805715. PMID 19516034.
5. Gatherer D, Kohl A. "Zika virus: a previously slow pandemic spreads rapidly through the Americas". Journal of General Virology. 2015;97(2):269-73. doi:10.1099/iav.0.000381. PMID 26684466.
6. Sikka V, Chattu, VK, Popli RK, et al. "The emergence of Zika virus as a global health security threat: A review and a consensus statement of the INDUSEM Joint working Group (JWG)". Journol of Global Infectious Diseases. 2016;8(1):3-15. doi:10.4103/0974-777X.176140. ISSN 0974-8245.
7. Dyer, Owen. "Zika virus spreads across Americas as concerns mount over birth defects". BMJ. 2015;351: h6983. doi.lO.1136/bmi.h6983. PMID. 26698165.
8. "Ministerio da Saude confirma 8 casos de zika virus noRNe8 na BA" [Ministry of Health confirms 8 cases of Zika virus in infants and 8 in BAl Ben Estar (in Portuguese). 14 May 2015.
9. Monitoramento dos casos de microcefalias no Brasil" [Monitoring cases of microcephaly in Brazil] (in Portuguese). Centro de Operagoes de Emergencias em Saude Publico sobre Microcefalias. 2015. Retrieved 24 December 2015.
10. "Governo confirma relacao entre Zika virus e epidemia de microcefalia" Government confirms relationship between Zika virus and epidemic microcephaly]. BBC Brasil (in Portuguese). 2015. Retrieved on 10 March 2016.
11. Oster, Alexandra M, Brooks, John T, Stryker, Jo Ellen, et al. "Interim Guidelines for Prevention of Sexual Transmission of Zika virus — United States. 2016". Morbidity and Mortality Weekly Report. 2016;65(5):120-1. doi:10.15585/mmwr. mm6505el. ISSN 0149-2195. PMID 26866485.
12. "CDC encourages following guidance to prevent sexual transmission of Zika virus". CDC Newsroom Releases. Centers for Disease Control and Prevention. 23 February 2016.
13. Hills, Susan L, Russell, Kate, Hennessey, Morgan, et al. "Transmission of Zika Virus through Sexual Contact with Travelers to Areas of Ongoing Transmission — Continental United States. 2016". Morbidity and Mortality Weekly Report. 2016;65(8). doi:10.15585/mmwr.mm6508e2er. ISSN 0149-2195.
14. Franchini M, Velati C. "Blood safety and zoonotic emerging pathogens: now it's the turn of Zika virus!". Blood Transfusion 2016;(14): 93-94. doi-.10.2450/2015.0187-15. PMID 26674809.
15. "*Aedes luteocephala*". Medically Important Mosquitoes. Walter Reed Biosystematics Unit. Retrieved 1 February 2016.
16. Grard, G, Caron M, Mom bo IM, Nkoghe D, Ondo SM, Jiolle D, Fontenille D, Paupy C, Leroy EM. "Zika Virus in Gabon (Central Africa), 2007: A New Threat from *Aedes albopictus*?." PLOS Negl Trop Dis. 2014 ;8(2):e2681. doi:10.137 1/Journal.ontd.0002681. ISSN 1935-2735. PMC 3916288 /PMID 24516683.
17. Wong PJ, Li MI, Chong C, Ng L, Tan C. "Aedes (Stegomyia) albopictus (Skuse): A Potential Vector of Zika Virus in Singapore". PLOS Negl Trop Dis. 2013;7(8): e2348. oi:10.1371/Journol.ontd.0002348. ISSN 1935-2735. PMC 3731215%. PMID 23936579.
18. Dupont-Rouzeyrol, Myrielle; Biron, Antoine; O'Connor, Olivia; etal. "Infectious Zika viral particles in breast milk". The Lancet. 387:1051. doi:10.1016/s0140-6736(16)00624-3.
19. "Symptoms, Diagnosis and Treatment of Zika Virus". Zika Virus Home. Centers for Disease Control and Prevention. Retrieved 29 April 2016.
20. Heang V, Yasuda, CY, Sovann Ly, et al. (2012). "Zika Virus Infection, Cambodia. 2010". Emerging Infectious Diseases. 18 (2): 349-351. doi:10.3201/eidl802.111224. ISSN 1080-6040. PMC 3310457%. PMID 22305269.
21. "Factsheet for health professionals". Zika virus infection. European Centre for Disease Prevention and Control. Retrieved 22 December 2015.
22. "First Zika virus-related death reported in US in Puerto Rico". Washington Post. Retrieved 29 April 2016.
23. Nayak, Shriddha; Lei, Jun; Pekosz, Andrew; Klein, Sabra; Burd, Irina. "Pathogenesis and Molecular Mechanisms of Zika Virus". Seminars in Reproductive Medicine. 2016;34:266-272. doi:10.1055/s-0036-1592071. ISSN 1526-8004.
24. "Zika virus". Retrieved 24 December 2015.
25. Fauci, Anthony S.; Morens, David M. "Zika Virus in the Americas – Yet Another Arbovirus Threat". New England Journal of Medicine. 2016;374:601-4. doi:10.1056/NEJMpl600297. PMID 26761185.
26. "Revised diagnostic testing for Zika, chikungunya, and dengue viruses in US Public Health Laboratories". Division of Vector-borne Diseases. Centers for Disease Control and Prevention. Retrieved 15 March 2016.
27. Chen LH, Hamer DH. "Zika Virus: Rapid Spread in the Western Hemisphere". Annals of Internal Medicine. 2016;164:613. doi:10.7326/M16-0150. ISSN 0003-4819. PMID 26832396.
28. Chen LH, Hamer DH. "Zika Virus: Rapid Spread in the Western Hemisphere". Annals of Internal Medicine. 2016;164:613. doi:10.7326/M16-0150. ISSN 0003-4819. PMID 26832396.
29. Petersen EE, Polen, KND, Meaney-Delman D; et al. "Update: Interim Guidance for Health Care Providers Carina for Women of Reproductive Age with Possible Zika Virus Exposure — United States. 2016". MMWR. Morbidity and Mortality Weekly Report. 2016;65(12):315-22. doi:10.15585/mmwr.mm6512e2. ISSN 0149-2195.
30. Lowes R. "CDC Issues Zika Travel Alert". Medscape Medical News. Retrieved 16 January 2016.
31. How to Protect Yourself". Centers for Disease Control and Prevention. Retrieved on 16 March 2016.
32. "CDC issues interim travel guidance related to Zika virus for 14 Countries and Territories in Central and South America and the Caribbean". CDC Newsroom Releases. Centers for Disease Control and Prevention. 15 January 2016.
33. "Surveillance and Control of *Aedes aegypti* and *Aedes albopictus* in the United States". Chikungunya Virus Home: Resources. Centers for Disease Control and Prevention. 10 March 2016.
34. "Help Control Mosquitoes that Spread Dengue, Chikungunya, and Zika viruses" . Chikungunya Virus Home: Fact-sheets and Posters. Centers for Disease Control and Prevention. August 2015.
35. https://\A^wxdc.gov/zika/prevention/prevent-mosquito-bites.html Permethrin-treated clothing will protect you after multiple washings.

36. *http://www.nvtimes.com/2016/04/05/health/zika-virus-deet-pregnant-women-safety.html* DEET Seen as Safe for Pregnant Women to Avoid Zika Despite Few Studies.
37. Fulginiti VA, Brunei I, Philip A, Cherry JD. et al. "Aspirin and Reye Syndrome". Pediatrics. 1982;69(6): 810-2. ISSN 1098-4275. PMID 7079050. Retrieved 11 March 2016.
38. Barzon L, Trevisan M, Sinigaglia A, Lavezzo E, Palu G. "Zika virus: from pathogenesis to disease control". FEMS Microbiology Letters. 2016;363(18): fnw202. dpi:10.1093/femsle/fnw202. ISSN 1574-6968. PMID 27549304.
39. Morrison C. "DNA vaccines against Zika virus speed into clinical trials". Nature Reviews Drug Discovery. 2016;15(8): 521-22. doi:10.1038/nrd.2016.159. ISSN 1474-1776.
40. Levy R, Weissman A, Blomberg G, Hagay ZJ. Infection by parvovirus B19 during pregnancy: a review. Obstet Gynecol Survey. 1997;52:254-9. .[PubMed]
41. Feldman DM, Timms D, Borgida F. Toxoplasmosis, parvovirus, and cytomegalovirus in pregnancy. Clin Lab Med. 2010 Sep;30(3):709-20.[PubMed].
42. Anderson LJ. Role of parvovirus B19 in human disease. Pediatr infect.1987;6:711-8.
43. Markenson GR, yancey MK. Parvovirus B12 infections in pregnancy. Semin Perinals 1998:22:309-17.
44. Adler S, Koch WC. Human parvovirus B19. In: Remington JS, Klein JO (Eds). Infectious diseases of the fetus and newborn infant. 7th edn. Philadelphia: Saunders. 2010:845-5.
45. Rodis JF. parvovirus infection. Clin Obstet Gynecol. 1999;42: 107-20.
46. Lamont RF, Sobel JD, Vaisbuch E, Kusanovic JP, Mazaki-Tovi S, Kim SK, et al. Parvovirus B19 infection in human pregnancy. BJOG. 2011;118:175-86. doi: 10.1111/j.1471-0528.2010.02749.x.
47. Centers for Disease Control (CDC). Risks associated with human parvovirus B19 infection. Morb Mortal Wkly Rep. 1989;38:81-8, 93-7.
48. Gillespie SM, Cartter ML, Asch S, Rokos JB, Gary GW, Tsou CJ, et al. Occupational risk of human parvovirus B19 infection for school and day-care personnel during an outbreak of erythema infectiosum. JAMA. 1990;263:2061-5.
49. Chorba T, Coccia P, Holman RC, Tattersall P, Anderson LJ, Sudman J, et al. The role of parvovirus B19 in aplastic crisis and erythema infectiosum (fifth disease). J Infect Dis 1986;154:383-3.
50. Plummer FA, Hammond GW, Forward K, Sekla L, Thompson LM, Jones SE, et al. An erythema infectiosum-like illness caused by human parvovirus infection. N Engl J Med. 1985;313:74-9. doi: 10.1056/NEJM198507113130203.
51. Chisaka H, Ito K, Niikura H, Sugawara J, Takano T, Murakami T, et al. Clinical manifestations and outcomes of parvovirus B19 infection during pregnancy in Japan. Tohoku J Exp Med 2006;209:277-83.
52. Miller E, Fairley CK, Cohen BJ, Seng C. Immediate and long-term outcome of human parvovirus B19 infection in pregnancy. Br J Obstet Gynaecol. 1998;105:174-8.
53. Public Health Laboratory Service Working Party on Fifth Disease. Prospective study of human parvovirus (B19) infection in pregnancy. BMJ. 1990;300:1166-70.
54. Gratacós E, Torres PJ, Vidal J, Antolín E, Costa J, Jiménez de Anta MT, et al. The incidence of human parvovirus B19 infection during pregnancy and its impact on perinatal outcome. J Infect Dis. 1995;171:1360-3.
55. Miller E, Fairley CK, Cohen BJ, Seng C. Immediate and long-term outcome of human parvovirus B19 infection in pregnancy. Br J Obstet Gynaecol. 1998;105:174-8.
56. Rodis JF, Quinn DL, Gary GW Jr, Anderson LJ, Rosengren S, Cartter ML, et al. Management and outcomes of pregnancies complicated by human B19 parvovirus infection: a prospective study. Am J Obstet Gynecol. 1990;163(4 Pt 1):1168-71.
57. Guidozzi F, Ballot D, Rothberg AD. Human B19 parvovirus infection in an obstetric population. A prospective study determining fetal outcome. J Reprod Med. 1994;39:36-8.
58. Komischke K, Searle K, Enders G. Maternal serum alphafetoprotein and human chorionic gonadotropin in pregnant women with acute parvovirus B19 infection with and without fetal complications. Prenat Diagn. 1997;17:1039-46
59. CarrcaT, Matiasa Brandao, Montenegro N. Early sign of cardiac failure—a clue for parvovirus infection screening in the first trimester? Fetal Diagn. Therapy. 2011;30:150-2s.
60. Eis-Hübinger AM, et al. Parvovirus B19 infection in pregnancy. Intervirology. 1998;41:178-84.
61. SOGC-December 2014 (Replaces no. 119, Sept 2002) 'SOGC Clinical Practice Guideline—Parvovirus B19 Infection in Pregnancy'. Jobstet Gynaecol Can. 2014;36(12):1107-16.
62. Tolfvenstam T, Broliden K. 'Parvovirus B19 infection', Seminars in Fetal and Neonatal Medicine, 2009;14(4), pp. 218–21. doi: 10.1016/j.siny.2009.01.007.
63. Health Protection Agency. General Information on Parvovirus. Available at: *http://webarchive.nationalarchives.gov.uk/20140714084352*.
64. Health Protection Agency. Laboratory Confirmed Reports of Parvovirus B19 Infection, England and Wales 1993-2004.
65. Ergaz Z, Ornoy A. 'Parvovirus B19 in pregnancy', Reproductive Toxicology (Elmsford, NY), 2006;21(4):421-35. doi: 10.1016/j.reprotox.2005.01.006.
66. De Jong EP, de Haan TR, Kroes ACM, Beersma MFC, Oepkes D, Walther FJ. 'Parvovirus B19 infection in pregnancy'. Journal of Clinical Virology: The Official Publication of the Pan American Society for Clinical Virology. 2006;36(1):1–7. doi: 10.1016/j.jcv.2006.01.004.

SECTION 8: FETAL DYSMATURITY AND DYSMORPHOLOGY

Chapter 45

Fetal Growth Restriction: Monitoring and Management

Geetha Balsarkar, Jagruti Murkey

INTRODUCTION

Fetal growth restriction (FGR) is defined by the American College of Obstetricians and Gynecologists (ACOG) as 'the failure of a fetus to achieve its individual potential. It is associated with high-risk for perinatal morbidity and mortality where the risk increases with severity of condition'.

Small for gestational age (SGA) fetus is defined as fetal abdominal circumference (AC) or estimated fetal weight (EFW) <10th centile. Almost 50–70% of small for gestation age fetuses are constitutionally small but healthy. Such a fetus is found to be growing along the lower percentile (10th or 5th), but maintaining its growth curve. This is often called as "low profile fetus". Approximately, 20% of SGA fetuses are classified as having 'true' FGR, and another 5–10% are associated with chromosomal anomalies, structural anomalies, or chronic intrauterine infection.

RULES OF FETAL GROWTH

- Every fetus has its own growth rate.
- Every fetus maintains its growth rate as long as it is growing normally.
- Younger fetus grow faster than older fetuses.

Hence, early and accurate dating with appropriate biometry is important in making the diagnosis of FGR. Fetal monitoring is then based on ultrasound estimation of biometry, Doppler flow and liquor assessment.

A protocol-based approach starting with detailed history is essential.

HISTORY

- Menstrual history (Regularity/duration of cycle).
- Mode of conception (natural/IUI/IVF). If ART – Date of embryo transfer.
- Date of pregnancy confirmation.
- Medical history and previous obstetric history.

EXAMINATION

- Parental height and weight.
- Symphysiofundal height at every visit.

Prior Scan Records

This helps to ascertain the gestational age with accuracy, (Transvaginal scans are more reliable for dating in early pregnancy).

MONITORING THE GROWTH RESTRICTED FETUS

Clinical methods such as identifying subnormal uterine size, followed by abdominal palpation and direct measurement of the symphysiofundal height detects only 30% of IUGR fetuses. Ultrasound is the benchmark of actual pregnancy dating and diagnosis of FGR. Abdominal circumference should be considered as the best single measurement to screen for FGR as it has good correlation with fetal weight. Although cut-off value for FGR is at the 10th centile, adverse outcomes are mainly confined to fetuses below 5th or 3rd centiles.

Placental dysfunction starts with abnormal tertiary villous vessels and ends with characteristic fetal multi-vessel cardiovascular manifestations. These effects can be documented with Doppler ultrasound examination by:

- Fetal umbilical arteries for the placenta.
- Middle cerebral artery (MCA) for preferential brain perfusion.
- Ductus venosus for the cardiac effects of placental dysfunction.

As growth restriction progresses, Doppler abnormalities in these vascular territories also deteriorate, suggesting a sequential pattern of disease progression. The presence of maternal disease such as pre-eclampsia or autoimmune diseases may cause a sudden and unpredictable worsening of this sequence.

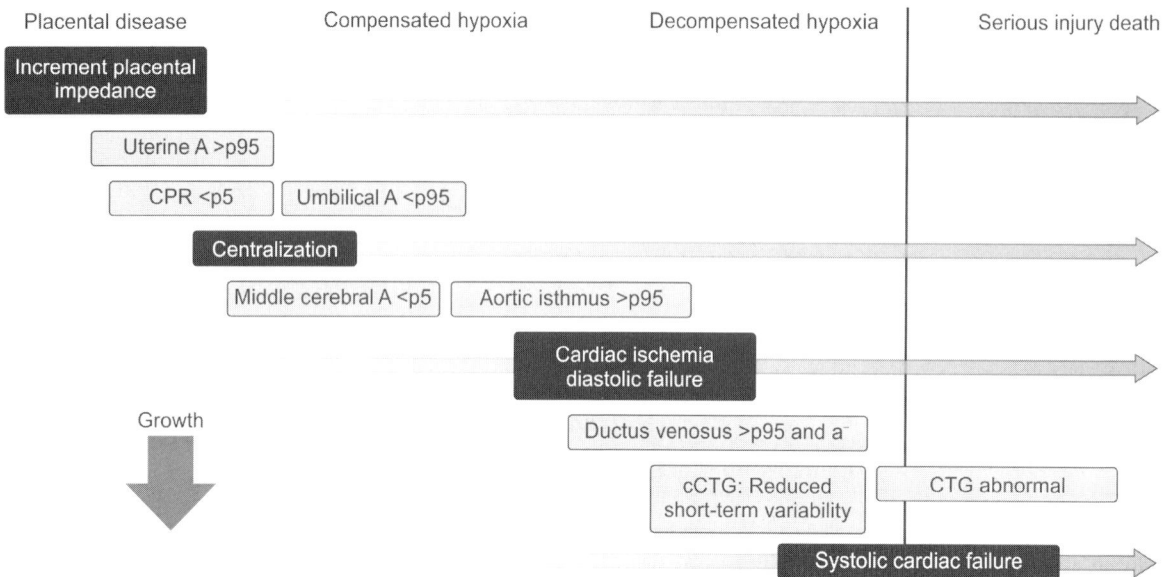

Fig. 45.1: Fetal deterioration in placental insufficiency

- Increased placental blood flow resistance indicates placental dysfunction as the underlying cause.
- Increased diastolic blood flow in the cerebral circulation indicates redistribution.
- As more placental vasculature is damaged, there is loss of diastolic flow in umbilical artery progressing to reversal.
- Progressive elevation in venous Doppler indices indicates alterations in cardiac function that precede deterioration of biophysical parameters in the fetus **(Fig. 45.1)**.

The first clinically relevant step is the distinction of 'true' fetal growth restriction (FGR), associated with signs of abnormal fetoplacental function and poorer perinatal outcome, from constitutional small-for-gestational age, with a near-normal perinatal outcome. Classifying a fetus as having true fetal growth restriction is clinically relevant, as these fetuses are associated with poorer perinatal outcome while constitutionally small fetuses have near normal perinatal outcome. Closer monitoring and appropriate delivery timing can be instituted which would then help reducing the incidence of perinatal insult.

According to recent recommendations, such a distinction should not be based solely on umbilical artery Doppler, since this index detects only early-onset severe forms. FGR should be diagnosed in the presence of any of the factors associated with a poorer perinatal outcome, including Doppler cerebroplacental ratio, uterine artery Doppler, a growth centile below the 5th centile.

FGR presents under two different phenotypes when the onset is early or late in gestation. In general, but not always, there is a correspondence between early-onset and the most severe forms of FGR. The cut-off to define early-versus late-onset FGR has commonly been set in an arbitrary fashion at about 32–34 weeks at diagnosis or 37 weeks at delivery. **Table 45.1** depicts the main differences between both clinical forms.

EARLY-ONSET FETAL GROWTH RESTRICTION

Early-onset FGR represents 20–30% of all FGRs. Early FGR presents in association with early pre-eclampsia (PE) in up to 50%. Early-onset FGR is highly associated with severe placental insufficiency and with chronic fetal hypoxia. This explains that UA Doppler is abnormal in a high proportion of cases. Early severe FGR is associated with severe injury and/or fetal death before term in many cases. Management is challenging and aims at achieving the best balance between the risks of leaving the fetus *in utero* versus the complications of prematurity.

LATE-ONSET FETAL GROWTH RESTRICTION

Late-onset FGR represents 70–80% of FGR. Its association with late pre-eclampsia (PE) is low, roughly 10%. In late onset FGR the degree of placental disease is mild, thus UA Doppler is normal in virtually all cases. Despite normal UA PI Doppler, there is a high association with abnormal CPR values. In addition, advanced brain vasodilation suggesting chronic hypoxia, as reflected by an MCA PI <p5, may occur in 25% of late FGR. Advanced signs of fetal deterioration with changes in the DV are virtually never observed.

Table 45.1: The main differences between early- and late-onset form

Early-onset FGR (1–2%)	Late-onset FGR (3–5%)
Problem: Management	*Problem:* Diagnosis
Placental disease: Severe (UA Doppler abnormal, high association with pre-eclampsia)	*Placental disease:* Mild (UA Doppler normal, low association with pre-eclampsia)
Hypoxia ++: Systemic cardiovascular adaptation	*Hypoxia +/–:* Central cardiovascular adaptation
Immature fetus = Higher tolerance to hypoxia = Natural history	Mature fetus = Lower tolerance to hypoxia = No (or very short) natural history
High mortality and morbidity; lower prevalence	Lower mortality (but common cause of late stillbirth); poor long-term outcome; affects large fraction of pregnancies

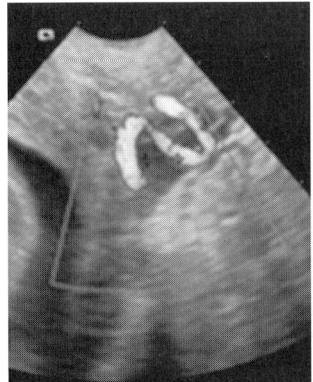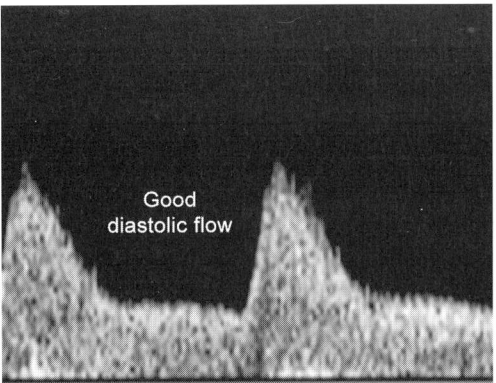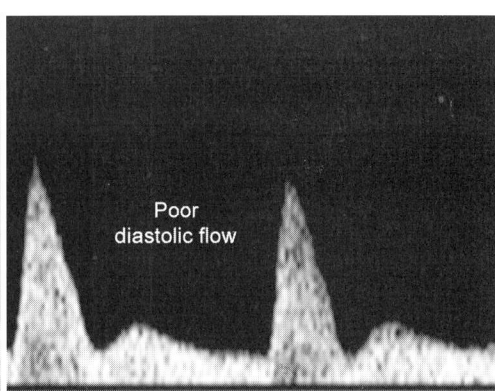

Fig. 45.2: Uterine artery Doppler

There is a risk of acute fetal deterioration before labor, as suggested by the high contribution to late-pregnancy mortality, and a high association with intrapartum fetal distress and neonatal acidosis. Thus, the cascade of sequential fetal deterioration described above does not occur in late FGR.

Once the diagnosis is established, late FGR does not represent a management challenge, as seen in early FGR. However, still undiagnosed late FGR contributes to a large share of late pregnancy stillbirths.

MONITORING IN FETAL GROWTH RESTRICTION

Uterine Artery Doppler (UtA) (Fig. 45.2)

Impaired trophoblastic invasion of the maternal spiral arteries results in high uterine artery PI and persistence of the uterine artery notch. In high-risk pregnancies uterine artery Doppler helps to identify patients at risk for pre-eclampsia and FGR.

Umbilical Artery Doppler (Fig. 45.3)

Umbilical artery (UA) Doppler provides both diagnostic and prognostic information for the management of FGR. The progression of UA Doppler patterns to absent or reverse end-diastolic flow correlates with the risks of injury or death and adverse perinatal outcome. Absent or reversed end-diastolic flow occurs when 60–70% of the placental villous tree is damaged. Use of UA Doppler in high-risk pregnancies (most of them SGA fetuses) improves perinatal outcomes, with a 29% reduction in perinatal deaths.

Middle Cerebral Artery Doppler

Middle cerebral artery (MCA) Doppler is valuable for the identification and prediction of adverse outcome among late-onset FGR, independently of the UA Doppler, which is often normal in these fetuses. MCA informs about the existence of brain vasodilation, a marker of hypoxia. Fetuses with abnormal MCA PI had a six-fold risk of emergency cesarean section for fetal distress when compared with SGA fetuses with normal MCA PI, which is particularly relevant because labor induction at term is the current standard of care of late-onset FGR **(Fig. 45.4)**.

Cerebroplacental Ratio

Cerebroplacental ratio (CPR) is emerging a important diagnostic index. The CPR improves remarkably the

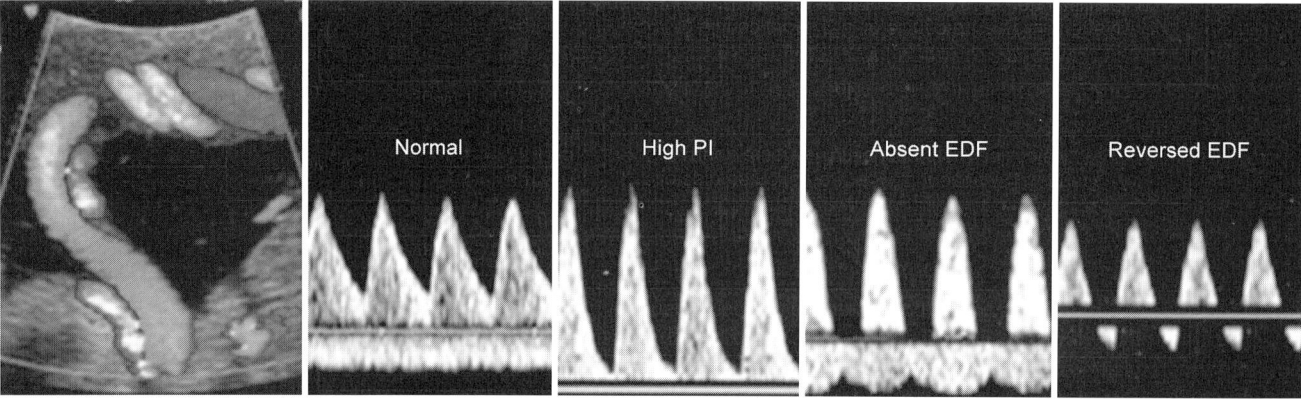

Fig. 45.3: Umbilical artery Doppler *(For color version, see Plate 3)*

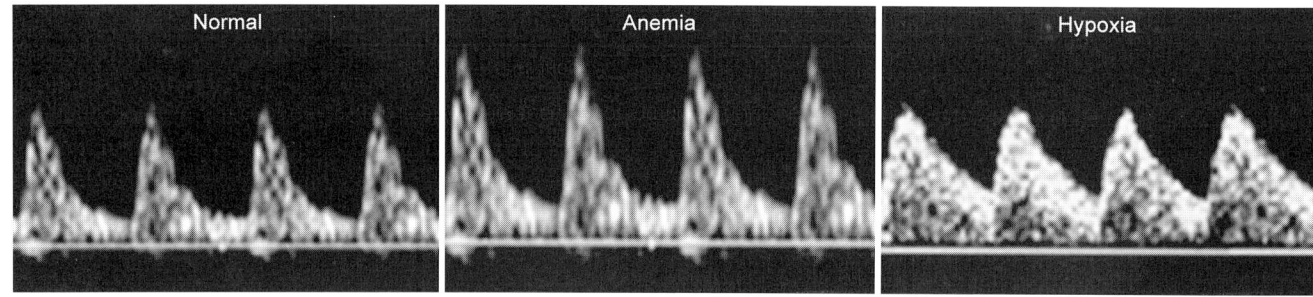

Fig. 45.4: Middle cerebral artery Doppler

sensitivity of UA and MCA alone, because increased placental impedance (UA) is often combined with reduced cerebral resistance (MCA). In late onset growth restriction, CPR may be abnormal before MCA PI becomes abnormal when there is still some forward flow in the umbilical artery. This deterioration in the CP ratio is associated with poorer neonatal neurodevelopmental outcomes.

Ductus Venosus Doppler

Ductus venosus (DV) Doppler is the strongest single Doppler parameter to predict the short-term risk of fetal death in early-onset FGR. DV flow waveforms become abnormal only in advanced stages of fetal compromise. The absent or reversed velocities during atrial contraction are associated with perinatal mortality independently of the gestational age at delivery. Thus, this sign is normally considered sufficient to recommend delivery at any gestational age, after of steroids administration **(Fig. 45.5)**.

Aortic Isthmus Doppler

This vessel reflects the balance between the impedance of the brain and systemic vascular systems. Reverse aortic isthmus (AoI) flow is a sign of advanced deterioration and a further step in the sequence starting with the UA and MCA Dopplers. The aortic isthmus Doppler is associated with increased fetal mortality and neurological morbidity in early-onset FGR.

Biophysical Profile

Biophysical profile (BPP) is calculated by combining ultrasound assessment of fetal tone, respiratory and body movements, with amniotic fluid index and a conventional CTG. Studies show an association between abnormal BPP and perinatal mortality and cerebral palsy. However, a high false-positive rate (50%) limits the clinical usefulness of the BPP. Evidence suggests that use of BPP in high-risk pregnancies does not reduce perinatal death. The use of BPP increases C section rates without improving perinatal outcome. Consequently, whenever Doppler expertise and/or cCTG are available, the incorporation of BPP in management protocols of FGR is questionable.

Management of FGR (Flow Chart 45.1)

The aim in clinical management of FGR should be:
- To distinguish FGR from SGA

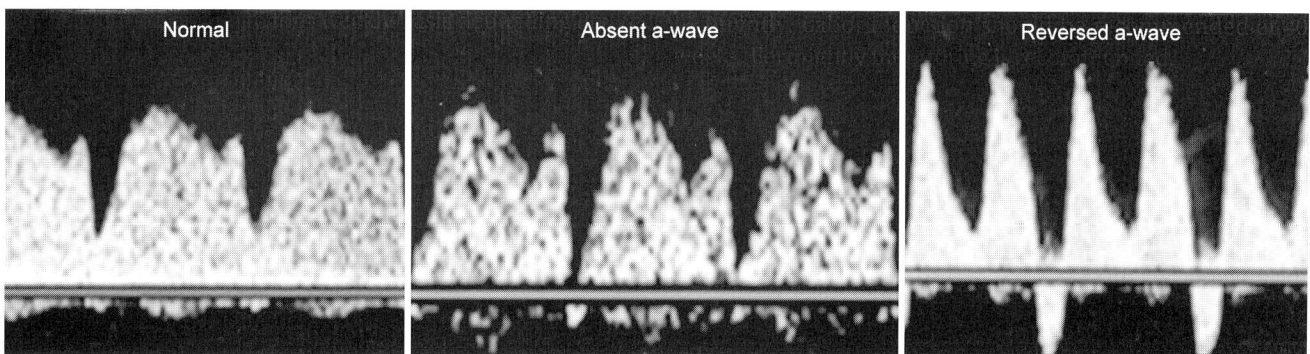

Fig. 45.5: Ductus venosus Doppler

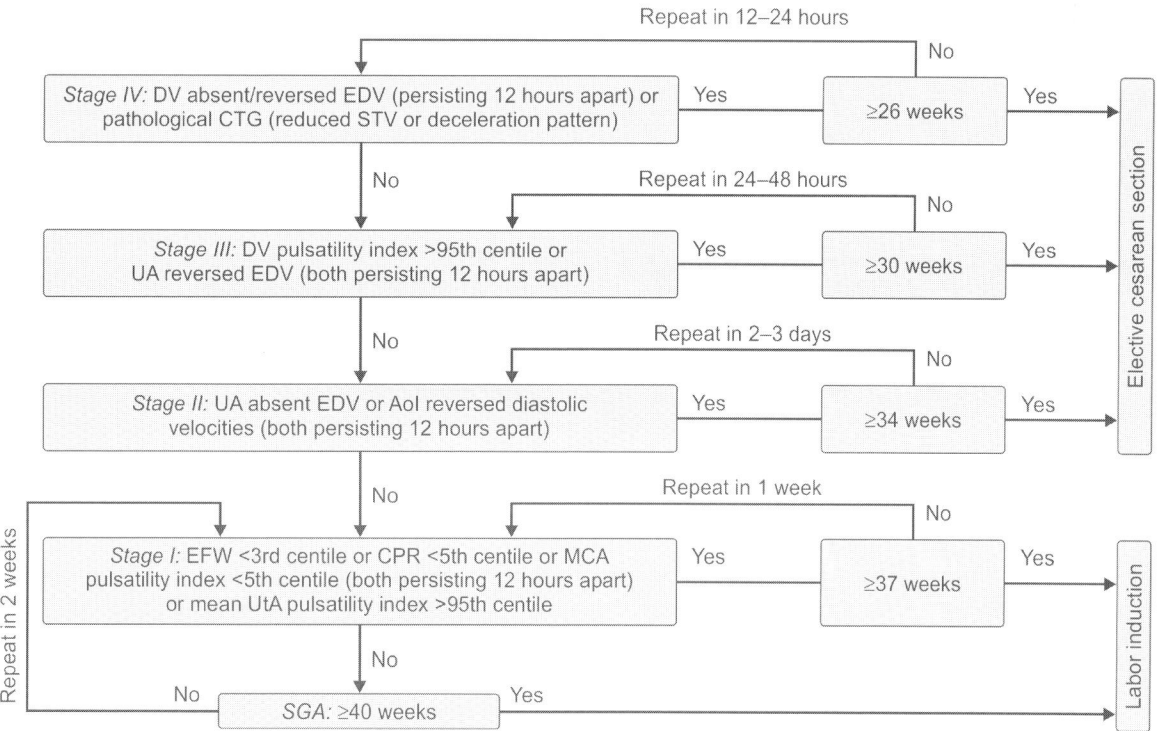

Flow chart 45.1: Stage-based decision algorithm for management of fetal growth restriction

- To monitor and identify the optimal time to deliver, balancing the *in utero* risks to the risks of prematurity and neonatal loss.

In the first step, once a small fetus (i.e. EFW <10th centile) has been identified, the Doppler study, i.e umbilical artery PI, middle cerebral artery PI, ductus venosus and the Cerebroplacental ratio (CPR) should be measured in order to classify FGR versus SGA. Once confirmed, growth assessment can be planned on two to four weekly basis depending on the gestational age.

In cases of FGR fetuses, changes in the UA, DV and AoI Doppler, and cCTG where available, are used to define stages of deterioration again depending on the gestational age.

Small-for-Gestational Age

Excluding infectious and genetic causes, the perinatal results are good.

Doppler and growth assessment is recommended fortnightly. Labor induction should be recommended at 40 weeks. Fortnightly monitoring is recommended.

STAGE-BASED CLASSIFICATION AND MANAGEMENT OF FGR (TABLE 45.2)

Stage I: Fetal Growth Restriction (Severe Smallness or Mild Placental Insufficiency)

Either UtA, UA or MCA Doppler, or the CPR are abnormal. In the absence of other abnormalities, evidence suggests a low risk of fetal deterioration before term. Labor induction beyond 37 weeks is acceptable, but the risk of intrapartum fetal distress is increased. Weekly monitoring recommended.

Stage II: Fetal Growth Restriction (Severe Placental Insufficiency)

This stage is defined by UA absent-end diastolic velocity (AEDV) or reverse AoI.

Delivery should be recommended after 34 weeks. The risk of emergency cesarean section at labor induction exceeds 50%, and, therefore, elective cesarean section is a reasonable option. Monitoring twice a week is recommended.

Stage III: Fetal Growth Restriction (Advanced Fetal Deterioration, Low-suspicion Signs of Fetal Acidosis)

The stage is defined by reverse absent-end diastolic velocity (REDV) or DV PI >95th centile. There is an association with a higher risk of stillbirth and poorer neurological outcome. However, since signs suggesting a very high risk of stillbirth within days are not present yet, it seems reasonable to delay elective delivery to reduce as possible the effects of severe prematurity. We suggest delivery should be recommended by cesarean section after 30 weeks.

Monitoring every 24–48 hour is recommended.

Stage IV: Fetal Growth Restriction (High-suspicion of Fetal Acidosis and High Risk of Fetal Death)

There are spontaneous FHR decelerations, reduced STV (<3 ms) in the cCTG, or reverse atrial flow in the DV Doppler. Spontaneous FHR deceleration is an ominous sign. The cCTG and DV are associated with very high risks of stillbirth within the next 3–7 days and disability. Deliver after 26 weeks by cesarean section at a tertiary care center under steroid treatment for lung maturation. Intact survival exceeds 50% only after 26–28 weeks, and before this threshold parents should be counseled by multidisciplinary teams. Monitoring every 12–24 hour until delivery is recommended.

BIBLIOGRAPHY

1. Alfirevic Z, Neilson JP. Biophysical profile for fetal assessment in high risk pregnancies. Cochrane Database Syst Rev. 2000:CD000038.

Table 45.2: Stage-based classification and management of FGR

Stage	Pathophysiological correlate	Criteria (any of)	Monitoring*	GA/mode of delivery
I	Severe smallness or mild placental insufficiency	EFW <3rd centile CPR <p5 UA PI > p95 MCA PI <p5 UtA PI >95	Weekly	37 weeks LI
II	Severe placental insufficiency	UA AEDV Reverse AoI	Biweekly	34 weeks CS
III	Low-suspicion fetal acidosis	UA REDV DV PI >p95	1–2 days	30 weeks CS
IV	High-suspicion fetal acidosis	DV reverse a flow cCTG <3 ms FHR decelerations	12 hours	26 weeks** CS

All Doppler signs described above should be confirmed at least twice, ideally at least 12 hours apart.

Abbreviations: GA = Gestational age; LI = Labor induction; CS = Cesarean section.

* Recommended intervals in the absence of severe pre-eclampsia. If FGR is accompanied by this complication, strict fetal monitoring is warranted regardless of the stage.

** Lower GA threshold recommended according to current literature figures reporting at least 50% intact survival. Threshold could be tailored according to parents' wishes or adjusted according to local statistics of intact survival.

2. Alfirevic Z, Stampalija T, Gyte GM. Fetal and umbilical Doppler ultrasound in high-risk pregnancies. Cochrane Database Syst Rev. 2010:CD007529.
3. Baschat AA, et al. Predictors of neonatal outcome in early-onset placental dysfunction. Obstet Gynecol. 2007;109:253–61.
4. Baschat AA, Gembruch U. The cerebroplacental Doppler ratio revisited. Ultrasound Obstet Gynecol. 2003;21:124–7.
5. Cruz-Martinez R, et al. Fetal brain Doppler to predict cesarean delivery for non-reassuring fetal status in term small-for-gestational-age fetuses. Obstet Gynecol. 2011;117:618–26.
6. Cruz-Martinez R, et al: Changes in myocardial performance index and aortic isthmus and ductus venosus Doppler in term, small for-gestational age fetuses with normal umbilical artery pulsatility index. Ultrasound Obstet Gynecol. 2011;38:400–5.
7. Figueras et al. Fetal Diagnosis and Therapy; January 2014. Update on Diagnosis and Classification of Fetal Growth Restriction and Proposal of a Stage-based Management protocol.
8. Figueroa-Diesel, et al. Doppler changes in the main fetal brain arteries at different stages of hemodynamic adaptation in severe growth restriction. Ultrasound in Obstetrics and Gynecology. 2007.
9. Fouron JC, et al. The relationship between an aortic isthmus blood flow velocity index and the postnatal neurodevelopmental status of fetuses with placental circulatory insufficiency. Am J Obstet Gynecol. 2005;192:497–503.
10. Hershkovitz R, et al: Fetal cerebral blood flow redistribution in late gestation: identification of compromise in small fetuses with normal umbilical artery Doppler. Ultrasound Obstet Gynecol. 2000;15:209–12.
11. Manual on Intrauterine Growth Restriction by Mediscan
12. Oros D, et al: Longitudinal changes in uterine, umbilical and fetal cerebral Doppler indices in late-onset small-for-gestational age fetuses. Ultrasound Obstet Gynecol. 2011;37: 191–5.
13. Schwarze A, et al. Qualitative venous Doppler flow waveform analysis in preterm intrauterine growth-restricted fetuses with ARED flow in the umbilical artery: correlation with short-term outcome. Ultrasound Obstet Gynecol. 2005;25:573–9.
14. Turan OM, et al: Progression of Doppler abnormalities in intrauterine growth restriction. Ultrasound Obstet Gynecol 2008; 32:160–7.

Chapter 46

Fetal Dysmorphology

Prachi Dixit, Madhuri Gawande, Shirish Vaidya

INTRODUCTION

Every couple conceives with the picture of healthy child in mind and a dysmorphic fetus can be the worst nightmare for them. According to the World Health Organization (WHO) fact-sheet an estimated 3,03,000 newborns die within 4 weeks of birth every year worldwide, due to congenital anomalies.[1] In India, the prevalence of congenital anomalies is 2.2% to 6.6%.[2] Keeping this fact in mind that 90% of the congenitally anomalous babies are born to women with no risk factor, antenatal screening and basic genetic sonography should be offered to every pregnant lady. An obstetrician should be able to timely detect congenital abnormality and should be able to answer questions pertaining to cause, management, prognosis and preventing recurrence in next pregnancy.

This chapter aims to provide key points about common fetal dysmorphic condition which can help to diagnose and communicate the information clearly and sensitively to the parents.

FETAL CRANIOSPINAL ABNORMALITIES

Central nervous system is the earliest organ system to develop. Teratogenic exposure in any form early in the developmental stage can affect CNS. For adequate visualization of central nervous system, three views of brain are used.
- *Transthalamic view:* Axial view through brain at the level of thalami, cavum septum pellucidum and falx cerebri.
- *Transventricular view:* Axial view above transthalamic view, including lateral ventricles and choroid plexus.
- *Transcerebellar view:* Through cerebellum, vermis, cistern magna.

Examination of spine is done in sagittal, transverse and coronal view.

OPEN NEURAL TUBE DEFECTS

Anencephaly, cephalocele and spina bifida: Neural tube closes at third to fourth week after fertilization. Head end is closed by 24th day and sacral end closes by 26th day postconception. Depending on the timing of interruption in closure of neural tube leads to various open neural tube defects (ONTD).

Open neural tube defects originate from multiple factors that can be genetic or environmental. Ultrasonography along with maternal serum alpha fetoprotein is used for screening of ONTD. 3D Ultrasonography and MRI scans can be used in high-risk patients. Neural tube defects (NTDs) are among the leading non-infectious birth defects with a worldwide prevalence of 1–2 per 1000 live births.[3] The overall birth prevalence of neural tube defects was found to be 4.5 per 1000 total births in a study conducted in eastern India India.[4] It is commonest congenital anomaly reported in India. Females are affected 4 times more frequently than males. Recurrence risk is 5% after 1st affected pregnancy and 13% after 2nd affected pregnancy.

Anencephaly

Bony calvaria of skull above orbits should be visualized by 10 weeks of gestation. Absence of cranial vault and cerebral hemispheres is called anencephaly **(Figs 46.1A to C)**. Forebrain and midbrain are replaced by a mass of thin-walled channels called "area cerebrovasculosa". Differential diagnoses are amniotic band syndrome, severe microcephaly, large encephalocele. Acrania is normally developed brain with absence of skull.

Cephalocele

Sac-like protrusion from the head not covered with bone is called cephalocele. Presence of brain in this sac is termed encephalocele. Occipital cephaloceles are most common. Others may be parietal, frontal or nasopharyngeal. Differential diagnoses are cystic hygroma, teratoma, and hemangioma.

Spina Bifida

On longitudinal view, a normal spine is seen to taper caudally. In case of vertebral defect, posterior ossification centers are more widely spaced than above and below vertebrae (splaying of posterior ossification center). Spina bifida is classified as

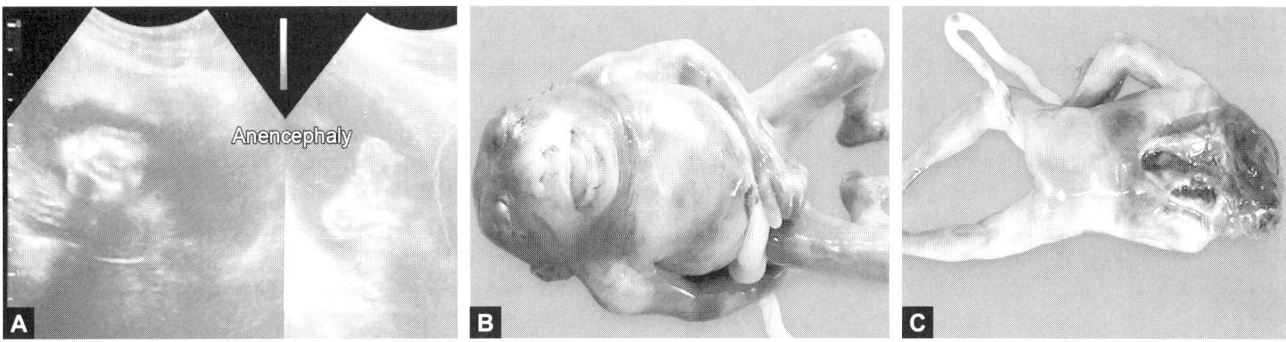

Figs 46.1A to C: Anencephaly *(For color version, see Plate 3)*

spina bifida occulta (covered by skin) or spina bifida aperta (not covered by skin). Defect may be covered by meningeal membranes appearing as cyst. When it contains spinal fluid, it is called meningocele. When it contains neural tissue, it is called meningomyelocele.

Spina bifida is commonly associated with Arnold-Chiari malformation (cerebellar vermis, fourth ventricle and medulla are displaced caudally). This malformation is associated with lemon and banana sign.[5] Caudal displacement of the cranial contents in a soft skull leads to scalloping of frontal bones that looks like lemon shape in transverse section. Cerebellar hemispheres are displaced in cisterna magna and are flattened rostrocaudally giving a banana shape ultrasonographic appearance. This picture is seen in second trimester in about 95% of fetuses with ONTD.[6]

Management

Prenatal

A detailed anomaly scan and fetal karyotyping is advised for open neural tube defects. There is high incidence of associated aneuploidy. Anencephaly is usually diagnosed early and should be advised termination.

The prognosis of cephaloceles depends on size, presence of brain matter in it and associated anomalies.

Spina bifida is associated with long-term disabilities like lower extremity paralysis, bladder and bowel incontinence. Still, early closure of the defect with ventriculoperitoneal shunting, surgery for fecal and urinary incontinence, dietary management, can improve the outcome.

In utero fetal surgeries for repair of meningomyelocele are under evaluation to prevent progression of damage to spinal cord from insults such as amniotic fluid trauma. They have been reported to decrease herniation of hind-brain and hydrocephalus.[7] In uterosurgeries have fallacies of prematurity and lethal pulmonary hypoplasia due to oligohydramnios. Long-term benefit in improving motor function in lower limb and bowel bladder incontinence is still under study.

Labor and Delivery

Anencephaly is associated with postmaturity. Fetal autopsy to be offered to see association with any genetic syndrome.

For cephalocele, cesarean section is to be done only for maternal indications. Large sacs may require decompression for vaginal delivery.

In isolated meningomyeloceles, elective cesarean section has been associated with better functional outcome.[8] Trauma and traction to the spine has to be avoided while delivery. Uterine incision should be retracted by assistant to avoid rubbing against the meningomyelocele.

Postnatal and prepregnancy: Recurrence risk is reduced by periconceptional administration of folate 4–5 mg 3 months prior to conception. Early registration and antenatal sonography at 11 weeks should be advised.

HYDROCEPHALUS

Abnormal increase in cerebral ventricular volume (ventriculomegaly) with increase in intracranial pressure and macrocephaly is termed hydrocephalus. Incidence of congenital hydrocephalus not associated with neural tube defect in the US is 5.8:10000 total births.[9] Risk of recurrence depends on associated anomaly. It is very low for sporadic chromosomal anomalies or congenital infections but very high for balanced translocations, X-linked conditions like aqueductal stenosis, autosomal recessive condition like Dandy Walker syndrome, autosomal dominant condition like achondropoplasia.[10,11]

Mechanism of increase in ventricular size:
- Obstruction to outflow tract (noncommunicating hydrocephalus)
- Decreased absorption of cerebrospinal fluid (CSF) by arachnoid granulations (communicating hydrocephalus)
- Increased synthesis of CSF by choroid papilloma.
- Relative increase in size of ventricles due to underdevelopment of cortical tissue.

Etiology

Hydrocephalus is associated with inherited malformations, congenital infections followed by scarring, infection followed by CSF obstruction, intraventricular hemorrhage, mass lesion, tumors. Most common conditions causing ventriculomegaly are aqueductal stenosis, Arnold-Chiari malformation secondary to spina bifida, Dandy Walker malformation, and holoprosencephaly. Sometimes, the etiology may remain unexplained.

Diagnosis

Diagnosis is made by measurement of width of atrium of lateral ventricles in transthalamic axial plane. Normally, the width of atrium remains constant throughout second and third trimester. Mean width is 7.6 mm, a value of 10 mm has been accepted as upper limit of normal. Choroid plexus is seen as dangling structures in ventriculomegaly. Fetal cortical mantle thickness may decrease but it does not correlate much with subsequent intelligence. Once diagnosed, serial scans are needed to assess prognosis. Differential diagnoses are alobar holoprosencephaly, hydranencephaly, porencephaly, arachnoid cyst, large aneurysm of vein of Galen.

Management

Prenatal

Once diagnosed, careful search for associated anomalies should be done and further management will depend on karyotype, gestational age, and infection screening. The placement of intrauterine ventriculoamniotic shunt is still under debate.[10]

Labor and Delivery

If serial ultrasound is showing worsening hydrocephalus, delivery can be considered at pulmonary maturity to prevent further cerebral damage. In cases of isolated disease with moderate-to-severe macrocephaly, elective cesarean section should be considered. For severe hydrocephalus with multiple anomalies, cephalocentesis should be planned with vaginal delivery.

Postnatal

If left untreated, isolated hydrocephalus may lead to massive enlargement of head, blindness, mental retardation. Some cases may also have spontaneous arrest of enlargement. Postnatal ventricular shunting has greatly improved the prognosis of isolated hydrocephalus. Neonatal deaths are usually seen with associated anomalies.

HOLOPROSENCEPHALY

The incomplete cleavage of primitive forebrain (prosencephalon) leads to several cerebral abnormalities which are called holoprosencephaly sequence. Based on degree of separation of cerebral hemispheres, it is divided into alobar (no cerebral cortical division), semilobar and lobar varieties. Development of midline cerebral structures like thalamus, corpus callosum, septum pellucidum is defective. Olfactory tract is absent (arhinencephaly). The incidence is about 1 in 10000 live births.[12]

Characteristic facial findings are:
- Cyclopia with one median orbit, proboscis from lower forehead, absent nose.
- Ethmocephaly with proboscis between two narrowly placed orbits and absent nose
- Cebocephaly (closely set eyes, single or absent nostril, flat nose) with microcephaly and rudimentary nose
- Hypotelorism, median cleft lip, flat nose
- Bilateral cleft lip.

This is one of the earliest diagnosed congenital anomalies ultrasonographically. It may be associated with trisomy 13 so karyotyping is offered. Prognosis is very poor. Neonatal death or severe mental retardation is seen. In absence of chromosomal abnormality, chances of recurrence are 6% to 14%.[13,14]

FACIAL CLEFTS

Cleft lip and palate are commonest congenital facial deformity. The birth prevalence of orofacial clefts in a study in India was found to be 1.3 per 1000 total births.[4] Failure of nasofrontal process to fuse with maxillary process leads to various varieties of cleft lip like unilateral, bilateral, complete or incomplete. Majority of cases are isolated but about 10% may be associated with genetic syndromes. Diagnosis is made by careful visualization in ultrasonography. 3D scan is very helpful. Karyotyping should be offered. Artificial palate may be required by infant to assist feeding. Isolated cases are excellently managed by corrective surgery.

DANDY-WALKER MALFORMATION

Complete or partial absence of cerebellar vermis and posterior fossa cyst continuous with 4th ventricle is called Dandy Walker malformation **(Fig. 46.2)**. Dandy Walker variant may have variable degree of hypoplasia of cerebellar vermis with or without enlargement of cerebellar fossa. Incidence is 1:30000 live births.[15] This condition is frequently associated with aneuploidies(around 50%) and other anomalies (68%). Prognosis is poor. Pregnancy termination should be offered. In isolated cases, recurrence risk may be 1–5%.[16]

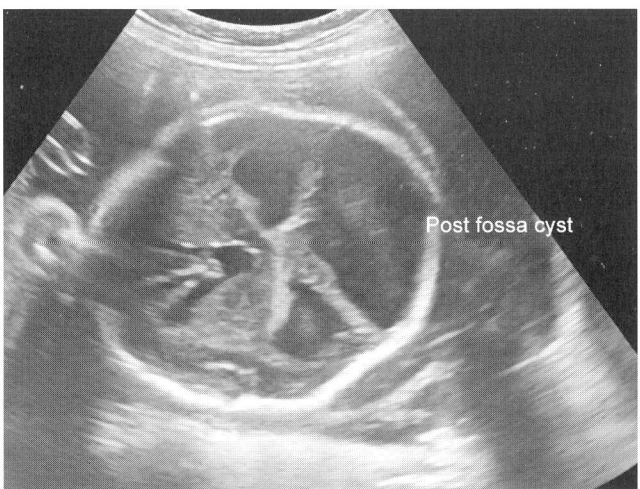

Fig. 46.2: Posterier fossa cyst (Dandy-Walker malformation)

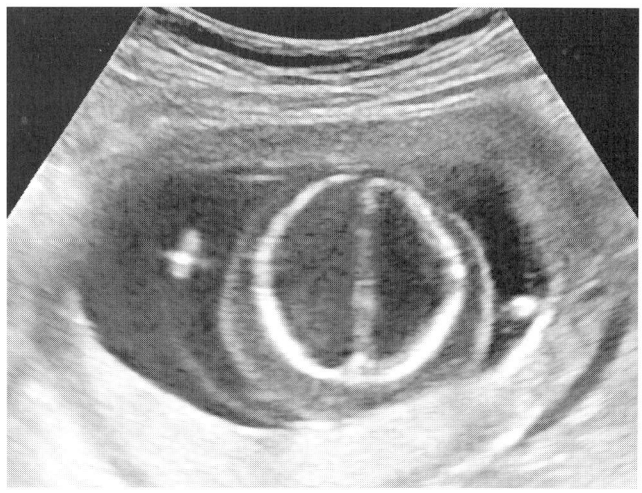

Fig. 46.3: Hydranencephaly

HYDRANENCEPHALY

Replacement of cerebral hemispheres with fluid covered by leptomeninges is called hydranencephaly **(Fig. 46.3)**. Skull is normally formed with few remnants of mesencephalon and basal ganglia. Subtentorial structures are normal. Bilateral internal carotid artery occlusion has been incriminated for pathogenesis of hydranencephaly. Prognosis is very poor. Pregnancy termination should be offered. Recurrence risk is negligible.

AGENESIS OF CORPUS CALLOSUM

Corpus callosum is plate of nerve fibers which connects the cortical hemispheres. It forms the roof of third ventricle. Corpus callosum agenesis can occur either as isolated condition or in combination with other anomalies. Prognosis depends on associated defects. Corpus callosum agenesis has been seen in normal intelligent people, therefore, counseling of parents should be done cautiously.

ABNORMALITY OF NECK-CYSTIC HYGROMA

Malformation of lymphatic system which form fluid-filled membranous cysts, lined by true epithelium in occipitocervical area is called cystic hygroma. This may be small and transient or large and persistent. Normally, lymphatics all over the body ultimately drain into two sacs lateral to jugular vein. These sacs develop connection with jugular vein at around 40 days of gestation. Cystic lymphatic collection in posterior triangle of neck results when the jugular lymphatic sacs fail to drain in jugular vein. This is called jugular lymphatic obstruction sequence (JLOS). Cystic hygroma can result from JLOS or sometimes can also be associated with generalized lymphatic hypoplasia. Mild varieties may resolve leaving behind webbed neck or peripheral edema.[17] Generalized lymphatic defect can lead to fetal hydrops.

Incidence of cystic hygroma is between 5–15 per 1000 live births. About 50–75% of fetuses with cystic hygroma are aneuploid. Turners syndrome is being commonest followed by trisomy 13, 18 and 21.[17,18,19] Mosaic pattern is also associated with cystic hygromas. Environmental exposures as fetal alcohol syndrome may also be seen with cystic hygroma. They are commonly associated with cardiac anomalies.

Diagnosis

Cystic hygromas can be easily identified by ultrasound seen as multiseptated cyst of varying size at the posterolateral portion of neck. Large hygromas have a dense midline septum across full thickness of hygroma. They should be differentiated from encephalocele, meningomyelocele, rarely teratoma. Features that are suggestive of cystic hygroma are intact skull and spine, lack of solid areas, presence of septas. Nuchal edema is mildest presentation of obstructed lymphatic channel **(Fig. 46.4)**.

Management

Once diagnosed, careful fetal anatomical survey for skin edema, ascites, pleural, and pericardial effusions, cardiac and renal anomalies should be done. Early diagnosed nondisappearing cystic hygromas have poor prognosis. Karyotyping is indicated. Depending on the karyotype report pregnancy termination should be offered. Nonseptated, isolated cystic hygromas have better survival rate. They are usually diagnosed after 30 weeks of gestation. Isolated cystic hygromas can be treated postnatally by surgery. *In utero* sclerotherapy is under study.[20] Postmortem examination is recommended.

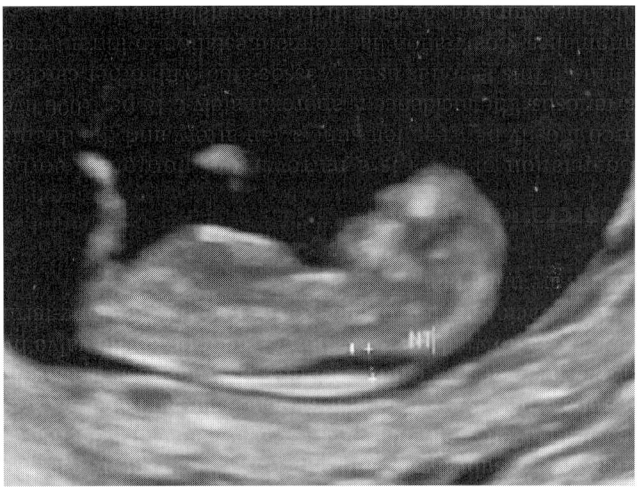

Fig. 46.4: Increased nuchal translucency

FETAL CARDIOVASCULAR ABNORMALITIES

The incidence of congenital heart disease (CHD) is approximately 0.4–1.1% of live births.[21] It might not be practical to screen every obstetric patient in Indian scenario but selective fetal echocardiography is indicated in certain cases which are divided in three groups familial, maternal and fetal.

Familial Indications

Previous child affected by CHD, CHD in maternal or paternal side, history of single gene disorder like Marfan syndrome, Noonan syndrome.

Maternal Indications

History of metabolic disorders like IDDM, phenylketonuria, connective tissue diseases. Exposure to teratogens like alcohol, valproic acid, phenytoin, lithium, isotretinoin, hydantoin. Maternal infections such as rubella, parvovirus, CMV.

Fetal Indications

Increased NT, abnormal tricuspid regurgitation (TR) or ductus venosus flow at 11–14 weeks scan and abnormal heart at 18–20 weeks scan.

The prevalence of major cardiac diseases is directly proportional to nuchal translucency, tricuspid regurgitation and abnormal ductus flow in early second trimester scan. Hence, study of both TR and ductus venosus flow is prognostic indicator of cardiac abnormalities at earlier scan.

Fetal echocardiography is recommended at 20–22 weeks of gestation as the sensitivity of earlier scan is only 60%.[22]

Fetal Echo is to be repeated even if earlier scan is normal in indicated cases.

Cardiac abnormalities in fetal life can be classified as—
- Structural cardiac disease
  - Shunt with balanced anatomy—ASD, VSD, overriding aorta, AV septal defects
  - Shunts with unbalanced anatomy
  - Hypoplastic valves or chambers
  - Discordant ventriculoarterial connection
  - Double discordancy
  - Isolated aortic or pulmonary stenosis—aortic stenosis, pulmonary stenosis
  - Ventricular or great arterial disproportion
- Cardiac arrhythmias

STRUCTURAL CARDIAC DISEASE

Septal Defects

Septal defects are most common CHDs with an incidence of 0.5 per 1000 live births.[21] Septal defect shunts are right to left or bidirectional in fetal life and usually become left to right as pulmonary pressure decreases after birth.

Ventricular Septal Defects

The VSD is most common septal defect **(Fig. 46.5)**. It can be isolated or associated with extracardiac abnormalities. VSD is classified according to the location as perimembranous, inlet, trabecular and outlet. Small to moderated size septal defects are not responsible for fetal compromise because the pressure in both the ventricles is similar in fetal life. Most of the VSDs close in intrauterine life and few get closed in first year of life. Very large defects are associated with massive shunts which can cause congestive cardiac failure at birth. Isolated VSD have good prognosis. If it is associated with other cardiac or other abnormalities, karyotyping is advised.

Atrioventricular Septal Defects

They are also called endocardial cushion defects. Atrioventricular (AV) septal defects are frequently associated with fetal aneuploidy (trisomy 21) and extracardiac anomalies. Once diagnosed, karyotyping should be offered before continuing pregnancy. Timely surgical correction can be associated with good prognosis.

Atrial Septal Defects

It is difficult to diagnose isolated ASD *in utero* because of presence of foramen ovale. There are two types of ASDs, primum and secundum. Absence of foramen ovale or reduction in size of foramen ovale (ostium secundum) seen during fetal echocardiography is diagnostic of ASD. ASDs do

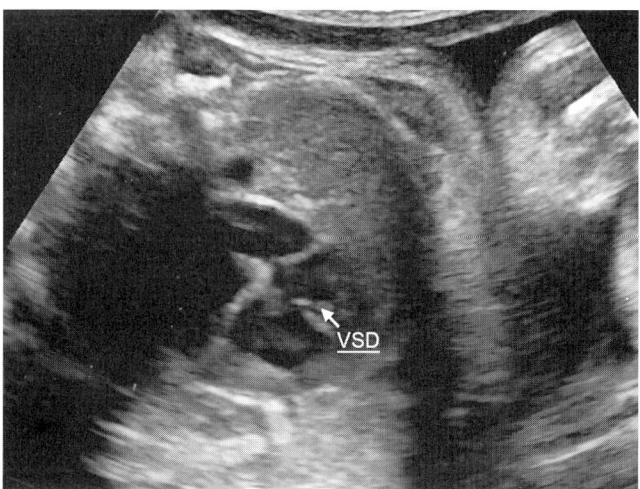

Fig. 46.5: Ventricular septal defect (VSD)

not affect fetal as well as neonatal cardiac function. But it can be associated with other cardiac abnormalities, an abnormal karyotype (trisomy 21) or genetic syndrome. The correction of defect should be planned before school age or whenever symptoms like breathlessness or failure to thrive occur. The surgical options are open technique with sternotomy or interventional catheter approach. Babies with less than 8 kg are considered unsuitable for surgery.

HYPOPLASTIC LEFT HEART SYNDROME

The characteristic of hypoplastic left heart syndrome is a small left ventricle secondary to mitral or aortic stenosis. Head and coronary artery receives blood supply by retrograde flow through ductus arteriosus and aortic arch. The incidence is 0.16 per 1000 live births.[23] It is usually diagnosed by ultrasound showing small left ventricle and hypoplastic ascending aorta. Hypoplastic left heart syndrome is well tolerated in uterine life but postnatal prognosis is poor. The treatment involves either cardiac transplantation or three-stage Norwood repair. The long-term prognosis is guarded.

OUTFLOW TRACT OBSTRUCTION

Tetralogy of Fallot

The tetralogy of Fallot (TOF) occurs 0.4 in 1000 live births.[21] The tetralogy consists of stenosis of the infundibulum of pulmonary artery, a ventricular septal defect, an aortic valve overriding the interventricular septum and hypertrophy of the right ventricle that usually develop in neonatal period. Cardiac failure in fetal life or postnatally is infrequent. In isolated cases the survival rate after corrective surgery is approximately 95%.[24] TOF can be associated with chromosomal abnormalities like DI George syndrome that is deletion of 22q11. Hence, karyotype should be offered. TOF requires correction in early postnatal life.

Transposition of Great Vessels

The prevalence of this abnormality is around 0.2 per 1000 live births.[21] The form having AV concordance and ventriculoarterial discordance is common. The pulmonary artery arises from left ventricle and aorta arises from right ventricle. About 50% cases of transposition of great vessels are associated with VSD and pulmonary stenosis. This cardiac abnormality is rarely associated with extracardiac abnormalities or abnormal karyotype. The hemodynamic compromise is unusual in utero. The newborns may be cyanotic and deteriorate rapidly after birth. If small foramen ovale is identified prenatally, it can be an indication of balloon atrial septotomy (Rash-Kind's procedure). Neonatal cardiac surgery involves switching of great arteries. The survival rate is 85–90%.[25]

Aortic Stenosis

The incidence of AS is 0.04 per 1000 live births.[21] The types are valvular, subvalvular and supravalvular. In severe cases, it can lead to left ventricular pressure overload which decreases coronary perfusion leading to subendocardial ischemia and in utero congestive cardiac failure. The diagnosis is usually by fetal Echo. Balloon dilatation of stenotic aortic valve by transthoracic puncture of fetus can be done but the long-term results are uncertain.

Coarctation of Aorta

Coarctation of aorta is a narrowing of portion of aortic arch mostly between left subclavian artery and the ductus arteriosus. The incidence is approximately 0.18 per 1000 live births.[21] This lesion is usually associated with other cardiac anomalies. Coarctation has no manifestation in intrauterine life. The symptoms develop in the neonatal period.

Pulmonary Stenosis

This lesion occurs in about 0.9 per 1000 live births.[21] The associated cardiac abnormalities are less common. It is present in Noonan's syndrome. The diagnosis is usually by fetal 2D ECHO. The prognosis is usually good and the only treatment required is postnatal balloon valvoplasty.

Management of Structural Congenital Heart Diseases

Once the cardiac defect is diagnosed, the multidisciplinary approach is used for counseling of couple. The associated extracardiac abnormalities are to be searched for. Abnormal karyotype is to be ruled out. The treatment is individualized according to the lesion. The progress of disease is to be followed by Doppler ultrasonography every 2–4 weeks. Timing of delivery should be mostly at term. Many fetuses with cardiac abnormalities tolerate normal labor and its presence is not an indication for termination of pregnancy or cesarean section. Delivery has to be planned in tertiary care center. In cases if fetal or neonatal demise occurs, a detailed postmortem is to be done by perinatal pathologist.

CARDIAC ARRHYTHMIAS

Normal fetal heart rate pattern is between 110 and 160 beats per minute with beat to beat variability. Any irregularity in cardiac rhythm or regular rhythm outside the normal range is called fetal arrhythymia. Frequency of fetal arrhythmias ranges from 1% to 3% of all pregnancies.[26,27] They are associated with significant morbidity and mortality. Transient arrhythymias in form of isolated ectopic beats go undiagnosed but sustained episodes can result in congestive cardiac failure and nonimmune hydrops. The most common fetal arrhythmias are extrasystole and tachycardias of which supraventricular tachycardia, atrial flutter and sinus tachycardia are commonest. Bradycardias are less common.

Diagnosis of fetal arrhythymia is made by simple auscultation, fetal Doppler, fetal electrocardiography or fetal echocardiography. Structural cardiac defects should be ruled out.

IRREGULAR HEART RATE

- *Premature atrial contractions:* Premature atrial contractions (PAC) are most common fetal dysrhythmias ranging from 1% to 3%.[28] They can be associated with illicit drug use, hyperthyroidism or trisomy 18.[29] Isolated PACs do not require treatment. Risk of structural heart disease does not increase. Patients are advised to avoid caffeine and beta adrenergic drugs.
- *Premature ventricular contractions:* PVCs are usually benign. Management involves avoidance of maternal stimulants like caffeine.

TACHYCARDIA

- *Sinus tachycardia:* It is defined as fetal heart rate between 160 and 210 beats per min with 1:1 atrio-ventricular conduction. It can be secondary to acidosis, anemia, myocarditis, infection, maternal drugs or maternal thyrotoxicosis. Management involves recognition and treatment of particular cause.
- *Supraventricular tachycardia (SVT)*
  They are of two types:
  1. AV node dependent supraventricular tachycardia
     - *Short ventriculoatrial tachycardia:* It is most common form of SVT. Heart rate ranges from 220 to 300 beats per min. Usually responds to transplacental digoxin or beta blocker therapy unless hydrops is already present. Medication to be continued for one year after birth.
     - *Long ventriculoatrial tachycardia:* It is incessant slow fetal SVT. The incidence is rare. It is relatively dangerous arrhythmia as can cause CCF or hydrops.
  2. AV node nondependent SVT
     - *Atrial flutter:* About one third of fetal tachycardia is atrial flutter.[29] This is rapid, regular atrial rhythm of 400–550 beats per min. Often diagnosed by fetal ECG. It can be isolated finding or associated with cardiac abnormalities. It can be managed by administration of maternal digoxin or sotalol. Prognosis is usually good if not associated with structural abnormalities or delivered at term. After successful conversion of rhythm, majority of children do not experience recurrence and require no treatment.
     - *Atrial fibrillation:* Atrial fibrillation is rare fetal arrhythmia and characterized by extremely rapid atrial rate of more than 500 beats/min. It is mostly associated with cardiac structural anomalies. The prognosis is variable. Maternal digoxin can be used for ventricular rate control. Postnatally, the newborn is converted to sinus rhythm through direct current cardioversion.
     - *Ventricular tachycardia:* VT is relatively rare form of fetal arrhythmias with the focus arising from ventricle. Sustained fast fetal VT with or without hydrops is often refractory to treatment which requires agents such as amiodarone and lidocaine.

BRADYCARDIA

Fetal bradycardia is usually defined as persistent heart rate below 100 beats per minutes and not associated with uterine contractions or decelerations. Usually presents as clinical dilemma in fetal life as can mimic fetal distress. The differential diagnosis can include sinus bradycardia, partial or complete heart block, long QT syndrome or atrial bigeminy, where the conduction of normal heart beat is halved leading to fetal heart rate between 60 and 70 beats per minute.[30] A maternal history, screening for connective tissue disorders, drug use, complete family history for arrhythmias, pacemakers, structural heart disease or congenital deafness in close family members, is warranted.

Sinus Bradycardia

It is associated with normal AV activation sequence, 1:1 conduction. The known causes can be fetal hypoxia, sinus node dysfunction, heterotaxy syndrome (two left atria). The management depends on causes. Close observation and postnatal ECG is required.

Atrioventricular Block

AV blocks define as failure of conduction of atrial impulses through AV node to the ventricles. Usually diagnosed by fetal echocardiography or electrocardiogram postnatally. Fetuses with tachyarrythmias usually have normal structural heart but with complete heart block can be associated with important heart malformations. The fetuses with isolated heart blocks do better. This complete heart block is usually due to transplacental transfer of anti-Ro/La antibodies. If cardiac function is good, these fetuses can survive till term. If heart rate goes below 55 in fetal life, maternal sympathomimetic like salbutamol may be helpful. But it is contraindicated in fetuses with long QT syndrome.[31] Steroids have also been used for prevention and treatment of complete atrioventricular block. The undergoing research suggests that immunoglobulin therapy can also be used in altering progression of block. Postnatally, pacing is advised for those children in whom heart rate falls below 55 for sustained period in 24 hours tape.

Management of Fetal Arrhythmias

We should balance the risks and benefits before initiating medical therapy for fetal arrhythmias. The best possible option is transplacental route. If this route is not possible, then direct drug therapy with drug infusion in umbilical vein, in amniotic fluid or intramuscular injections, can be used. Pregnancies close to term should be delivered. Most antiarrhythmic drugs require close monitoring except beta blockers. Perinatal mortality rate for arrhythmias ranges from 3.5% to 30% rate.[32]

FETAL GASTROINTESTINAL ABNORMALITIES

Most common gastrointestinal abnormalities detected antenatally are omphalocele, gastroschisis and diaphragmatic hernia.

Omphalocele (Exomphalos)

Omphalocele is herniation of abdominal contents into the base of umbilical cord due to arrest of migration of ventromedial dermatomyotomes.

Incidence is 1:2500 to 1:5000 pregnancies.[33] 1 out of 6 fetuses with omphalocele is chromosomally abnormal. Association with other congenital malformations is seen in 60-80% fetuses.[34]

Diagnosis

Omphalocele is easily diagnosed by ultrasound. It is seen as persistent of extra-abdominal viscera at the base of umbilical cord after 11 weeks of gestation. Umbilical cord is seen to insert in this mass rather than the abdominal wall. The contents of omphalocele are in a membrane which may rupture spontaneously. When the base of abdominal wall defect is greater than 6 cm, it is called " Giant Omphalocele." Giant defects, or those with ruptured membranes, may be associated defective thoracic cage, giant hypoplasia and postnatal respiratory complications.

Omphalocele produces a very high maternal serum alpha-fetoprotein concentration during second trimester.

Management

Prenatal: As it is frequently associated with other anomalies, a detailed ultrasonographic examination, fetal echocardiogram, karyotype should be done. Omphalocele is associated with cardiac defects in 45% of cases.[35] Isolated omphalocele has good prognosis. Parents should be counseled about issues of prolonged hospitalization, repeat surgeries, prematurity, sepsis, short gut syndrome which will help in decision making. Recurrence in next pregnancy in absence of other anomalies is extremely low.

Labor and Delivery

Delivery should be planned in a center equipped with pediatric surgery unit. Elective cesarean section has not been shown to be beneficial over vaginal delivery.

Postnatal: Maintaining hydration, asepsis, preventing hypothermia are important immediate concerns. Baby is put in a sterile bag containing Ringer lactate, stable plasma and penicillin, the bag is tied around axilla. Conservative management is preferred in neonates with other lethal malformations. Primary closure is considered in defects less than 4 cm. Large defects are covered with silastic silo and gradual decompression is done. Average hospital stay may be 3 weeks to 3 months. Long-term complications may be in form of adhesive small bowel obstruction, pain and constipation.[36]

Gastroschisis

Gastroschisis is a paraumbilical defect lateral to the umbilical vessels commonly on right side of abdominal wall.

Incidence is 1:2500 to 1:3000 live births. About 10% of large defects are found to be associated with other anomalies mostly cardiac.[37] Risk of abnormal karyotype is 1–3% commonest being trisomy 18.

Etiology

It is a congenital malformation with some studies suggesting association with recreational drugs, vasoactive substances, and aspirin.[38]

Diagnosis

Ultrasonography shows free-floating bowel loops with no covering membrane.

Management

Prenatal: A thorough search for other anomalies is recommended. In isolated gastroschisis, karyotyping is not needed. Serial ultrasound to look for amniotic fluid, fetal growth, bowel appearance, presence of other viscera like liver, uterus and testis in gastroschisis should be done. Complications are in form of bowel torsion, intestinal atresia, perivisceritis. Perivisceritis or peel is hypothesized to be because of chemical peritonitis caused by amniotic fluid. This may lead to ultrasonographic picture of increased echogenicity and thickening of bowel wall after 28 weeks representing a fibrinous peel binding together loops of bowel. Venous and lymphatic obstruction is another explanation for peel formation. Presence of peel does not affect surgical outcome. Prognosis is usually good with 60% primary closure and 90% survival. Recurrence in next pregnancy in absence of other anomalies is extremely low.

Labor and Delivery

In absence of other complications, vaginal delivery should be planned in a well-equipped center.

Postnatal: Immediate management is like omphalocele but more aggressive care is needed as bowel is not covered by any membrane. Mortality rate is 3–5% associated with prematurity, intestinal ischemia, necrosis, sepsis, etc.

Congenital Diaphragmatic Hernia

Congenital diaphragmatic hernia (CDH) is an anatomical defect in diaphragm which leads to herniation of abdominal contents into thoracic cavity. Site of herniation can be foramen of bochdalek (posterolateral defect in pleuroperitoneal canal), retrosternal hernia of Morgagni (defect in sternocostal hiatus), hiatus hernia (defect in central tendon of diaphragm) or complete eventration of diaphragm.

Incidence is 1:3500 live births, with about 50% having associated abnormalities, and 18% having aneuploidy.[39,40]

Associated Syndromes

Beckwith Wiedemann, Pierre Robin, Fryns, trisomy 13, 18, deletion 9p.

Diagnosis

Diagnosis of CDH is difficult in early gestation. Ultrasonographic diagnostic features are thoracic location of liver, bowel or stomach seen at level of heart, absence of stomach

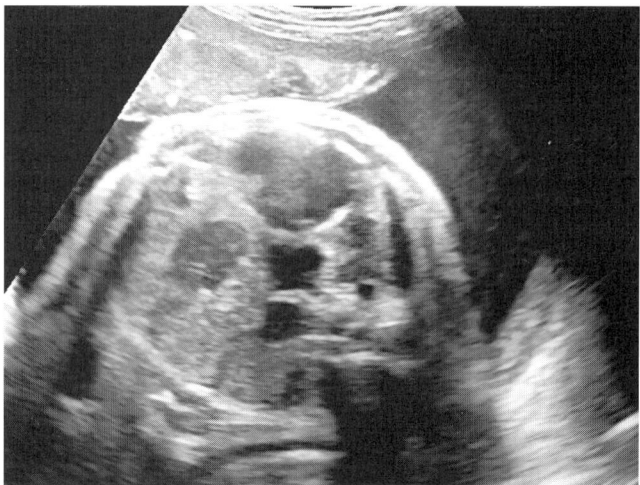

Fig. 46.6: Congenital diaphragmatic hernia

in abdomen and hydramnios (**Fig. 46.6**). By the time these findings are detected, pulmonary hypoplasia already sets in. Right-sided hernia is more difficult to identify as liver and lungs have same echogenicity in early gestation.

Early onset cyanosis, scaphoid abdomen, barrel-shaped chest, dextrocardia are signs seen postnatally.

Management

Prenatal: When CDH is seen on ultrasonography other abnormalities are thoroughly looked for. Karyotyping is advised. With associated anomalies, termination of pregnancy should be considered. Isolated CDH without any genetic syndrome has very low recurrence risk in next pregnancy.

Factors which have been found to adversely affect prognosis of CDH are:[41]

- Diagnosis before 25 weeks.
- Presence of liver in chest
- Right-sided CDH
- Ratio of fetal lung to head circumference
- Ratio of fetal lung to heart
- Decreased lung volume

Labor and delivery: There is no evidence of better outcome on elective cesarean section. Delivery should be planned in well-equipped centre.

Postnatal: Immediate aggressive management with intubation and artificial ventilation is required for the neonate. Long-term morbidity secondary to bronchopulmonary dysplasia may be seen in survivors after postnatal repair of CDH.

BODY STALK ANOMALY

This is an early embryonic maldevelopment due to abnormal folding of trilaminar disk. Amnion forms a continuous sheet between anterior abdominal wall and placenta. Fetus appears attached to placenta. Incidence is 1:7500 to 1:42000 pregnancies.

This condition is lethal and associated with neural tube, spine and lower limb deformities.

Karyotype is normal hence when confirmed sonologically, no need for amniocentesis. Pregnancy termination should be opted. Recurrence risk is extremely low.

BLADDER AND CLOACAL EXSTROPHIES

Incidence of bladder exstrophy is 4 times more frequent than cloacal exstrophy being 1:35000 and 1:200000 pregnancies respectively.[42] Rare cases of familial recurrence are seen. Cloacal exstrophy occurs commonly with omphalocele, imperforate anus and spina bifida called OEIS. Etiology is believed to be failure of development of caudal fold of anterior abdominal wall leading to a common cloaca with urogenital and spinal abnormality.

Diagnosis

In bladder exstrophy, the fetal bladder is not seen within the abdomen. In severe cases even the pubic symphysis will be wide apart and associated genital anomalies are present. Ultrasound features of cloacal exstrophy are low insertion of umbilical cord, defect in low anterior abdominal wall, omphalocele and bladder exstrophy. Herniation of ileum from bladder is seen as "elephant's trunk"

Long-term morbidities like incontinence, abnormal sexual and reproductive function may exist in majority of cases even after advanced multiple surgeries and hospitalizations. Hence, option of termination of pregnancy should be given.

ESOPHAGEAL ATRESIA

There are many types of esophageal atresia, commonest being proximal atresia with distal.

Etiology

During development separation of GI tract and respiratory tract occurs at 3–5 weeks of gestation. Failure to do so leads to tracheoesophageal fistula.

Incidence is 1:3500 live births.[43] 50% of these are isolated and about 50% being associated with syndromes like VATER or VACTREL (vertebral anomalies, anal atresia, cardiac anomalies, tracheoesophageal fistula, renal agenesis, limb defects). Recurrence risk is present in next pregnancy as few familial forms are known.

Diagnosis

Fetal swallowing movements begin after 16 weeks of gestation hence stomach bubble should be visualized after 16–20 weeks, failure to do so with polyhydramnios should create suspicion of tracheoesophageal fistula.

Differential diagnosis for nonvisualization of fetal stomach:
- Esophageal atresia
- Congenital diaphragmatic hernia
- Neurological impaired swallowing
- Cleft lip and palate

In few variants, a small stomach bubble may be seen, so diagnosis should be suspected in all cases of polyhydramnios.

Management

Prenatal

As this condition is associated with many syndromes, hence thorough search for any other anomaly should be made. Karyotyping should be advised. In absence of other anomalies and baby weight greater than 1500 gm, survival rate is 100% after end-to-end esophageal anastomosis.

Labor and Delivery

Decision about mode of delivery is not influenced by this malformation.

Postnatal

Presence of breathing difficulties, cyanosis, excessive respiratory secretions in a newborn are suggestive of this anomaly. Oral feeds should not be given to prevent aspiration. Definitive surgery is done after stabilizing the neonate.

DUODENAL ATRESIA

Etiology

Failure of canalization of duodenum, due to some insult either proximal or distal to ampulla of Vater at 11 weeks of gestation, leads to duodenal atresia. Incidence is 1:6000 live births. 30% of isolated atresias are associated with Down's syndrome. Around 50% have associated cardiac, tracheal, esophageal, renal, hepatobiliary and pancreatic ductal anomalies. Ultrasonographic finding of hydramnios with presence of "double bubble sign" late in second trimester scan is suggestive of duodenal atresia **(Fig. 46.7)**.

Diagnosis is done by postnatally passing nasogastric tube from oral cavity up to the level of duodenum and taking abdominal radiograph. Differential diagnoses are annular pancreas, choledochal or duplication cyst, more distal atresias. Prognosis is good for isolated condition and recurrence is low.

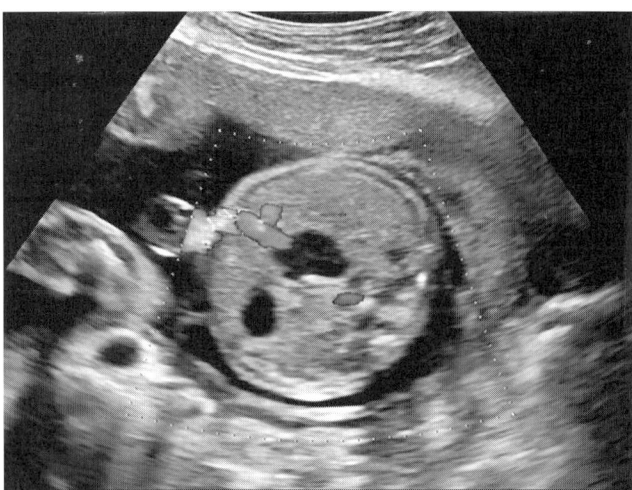

Fig. 46.7: Duodenal atresia (double bubble sign)
(For color version, see Plate 3)

JEJUNAL AND ILEAL ATRESIA

These atresias occur after completion of organogenesis due to vascular compromise. Less commonly are associated with other anomalies. Ultrasound picture is suggestive of multiple distended bowel loops. Post repair prognosis is good.

ANAL ATRESIA, IMPERFORATE ANUS

Incidence is 1:2500 live births. Associated with multiple anomalies in 85% cases including VACTREL.

Long-term morbidities like fecal incontinence, constipation are common after surgical correction of defect.

HYPERECHOGENIC BOWEL

Echogenicity equal to surrounding bone is termed as hyperechogenic bowel. It is an important soft marker of aneuploidies. It occurs in 0.1-0.8% of pregnancies. This condition may be associated with bowel obstruction, cystic fibrosis, meconium ileus, viral infection or aneuploidy. Unexplained death is reported in 5% of cases with second trimester echogenic bowel.

Screening for cystic fibrosis should be offered if meconium ileus is suspected. Diagnosed bowel obstruction or perforation may be an indication of preterm intervention in form of drainage of fetal ascites or preterm delivery.

Infants with meconium ileus become symptomatic in 24-48 hours of life in form of abdominal distension or delayed passage of meconium.

FETAL GENITOURINARY ABNORMALITIES

Uronephrologic abnormalities are common with prevalence of 1 in 250 to 1 in 1000 deliveries. These abnormalities can be detected in second trimester ultrasound as they are associated with early onset oligohydramnios.

FETAL UROPATHIES

According to pathophysiology, fetal uropathies can be classified as:
- Upper urinary tract dilation
  - Ureteropelvic junction obstruction
- Mid-level dilation
  - Megaureter (ureterovesical junction obstruction)
  - Ureterocele (cystic dilation of intravesicle ureter)
- Lower urinary tract obstruction
  - Bladder outlet obstruction
  - Reflux

Prune belly sequence is an abnormality characterized by deficient abdominal wall, bladder distension, renal dysplasia, absence or hypoplasia of prostrate and cryptorchidism.

Diagnosis

Upper Urinary Tract Obstruction

Pyelectasis: Moderate dilatation of renal pelvis without involvement of calyces is defined as pyelectasis. AP diameter of more than 4-7 mm in second trimester and 8-10 mm in third trimester is designated as pyelectasis.[44,45] Serial follow-up is required to see advancement of pathology with gestational age.

Hydronephrosis: Anteroposterior pelvic diameter of more than 1.5 cm at term or calyceal dilatation is called hydronephrosis. Initially, the calyces may retain their shape but later they may become irregular in shape and ultimately merge with pelvis forming single sonolucent area. Renal parenchymal thinning is defined as parenchyma thinner than 3 mm.

Pyelectasis and hydronephrosis are seen with upper urinary tract obstruction. Ureteropelvic junction (UPJ) obstruction is most common congenital malformation of urinary tract accounting for 20-50% of cases. It leads to pyelectasis and hydronephrosis **(Fig. 46.8)**. Incidence of UPJ obstruction is 1 in 1200 live births. Males are commonly affected and condition is mostly unilateral (70%). Etiology is mechanical obstruction at ureteropelvic junction due to adhesions, valves, aberrant vessel or duplicate ureter. Abnormality in arrangement of longitudinal muscle fibers of ureter can also lead to UPJ obstruction. When isolated, this entity has good prognosis as irreversible renal parenchymal damage is rare. In 27% of cases, it can be associated with other renal anomalies or anomalies of other systems.

Mid-level Dilation

Hydroureter: Normally ureter is not visualized in fetal scan. Dilated ureter which can be seen as convoluted peristaltic

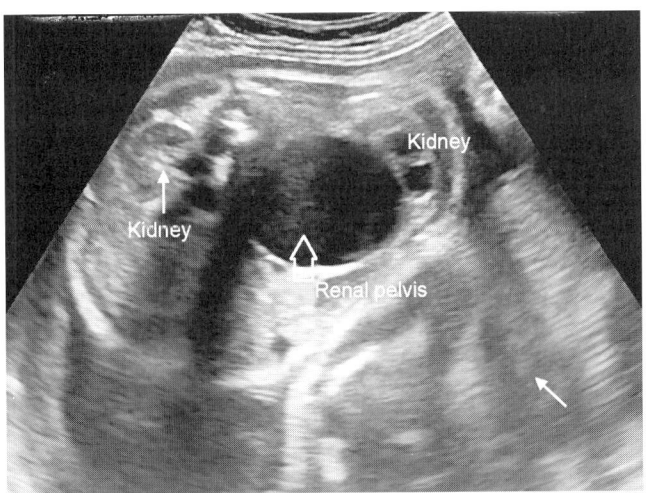

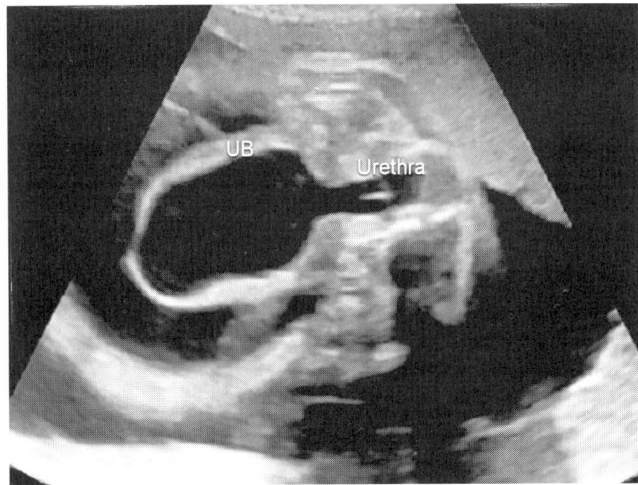

Fig. 46.8: Ureteropelvic junction (UPJ) obstruction

Fig. 46.9: Key hole sign-bladder outlet obstruction (posterior urethral valve)

structure is defined as hydroureter or megaureter seen in mid-level dilation ureterovesical junction obstruction is the cause of hydroureter and it is second most common cause of fetal uropathy. It results from ureterocele or physiological dysfunction of distal ureter. Gradually it progresses to dilated pelvicalyceal system and hydronephrosis. As it is mostly unilateral and amniotic fluid is normal.

Vesicoureteral reflux (VUR) is another common cause of hydroureter. It is commonly seen in females. Etiology is defective flap valve mechanism at intravesical portion of ureter which leads to reflux of urine from bladder to ureter. Bladder pressure is transmitted to the kidneys. Children with VUR are prone to urinary tract infection, pyelonephritis, hypertension and end-stage renal disease. It cannot be diagnosed by ultrasound alone. Color Doppler or dynamic imaging of reflux can be helpful in diagnosis.

Low-level Dilation

Obstructive uropathy refers to conditions which cause complete obstruction to urine flow. This leads to gradual retrograde dilation of urinary tract. This ultimately leads to irreversible renal damage. Conditions associated with obstructive uropathy are posterior urethral valve, urethral stricture, urethral agenesis. Dilated urinary bladder which does not empty during course of ultrasound examination is suggestive of bladder outlet obstruction. Gradually bladder muscular wall may get hypertrophied assuming thickness greater than 3 mm. Dilated urethra is also seen in case of posterior urethral valves. This gives a "key hole" appearance at lower part of bladder **(Fig. 46.9)**. Posterior urethral valves are membranous folds located in posterior wall of urethra. They are sporadic disorders affecting males.

Obstructive uropathy in females is associated with urethral atresia and cloacal malformation. These conditions are associated with poor prognosis.

Management

Prenatal

When observing a dilated fetal urinary tract in ultrasonography other associated anomalies should be looked for. Fetal karyotyping should be considered as 12% of genitourinary defects may be associated with chromosomal anomalies.[46] However, chances of aneuploidy are very rare with isolated uropathy like posterior urethral valve or hydronephrosis. Anomalies which may lead to severe oligohydramnios from 16 weeks onwards may preclude pulmonary development and cause pulmonary hypoplasia characterized by decreased lung size, decreased branching and hyperplastic vasculature. The period between 16 and 25 weeks of gestational age is crucial as this is canalicular phase of lung development. If mean vertical pocket before 25 weeks of gestation is less than 10 mm, then it is associated with pulmonary hypoplasia and neonatal mortality in 90% cases.[47]

In low urinary tract obstruction with bilateral renal involvement, it is important to assess postnatal renal function and prognosis. Renal ultrasound for renal parenchyma, fetal urine analysis and fetal blood sampling is done to assess renal function. High fetal urine concentration of sodium (>100 mmol/L) and beta 2 microglobulin (>6 mg/L) is suggestive of renal failure.[48] These fetuses have high incidence of postnatal renal failure.

When there is terminal failure or multiple anomalies, pregnancy termination can be considered. Isolated uropathies which may have good postnatal renal function on timely intervention are posterior urethral valve, obstructive ureterocele, bilateral pelviureteric junction obstruction. Fetal intervention is advised only when there is bilateral involvement with abnormal renal parenchyma and abnormal renal function. Before fetal intervention, it should be ensured that there is no associated life-threatening anomaly, karyotype is normal, no renal dysplasia and renal function should be preserved. Fetal therapies in form of open fetal surgery, endoscopic ablation of posterior urethral valve, ultrasound-guided percutaneous vesicoamniotic shunting, serial vesicocentesis, percutaneous fetal cystoscopy have been tried. In a randomized control trial on percutaneous shunting in lower urinary tract obstruction (PLUTO) no conclusive evidence could be drawn to prove benefit of vesicoamniotic shunting.[49] Complications like chorioamnionitis, PPROM are known to occur with this procedure.

KIDNEY ABNORMALITIES

Fetal renal anomalies can be classified as—
- *Anomalies of number:*
  - *Renal agenesis:* Renal agenesis results due to early degeneration of ureteric bud. It may be unilateral or bilateral. Ipsilateral genital abnormalities like duplicated or hypoplastic ureter, absent fallopian tube, absent vas deferens, absent epididymis may be associated. Bilateral agenesis is lethal whereas isolated unilateral renal agenesis remains symptom-free **(Fig. 46.10)**.
  - *Renal duplication:* Renal duplication results due to premature division of ureteric bud before it connects to nephrogenic mesoderm. It is associated with double ureter. Upper kidney is associated with some amount of dysplasia or outflow obstruction. The upper ureter enters bladder more caudally. It is commonly associated with ureterocele and may have ectopic insertions in urethra, vagina or seminal vesicle.
- *Anomalies of location:*
  - *Ectopic kidney:* Usually located caudally
  - *Crossed renal ectopia:* Both kidneys on same side
  - *Horseshoe kidney:* Lower poles of the kidneys fuse
- *Anomalies of size and structure:*
  - *Renal hypoplasia:* When kidney mass is 2 SD below the mean, it is called renal hypoplasia.
  - *Multicystic dysplasia (Potter's type II):* Multicystic dysplasia is characterized by presence of multiple cysts (macrocysts) in kidney varying in size from 0.5 cm to 3 cm. Developmental failure of mesonephric blastema leads to formation of cysts. The cysts are neither connected to each other nor to the urinary tract. These kidneys lose their normal shape. This disorder is usually unilateral but when bilateral, this condition is lethal. Isolated unilateral condition has good prognosis. When unilateral, the opposite kidney is affected with other anomalies like 50% of times.
  - *Autosomal recessive polycystic kidney disease (infantile polycystic disease or Potter's type I):* This condition leads to enlarged, spongy kidneys which have retained their shape. Characterized by presence of microcysts (1-2 mm) extending radially from medulla to cortex. These cysts are dilated collecting ducts.[50,51] This is an autosomal recessive condition with 25% recurrence risk. In ultrasonology, they are either seen as hyperechoic enlarged kidney with no corticomedullary differentiation **(Fig. 46.11)** or seen as normal kidney where it is difficult to diagnose the condition antenatally. They are always associated with portal fibrosis and proliferation of bile duct in liver with cystic

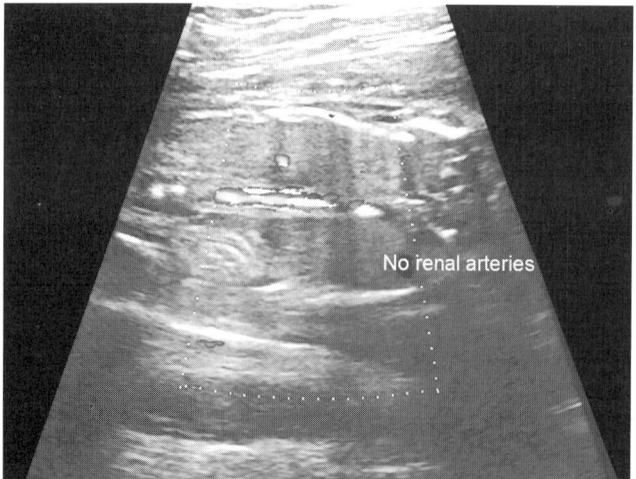

Fig. 46.10: Bilateral renal agenesis—no renal arteries
(For color version, see Plate 3)

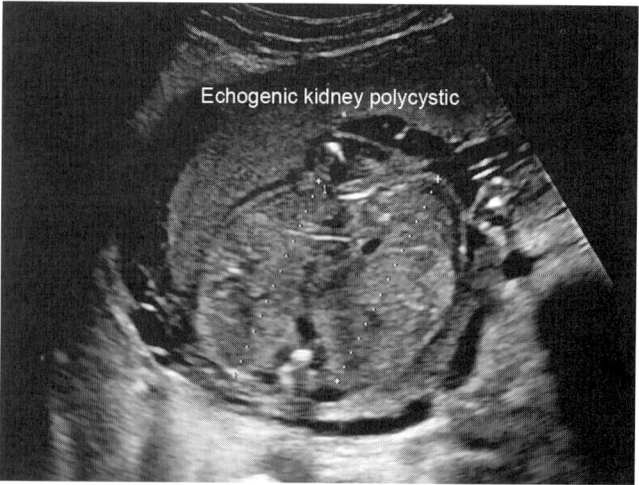

Fig. 46.11: Bilateral dysplastic echogenic kidney

changes. When diagnosed antenatally, they present in second trimester as anuria and absent amniotic fluid. These fetuses do not have other associated congenital malformations but the renal disease itself has very poor prognosis.

- *Autosomal dominant polycystic kidney disease (adult polycystic kidney disease ADPKD, Potter's type III):* Most of the cases have clinical onset in adult life hence it is also called adult onset polycystic kidney disease. This is a common cause of enlarged hyperechoic kidney as they have high frequency of mutation in general population.[52] Fetal ADPKD presents as hyperechogenic kidney with increased corticomedullary differentiation with normal amniotic fluid. This genetic condition has variable expressivity ranging from lethal neonatal disease to an incidental autopsy finding in adults. Commonly, it is first diagnosed in fourth decade of life. There are no adequate prognostic guidelines when the disease is diagnosed in utero.
- *Transient nephromegaly:* It is a poorly understood condition characterized by renal enlargement with corticomedullary differentiaton. Renal function is not altered. Regress during first year of life and has good prognosis.

Management of Renal Anomalies

Isolated unilateral renal anomalies have invariably good prognosis. Prognosis is mostly poor in bilateral disease associated with severe oligohydramnios in second trimester. The biochemical markers used in fetal uropathies like urine sodium or beta 2 microglobulin play no role in nephropathies. In borderline case, it is difficult to diagnose etiology of hyperechogenic kidney including ARPKD, ADPKD and transient nephromegaly on ultrasound. The outcome of all these are quiet variable. Even in same etiologic groups outcome may vary hence parental counseling is difficult. For every stillborn or terminated fetus with renal anomaly, histopathologic diagnosis and DNA analysis is important for proper genetic counseling for future pregnancies.

FETAL SKELETAL ABNORMALITIES

The incidence of congenital skeletal anomalies is around 2–7 in 10,000.[53] Of these, most can be detected with antenatal ultrasound. Most skeletal structures can be identified sonographically by 14–15 weeks. Skeletal dysplasia can be of two types, generalized affecting all the bones or localized limb anomalies which may or may not be part of a genetic syndrome.

Skeletal dysplasias are associated with wide range of genetic syndromes and hence involvement of geneticists, radiologists and orthopedic surgeons is necessary to define

Table 46.1: Terminology used to describe skeletal abnormalities

Achiria	Absent hand
Apodia	Absent feet
Acromelia	Shortening of distal segments of limbs hands and feet
Amelia	Complete absence of limb from shoulder or pelvic girdle
Apodia	Absent foot
Arthrogryposis	Joint contractures
Camptomelia	Bent limbs or fingers
Clinodactyly	Incurved 5th finger
Ectrodactyly	Split hands or feet
Hemimelia	Absent distal arm or leg below elbow or knee
Meromelia	Partial absence of limbs
Mesomelia	Shortening of middle segment of limb (radius/ulna) and (tibia/fibula)
Micromelia	Shortening of long bones
Phocomelia	Hands or feet attached to shortened arms or legs
Platyspondyly	Flattening of the vertebra bodies
Rhizomelia	Shortening of the proximal long bones
Syndactyly	Fused digits
Talipes	Club foot

both diagnosis and prognosis for proper parental counseling. For doing this efficiently, a good understanding of few terminologies is required **(Table 46.1)**.

CONDITIONS ASSOCIATED WITH EARLY ONSET SEVERE SYMMETRICAL SHORTENING OF LONG BONES

Achondrogenesis

It is a lethal condition. Achondrogenesis is a dominant mutation. DNA analysis should be offered.
- *Type 1 (Parenti-Fraccaro syndrome):* Long bones have extreme micromelia. Calvarium and vertebral column are hypomineralized.[54]
- *Type 2 (Langer Salindo syndrome):* Long bones are short thin and straight. Calvarium is normal but spine is hypomineralized.

Thanatophoric Dysplasia

This is most common lethal skeletal dysplasia. Long bones are very small with thickening of metaphyses. "Trident hand" abnormality is seen which means presence of short splayed fingers. Small ribs produce small thorax producing a truncal "champagne cork" appearance. Skull is normally ossified. Some variants show "cloverleaf deformity" of skull with prominence of parietal bones.[55-58] Frontal bossing and depressed nasal bridge is seen.

It is a dominant sporadic condition which results from mutation in fibroblast growth factor gene.[59] Recurrence risk is very low in next pregnancy.

CONDITIONS ASSOCIATED WITH BOWED OR FRACTURED LIMBS

Campomelic Dysplasia

Characterstic features are bowed femur, bowed short tibia, hypoplastic fibula, marked talipes.[60,61] Ribs are short. Brachycephaly, micrognathia and short clavicles can be detected. May have associated cardiovascular septal defects.

This condition is associated with very high mortality in infancy. Termination of pregnancy can be offered after confirming the condition with karyotyping in antenatal period. Recurrence risk in next pregnancy is 5%.[60]

Osteogenesis Imperfecta

Osteogenesis imperfecta is a disorder of poor bone mineralization with an incidence of 1 in 10,000. It is classified in four clinical types.[62] Type I is an autosomal dominant disorder. Others may show gonadal mosaicism hence have a recurrence risk of around 5-7%.[63,64]

Type II and III are mostly lethal and can be diagnosed before 22 weeks of gestation by ultrasound hence termination of pregnancy should be offered.[65-73] Recognized in sonography as long bones having severe micromelia. Skull bones are severely hypomineralized that they produce no acoustic shadow.[55-74] Head can be deformed even by the pressure of ultrasound probe even in late pregnancy.

Type I and IV may not be detected antenatally. They show variable fracturing at birth.

Hypophosphatasia

Hypomineralization results due to deficiency of alkaline phosphatase. Severity of condition may vary from mild to lethal forms. In severe forms, ultrasound features are similar to that of osteogenesis imperfecta type II. Diagnosis is confirmed by measuring cellular alkaline phosphatase in chorionic villous sample.[74] Autosomal recessive forms are usually lethal and termination of pregnancy can be offered.

Milder forms are autosomal dominant and maldevelopment tends to improve with age.

CONDITIONS ASSOCIATED WITH MILD-TO-MODERATE SYMMETRICAL SHORTENING OF LONG BONES

Jeune's Thoracic Dystrophy (Asphyxiating Thoracic Dystrophy)

This is a familial condition in which the chest is reduced in anteroposterier diameter and protrusion of anterior abdominal wall. This is associated with limb shortening, postaxial polydactyly and renal, pulmonary, hepatic and pancreatic dysplasias.

Neonatal mortality is around 70%. It is autosomal recessive disorder with recurrence rate of 25%.

Short Ribbed Polydactyly Syndrome

It is a spectrum of disorders characterized by micromelia, short ribs, small thorax cleft lip/palate, short tibiae with pointed ends, bowed forearms, talipes, may have clover leaf skull and exomphalos.

This condition is lethal because of pulmonary hypoplasia. These are autosomal recessive disorder with 25% recurrence risk.

Ellis-van Creveld Syndrome (Chondroectodermal Dysplasia)

Small thorax associated with shortening of middle segment of the limb (mesomelia), polydactyly, atrial septal defect.

It is an autosomal recessive disorder with mortality of around 33% in infancy.

ACHONDROPLASIA

It is most common nonlethal skeletal dysplasia with an incidence of 5-15 per 1,00,000 births. Majorly, its a sporadic condition caused by mutation in FGFR3 gene. Shortening of long bones manifests after 24 weeks of gestation.

Characteristic features are short middle and distal segments of limb (acromesomelia), frontal bossing, depressed nasal bridge, small thorax, nonprogressive hydrocephaly.

Life expectancy and intelligence are normal. Few orthopedic surgeries might be required for deformity corrections.

Recurrence risk is very low.

JOINT DEFORMITIES

Talipes

Talipes as isolated deformity occurs in 1:1200 births. It can also occur along with genetic syndromes. A careful search for other anomaly is mandatory. Karyotyping is recommended only when other markers of aneuploidy are seen **(Fig. 46.12)**.

Rocker Bottom Feet

Posterior prominent heel and convexity of normal cancave plantar arch. This condition may be associated with trisomy 18, 13 and other syndromes.

ABNORMALITIES OF AMNIOTIC FLUID

After few weeks of gestation, the fetus is sorrounded by a protective fluid filled in amniotic membrane called amniotic fluid (AF). This provides nutrition to fetus, helps in proper development of lungs, musculoskeletal and gastrointestinal organ and provides space to fetus preventing cord compression. Quantification of amniotic fluid is done by dye dilution technique but in usual clinical practice, amniotic fluid is assessed by ultrasound. Two commonly used methods are amniotic fluid index (AFI) and single deepest pocket (SDP). Amniotic fluid index is summation of loop-free deepest pocket of amniotic fluid in four quadrants of uterus in supine position. SDP is single deepest measurement obtained in same way.

Oligohydramnios

Decreased amount of amniotic fluid is called oligohydramnios. Oligohydramnios is defined as AFI of less than 5 cm or SDP of less than 2 cm. Incidence of oligohydramnios is 3–5% of pregnancy.[75]

Etiopathogenesis

Early onset oligohydramnios are mostly due to fetal nephrouropathies. Decreased urine production from fetal kidneys due to any cause leads to reduced amniotic fluid. This may occur in reduced renal perfusion as in IUGR or obstruction to urine outflow tract or dysplastic kidneys **Table 46.2** shows common causes of oligohydroamnios.

Investigations

- Detailed fetal anomaly scan
- MRI if severe oligohydramnios making ultrasonography difficult
- Doppler ultrasound for renal arteries
- Fetal karyotype
- Fetal urine analysis in obstructive uropathy
- Vaginal pH to confirm rupture of amniotic membranes

Maternal Risks

There is increased risk of chorioamnionitis in case of rupture of membranes which is an important cause of oligohydramnios. Risk of operative delivery and cesarean section increases due to high incidence of fetal distress.

Fetal Risks

In early pregnancy, there is high risk of fetal death, especially when associated with abnormal karyotype or renal anomaly. In preterm premature rupture of membranes, prognosis depends on the severity of oligohydramnios and gestational age. Severe oligohydramnios before 23 weeks has high chances of pulmonary hypoplasia and Potter sequence. Potter sequence is characterized by skeletal deformities, contractures depressed nose, wrinkled skin and pulmonary hypoplasia.

Mild-to-moderate third trimester oligohydramnios has high chances of meconium aspiration, fetal distress and NICU admissions but have relatively better prognosis than early onset oligohydramnios.

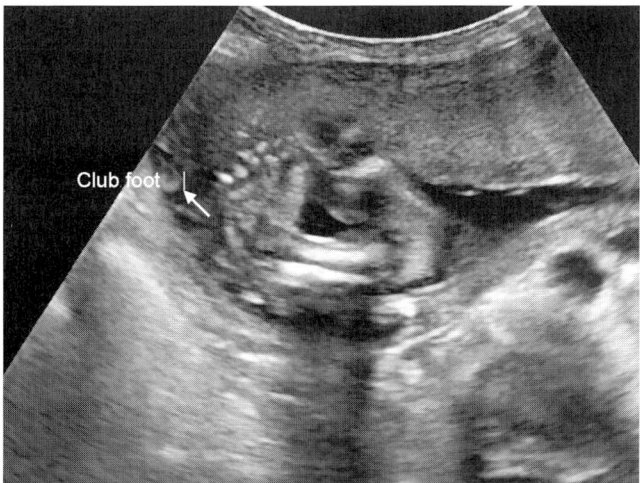

Fig. 46.12: Club foot

Table 46.2: Causes of oligohydramnios
Maternal
• Premature rupture of membranes
• Intrauterine growth restriction
• Maternal dehydration
• Postmaturity
Fetal
• Chromosomal anomalies
• Fetal nephrouropathies

Management

Maternal hydration with hypotonic solutions as 5% dextrose or oral water intake has shown to improve AFI.[73] Isotonic saline infusion has not been found to be beneficial. Amnioinfusion has been shown to improve perinatal survival in PROM.

Polyhydramnios

AFI of 25 cm or more or SDP of greater than 8 cm is called polyhydramnios. The incidence of polyhydroamnios is 1–3% of all pregnancies.

Etiopathogenesis

Polyhydramnios is caused either by decreased absorption as in conditions leading to defective swallowing or increased production of fetal urine as in conditions with high cardiac output. Increased urine output is also a rare cause of polyhydramnios as seen in Bartter syndrome, an autosomal recessive disorder of defective salt absorption. **Table 46.3** shows common causes of polyhydroamnios.

Maternal Risks

Moderate-to-severe polyhydramnios is associated with abdominal discomfort and dyspnea. Hyperplacentosis associated with polyhydramnios can cause severe pre-eclampsia-like disorder (maternal mirror syndrome). Overstretching of uterus leads to preterm labor. Sudden decompression on rupture of membranes can cause placental abruption or amniotic fluid embolism. It is also associated with postpartum uterine atony and hemorrhage.

Fetal Risks

Whenever moderate-to-severe polyhydramnios is observed congenital anomaly should always be suspected. Prematurity due to preterm labor adds to morbidity.

Table 46.3: Causes of polyhydramnios

Maternal
Maternal diabetes
Fetal
- Twin-twin transfusion syndrome
- Congenital infections
- Fetal hydrops
- CNS abnormalities
- Myotonic dystrophy
- Esophageal atresia or upper gastrointestinal obstruction
- Placental or fetal tumors.

Investigations

- Detailed anomaly scan
- Karyotype if other anomalies seen
- Maternal diabetes testing
- Blood grouping
- Infection screening

Management

Specific conditions have to be targeted for treatment of polyhydramnios. Maternal blood sugar control prevents progress in gestational diabetes. Laser ablation of vessels in twin-twin transfusion syndrome.

For symptomatic improvement, in case of maternal dyspnea prostaglandin inhibitors have been used. Indomethacin acts by resorbing water in renal tubule by prostaglandin inhibition. Dose is 25 mg every 6 hours up to 34 weeks of gestation. Side effects are seen in form of oligohydramnios and fetal ductal arteriosus obstruction. Weekly monitoring with fetal echocardiography is recommended when administering indomethacin.

Amnioreduction can be done in severe polyhydramnios to reduce maternal discomfort.

Nonimmune Hydrops Fetalis

Hydrops fetalis is accumulation of fluid in at least two body cavities. It is associated with high rates of perinatal mortality and neonatal morbidity. On etiological basis, it is classified as immune and nonimmune hydrops. When investigated thoroughly etiology can be identified in 80% cases.

Prevalance of nonimmune hydrops is roughly estimated as 1:2000, but to be specific, it is regionally dependent (alpha thalassemia) and subject to seasonal variation (parvovirus endemics).[76]

Diagnosis

Recognition of fluid in two or more cavities, including the abdomen (ascites, **Fig. 46.13**), thorax (pleural or pericardial effusion), or skin (scalp edema, **Fig. 46.14**) is diagnostic of hydrops fetalis. These features may be seen in routine second or third trimester scan. Sometimes, hydrops is identified in scan done for decreased fetal movements or polyhydramnios. Pattern of fluid distribution in cavities may guide towards the diagnosis, viz. Anemic fetus will develop ascites first followed by subcutaneous edema with insignificant thoracic fluid.

Ascites can be identified by echolucent collection of fluid that outlines the abdominal viscera. Pleural fluid may be unilateral or bilateral initially outlining the lungs and mediastinal structures. Minimal (less than 2 mm) pericardial fluid may be normal finding but more collection is suggestive of pericardial effusion. Subcutaneous edema is best seen in

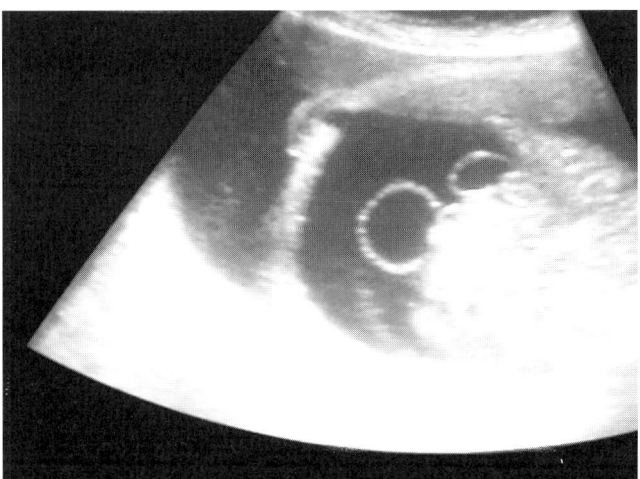

Fig. 46.13: Hydrops fetalis (ascites)

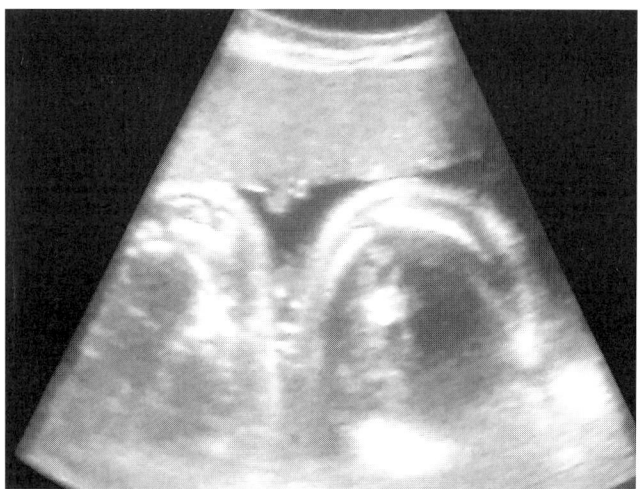

Fig. 46.14: Hydrops fetalis (scalp edema)

scalp region or nuchal region. Placenta may also become edematous with thickness of greater than 5 cm and ground glass appearance.

Pathophysiology

An imbalance in the production and absorption of fluid can lead to hydrops fetalis. Hydrops is a consequence of different disease processes and mostly a sign of end-stage disease. Common conditions associated with non-immune hydrops are enlisted in **Table 46.4**.

In cardiovascular abnormalities, obstruction to outflow will lead to increased backward pressures, which leads to increased venous and lymphatic pressure and ultimately lead to hydrops. Hyperdynamic circulation due to arteriovenous shunts can conclude in fetal hydrops.

A space-occupying lesion in thorax can lead to increased central venous pressure and obstruction to venous and lymphatic drainage.

Anemia and other hematological disorders cause capillary and tissue hypoxia with extravasation of proteins which can retain fluid and cause hydrops. Also, compensatory mechanism for anemia can lead to high output cardiac failure.

Infectious conditions like parvovirus, cytomegalovirus, toxoplasmosis may cause fetal anemia due to their affect on erythroid precursors. Herpes simplex, coxsackie virus and adenovirus can rarely lead to fetal myocarditis and end as hydrops.

In chromosomally abnormal fetuses-lymphatic channel abnormalities have been found to be associated with hydrops. Hence, karyotyping should be offered which should include culture to detect even the rarer chromosomal arrangements.

For genetic conditions like skeletal dysplasias, neuromuscular disorders or lysosomal storage diseases appropriate fetal samples (cultured fibroblast, white cells, serum) need to be collected for proper diagnosis.

Table 46.4: Conditions associated with nonimmune hydrops

Abnormalities associated with nonimmune hydrops

- Chromosomal abnormalities (11–33%)
  - Turner's syndrome
  - Rarely other aneuploidies
- Genetic conditions (3%)
  - Wide varieties of skeletal dysplasias
    - Thanatophoric dysplasia
    - Jeune thoracic asphyxiating dystrophy
    - Short rib polydactyly syndrome
  - Neuromuscular disorders
  - Inborn errors of metabolism
  - lysosomal storage disease
- Cardiovascular abnormalities (25%)
  - Fetal arrhythmia
  - Obstructive right or left heart lesions
  - Large atrioventricular defect
  - Fetal or placental arteriovenous shunts as in sacrococcygeal teratomas, vein of galen aneurysm, placental chorioangioma
- Thoracic abnormalities (8%)
  - Space-occupying lesion like chylothorax
  - Congenital cystic adenomatoid malformation
  - Pulmonary sequestration
  - Diaphragmatic hernia
- Hematological causes (17%)
  - Alpha thalessemia
  - Glucose-6-phosphate dehydrogenase deficiency
  - Failed anemia
  - Congenital leukemia
  - Myeloproliferative disorders
- Infectious causes (4%)
  - Parvovirus B19
  - Cytomegalovirus
  - Syphilis
  - Toxoplasmosis
  - Coxsackie, herpes, adenovirus

Clinical Evaluation of Hydropic Fetus

In general, onset of hydrops at <20 weeks is highly associated with chromosomal abnormality and poor prognosis. Systemic evaluation of fetal anatomy should be performed including measurement of placental thickness. Fetal echocardiography should be done for cardiac anomaly or arrhythmia. Fetal Doppler should be done to look for any arteriovenous malformations, or hyperdynamic circulation. Fetal anemia can be investigated by middle cerebral artery peak velocity.

Detailed family history for genetic diseases. Amniocentesis for detection of chromosomal abnormality as well as fetal infections. Cordocentesis for hemoglobinopathies, anemia. While performing cordocentesis, one should be aware that there can be associated thrombocytopenia which can make the procedure more hazardous. Hence blood and platelets should be available for transfusion.

A detailed workup and systematic approach can help determine the etiology in majority of cases. In case of a still born, postmortem can provide valuable information.

This exhaustive workup can help the clinician to discuss with parents the plan of management and risk of recurrence in the next pregnancy.

Obstetric Management

Sometimes, associated hyperplacentosis and polyhydramnios can be the cause of significant maternal illness, described as maternal mirror syndrome. Large placental mass with associated dysfunction such as impaired oxygen exchange, increased angiogenic factors, villous edema is termed hyperplacentosis. This resembles severe pre-eclampsia and maternal monitoring is required as for pre-eclampsia. A preterm delivery may be needed due to maternal indications.

Delivery should be planned in a tertiary care center with well-equipped neonatal support.

POSTNATAL EXAMINATION OF A STILLBORN OR ANOMALOUS NEONATE

It is important to emphasize about the importance of screening a terminated or sponataneous stillbirth because in busy labor rooms often no further investigations are done and corpse is disposed. This leads to missing only opportunity for suffering parents to get an idea about cause of mishap and how could they prevent it to recur.

Complete evaluation consists of:
- Clinical examination (recorded details and photograph)
- Radiographic study (anterior and lateral whole body X-ray)
- Chromosomal study (heparinized blood sample from cord or fetal heart)
- Fetal autopsy (can be stored in 10% formalin for transportation)
- Histopathology of target organs, e.g. Kidney, skin, muscle
- Examination of placenta and cord (placental histology for infections)

REFERENCES

1. World Health Organization. Congenital anomalies (Factsheet). Retrived from *http://www.who.int/mediacentre/factsheets/fs370/en/*. 2016
2. Sarkar S, Patra C, Dasgupta MK, et al. Prevalence of Congenital Anomalies in Neonates and Associated Risk Factors in a Tertiary Care Hospital in Eastern India. J Clin Neonatol. 2013;2(3):131-4.
3. Greene ND, Copp AJ. Development of the vertebrate central nervous system: Formation of the neural tube. Prenat Diagn. 2009;29:303-11.
4. Allagh KP, Shamanna BR, Murthy GVS, et al. Birth Prevalence of Neural Tube Defects and Orofacial Clefts in India: A Systematic Review and Meta-analysis. PLoS One. 2015;10(3):21.
5. Nicolaides KH, Campbell S, Gabbe SG, Guidetti R. Ultrasound screening for spina bifida. Cranial and cerebellar signs. Lancet. 1986;ii:72-4.
6. Van den Hof MC, Nicolaides KH, Campbell J, Campbell S. Evaluation of the lemon and banana signs in one hundred thirty fetuses with open spina bifida. Am J Obstet Gynecol. 1990;162:322-7.
7. Tubbs RS, Chambers MR, Smyth MD, et al. Late gestational intrauterine myelomeningocele repair does not improve lower extremity function. Pediatr Neurosurg. 2003;38:128-32.
8. Luthy DA, Wardinsky T, Shurtleff DB, et al. Cesarean section before the onset of labor and subsequent motor function in infants with meningomyelocele diagnosed antenatally. N Engl J Med. 1991;324:662-6.
9. Drugan A, Krause B, Canady A, et al. The natural history of prenatally-diagnosed ventriculomegaly. JAMA. 1989;261:1785-8.
10. In Jones KL (Eds). Smith's Recognizable Patterns of Human Malformation, 5th edn. Philadelphia: Elsevier Saunders; 2006:870.
11. Lorber J, De NC. Family history of congenital hydrocephalus. Dev Med Child Neurol. 1970;22:94-100.
12. Bullen PJ, Rankin JM, Robson S. Investigation of the epidemiology and prenatal diagnosis of holoprosencephaly in the North of England. Am J Obstet Gynecol. 2001;184:1256-62.
13. Roach E, Demyer W, Conneally PM, et al. Holoprosencephaly: Birth data, genetic and demographic analyses of 30 families. Birth Defects Orig Artic Ser. 1975;11:294-313.
14. Odent S, Le Marec B, Munnich A, et al. Segregation analysis in nonsyndromic holoprosencephaly. Am J Med Genet. 1998;77:139-43.
15. Ecker JL, Shipp TD, Bromley B, Benacerraf B. The sonographic diagnosis of Dandy-Walker and Dandy-Walker variant: Associated findings and outcomes. Prenat Diagn. 2000;20:328-32.
16. Murray JC, Johnson JA, Bird TD. Dandy-Walker malformation: Etiologic heterogeneity and empiric recurrence risks. Clin Genet. 1985;28:272-83.
17. Chervenak FA, Isaacson G, Blakemore KJ, et al. Fetal cystic hygroma. Cause and natural history. N Engl J Med. 1983;309:822-5.

18. Abramowicz JS, Warsof SL, Doyle DL, et al. Congenital cystic hygroma of the neck diagnosed prenatally: Outcome with normal and abnormal karyotype. Prenat Diagn. 1989;9:321-7.
19. Allanson J. Lymphatic circulation. In: Stevenson R, Hall J, Goodman R (Eds). Human Malformations and Related Anomalies. New York: Oxford University Press; 1993. pp. 145-81.
20. Ogita K, Sutia S, Taguchi T, et al. Outcome of fetal cystic hygroma and experience of intrauterine treatment. Fetal Diagn Ther. 2001;16:105-10.
21. Hoffman JIE, Kaplan S. The incidence of congenital heart disease: Incidence and inheritance. J Am Coll Cardiol. 2002;39:1890-900.
22. Westin M, Saltvedt S, Bergman G, et al. Routine ultrasound examination at 12 or 18 gestational weeks for prenatal detection of major congenital heart malformations? A randomised controlled trial comprising 36,299 fetuses. BJOG. 2006;113:675-82.
23. Fyler DC, Buckley LP, Hellembrand WE, et al. Report of the New England Regional Cardiac program. Pediatrics. 1980;65:375-461.
24. Poon LC, Huggon IC, Zidere V, Allan LD. Tetralogy of Fallot in the fetus in the current era. Ultrasound Obstet Gynecol. 2007;29:625-7.
25. Bonnet D, Coltri A, Butera G, et al. Detection of transposition of the great arteries in fetuses reduces neonatal morbidity and mortality. Circulation. 1999;99:916-8.
26. Cameron A, Nimrod C, Nicholson S, et al. Evaluation of fetal cardiac dysrhythmias with two-dimensional, M-mode, and pulsed Doppler ultrasonography. Am J Obstet Gynecol. 1998;158:286.
27. Reed K. Fetal arrhythmias: Etiology, diagnosis, pathophysiology, and treatment. Semin Perinatol. 1989;13:294.
28. Shenker L. Fetal cardiac arrhythmias. Obstet Gynecol Surv. 1979;34:561-72.
29. Ferrer PL. Fetal arrhythmias. In: Deal BJ, Wolff GS, Gelband H (Eds). Current Concepts in Diagnosis and Management of Arrhythmias in Infants and Children. Armonk, NY: Futura; 1998. pp. 17-63.
30. Donofrio MT, Gullquist Sd, Mehta ID, et al. Congenital complete heart block:fetal management protocol, review of the literature, and report of smallest successful pacemaker implantation. J Perinatol. 2004;24(2):112-7.
31. Duke C, Stuart G, Simpson JM. Ventricular tachycardia secondary to prolongation of the QT interval in a fetus with autoimmune medicated congenital heart block. Cardiol Young. 2005;15(3):319-21.
32. Simpson JM, Sharland GK. Fetal tachycardias: Management and outcome of 127 cases. Heart. 1998;79:576-81.
33. Mann S, Blinman TA, Wilson D. Prenatal and postnatal management of omphalocele. Prenat Diagn. 2008;28:626-32.
34. Stoll C, Alembik Y, Dott B, Roth MP. Omphalocele and gastroschisis and associated malformations. Am J Med Genet. 2008;146A:1280-5.
35. Gibbin C, Touch S, Broth RE, Berghella V. Abdominal wall defects and congenital heart disease. Ultrasound Obstet Gynaecol. 2003;21:334-7.
36. loortje C, van Eijcka L, Rene MH, van Goora H. The incidence and morbidity of adhesions after treatment of neonates with gastroschisis and omphalocele: A 30-year review. J Pediatr Surg. 2008;43:479-83.
37. Mastroiacovo P, Lisi A, Castilla EE, et al. Gastroschisis and associated defects: An international study. Am J Med Genet. 2007;143A:660-71.
38. Draper ES, Rankin J, Tonks AM, et al. Recreational drug use: A major risk factor for gastroschisis? Am J Epidemiol. 2008;167:485-91.
39. Kalache K, Wauer R, Mau H, et al. Associated malformations and chromosomal defects in congenital diaphragmatic hernia. Fetal Diagn Ther. 1995;10:52-9.
40. Jesudason EC. Challenging embryological theories on congenital diaphragmatic hernia: Future therapeutic implications for paediatric surgery. Ann R Coll Surg Engl. 2002;84:252-9.
41. Metkus AP, Filly RA, Stringer MD, et al. Sonographic predictors of survival in fetal diaphragmatic hernia. J Pediatr Surg. 1996;31:148-51.
42. Martinez-Frias ML, Bermejo E, Rodriquez-Pinilla E, Frias J. Exstrophy of the cloaca and exstrophy of the bladder: Two different expressions of a primary developmental field defect. Am J Med Genet. 2001;99:261-9.
43. Shaw-Smith C. Oesophageal atresia, tracheoesophageal fistula, and the VACTERL association: Review of genetics and epidemiology. J Med Genet. 2006;43:545-54.
44. Anderson N, Clautice-Engle T, Allan R, et al. Detection of obstructive uropathy in the fetus: Predictive value of sonographic measurements of renal pelvic diameter at various gestational ages. Am J Roentgenol. 1995;164:719-23.
45. Thornburg LL, Pressman EK, Chelamkuri S, et al. Third trimester ultrasound of fetal pyelectasis: Predictor for postnatal surgery. J Pediatr Urol. 2008;4:51-4.
46. Nicolaides KH, Cheng HH, Abbas A, et al. Fetal renal defects: Associated malformations and chromosomal defects. Fetal Diagn Ther. 1992;7:1-11.
47. Kilbride HW, Yeast J, Thibeault DW. Defining limits of survival: Lethal pulmonary hypoplasia after midtrimester premature rupture of membranes. Am J Obstet Gynecol. 1996;175:675-81.
48. Daikha-Dahmane F, Dommergues M, Muller F, et al. Development of human fetal kidney in obstructive uropathy: Correlations with ultrasonography and urine biochemistry. Kidney Int. 1997;52:21-32.
49. Quintero RA, Morales WJ, Allen MH, et al. Fetal hydrolaparoscopy and endoscopic cystotomy in complicated cases of lower urinary tract obstruction. Am J Obstet Gynecol. 2000;183:324-30.
50. Johnson MP, Freedman AL. Fetal uropathy. Curr Opin Obstet Gynecol. 1999;11:185-94.
51. Clark TJ, Martin WL, Divakaran TG, et al. Prenatal bladder drainage in the management of fetal lower urinary tract obstruction: A systematic review and meta-analysis. Obstet Gynecol. 2003;102:367-82.
52. Tsatsaris V, Gagnadoux MF, Aubry MC, et al. Prenatal diagnosis of bilateral isolated hyperechogenic kidneys. Is it possible to predict long-term outcome? BJOG. 2002;109:1388-93.
53. Orioli IM, Castilla EE, Barbosa-Netos JG. The birth prevalence rates for the skeletal dysplasias. J Med Genet. 1986;23:328-32.
54. Glenn LW, Teng SSK. In utero sonographic diagnosis of achondrogenesis. J Clin Ultrasound. 1985;13:195-8.

55. Tan AWC, Chitty LS. Early onset skeletal dysplasias: Differentiating lethal from non-lethal. J Obstet Gynaecol. 2006;26:S62.
56. Chervenak FA, Blakemore KJ, Isaacson G, et al. Antenatal sonographic findings of thanatophoric dysplasia with cloverleaf skull. Am J Obstet Gynecol. 1983;146:984-5.
57. Burrows PE, Stannard MW, Pearrow J, et al. Early antenatal sonographic recognition of thanatophoric dysplasia with cloverleaf skull deformity. Am J Roentgenol. 1984;143:841-3.
58. Weiner CP, Williamson RA, Bonsib SM. Sonographic diagnosis of cloverleaf skull and thanatophoric dysplasia in the second trimester. J Clin Ultrasound. 1986;14:463-5.
59. Tavormina PL, Shiang R, Thompson LM, et al. Thanatophoric dysplasia (types I and II) caused by distinct mutations in fibroblast growth factor receptor 3. Nat Genet. 1995;9: 321-8.
60. Mansour S, Hall CM, Pembrey ME, Young ID. A clinical and genetic study of campomelic dysplasia. J Med Genet. 1995;32:415-20.
61. Mansour S, Offiah AC, McDowall S, et al. The phenotype of survivors of campomelic dysplasia. J Med Genet. 2002;39:597-602.
62. Sillence DO, Senn A, Danks DM. Genetic heterogeneity in osteogenesis imperfecta. J Med Genet. 1979;16:101-16.
63. Thompson EM, Young ID, Hall CM, Pembrey ME. Recurrence risks and prognosis in severe sporadic osteogenesis imperfecta. J Med Genet. 1987;24:390-405.
64. Cole WG, Dalgleish R. Syndrome of the month. Perinatal lethal osteogenesis imperfecta. J Med Genet. 1995;32:284-9.
65. Dinno ND, Yacuob US, Kadlec JF, Garver KL. Midtrimester diagnosis of osteogenesis imperfecta, type II. Birth Defects. 1982;18:125-32.
66. Milsom I, Mattsson LA, Dahlen-Nilsson I. Antenatal diagnosis of osteogenesis imperfecta by real-time ultrasound: Two-case reports. Br J Radiol. 1982;55:310-2.
67. Shapiro JE, Phillips JA, Byers PH, et al. Prenatal diagnosis of lethal osteogenesis imperfecta (OI type II). J Paediatr. 1982;100:127-33.
68. Elejalde BR, de Elejalde MM. Prenatal diagnosis of perinatally lethal osteogenesis imperfecta. Am J Med Genet. 1983;14:353-9.
69. Aylsworth AS, Seeds JW, Guilford WB, et al. Prenatal diagnosis of a severe deforming type of osteogenesis imperfecta. Am J Med Genet. 1984;19:707-14.
70. Brons JTJ, van der Harten JJ, Wladimiroff JW, et al. Prenatal ultrasonographic diagnosis of osteogenesis imperfecta. Am J Obstet Gynecol. 1988;159:176-81.
71. Constantine G, McCormack J, McHugo J, Fowlie A. Prenatal diagnosis of severe osteogenesis imperfecta. Prenat Diagn. 1991;11:103-10.
72. Munoz C, Filly R, Golbus MS. Osteogenesis imperfecta a type II:Prenatal sonographic diagnosis. Radiology. 1990;174:181-5.
73. Robinson LP, Worthen NJ, Lachman RS, et al. Prenatal diagnosis of osteogenesis imperfecta type III. Prenat Diagn; 1987. pp. 7-15.
74. Mulivor RA, Mennuti M, Zackai EH, Harris H. Prenatal diagnosis of hypophosphatasia:Genetic, biochemical and clinical studies. Am J Hum Genet. 1978;30:271-82.
75. Volante E, Gramellini D, Moretti S, et al. Alteration of the amniotic fluid and neonatal outcome. Acta Biomed. 2004;75:71-5.
76. Smoleniec JS, Pillai M, Caul EO, Usher J. Subclinical transplacental parvovirus B19 infection:An increased fetal risk? Lancet. 1994;343:1100.

SECTION 9: AUTOIMMUNE DISEASES AND OTHER DISORDERS DURING PREGNANCY

Chapter 47

Systemic Lupus Erythematosus in Pregnancy

Anupama B Solanki, Shashi Khare

INTRODUCTION

Systemic lupus erythematosus (SLE) is an autoimmune disease with significant female predominance. Almost 90% of lupus cases are in women and its prevalence in those of childbearing age is approximately 1 in 500. Improved survival, has led to increased numbers of pregnancies in SLE. The pregnancy outcomes have also significantly improved. The rate of pregnancy loss has decreased from 43% to 17% in recent years.[1] Lupus is a autoimmune disease with a complex pathogenesis that results in interaction between susceptible genes and environmental factors.[2] Immune system abnormalities include B lymphocytes that are responsible for autoantibody production. These result in tissue and cellular damage when autoantibodies or immune complexes are directed at one or more cellular nuclear components.[2] In addition, immunosuppression is impaired, including regulatory T-cell function. Genetic influences are implicated by a higher concordance with monozygotic compared with dizygotic 25 versus 2% respectively. The relative risk of disease is increased, if there is inheritance of the "autoimmunity" gene on chromosome 16.[3]

INCIDENCE AND PREVALENCE

Systemic lupus erythematosus is rare in India. It affects predominantly women in their reproductive years. The median age of onset in Indian is 24.5 years and the sex ratio (F:M) is 11:1. A prevalence study in India (carried out in a rural population near New Delhi) found a point prevalence of 3 per 100,000.[4] This is a much lower figure than reported from the west (varying from 12.5 per100,000 adults in England 3 to 39 per 100,000 in Finland 4 and 124 per 100,000 in USA.[4]

CLINICAL MANIFESTATIONS OF SLE

- Systemic—fatigue, malaise, fever, weight loss
- Musculoskeletal—arthralgia, myalgia, polyarthritis, myopathy
- Hematological—anemia, hemolysis, leukopenia, thrombocytopenia, splenomegaly
- Cutaneous—malar (butterfly) rash, discoid rash, photosensitivity, oral ulcers, alopecia, skin rashes
- Neurological—cognitive dysfunction, mood disorder, headache, seizures
- Cardiopulmonary—pleuritis, pericarditis, myocarditis, endocarditis, pneumonitis, pulmonary hypertension
- Renal—proteinuria, casts, nephrotic syndrome, renal failure
- Gastrointestinal—nausea, pain, diarrhea, abnormal liver enzymes levels
- Vascular—arterial and venous thrombosis
- Ocular—conjunctivitis

DIAGNOSIS OF SYSTEMIC LUPUS ERYTHEMATOSUS

The patients with 4 points out of 16, have definite diagnosis of SLE. With 3 points highly suggestive of SLE, with 2 points probable SLE and with one-point possible SLE **(Table 47.1)**.

Serology in SLE[4]

Since SLE is associated with a number of autoantibodies, it is important to understand their relevance in clinical practice. Some of these are useful as diagnostic markers, others help in quantifying disease activity and still others are primarily of research interest, making no contribution to patient care. A brief discussion follows:

- *Antinuclear antibody (ANA):* ANA is a good screening test for SLE because 95% of cases show a high titer (1:80 or more) of this autoantibody.

  A negative test result makes the diagnosis highly improbable. ANA may be positive in other rheumatic disorders such as systemic sclerosis, Sjögren's syndrome, overlap syndrome, antiphospholipid syndrome, polymyositis and rheumatoid arthritis. Like the rheumatoid factor test, ANA may also be positive in chronic infections, malignancies and in normal individuals.

  Thus, the specificity of ANA for diagnosis of SLE is quite low (approx 40% only).

Table 47.1: 2015 ACR/SLICC revised criteria for diagnosis of SLE[5]

Acute/subacute cutaneous lupus rash	Up to 2 points
• Malar rash	2.p
• Subacute cutaneous lupus erythematosus rash	1.p
• Palapable pupura or urticarial vasculitis	1.p
• Photosensitivity	1.p
Discoid lupus erythematosus (DLE) rash or hypertrophic Lupus rash	1.p
Non-scarring frank alopecia	1.p
Oral/nasal ulcers	1.p
Joint disease	1.p
Pleurisy and/or pericarditis	1.p
Psychosis and/or seizure and/or acute confusion	1.p
Kidney involvement	Up to 2 points
• Proteinuria≥ 3+ or ≥ 500 mg/day or urinary casts	1.p
• Biopsy-proven nephritis compatible with SLE	2.p
Hematologic	Up to 3 points
• WBC count < 4000/mm³ or lymphocyte count < 1500/mm³ on ≥ 2 occasions or WBC count < 4000/mm³ along with lymphocyte count < 1500/mm³ in one occasion	1.p
• Thrombocytopenia < 100,000/mm³	1.p
• Hemolytic Anemia	1.p
Serologic tests	Up to 3 points
• Low titer positive ANA	1.p
• High titer FANA with homogenous or rim pattern	2.p
• Positive anti-ds DNA	2.p
• Positive anti-Sm	2.p
• Anti-phospholipid antibodies (aPLs)	1.p
• Low serum complement (C3 and/or C4 and/or CH50)	1.p

Although many laboratories use ELISA technique for the sake of convenience and economy, the gold standard method for testing and reporting ANA is the indirect immunofluorescence method.

Performing serial titers of ANA in a diagnosed case of SLE is of no clinical value because it does not correlate well with disease activity. It can remain positive for long periods in the absence of any disease activity. What we treat is disease and not ANA.

ANAs are actually a family of autoantibodies, which may be directed against any one of the following nuclear antigens:
– Double stranded—DNA
– Extractable nuclear antigens (ENA)
– Histones
– Nuclear RNA

Anti-double-stranded DNA antibody (anti-dsDNA): This test has high specificity for SLE. The positivity of anti-dsDNA in SLE at the time of presentation is in the range of 60% (although the cumulative positivity during the course of disease may approach 90%). Hence, anti-dsDNA cannot be a good screening test for SLE. When positive, the test establishes the diagnosis of SLE. The anti-dsDNA titers most often correlate with disease activity.

Antibodies to extractable nuclear antigens (anti-ENA): These include anti-Sm, anti-UIRNP, anti-Ro and anti-La antibodies. Anti-Sm antibody is quite specific for SLE but it is found only in 10–30% of patients. Anti-Ro is associated with ANA negative SLE, Sjögren's syndrome, congenital heart block, neonatal SLE and subacute cutaneous lupus erythematosus.

Anti-La is associated with SLE and Sjögren's syndrome. Antihistone antibodies are associated with drug-induced SLE.

Complement levels (C3 and C4): These two complement components are useful in the diagnosis and follow-up of SLE. Their levels drop because of consumption. C3 and C4 levels are negatively correlated with lupus activity.

Differential diagnosis of SLE:[4]
The following conditions need to be considered in differential diagnosis of SLE
• Undifferentiated connective tissue disease
• Primary Sjögren's syndrome
• Primary antiphospholipid syndrome
• Fibromyalgia with positive ANA
• Idiopathic thrombocytopenic purpura
• Drug-induced lupus
• Early RA

Prepregnancy Counseling

Active SLE at the time of conception is known to be the strongest predictor of adverse pregnancy outcomes.[5] Hence, ideally, all pregnancies in women with SLE should be planned during periods of disease control. All patients should be counseled about the possible issues including risk of disease flares, higher rates of pregnancy complications, suboptimal obstetric outcomes, and the risk of neonatal lupus syndromes. The need for optimal disease control with safe medications during pregnancy should be explained. The incidence of flare during pregnancy with conception while in remission is less than 10%. It is strongly recommended that the disease should be in clinical remission for at least 6 months before the patient plans for pregnancy.[5] The best time for conception is after 6-12 months of remission with hydroxychloroquine but no cytotoxic drugs. At the onset of pregnancy, a complete assessment of disease activity and severity should be made. The spouse and other family members should be counseled. Childbearing should not be contemplated in women with pulmonary hypertension, and those with lupus nephritis with a baseline serum creatinine >250 µmol/L.[6]

Evaluation at first visit: Initial evaluation should be based on thorough history taking and physical examination along with careful BP measurement.[7]

Investigations during first visit:
- Routine urine analysis
- Hb%, ESR, total WBC count, differential count and platelet count
- Serum creatinine
- 24-hour urinary total protein (creatinine clearance test, if possible)
- Anti-ds-DNA (raised level indicates active SLE or impending flare).
- Anti-Ro (SS-A) and Anti-La (SS-B), Anti-phospholipid Antibodies (Anticardolipin Ab and lupus anticoagulant).
- Serum C3 and C4 level (low C3 indicates active SLE or impending flare in over 80% of patients).[2]
- Fasting blood glucose, if at high risk
- Serum lipids, if the patient is nephrotic or on steroids
- Coombs test
- Ultrasound examination (Should be selective rather than routine)
- *Others:* Hepatitis B and C serology, Anti-HIV screening, syphilis serology (as a part of routine antenatal tests)

Follow-up at subsequent visits: History and clinical examinations should be focused on identification of disease flares and pregnancy-related complications.

Laboratory assessment includes:
- Blood counts including platelet, Hb%, ESR
- Routine urine analysis
- Serum creatinine, urinary protein:creatinine ratio
- Fasting blood glucose (FBG)/Modified oral glucose tolerance test (OGTT) 24 to 28 weeks
- anti-dsDNA and C3 {At the end of each trimester}
- Biophysical profile (BPP) scoring from 28 weeks
- Women detected to have either anti-Ro or anti-La antibodies should be offered serial fetal echocardiograms between 16 weeks and 24 weeks of gestation[6]

General principles of treatment of lupus pregnancy: Antenatal management of pregnant patients will SLE requires close collaboration between rheumatologist and obstetrician. The monitoring should be more frequent and detailed than the usual standard of care. Each visit should include thorough physical examination, routine laboratory tests and specific investigations, tailored to the risk profile of the particular pregnancy. Objective should be to maintain good health, prevent complications and early detection and rapid treatment of flares.

General Advice[7]

Avoiding sun exposure is very important to prevent flares. Mother should take low salt diet containing adequate amount of vitamins and minerals. Treatment when there is no sign of flares or complications:

Drugs those can be used safely during pregnancy:
- Folic acid (this is recommended)
- Hydroxychloroquine
- Low dose Aspirin (75 mg/day) if antiphospholipid antibodies present, in high risk patient or presence of nephritis for prevention of pre-eclampsia,[5]

Arthralgia and serositis can be managed by occasional dose of NSAIDs. However, chronic or large intermittent dosing is avoided due to side effects. Non-steroidal anti-inflammatory drugs (NSAIDs) were considered safe during the first and second trimesters. However, moderate associations between NSAID use in first trimester and specific birth defects were recently reported.[8] There is also an increased risk of impaired fetal renal function with use after 20 weeks of gestation. Hence, caution needs to be exercised when using NSAIDs during early pregnancy. Continued use after the 32 week of gestation can increase the risk of premature closure of the ductus arteriosus by almost 15-fold, and should be avoided.[9] The data on the cyclooxygenase 2 inhibitors in pregnancy is very limited, and they are best avoided during pregnancy.

There are many controversies of using steroid in this group of patient to prevent flares as flare prophylaxis. Use of steroid increases the risk of fetal cleft palate, IUGR, PROM, DM, pre-eclampsia. Steroid exposure should be limited to a minimum during the pregnancy. High doses during pregnancy are associated with an increased risk of diabetes, hypertension, pre-eclampsia and premature rupture of membranes.[10] However, in the case of disease flares, short courses of high doses and/or intravenous pulse methylprednisolone can be used. Patients on long-term steroid therapy should also receive stress doses at the time of delivery. Severe disease is managed with corticosteroids such as prednisone, 1 to 2 mg/kg orally per day. After the disease is controlled, this dose is tapered to a daily morning dose of 10-15 mg. Use of fluorinated compounds, such as dexamethasone and betamethasone should be limited to a single course for fetal lung maturity, in cases of premature delivery. Repeated use has been associated with impaired neuropsychological development of the child in later life, and should be avoided.[5]

Hydroxychloroquine should be continued in all pregnant women with SLE. Multiple studies have proven the beneficial effects of hydroxychloroquine in SLE, including during pregnancy. Reduction in disease activity was noted with no harmful effects on the baby with use during pregnancy, while discontinuation led to an increase in disease flares.[5] The risk of congenital heart block (CHB) and neonatal lupus syndromes was also significantly reduced in at-risk pregnancies with sustained use of hydroxychloroquine

Immunosuppressive agents are beneficial in controlling active disease. Azathioprine is one of the only few immunosuppressive agents that has documented safety during pregnancy.[10] The dose should be limited to maximum of 2 mg/kg/day, to avoid risk of fetal cytopenias and immune suppression.[10] Most other agents, such as cyclophosphamide, methotrexate, and mycophenolate, are contraindicated during pregnancy and should be discontinued at least 3 months before conception.

Disease Flares

SLE may flare during pregnancy or in the postpartum period. Widely variable rates of flares during pregnancy, from 25–65%, have been reported.[11] The heterogeneous study designs, different patient ethnicities, diverse control groups, and variable definitions of flares used in these studies, are likely responsible for the disparate results. Defining SLE disease activity in pregnancy can be difficult. Physiological changes in pregnancy, such as joint pain, rash, and constitutional symptoms can overlap with the signs of disease activity. Mild variations in common laboratory tests, including mild anemia, mild thrombocytopenia, and mild proteinuria, can occur in normal pregnancy. Pregnancy-specific disease activity scales (SLEPDAI, LAIP) have been developed, but mostly remain as research tools. In practice, the sound clinical judgment of an experienced clinician remains the gold standard.

Active disease at the time of conception is a strong predictor of continued activity and flares during pregnancy, increasing the fetal and maternal risk by threefold to fourfold.[12] Presence of lupus nephritis increased overall and renal flares during pregnancy by two-fold to three-fold.[12] Most of the flares in pregnancy are mild-to-moderate in severity, severe flares being reported in 10–40% of the patients.[11] The majority of the flares involve renal, musculoskeletal, and hematological systems.

Treatment for Lupus Flares

Lupus flares should be treated with the appropriate steroid (usually prednisolone) dose. Azathioprine and cyclosporine can be used in pregnancy with active SLE. Cytotoxic drugs such as cyclophosphamide should be avoided during first trimester except in rare circumstances such as pulmonary alveolar hemorrhage or class IV nephritis due to SLE. These drugs have some side effects over pregnancy and fetus. Cyclophosphamide and Methotrexate are the most teratogenic among them and should be avoided in pregnancy. More safety data are needed for the use of mycophenolate mofetil.

Delivery

Women who have required glucocorticoids (e.g., prednisone) to control systemic lupus erythematosus during pregnancy need an increased dose, called a stress dose, during delivery.[13] The increased dose helps the body respond normally to the physical stresses of childbirth. Delivery should be done in such hospital where pediatric care is available; if possible in a hospital where Neonatal ICU is available. Indication of cesarean section same as normal pregnancy.

Indications for Cesarean Section

Include maternal reasons (avascular necrosis of the hips with inadequate hip abduction) or fetal reasons (fetal distress, abnormal nonstress test, cephalopelvic disproportion and transverse presentation, etc.)

Neonatal Care

After delivery heart rate of the baby should be counted and also there should be a search for any cutaneous lesion. Treatment of established congenital heart block (CHB) is difficult.[14] Therefore, it is better to prevent during pregnancy. Most of the time cutaneous lesion can be treated with topical steroids.

Issues of Breastfeeding

Majority of drugs are excreted in human milk in variable amounts. From neonatal perspective, maternal intake of prednisolone less than or up to 30 mg/day, warfarin, cyclosporine in standard doses and weekly chloroquine for malaria prophylaxis are considered safe. If the dose of prednisolone is greater than 30 mg/day, feeding should be avoided for 4 hours after ingestion of the morning dose of steroid. By this time, the blood levels are quite low and very limited amounts are secreted into the milk. However, breastfeeding is contraindicated, if mother is on cyclophosphamide, azathioprine, hydroxychloroquine for SLE.

Advice of Contraception

Several conditions in SLE may require effective contraception such as very active disease, severe organ involvement or damage, and the use of embryotoxic/fetotoxic drugs. Therefore, contraceptive counseling is essential in clinical rheumatology, although many women still do not receive adequate information in clinical practice.[15] A common misconception among women with SLE is that they "cannot use birth control", since the "classical" estrogen-containing pill is generally contraindicated. The message should be that women with SLE should be considered good candidates for many contraceptive methods, including hormonal contraceptives, and the most suitable choice should be made individually the safety of low-dose combined OC in a well-defined population of stable SLE patients with inactive or stable active disease with respect to the risk of lupus flares.

OCP should be avoided in antiphospholipid syndrome, other thromboembolic diseases, highly active disease, migraine, nephritis Raynaud's phenomenon.[15] Progestin-only preparations (daily oral pill, depot medroxyprogesterone, and subcutaneous implants) do not appear to increase immune activity and are not associated with increased rates of flares, and the dose of progestin does not increase the risk of thrombosis.[15]

Barrier methods are the safest method for contraception. Use of intrauterine devices is controversial because it causes infections such as endometritis, PID, etc.

Pregnancy Complications

Pregnancy in the setting of SLE is associated with a higher risk of complications, compared to normal. Women deliveries reported manyfold increased risk of maternal death, pre-eclampsia, preterm labor, thrombosis, infection, and hematologic complications during SLE pregnancy.[16] The biggest issue is the 3–5 times higher risk of pre-eclampsia, complicating 16–30% of SLE pregnancies.[13] The predisposing factors for pre-eclampsia include advanced maternal age, previous personal or family history of pre-eclampsia, pre-existing hypertension or diabetes mellitus, and obesity. In SLE, additional specific risk factors include active or history of lupus nephritis, presence of anti-phospholipid antibodies, declining complement levels, and thrombocytopenia.

Obstetric Outcome

The main obstetric issues in SLE pregnancy are higher rates of fetal loss, preterm birth, intrauterine growth restriction (IUGR), and neonatal lupus syndromes. However, the rate of fetal loss has declined and live births rates of 80–90% have recently been reported.[11] Active disease and lupus nephritis increase the risk of fetal loss and other adverse outcomes.[17] Proteinuria, hypertension, thrombocytopenia, and presence of antiphospholipid antibodies are other negative predictors for fetal survival.

Neonatal Lupus Syndromes

Neonatal lupus syndromes (NLS) is a form of passively acquired fetal autoimmunity from maternal antibodies, anti-Ro and anti-La antibodies. Majority of the manifestations, such as rash, hematologic and hepatic abnormalities, parallel the presence of maternal antibodies in the neonatal circulation. They tend to resolve with the clearance of the antibodies by six to eight months of life. In contrast, cardiac complications are a result of permanent damage to the fetal cardiac conduction system by maternal antibodies.

The cardiac manifestations of NLS include conduction defects, structural abnormalities, cardiomyopathy and congestive cardiac failure.[18] However, the most common issue is congenital heart block (CHB). CHB results from diffuse myocarditis and fibrosis in the region between atrioventricular node and bundle of His fetal echo should be performed between 18 and 26 weeks. CHB leads to high fetal mortality; rates of 15–30% have been reported. The majority of survivors require pacemakers, adding to the significant morbidity.

CONCLUSION

Systemic lupus erythematosus is a multisystem disease. Therefore, interdisciplinary approach is needed to treat the disease. Doctor, patient and her family should work together for planning of pregnancy and during pregnancy to overcome the complications. Pregnancy in women with SLE is a high-risk condition. Despite considerable improvement in success rates, substantially high maternal and fetal morbidity and mortality still remain a cause for concern. Disease activity may worsen during the pregnancy and in turn may increase the risk of other maternal and fetal complications. The key to success lies in the multidisciplinary care with close monitoring. Early detection of threats to maternal and fetal well-being, with judicious use of appropriate medications, is essential to achieve good outcomes.

KEY POINTS

- Pregnancy in the setting of SLE remains a high-risk situation.
- Multidisciplinary care with close monitoring is essential for good outcomes.
- Active disease at conception is associated with adverse maternal and fetal outcomes.
- Pregnancy should be planned at times of disease quiescence with effective use of contraception.
- Preconception assessment should be done prior to the planned pregnancy.
- Specific monitoring and treatment protocols are required in high-risk situations such as presence of specific antibodies (aPL and anti-Ro).
- Disease flares, pre-eclampsia, fetal loss, prematurity, intra-uterine growth restriction and neonatal lupus syndromes (including CHB) remain the main issues.
- Safe treatment options exist and should be appropriately used for disease activity during pregnancy.

REFERENCES

1. Clark CA, Spitzer KA, Laskin CA. Decrease in pregnancy loss rates in patients with systemic lupus erythematosus over a 40-year period. J Rheumatol. 2005;32(9):1709-12.
2. Tsokos GC. Systemic lupus erythematosus. N Engl J Med. 2011; 365(22):2110.
3. Hahn BH. systemic lupus erythematosus. In: longo DL, Fauci AS, Kasper DL, et al (Eds). Harrison's Principle of Internal Medicine, 18th edn. New York, McGraw-Hill, 2012.
4. Kumar A. Indian Guidelines on the Management of SLE. Indian J Rheumato Assoc. 2002;10:80-96.
5. Lateef A, Petri M. Management of pregnancy in systemic lupus erythematosus. Nat Rev Rheumatol. 2012;8(12):710-8. [PubMed] .
6. Motha MBC, Wijesinghe PS. Systemic lupus erythematosus and pregnancy: a challenge to the clinician. Ceylon J Med. 2009;54(4):107-9.
7. Roy JS, Das PP. SLE in Pregnancy. [BSMMU J]. 2010;3(1):54-9.
8. Adams K, Bombardier C, van der Heijde DM. Safety of pain therapy during pregnancy and lactation in patients with inflammatory arthritis: a systematic literature review. J Rheumatol Suppl. 2012;90:59-61.[PubMed]
9. Koren G, Florescu A, Costei AM, Boskovic R, Moretti ME. Nonsteroidal antiinflammatory drugs during third trimester and the risk of premature closure of the ductus arteriosus: a meta-analysis. Ann Pharmacother. 2006;40(5):824-9. [PubMed]
10. Ostensen M, Khamashta M, Lockshin M, Parke A, Brucato A, Carp H, Doria A, Rai R, Meroni P, Cetin I, et al. Anti-inflammatory and immunosuppressive drugs and reproduction. Arthritis Res Ther. 2006;8(3):209. [PMC free article] [PubMed]
11. Carvalheiras G, Vita P, Marta S, Trovao R, Farinha F, Braga J, Rocha G, Almeida I, Marinho A, Mendonca T, et al. Pregnancy and systemic lupus erythematosus: review of clinical features and outcome of 51 pregnancies at a single institution. Clin Rev Allergy Immunol. 2010;38(2-3):302-6. [PubMed]
12. Saavedra MA, Cruz-Reyes C, Vera-Lastra O, Romero GT, Cruz-Cruz P, Arias-Flores R, Jara LJ. Impact of previous lupus nephritis on maternal and fetal outcomes during pregnancy. Clinical Rheumatology. 2012;31(5):813-9.
13. Mittal G, Sule A, Pathan E, Gaitonde S, Samant R, Joshi VR.Pregnancy in lupus: analysis of 25 cases. Indian J Rheumato Assoc. 2001;9:69-71.
14. Bandyopadhyay D, Singh S, Kumari R. Pregnancy with SLE and fetal congenital heart block. Indian J Obstet Gynecol. 2006;56(6):532-31.
15. Yazdany J, Trupin L, Kaiser R, et al. Contraceptive counseling and use among women with systemic lupus erythematosus: a gap in health care quality? Arthritis Care and Research. 2011;63(3):358-65.
16. Clowse ME, Jamison M, Myers E, James AH. A national study of the complications of lupus in pregnancy. Am J Obstet Gynecol. 2008;199(2):127, e121-12629.
17. Wagner SJ, Craici I, Reed D, Norby S, Bailey K, Wiste HJ, Wood CM, Moder KG, Liang KP, Liang KV, et al. Maternal and foetal outcomes in pregnant patients with active lupus nephritis. Lupus. 2009;18(4):342-7.
18. Hornberger LK, Al Rajaa N. Spectrum of cardiac involvement in neonatal lupus. Scand J Immunol. 2010;72(3):189-97.

Chapter 48

Antiphospholipid Antibody Syndrome

Deepti Shrivastava

INTRODUCTION

Antiphospholipid antibody syndrome is an inherent autoimmune thrombophilic condition that is marked by presence of antibodies in the blood that recognize and attack phospholipid-binding proteins, also known as Hughes syndrome.[1,2]

Lupus anticoagulant syndrome is a misnomer as it may be found secondarily associated with systemic lupus erythematosis (SLE).

The clinical manifestations of APLA syndrome are due to vascular thrombosis and exhibit as bad obstetric history with fetal demise at different gestational ages[2] especially recurrent spontaneous miscarriages and less frequently, maternal thrombosis.[3] Many other clinical manifestations may occur.[4,5] Women with the clinical features of APLA syndrome should be tested for 3 antiphospholipid antibodies that have proven association with the diagnosis of APLA: lupus anticoagulant (LA), anticardiolipin antibody (ACA), and antibeta-2 glycoprotein 1 antibody.

These antibodies predispose to clotting in vivo, predominantly by interfering with the antithrombotic role of phospholipids. The antiphospholipid (APL) autoantibodies bind moieties on negatively charged phospholipids or moieties formed by the interaction of negatively charged phospholipids with other lipids, phospholipids or proteins.

There are three types of APLA syndrome:
1. *Primary* APLA syndrome is diagnosed in patients demonstrating the clinical and laboratory criteria for the disease without other recognized autoimmune disease.
2. *Secondary* APLA syndrome is diagnosed in patients with other autoimmune disorders, such as systemic lupus erythematosus (SLE)
3. *Catastrophic* antiphospholipid syndrome (CAPS) represents the severe end of the spectrum with multiple organ thromboses in a rapid period of time. Multiorgan failure has been described during pregnancy by Asherson[6] and during postpartum by Kochenour.[7]

Obstetric features of APLA syndrome: Unexplained fetal death or stillbirth.

Recurrent pregnancy loss 3 or more spontaneous abortions with no more than 1 live birth:
- Unexplained second or third trimester fetal death
- Severe pre-eclampsia at less than 34 weeks gestation
- Unexplained severe fetal growth restriction
- Chorea gravidarum.

Nonobstetric features of APS are as follows:
- Nontraumatic thrombosis or thromboembolism (venous or arterial)
- Stroke, especially in individuals aged 24–50 years
- Unexplained transient ischemic attack
- Unexplained amaurosis fugax
- Autoimmune thrombocytopenia
- Autoimmune hemolytic anemia
- Unexplained prolongation of a clotting assay
- Livedo reticularis
- SLE or other connective tissue disorder
- False-positive serologic test result for syphilis.

EPIDEMIOLOGY

In normal healthy populations prevalence of APLA syndrome is 2–4% in general.
- ACA range between 1.0% and 5.6%
- LA has been reported to range between 1.0% and 3.6%.[8-10]

The prevalence of elevated aPL antibodies may also increase with age.[11] About one-third of SLE patients are ACA positive. LA prevalence is about 15% in SLE patients. A positive LA appears to be more specific for APS than an elevated ACA.

Primarily, ACA are not as strong a risk factor for thrombosis as LA. Lupus anticoagulant is consistently the most powerful predictor of thrombosis.[12-14]

Approximately 40% of patients with systemic lupus erythematosus have antiphospholipid antibodies,[13] but less than 40% of them are predisposed to have thrombotic events.[15] However, thrombotic antiphospholipid syndrome is regarded as a major adverse prognostic factor in patients with lupus.[16]

OBSTETRIC IMPLICATIONS

- Recurrent pregnancy loss 25%. Usually in 15% at 1st trimester after the establishment of FHR-activity.
- *Pre-eclampsia:* About 15–50%. 15% of severe pre-eclampsia, before 34 weeks have APL Ab
- IUGR: 30%
- Preterm labor
- Maternal thrombosis (including strokes).

Antiphospholipid Antibodies and Infertility

The APLA is responsible for implantation failure in 23% females referred for IVF (Chilcott et al, 2000).

Postpartum syndrome are rare such as pleuropulmonary disease, fever, cardiac manifestations.

ETIOPATHOGENESIS

Pathophysiology

Basic 3 types of antibodies detected are:
1. *LA:* Risk of arterial thrombosis, leading to stroke.
2. *ACA:* Risk of venous thrombosis.
3. *Anti-β_2 GP1:* For other manifestations along with.

All these antibodies have major specificity for β_2-glycoprotein 1 (2GP1).[16,17] Other antigenic targets for them are proteins C and S, prothrombin and annexin V.[18] Whether these antibodies themselves are etiological factors or epiphenomenon, is uncertain.

Autoantibodies for β_2-glycoprotein 1, also known as apolipoprotein H, a member of the complement control protein. Antiphospholipid antibodies activate platelets that increase expression of synthesis of thromboxane A2. The activation of endothelial cells, monocytes, and platelets by antiphospholipid antibodies, conducting to the increased synthesis of tissue factor and thromboxane A2, induce a procoagulant state.[19-21]

Interaction of antiphospholipid antibodies with proteins implicated in clotting regulation, such as prothrombin, factor X, protein C and S,[22] and plasmin,[23] tissue factor pathway inhibitor, might hinder inactivation of procoagulant factors and impede fibrinolysis.[24]

Interference with annexin A5, a natural anticoagulant that binds to phosphatidylserine exposed during trophoblast syncytium formation, favor a more direct effect on placental structures, promoting placental thrombosis and fetal loss.[25]

Activation of the complement cascade also provoke thrombosis and fetal loss.[26] This occurs often in presence of a second hit due to some trigger factor.[18] Traditional cardiovascular risk factors such as tobacco, inflammation or estrogens might have an important role at this point, in fact such risk factors are present in more than 50% of patients with antiphospholipid syndrome.

Possible Etiological Factors

Absolute cause is not known. There is genetic predisposition for HLA-DR2, HLA-DR53, and HLA-DR4 positive individuals. Possible triggers identified and stratified accordingly. It is found associated with positive family history to the extent of 33%, some other autoimmune disorders are also found associated with anti-phospholipid antibodies. Currently accepted "second-hit" hypothesis, a trigger event-such as cigarette smoking, oral contraceptives, chlorpromazine and other phenothiazines, surgical procedures, prolonged immobilization, or a genetic prothrombotic state-may increase the likelihood of an APLA positive patient developing a vascular event. Women with pregnancy events alone have a high likelihood of developing thrombosis in later years.[27]

APLA can be stimulated by infections also, in 2 ways:
1. *Without associated thrombosis:* Commonly along with some viruses, such as cytomegalovirus, Epstein-Barr virus, adenoviruses, bacterial (e.g. *bacterial endocarditis*, tuberculosis, *Mycoplasma pneumoniae*, spirochetal (e.g. syphilis, leptospirosis, Lyme disease), and parasitic (e.g. malaria infection) infections.
2. *Possible association with thrombosis:* Like in varicella, HIV, hepatitis C.

Pathology

Exactly unknown but mainly defect in cellular apoptosis is there due to exposure of membrane phospholipids to the binding of various plasma proteins, $\beta_2$gp1 are main targets for autoantibodies. There is imbalance of homeostatic regulation, production of antibodies against prothrombin, protein C, S annexins, activation of platelets to enhance endothelial adherence, activation of vascular endothelium—platelet and monocyte binding, antibodies against oxidized LDL—atherosclerosis in elderly patients. Complement activation also has been increasingly recognized as a possible significant role in the pathogenesis of APLA Syndrome **(Fig. 48.1)**.

DIAGNOSIS

According to international consensus statement 2006 on revised criteria for classification of APLA syndrome: Diagnosis of APLA syndrome is made when *at least one clinical and at least one laboratory criteria* are met.

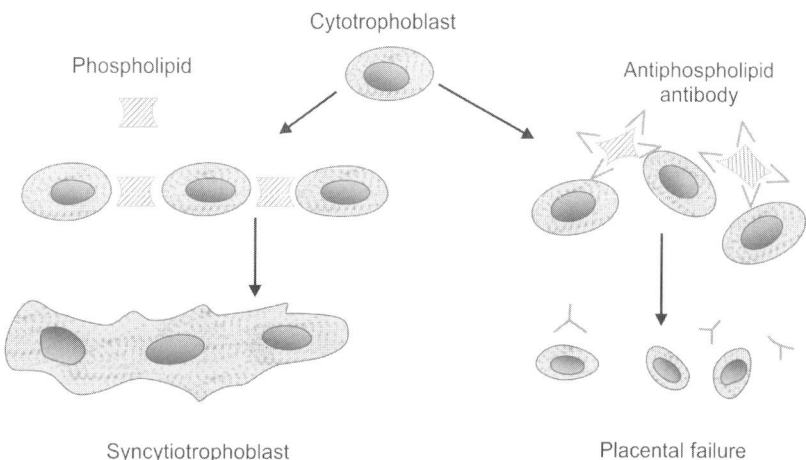

Fig. 48.1: Placental failure in APLA syndrome

Clinical Criteria

Vascular Thrombosis

- One or more clinical episodes of arterial, venous or small-vessel thrombosis in any tissue or organ.
- Thrombosis must be confirmed by imaging or Doppler studies.

Pregnancy Morbidity

- One or more unexplained deaths of a morphologically normal fetus at or beyond the 10th week of gestation
- One or more premature births of a morphologically normal neonate at or before the 34th week of gestation due to pre-eclampsia, eclampsia or placental insufficiency
- Three or more unexplained consecutive spontaneous abortions before the 10th week of gestation with maternal anatomic or hormonal abnormalities.

Laboratory Criteria

- *ACA of IgG* and/or *IgM* isotype in serum or plasma present in medium [>40 GPL or MPL] or high titer [>99th percentile]
  Also measured by ELISA for β_2GP1-dependent anti-cardiolipin Ab
- LA in serum (detected in following steps)
  - Prolonged phospholipid dependent coagulation demonstrated on a screening test [e.g. aPTT, dRVVT, dilute prothrombin time)
  - Failure to correct the prolonged coagulation time by mixing with normal platelet plasma
  - Shortening/correction of the prolonged coagulation time by adding excess phospholipid
  - Exclusion of other coagulopathies [Factor VIII inhibitor or heparin]
- *Anti-B_2 GPI antibody* of IgG and/or IgM isotype in serum or plasma (in titer >99th percentile]
  Measured by standardized ELISA, on two or more occasions at least 12 weeks apart.

Other manifestations are:
- Cardiac valve disease
- Livedo reticularis
- Thrombocytopenia
- Renal thrombotic microangiopathy
- Neurological manifestations-chorea

Noncriteria antibodies may also present such as:
- Antiphosphatidylserine antibodies
- Antiphosphatidylethanolamine antibodies
- Antibodies against prothrombin alone
- Antibodies to phosphatidylserine-prothrombin complex.

The reference ranges of serum ACA are as follows:
- <10.0 MPL (negative)
- 10.0–14.9 MPL (borderline)
- 15.0–39.9 MPL (weakly positive)
- 40.00–79.9 MPL (positive)
- >or = 80.0 MPL (strongly positive)

MPL refers to IgM phospholipid units. One MPL unit is 1 microgram of IgM antibody.
Reference values apply to all ages.

In Short

- *Low positive:* Fewer than 20 G phospholipids (GPL), M phospholipids (MPL), A phospholipids (APL) units
- *Medium positive*: 20 or more but fewer than 80 GPL, MPL, APL units

Table 48.1: Historical development of classification criteria of APLA syndrome

Comparison of laboratory criteria of APLA Syndrome Test	Sapporo criteria (1999)	Sydney criteria (2006)
LA	Screening, mixing, and confirmation tests Two or more occasions at least 6 weeks apart	Screening, mixing, and confirmation tests Two or more occasions at least 12 weeks apart
ACA	Detected by standardized ELISA IgG and/or IgM Medium or high titer Two or more occasions at least 6 w apart	Detected by standardized ELISA IgG and/or IgM Medium or high titer (>40 units titer or >99th percentile) Two or more occasions at least 12 w apart
Anti-β2GPI Ab		IgG and/or IgM Titer >99th percentile Two or more occasions at least 12 weeks apart

- *High positive*: 80 or more GPL, MPL, APL units (APL, GPL, and MPL units refer to arbitrary units. The abbreviation APL denotes the result is from the IgA isotype, the abbreviation GPL denotes the result is from the IgG isotype and the abbreviation MPL denotes the result is from the IgM isotype. The letters "PL" denote specificity for phospholipid antigens).

There are so many advances in criteria since 1999. Sapporo[28] JAPAN consensus conference criteria were practiced. Later on it was revised in 2006 as Sydney conference.[29-32]

Numerous modifications were made to the initial statement and better defining of clinical criteria was made by confirmation (*see* Table 48.1).

DIFFERENTIAL DIAGNOSIS[33-36]

Common autoimmune diseases associated with APLA are:
- SLE—25–50%
- Sjögren's—42%
- Rheumatoid arthritis—33%
- Autoimmune thrombocytic purpura—30%
- Autoimmune hemolytic anemia—unknown
- Behçet syndrome—20%.

TREATMENT

Obstetric indications for laboratory tests are:
- Unexplained stillbirth
- Recurrent pregnancy loss
- Unexplained 2nd or 3rd trimester fetal death
- IUGR
- Severe pre-eclampsia at <34 weeks
- Placental abruption.

The goals of treatment in pregnant women with antiphospholipid syndrome are to improve maternal and fetal-neonatal outcomes by keeping to a minimum the risks of the recognized complications of the disorder, including maternal thrombosis, fetal loss, pre-eclampsia, placental insufficiency, and fetal growth restriction, and the need for iatrogenic preterm birth.[37]

The optimal treatment of woman with infertility and pregnant women with Antiphospholipid antibodies and 1 or more fetal losses after 10 weeks gestation without thrombosis is controversial.[38]

Before Pregnancy

Preconceptional counseling:
- *Clinical:* Review medical and obstetric history, assess any other risk factors, obesity, age
- *Laboratory:* Confirm persistent APLA Ab, assess renal functions, CBC for anemia and thrombocytopenia
- Advice to postpone pregnancy if thrombotic event is within 6 month.
- Start low dose aspirin preconceptionally.

During Pregnancy

- Confirm live embryo at 6 weeks by TVS
- Continue low dose aspirin, start LMWH heparin
- Antenatal visits every 4 weeks until 20 weeks then weekly. Monitor for missed abortion, early onset pregnancy induced hypertension.
- USG and color Doppler every 4 weekly after 20 weeks to assess fetal growth and amniotic fluid index. If early diastolic notch present then do 2 weekly growth scans due to high risk of IUGR. Weekly NST and platelet counts.

Postpartum in Presence of History of Thrombosis

Warfarin thromboprophylaxis as soon as the patient is clinically stable after delivery (International normalized ratio (INR) of 3 is desirable). If there is no history of thrombosis:

then heparin for 5 days and oral anticoagulant for 6 weeks. Heparin and warfarin are safe with breast feeding. Estrogen-containing contraception are contraindicated.

For women who are refractory to aspirin and heparin: Full anticoagulation in the next pregnancy if failed: IV immunoglobulin: (anti-idiotypic down regulation of auto-antibody production) can be tried.

Earliest treatment for recurrent pregnancy loss associated with APLA is a combination of high dose prednisone and low-dose aspirin, with 75% success in outcome. Although high maternal and fetal morbidity, in terms of gestational diabetes, hypertension, and premature rupture of membranes are there. A randomized controlled study of prednisone and aspirin as compared with heparin and aspirin showed low-dose subcutaneous heparin with low-dose aspirin to be equally efficacious with less morbidity.[39] Moreover, a Cochrane analysis concluded that intravenous immunoglobulins were associated with an increased risk of pregnancy loss or premature birth, compared with heparin and low-dose aspirin.[40]

Heparin is the anticoagulant drug of choice during pregnancy.[41] Heparin does not cross the placenta and is widely considered safe for the embryo-fetus. Of the 2 clinically available forms, the low molecular weight heparin (LMWH) preparations offer some advantages over unfractionated heparin (UFH). Both UFH and LMWH act primarily by binding to antithrombin to catalyze the molecule binding to and altering the activity of serine protease procoagulants. UFH enhances the activity of antithrombin for Factor Xa and thrombin, whereas the predominant effect of LMWH is via antithrombin-mediated anti-Factor Xa activity. UFH has complex pharmacokinetics that ultimately leads to a somewhat unpredictable anticoagulant response. Also, the bioavailability of the UFH after subcutaneous injection is reduced compared with intravenous infusion.

Heparin is the anticoagulant drug of choice during pregnancy.[42] Heparin does not cross the placenta and is widely considered safe for the embryo-fetus. Of the 2 clinically available forms, the low molecular weight heparin (LMWH) preparations offer some advantages over unfractionated heparin (UFH). Both UFH and LMWH act primarily by binding to antithrombin to catalyze the molecule binding to and altering the activity of serine protease procoagulants. UFH enhances the activity of antithrombin for factor Xa and thrombin, whereas the predominant effect of LMWH is via antithrombin-mediated anti-factor Xa activity. UFH has complex pharmacokinetics that ultimately leads to a somewhat unpredictable anticoagulant response. Also, the bioavailability of the UFH after subcutaneous (SC) injection is reduced compared with intravenous infusion.

To summarize, low-dose aspirin (75 mg) in combination with heparin is the first line treatment start with the positive pregnancy test till 34 weeks. It is documented with success of 70% (Rai et al. 1997) and reduces the miscarriage rate by 54% (Empson et al, Cochrane Database Syst Rev, 2005 *Complications of heparin* are hemorrhage, thrombocytopenia and osteopenia. Advantages of LMWH is that it requires once daily dose, causes less thrombocytopenia and osteopenia. Dosage for standard heparin in first trimester is 5000–10000 units subcutaneous per 12 hours and in 2nd and 3rd trimester is 10000 units per 12 hours. For *LMWH* enoxaparin 20 mg once daily and dalteparin 5000 U once daily.

With history of thrombosis: IV immunoglobulin are documented to have no benefit relative to heparin and low dose aspirin. They should be reserved for cases refractory to aspirin and heparin (Jivaraj and Rai, 2003).

Corticosteroids (prednisone): They are also abandoned (do not improve the live birth significant maternal and fetal morbidity) (Laskin et al. 1997).

Warfarin is suitable for thromboprophylaxis in puerperium and in whom history of recurrent thrombosis or cerebral thrombosis (Branch et al. 2003).

Prognosis

APLA is one of the major causes of thrombosis and its complications in women with arterial thrombosis. Coronary artery occlusions and venous thrombosis being reported in patients with this syndrome. Previous thrombosis may have a recurrence rate of 25% per year in untreated patients.

A 2015 retrospective analysis by the European Registry on Obstetric Antiphospholipid Syndrome (EUROAPS) found very good maternal-fetal outcomes in women whose obstetric APLA was treated but previous fetal loss appears to be a risk factor for fetal loss, pre-eclampsia, premature birth, and placenta-mediated complications in women with pure APLA. According to the Nimes Obstetricians and Hematologists Antiphospholipid Syndrome (NOH-APS)[43] study, the incidence of such late-pregnancy complications were greater in the treated women with pure APLA compared to nontreated women negative for antiphospholipid antibodies, in spite of treatment included low molecular weight heparin (LMWH) and low-dose aspirin (LDA).

Maternal Morbidity

Thrombosis, especially in patients with APLA and a history of thrombosis, is a major concern. Morbidity may be directly due to thrombotic events or it may be because of severe pre-eclampsia requiring premature delivery. It is also associated with anticoagulation in patients treated with heparin or low-molecular-weight heparins in pregnancy.

Landry-Guillain-Barré-Strohl syndrome of acute inflammatory demyelinating polyradiculoneuropathy is very rarely associated with the patients and usually present with progressive bilateral and symmetrical muscle weakness accompanied by mild sensory symptoms, including paresthesia, numbness, and tingling. The disease can progress to involve the respiratory muscles, resulting in respiratory failure. Two thirds of the patients have a history of viral-like infections 1–3 weeks prior to the onset of symptoms. CMV infection has been incriminated as a potential etiologic agent in some pregnant patients presenting with LGBSS.

Maternal Mortality

Mortality rates during pregnancy are not well characterized. Multiorgan failure due to disturbance in homeostasis of body has been described during pregnancy by Asherson and during postpartum by Kochenour. Complications secondary to severe pre-eclampsia may be life-threatening.

Perinatal Morbidity

About 10–15% of women are at high risk for fetal growth restriction. Neonatal morbidity and mortality may be influenced by indicated preterm delivery for maternal severe pre-eclampsia or fetal growth restriction. Neonatal lupus dermatitis, a variety of systemic and hematologic abnormalities, and isolated congenital heart block have been associated with APLA and SLE.

Perinatal Mortality

Fetal deaths at or beyond 20 weeks' gestation may be attributable to APLA involvement. The rate of fetal loss may exceed 90% in untreated patients with APLA. Therapy (including aspirin and heparin) can reduce the rate of fetal loss to 25%, as described by Cowchock et al.

Recent Advances in Treatment

Most of the future therapies (clopidogrel, rivaroxaban, statins, rituximab, and other new anticoagulant drugs) are for non-pregnant patients. The only new drugs for APLA that pregnant women can use are dipyridamole and hydroxychloroquine.

Combination treatment with aspirin plus dipyridamole have shown higher efficacy than has aspirin alone in patients with stroke. Such combination might be considered in selected patients with antiphospholipid syndrome in whom warfarin is not effective or safe. Observational studies have suggested an antithrombotic effect of hydroxychloroquine in patients with antiphospholipid antibodies, most of whom have systemic lupus erythematosus.[44,45]

Furthermore, results from basic studies have shown a dose-dependent reduction by hydroxychloroquine of platelet activation and clotting induced by antiphospholipid antibodies.[46,47] Hydroxychloroquine directly inhibits the binding of antiphospholipid antibody-2-glycoprotein-1 complexes to phospholipid surfaces.[48] An additional and previously unrecognized role of hydroxychloroquine in prevention of pregnancy loss is suggested by the description of its protective effect of the annexin A5 shield formed over phospholipid bilayers from damage induced by antiphospholipid antibodies.[49] In view of the excellent safety profile, including the absence of any adverse effects on the fetus-neonate,[50] and the absence of associated bleeding, hydroxychloroquine should be considered for an adjuvant antithrombotic role in patients with systemic lupus erythematosus who are positive for antiphospholipid antibodies. Patients with primary antiphospholipid syndrome and recurrent thrombosis despite adequate anticoagulation, who have difficulty maintaining adequate anticoagulation intensity, or have a high-risk profile for major hemorrhage, might also benefit from hydroxychloroquine treatment.

Furthermore, recent data from an experimental model of APL antibody-induced pregnancy losses in mice[51] suggest that the therapeutic effect of heparin in the disorder might be due to the inhibition of complement rather than its inhibition of coagulation. These data, if generalizable to human APLA related pregnancy losses, have raised the intriguing possibility of novel non anticoagulant approaches to treatment

CONCLUSION

Thrombosis and the related pregnancy complications associated with APLA syndrome are preventable to some extent. Identification of at risk patients, determination of a candidate for thrombophilia screening, and who may warrant thromboprophylaxis. Various thromboprophylaxis regimens and peripartum anticoagulant management are effective up to 75% in prevention of severe life-threatening complications. Although optimal treatment of patients with antiphospholipid antibodies is not well standardized yet to make universal recommendations but low-dose aspirin and low molecular weight heparin have main role along with close monitoring for development of severe pre-eclampsia and severe IUGR by color Doppler and NST, along with good neonatal care for early termination of pregnancy are mainstay of treatment. In order to reduce the risk of postpartum deep vein thrombosis, antithrombotic coverage of the postpartum period is recommended in all women with antiphospholipid syndrome, with or without previous thrombosis. Generally, women with previous thrombosis will need long-term anticoagulation, and most experts prefer switching the treatment to warfarin, as soon as the patient is clinically stable after delivery, to limit further risk of heparin-induced osteoporosis and bone fracture.

ABBREVIATIONS

- ACA: Anticardiolipin antibody
- APLA: Antiphospholipid antibody syndrome
- aPTT: Activated partial thromboplastin time

- CAPS: Catastrophic antiphospholipid syndrome
- CBC: Complete blood count.
- CMV: Cytomegalovirus
- dRVVT: Dilute Russell's viper venom testing
- ELISA: Enzyme-linked immunosorbent assay
- EUROAPS: The European Registry on Obstetric Antiphospholipid Syndrome
- GPL: IgG antiphopholipid
- IUGR: Intrauterine growth retardation
- LA: Lupus anticoagulant
- LDA: Low dose aspirin
- LGBSS: Landry-Guillain-Barré-Strohl syndrome
- LMWH: Low molecular weight heparin
- MPL: Ig M antiphospholipid
- NOH-APS: The Nimes Obstetricians and Hematologists Antiphospholipid Syndrome
- NST: Nonstress test
- SLE: Systemic lupus erythematosus
- TVS: Transvaginal sonography
- UFH: Unfractionated heparin

REFERENCES

1. Hughes GR. Thrombosis, abortion, cerebral disease and the lupus anticoagulant. BMJ. 1983;287:1088-9. [PMC free article] [PubMed]
2. Hughes GRV. The antiphospholipid syndrome: ten years on. Lancet. 1993;342:341-4. [PubMed]
3. Roubey RAS, Hoffman M. From antiphospholipid syndrome to antibody-mediated thrombosis. Lancet. 1997;350:1491-3. [PubMed]
4. Khamashta MA, Cervera R, Asherson RA, Font J, Gil A, Coltart DJ, Vázquez JJ, Paré C, Ingelmo M, Oliver J, et al. Association of antibodies against phospholipids with heart valve disease in systemic lupus erythematosus. Lancet. 1990;335:1541-4. [PubMed]
5. Mialdea M, Sangle SR, D'Cruz DP. Antiphospholipid (Hughes) syndrome: beyond pregnancy morbidity and thrombosis. Journal of Autoimmune Diseases. 2009;19:6. [PMC free article] [PubMed]
6. Asherson RA, Khamashta MA, Ordi-Ros J, Derksen RH, Machin SJ, Barquinero J, et al. The "primary" antiphospholipid syndrome: major clinical and serological features. Medicine (Baltimore). 1989;68(6):366-74. [PubMed]
7. Kochenour NK, Branch DW, Rote NS, et al. A new postpartum syndrome associated with antiphospholipid antibodies. Obstet Gynecol. 1987;69(3 Pt 2):460-8. [PubMed]
8. De Groot PG, Lutters B, Derksen RH, Lisman T, Meijers JC, Rosendaal FR. Lupus anticoagulants and the risk of a first episode of deep venous thrombosis. J Thromb Haemost. 2005;3:1993-7. [PubMed]
9. Petri M. Classification and epidemiology of the antiphospholipid syndrome In: Asherson RA, Cervera R, Piette JC, Shoenfeld Y (Eds). The Antiphospholipid Syndrome II. Elsevier. 2002;11:22.
10. Shi W, Krilis SA, Chong BH, Gordon S, Chesterman CN. Prevalence of lupus anticoagulant and anticardiolipin antibodies in a healthy population. Aust N Z J Med. 1990;20:231-6. [PubMed]
11. Richaud-Patin Y, Cabiedes J, Jakez-Ocampo J, Vidaller A, Llorente L. High prevalence of protein-dependent and protein-independent antiphospholipid. Thromb. Res. 2000;99:129-33. [PubMed]
12. Tektonidou MG, Laskari K, Panagiotakos DB, Moutsopoulos HM. Risk factors for thrombosis and primary thrombosis prevention in patients with systemic lupus erythematosus with or without antiphospholipid antibodies. Arthritis Rheum. 2009;61:29-36. [PubMed]
13. Galli M, Luciani D, Bertolini G, Barbui T. Lupus anticoagulants are stronger risk factors for thrombosis than anticardiolipin antibodies in the antiphospholipid syndrome: a systematic review of the literature. Blood. 2003;101:1827-32. [PubMed]
14. Martinez-Berriotxoa A, Ruiz-Irastorza G, Egurbide MV, et al. Transiently positive anticardiolipin antibodies do not increase the risk of thrombosis in patients with systemic lupus erythematosus. Lupus. 2007;16:810-6. [PubMed]
15. Martinez-Berriotxoa A, Ruiz-Irastorza G, Egurbide MV, et al. Transiently positive anticardiolipin antibodies do not increase the risk of thrombosis in patients with systemic lupus erythematosus. Lupus. 2007;16:810-6. [PubMed]
16. Mok CC, Tang S, To C, Petri M. Incidence and risk factors of thromboembolism in systemic lupus erythe-matosus: a comparison of three ethnic groups. Arthritis Rheum. 2005;52:2774-82. [PubMed]
17. Ruiz-Irastorza G, Egurbide MV, Ugalde J, Aguirre C. High impact of antiphospholipid syndrome on irreversible organ damage and survival of patients with systemic lupus erythematosus. Arch Intern Med. 2004;164:77-82. [PubMed]
18. De Groot PG, Horbach DA, Simmelink MJ, Van Oort E, Derksen RH. Antiprothrombin antibodies and their relation with thrombosis and lupus anticoagulant. Lupus. 1998;7(Suppl 2):S32-S36. [PubMed]
19. Satoh A, Suzuki K, Takayama E, et al. Detection of anti-annexin IV and V antibodies in patients with antiphospholipid syndrome and systemic lupus erythematosus. J Rheumatol. 1999;26:1715-20.[PubMed]
20. Girardi G, Redecha P, Salmon JE. Heparin prevents antiphospholipid antibody-induced fetal loss by inhibiting complement activation. Nat Med. 2004;10:1222-6. [PubMed]
21. Pierangeli SS, Chen PP, Gonzalez EB. Antiphospholipid antibodies and the antiphospholipid syndrome: an update on treatment and pathogenic mechanisms. Curr Opin Hematol. 2006;13:366-75. [PubMed]
22. Riboldi P, Gerosa M, Raschi E, Testoni C, Meroni PL. Endothelium as a target for antiphospholipid antibodies. Immunobiology. 2003;207:29-36. [PubMed]
23. Esmon NL, Safa O, Smirnov MD, Esmon CT. Antiphospholipid antibodies and the protein C pathway. J Autoimmun. 2000;15:221-5.[PubMed]
24. Lin WS, Chen PC, Yang CD, et al. Some antiphospholipid antibodies recognize conformational epitopes shared by beta2-glycoprotein I and the homologous catalytic domains of several serine proteases. Arthritis Rheum. 2007;56:1638-47. [PMC free article] [PubMed]
25. Rand JH, Wu XX, Quinn AS, et al. Human monoclonal antiphospholipid antibodies disrupt the annexin A5 anticoagulant crystal shield on phospholipid bilayers:

evidence from atomic force microscopy and functional assay. Am J Pathol. 2003;163:1193-200.[PMC free article] [PubMed]
26. Salmon JE, Girardi G. Antiphospholipid antibodies and pregnancy loss: a disorder of inflammation. J ReprodImmunol. 2007 Epub ahead of print, PMID: 17418423. [PMC free article] [PubMed]
27. Erkan D, Merrill JT, Yazici Y, et al. High thrombosis rate after fetal loss in antiphospholipid syndrome: effective prophylaxis with aspirin. Arthritis Rheum. 2001;44:1466-7. [PubMed]
28. Lockshin MD, Sammaritano LR, Schwartzman S. Validation of the Sapporo criteria for antiphospholipid syndrome. Arthritis Rheum. 2000;43:440-3.
29. Wilson A, Gharavi AE, Koike T, et al. International consensus statement on preliminary classification criteria for definite antiphospholipid syndrome. Arthritis Rheum. 1999;42:1309-11.[PubMed]
30. Miyakis S, Lockshin MD, Atsumi T, et al. International consensus statement on an update of the classification criteria for definite antiphospholipid syndrome (APS) J ThrombHaemost. 2006;4:295-306.[PubMed]
31. The American College of Obstetricians and Gynecologists. Antiphospholipid Syndrome. January/2011;118:1-8. ACOG Practice Bulletin. 2011;118:1-8.
32. Lackner KJ, Peetz D, von Landenberg P. Revision of the Sapporo criteria for the antiphospholipid syndrome-coming to grips with evidence and Thomas Bayes? Thromb Haemost. 2006;95:917-19. [PubMed]
33. Perez MC, Wilson WA, Brown HL, Scopelitis E. Anticardiolipin antibodies in unselected pregnant women in relationship to fetal outcome. J Perinatol. 1991;11:33-6.
34. Rix P, Stentoft J, Aunsholt NA, Dueholm M, Tilma KA, Hoier-Madsen M. Lupus anticoagulant and anticardiolipin antibodies in an obstetric population. Acta Obstet Gynecol Scand. 1992;71:605-9.
35. Pattison NS, Chamley LW, McKay EJ, Liggins GC, Butler WS. Antiphospholipid antibodies in pregnancy: prevalence and clinical associations. Br J Obstet Gynaecol.1993;100:909-13.
36. Phadke KV, Phillips RA, Clarke DT, Jones M, Naish P, Carson P. Anticardiolipin antibodies in ischaemic heart disease: marker or myth? Br Heart J. 1993;69:391-4.
37. Branch DW, Khamashta MA. Antiphospholipid syndrome: obstetric diagnosis, management, and controversies. Obstet Gynecol. 2003;101:1333-44. [PubMed].
38. Lim W, Crowther MA, Eikelboom JW. Management of antiphospholipid antibody syndrome. A systematic Review. JAMA. 2006;295(9).
39. Cowchock FS, Reece EA, Baldan D, et al. Repeated fetal losses associated with antiphospholipid antibodies: a collaborative randomized trial comparing prednisone with low dose heparin treatment. Am J Obstet Gynecol. 1992;166:1318-27. [PubMed]
40. Empson M, Lassere M, Craig J, Scott J. Prevention of recurrent miscarriage for women with antiphospholipid antibody or lupus anticoagulant. Cochrane Database Syst Rev. 2005;CD002859 [PubMed]
41. Rai R, Cohen H, Dave M, Regan L. Randomised controlled trial of aspirin and aspirin plus heparin in pregnant women with recurrent miscarriage associated with phospholipid antibodies (or antiphospholipid antibodies) BMJ. 1997;314:253-57. [PMC free article] [PubMed].
42. Davis SM, Branch DW. Thromboprophylaxis in Pregnancy: Who and How? Obstet Gynecol Clin N Am. 2010;37:333-43. [PubMed].
43. Gris JC, Quire I, Monpeyroux F, et al. Case-control study of the frequency of thrombophilic disorders in couples with late foetal loss and no thrombotic antecedent-the Nimes obstetricians and hematologists study 5 (NOHA 5) Thrombosis Haemostasis. 1999;81:891-9. [PubMed]
44. Erkan D, Yazici Y, Peterson MG, Sammaritano L, Lockshin MD. A cross-sectional study of clinical thrombotic risk factors and preventive treatments in antiphospholipid syndrome. Rheumatology (Oxford). 2002;41:924-9. [PubMed]
45. Kaiser R, Cleveland C, Criswell L. Risk and protective factors for thrombosis in systemic lupus erythematosus: results from a large, multiethnic cohort. Ann Rheum Dis. 2009;68:238-41. [PMC free article][PubMed]
46. Espinola RG, Pierangeli SS, Gharavi AE, Harris EN. Hydroxychloroquine reverses platelet activation induced by human IgG antiphospholipid antibodies. Thromb Haemost. 2002;87:518-22. [PubMed]
47. Edwards MH, Pierangeli S, Liu X, Barker JH, Anderson G, Harris EN. Hydroxychloroquine reverses thrombogenic properties of antiphospholipid antibodies in mice. Circulation. 1997;96:4380-4.[PubMed]
48. Rand J, Wu X, Quinn A, Chen P, Hathcock J, Taatjes D. Hydroxychloroquine directly reduces the binding of antiphospholipid antibody-β2-glycoprotein I complexes to phospholipid bilayers. Blood. 2008;112:1687-95. [PMC free article] [PubMed]
49. Rand JH, Wu XX, Quinn AS, et al. Hydroxychloroquine protects the annexin A5 anticoagulant shield from disruption by antiphospholipid antibodies: evidence for a novel effect for an old antimalarial drug. Blood. 2010;115:2292-9. [PMC free article]
50. Ruiz-Irastorza G, Ramos-Casals M, Brito-Zeron P, Khamashta MA. Clinical efficacy and side effects of antimalarials in systemic lupus erythematosus: a systematic review. Ann Rheum Dis. 2010;69:20-8.[PubMed]
51. Salmon JE, Girardi G. Antiphospholipid antibodies and pregnancy loss: a disorder of inflammation. J ReprodImmunol. 2007 Epub ahead of print, PMID: 17418423. [PMC free article] [PubMed]

Chapter 49

Dermatological Disorders in Pregnancy

Ritu Choubey, Pushpa Pandey

INTRODUCTION

During pregnancy, the body undergoes multiple hormonal, immunological[1] and metabolic changes which manifest as alterations on the skin. As a result of these changes, the skin develops certain physiological changes and sometimes pregnancy-specific skin conditions (*dermatoses*). Pregnancy also affects the pre-existing skin disorders while certain skin infections are common due to the immunological changes. To understand these clearly, the common skin disorders in pregnancy can be categorized broadly into following three categories:
1. Physiological skin changes
2. Infections and pre-existing skin disorders
3. Pregnancy-specific dermatoses.

PHYSIOLOGICAL SKIN CHANGES

It is imperative to understand the normal physiological changes[2] that occur during gestation as it helps in differentiating between pathological skin conditions and to avoid any undue therapeutic interventions. Due to the profound hormonal, immunological and metabolic changes[3] there are a variety of skin diseases which manifest for the first time in pregnancy while some pre-existing skin disorders or conditions show exacerbation or go into remission.

Most of the physiological changes reverse postpartum and pose no maternal or fetal risk.

Some of the most common physiological changes are listed below in **Table 49.1**.

Table 49.1: Physiological skin changes during pregnancy
- Pigmentary changes
- Hair and nail changes
- Vascular changes
- Glandular changes
- Connective tissue changes
- Mucosal changes

PIGMENTARY CHANGES

Pigmentary changes occur in 90% women[2] of every race during pregnancy. This is due to the raised levels of MSH (melanocyte-stimulating hormone), estrogens and progesterone.

Hyperpigmentation may manifest as diffuse or selective. Selective hyperpigmentation occurs in the already pigmented areas like areola, groins and axillae. Linea nigra is an example of selective hyperpigmentation. It is a linear pigmented band in the midline of abdominal wall.

Melasma, also known as chloasma or mask of pregnancy, is very common in Indian women. It is an irregular hyperpigmented symmetrical macular pigmentation that develops on the face. It can be centrofacial (involving the central part of the face on the cheeks, malar areas, above eyebrows and upper lip), malar (cheeks and nose) or mandibular in distribution. Estrogens are believed to play a role in the development of melasma. Melasma, sometimes, improves spontaneously during pregnancy or may remain unchanged after delivery. Treatment of melasma is not recommended during pregnancy and the woman should only be advised a good sunscreen to prevent further darkening of the lesions by ultraviolet radiations.

There is darkening of moles and ephelides (*freckles*) seen during pregnancy but any major change in the size or surface of a mole warrants careful evaluation and intervention. Some women develop vulval melanosis which is pigmented macular lesions on the vulva.

Other pigmentary changes are worsening of acanthosis nigricans, especially in women who develop gestational diabetes while some show pseudoacanthotic changes. Pseudoacanthotic changes are hyperpigmented velvety plaques on the neck, groins, axillae, popliteal and antecubital fossa **(see Fig. 49.2)**. These changes involute spontaneously postpartum.

HAIR AND NAIL CHANGES

There is a change in the hair cycle during pregnancy due to the effect of estrogens. Some women develop mild to moderate hirsutism which may or may not resolve after delivery. If the extent of hirsutism is more than expected and associated with acne and other signs of virilization, polycystic ovaries, ovarian tumors, etc. should be ruled out. Some women only develop hypertrichosis. The fine hair usually resolve within 6 months of delivery.

The terminal coarse hair can be treated with laser six months after delivery but can recur in subsequent pregnancies.

Some women experience hair thinning during pregnancy[3,4] especially in the temporoparietal region but majority of them, experience hair shedding after delivery (known as *telogen effluvium*) which can be very distressing and can take up to one year for recovery.

Nail changes during pregnancy include increased growth, brittleness, softening and in some cases, onycholysis. Other nail changes include longitudinal melanonychia, transverse grooves on the nail plate or tumors like granuloma gravidarum (discussed under vascular changes).

All these changes usually resolve postpartum. The pregnant woman should be counseled about the transient nature of these changes. Etiologies like thyrotoxicosis (in onycholysis), vitamin deficiencies should be ruled out. The woman should be advised to keep the nails short and to avoid use of nail paints and removers.

VASCULAR CHANGES

Vascular changes include increased vascularity[2] as a result of hormonal changes. These manifest as palmar erythema, nonpitting edema of the face and extremities, spider nevi and dilated capillaries, telangiectasia at various sites.

Sometimes, women develop a soft, friable, deep red nodular lesion which can arise on the mucosal surface like the gingiva or any other nonmucosal sites like face, extremities or nail bed. This is known as pyogenic granuloma, also known as granuloma gravidarum (**Fig. 49.1**). It is a benign vascular lesion which can bleed with trivial trauma or ulcerate and become painful. It usually regresses after delivery but can be cauterized using electrocautery or radiocautery in the second trimester if it becomes symptomatic.

Varicosities and hemorrhoids occur quite often in pregnant women for which the pregnant women are advised leg elevation and left lateral position for sleeping.

Petechial or purpuric spots, especially on the lower extremities are, sometimes, seen in pregnant women which resolve after child birth.

Hemangiomas may also develop during pregnancy and can be treated with laser after delivery if they do not undergo spontaneous regression.

CONNECTIVE TISSUE CHANGES

These include development of striae, skin tags, increase in the size of pre-existing keloids or hypertrophic scars.

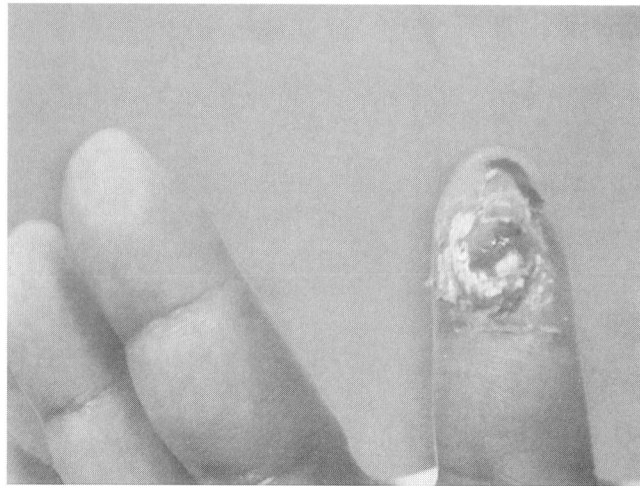

Fig. 49.1: Depicting granuloma gravidarum (pyogenic granuloma on the index finger) *(For color version, see Plate 4)*

Striae distensae (stretch marks) develop as a result of the connective tissue changes.[2] These are atrophic scars which are pinkish red (striae rubra) initially and later become white (striae alba). Striae run parallel to the skin tension lines and predominantly appear on the abdomen, breast, buttocks and thighs. The woman can experience pruritus initially on the stretch marks.

Skin tags (also known as *acrochordons*) are benign outgrowths of skin commonly appearing on the neck, axillae and groins (**Fig. 49.2**).

All these conditions can be treated postpartum for cosmetic purposes.

GLANDULAR CHANGES

Different glands like the apocrine, eccrine and sebaceous glands undergo changes in their functioning during pregnancy. Due to the sebaceous gland activity some patients develop acne for the first time during pregnancy while some with pre-existing acne may show an exacerbation. Rosacea may have an unpredictable course while some women develop perioral dermatitis (**Fig. 49.3**).

Due to the changes in the eccrine gland activity some women develop hyperhidrosis and develop miliaria (*prickly heat*) while some show reduced palmar sweating. Those with fox Fordyce's disease[5] also known as apocrine miliaria (**Fig. 49.4**) often show improvement in pregnancy.

MUCOSAL CHANGES

There is increased vascularity[2] of the mucosal surfaces leading to gingival edema and hypertrophy. Gingivitis and periodontitis may develop in some women while some develop pyogenic granuloma.

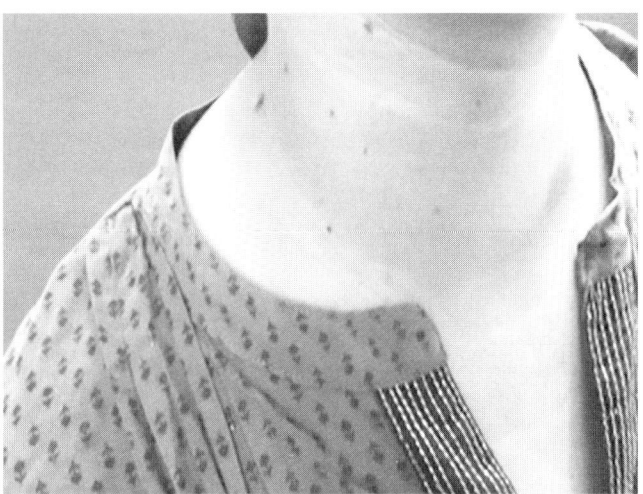

Fig. 49.2: Pseudoacanthotic changes on the neck with skin tags *(For color version, see Plate 4)*

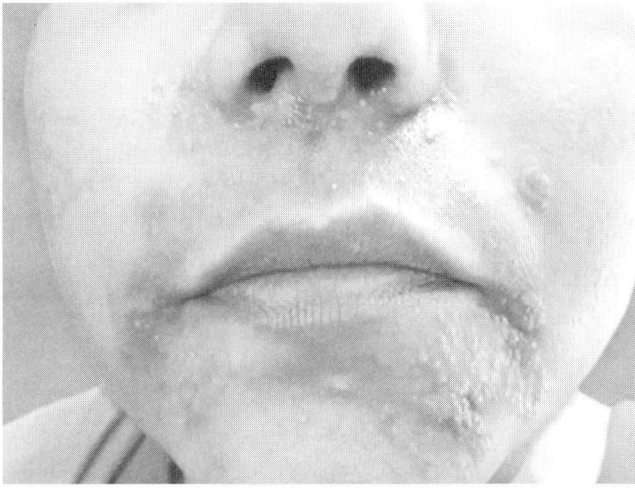

Fig. 49.3: Perioral dermatitis *(For color version, see Plate 4)*

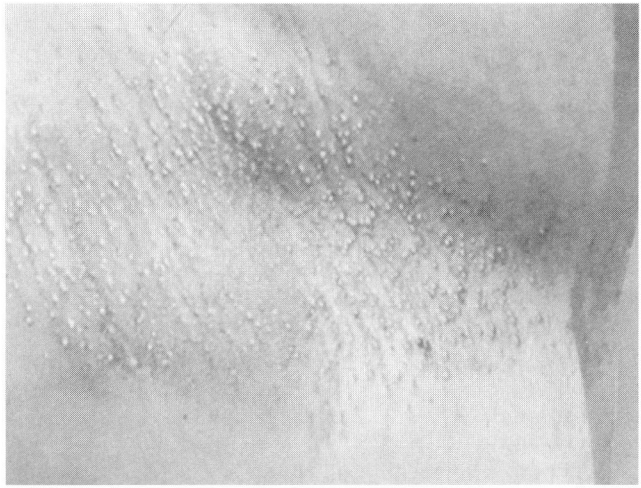

Fig. 49.4: Fox Fordyce's disease (axilla) *(For color version, see Plate 4)*

SKIN INFECTIONS AND PRE-EXISTING SKIN DISORDERS IN PREGNANCY

The cell-mediated immunity is lowered[1,3] during pregnancy because of which pregnant women are more prone to developing certain skin infections and there may be an exacerbation of certain pre-existing skin disorders. Some of the common skin infections during pregnancy are categorized in **Table 49.2**.

Bacterial Infections

Some of the commonest bacterial infections seen during pregnancy are skin and soft tissue infections (SSTIs) like folliculitis, abscesses, cellulitis, impetigo caused by *Staphylococcus aureus, Streptococcus.*

These infections can be treated with appropriate topical antibiotics like mupirocin and clindamycin and, if required, systemic antibiotics-like penicillins or cephalosporins can be used which are safe in pregnancy.

Fungal Infections

Superficial dermatophytic infection (like tinea cruris and corporis), pityriasis versicolor, candidiasis (discussed under sexually transmitted diseases) are commonly seen, especially in tropical countries.

Today, there is a rising trend of fungal infections. Newer molecules like eberconazole, oxiconazole, luliconazole, butenafine may be used. Systemic terbinafine may be used.[6] Safety of the other systemic antifungal is highlighted in **Table 49.3**.

Viral Infections

Herpes simplex, herpes zoster, varicella and HPV (human papilloma virus) infection (condylomata acuminata) are some of the viral infections seen in pregnancy. Herpes simplex and varicella infections can affect the fetal outcome so these should be promptly treated.

Table 49.2: Skin infections during pregnancy

- *Bacterial infections:* SSTIs (skin and soft tissue infections), impetigo
- *Fungal infections:* Superficial dermatophytosis, candidiasis
- *Viral infections:* Herpes simplex, herpes zoster, varicella and HPV infections
- *Mycobacterium infections:* Leprosy, cutaneous tuberculosis (rare)
- *Sexually transmitted diseases:* Syphilis, gonorrhea, candidiasis, trichomoniasis, vaginosis
- *Parasitic infections:* Scabies and pediculosis

Table 49.3: US-FDA prescribing categories

Categories	Description
A	Controlled studies show no fetal risk
B	No fetal risk despite possible animal risk or animal studies don't show fetal risk and human studies are lacking
C	Risk cannot be ruled out, human and animal studies are lacking
D	Human studies show positive evidence for fetal risk
X	Contraindicated in pregnancy. Data show fetal risk that outweigh any benefit

Herpes simplex infection could be a primary infection or recurrence. Genital herpes is caused by HSV-2 (Herpes Simplex Virus) while orolabial herpes is caused by HSV-1. These present with grouped vesicular lesions on erythematous base which are painful and may or may not be associated with lymphadenopathy. Diagnosing genital herpes may be challenging as they may not present as classical vesicular lesions but as ulcerations. These can be treated with systemic acyclovir[7] which is safe in pregnancy.

Herpes zoster is a varicella zoster virus infection which manifests as grouped vesicular lesions unilaterally in dermatomal distribution and associated with pain and burning. This can be treated with systemic acyclovir.

Varicella infection (chicken pox) carries the risk of congenital varicella syndrome in the child, especially if it occurs within the first 20 weeks. Acyclovir can be used safely.

HPV infections like genital warts (*condylomata acuminata*) usually become bigger in size and number and can infect the child. These can be treated with destructive therapies like electrocautery or radiocautery or cryotherapy. Agents like podophyllin and 5-fluorouracil are contraindicated in pregnancy.

Mycobacterial Infections

Leprosy and cutaneous tuberculosis (very rare) are commonly seen mycobacterial infections in India.

Due to the reduced cellular immunity[1,3] the course of leprosy is adversely affected during pregnancy.[8] There can be a relapse of leprosy or women with pre-existing leprosy infection may develop lepra reactions. Multidrug therapy with rifampicin, dapsone and clofazimine should be continued during pregnancy and systemic corticosteroids are used to control the lepra reactions.

Sexually Transmitted Diseases

Bacterial vaginosis, vaginal candidiasis, trichomoniasis, Chlamydia infection, syphilis, gonorrhea are some of the commonest sexually transmitted diseases.

Universal screening during the prenatal visit for sexually transmitted diseases is recommended.[9] Treatment recommended for these sexually transmitted diseases (STDs) is highlighted below in **Table 49.4**.

Table 49.4: Treatment recommendation for STDs

• Candidiasis	Clotrimazole 1% or miconazole 2% cream daily for 7 days
• Bacterial vaginosis	Oral metronidazole 500 mg twice daily for 7 days
• Trichomoniasis	Oral metronidazole 2 g orally
• Chlamydia	Oral azithromycin 1 g orally single dose or amoxicillin 500 mg thrice daily for 7 days
• Gonorrhea	Injection ceftriaxone 250 mg intra-muscularly
• Syphilis	Primary, secondary and early latent (acquired less than 1 year) inj benzathine penicillin 2.4 million units intramuscularly as a single dose. In cases of late syphilis to be repeated weekly for 3 weeks. In penicillin allergic patients, doxycycline 100 mg be given twice daily for 2 weeks.

Parasitic Infections

Scabies and pediculosis are commonly seen amongst the rural population of India. Scabies is a common differential diagnosis for pregnancy-specific dermatoses. These are treated with single application of topical permethrin cream.

Other than the above mentioned infections, some patients have pre-existing disorders which may have an unpredictable course during pregnancy. Women with pre-existing psoriasis may show worsening of the lesions during pregnancy. Connective tissue disorders like systemic lupus erythematosus (SLE) may worsen during pregnancy while systemic sclerosis may show improvement during pregnancy and then worsen postpartum.[10]

PREGNANCY-SPECIFIC DERMATOSES

Pregnancy-specific dermatoses[11-13] are a group of hetero-geneous inflammatory pruritic disorders attributed to pregnancy. These disorders share a common symptom of pruritus. Some of these are distressing for the patient due to profound itching while some are associated with adverse maternal and fetal outcome.

There are many different classifications for pregnancy-specific dermatoses but for practical purposes these can be broadly classified into **Table 49.5**.

ATOPIC ERUPTION OF PREGNANCY

These account for 50% of the pregnancy associated pruritic disorders[14] with an incidence of 1:10.

Synonyms

Prurigo gestationis (Besnier), papular dermatitis of pregnancy, early onset prurigo of pregnancy, pruritic folliculitis of pregnancy, papular dermatitis of Spangler.

Table 49.5: Pregnancy-specific dermatosis

Dermatoses without fetal risk	Dermatoses with fetal risk
Atopic eruption of pregnancy (AEP)	Pemphigoid gestationis
Polymorphic eruption of pregnancy (PEP)	Pustular psoriasis
Intrahepatic cholestasis of pregnancy (ICP)	

Etiology

Pregnancy-induced alterations in the Th1 and Th2 cytokine balance with dominant Th2 response are believed to be responsible. There is usually a family or personal history of atopy although the skin manifestations may occur for the first time in pregnancy. Approach to a pregnant patient presenting with pruritus is shown in **Flow chart 49.1**.

Clinical Presentation

It occurs early in the pregnancy (often first trimester). Almost all patients present with pruritic papules and eczematous lesions with excoriations at the classical sites of atopic dermatitis (like the antecubital, popliteal fossa, nape of the neck, face). Some may develop follicular papules or pustules[15] on the trunk which may involve the extremities. Those women with pre-existing atopic dermatitis may show worsening of the lesions. There is marked xerosis associated with pruritus. This condition does not affect the fetal outcome and responds well to the treatment.

Laboratory Findings

Elevated levels of serum IgE are seen in the majority of the patients.

Flow chart 49.1: Algorithmic approach for pruritus in pregnancy

```
                        Pruritus in pregnancy
                    ┌────────────┴────────────┐
           Pruritus with skin lesions    Pruritus without skin
                                         lesions (only excoriations)
        ┌──────────┴──────────┐           ┌──────────┴──────────┐
   Any trimester          3rd trimester   Raised            Laboratory
                                          serum bile        findings
                                          acids             normal
  ┌─────────┴─────────┐                     │                  │
- History of atopy +/-  - No history of atopy  ICP***      Rule out other
- Eczematous lesions    - Laboratory findings               causes like
  on the typical sites    normal                            contact
  of atopic dermatitis                                      dermatitis,
- Raised IgE levels                                         infections and
        │                  │                                drug eruptions
        │                  │           ┌─────────┴─────────┐
      AEP*         Rule out other    - Periumbilical     - Papular and/or bullous
                   causes like         papular lesions     lesions
                   contact dermatitis, - Laboratory       - Skin biopsy with DIF***
                   infections,          findings normal     confirms the diagnosis
                   drug eruptions          │                  │
                                         PEP**              PG****
```

AEP*   - Atopic eruption of pregnancy
PEP**   - Polymorphic eruption of pregnancy
ICP*** - Intrahepatic cholestasis of pregnancy
PG**** - Pemphigoid gestationis

Prognosis

No maternal or fetal risk. The condition responds to therapy and recurrences are seen in subsequent pregnancies.

Differential Diagnosis

Polymorphic eruption of pregnancy, intrahepatic cholestasis, scabies and other causes of dermatitis not associated with pregnancy.

Treatment

Treatment is aimed at relieving the itching. Patients are advised to avoid excessive use of soaps. Topical emollients, topical low to mid potent steroids, systemic antihistaminics are used. The patient should be advised to use topical steroids only under supervision. Treatment of secondary infection and, in some cases, UVB (ultraviolet B) therapy may be necessary.

First-line
- Topical emollients
- Topical steroids
- Oral antihistaminics

Second-line
- Narrow band UVB therapy

Third-line
- Systemic steroids

Salient Points

- Pruritic skin lesions on the typical atopic dermatitis sites
- There may or may not be a history of atopy
- Majority of patients have raised levels of IgE levels
- Does not affect the maternal or fetal outcome
- Responds well to the treatment

POLYMORPHIC ERUPTION OF PREGNANCY (PEP)

This is the second most common dermatoses[12,13] in pregnancy with an incidence of 1:160–200.

Synonyms

Pruritic urticarial papules and plaques of pregnancy (PUPP), late onset prurigo of pregnancy, toxemic rash of pregnancy.

Etiology

Unknown. Antigenic stimulation leading to allergic reaction from skin stretching is suggested as a trigger. Excessive weight gain and multiple gestation pregnancies are the risk factors.

Clinical Presentation

It occurs most often in the primiparous women and tends to occur late in the third trimester (particularly last few weeks) of pregnancy. The eruption is associated with severe pruritus and consists of wide spread erythema and urticarial papules and plaques (sometimes vesicles or targetoid lesions) *sparing the umbilicus.*[16] The lesions typically appear first in the striae and later spread to the buttocks, lateral part of the trunk and extremities. Unlike AEP, face is rarely involved **(Figs 49.5A and B)**.

Laboratory Findings

Normal.

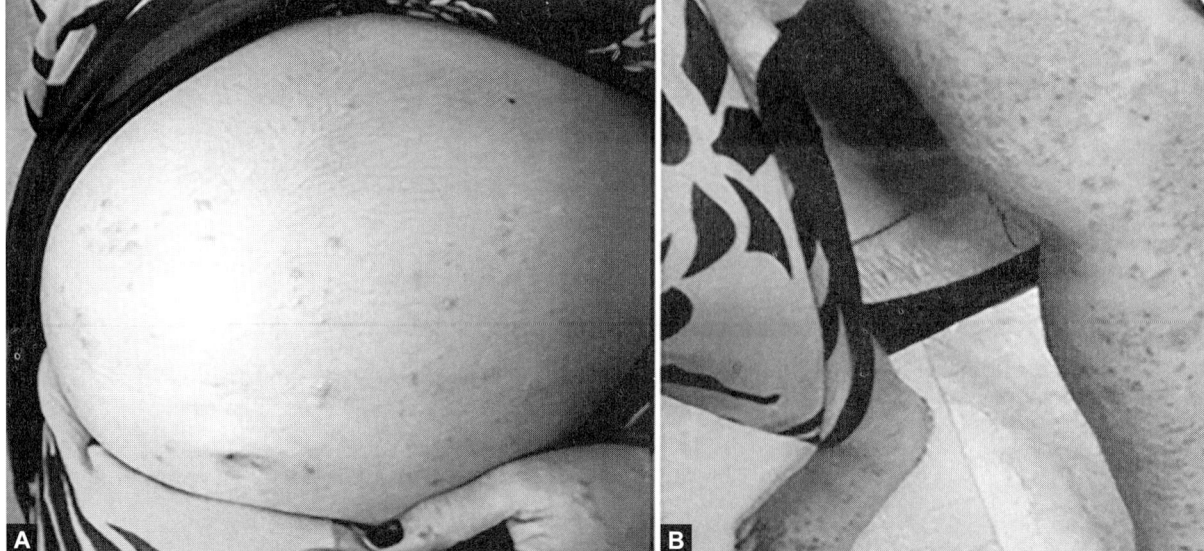

Figs 49.5A and B: (A) Pruritic papular lesions (periumbilical) of PEP; (B) Erythematous papules and plaques with targetoid lesions on the lower extremity of PEP *(For color version, see Plate 4)*

Prognosis

No maternal or fetal risk associated with this condition. Lesions resolve within 4 weeks postpartum. This condition usually does not recur in subsequent pregnancies.

Differential Diagnosis

Drug eruption, erythema multiforme, scabies, allergic contact dermatitis and pemphigoid gestationis (discussed later). See **Flow chart 49.1**.

Treatment

Topical corticosteroids and systemic antihistaminics are the mainstay of the treatment; while in severe cases, systemic steroids (prednisolone) can be used.

First-line
- Topical emollients
- Topical steroids
- Oral antihistamines

Second-line
- Systemic steroids

Salient Points

- Manifests late in pregnancy (usually late third trimester)
- Lesions comprise pruritic urticarial papules and plaques sparing the umbilicus
- No adverse maternal or fetal outcome.

INTRAHEPATIC CHOLESTASIS OF PREGNANCY

This condition has an incidence of 0.02–27%. This may or may not be associated with jaundice[17] but pruritus is quite severe. This dermatoses of pregnancy may be associated with adverse fetal outcomes. Timely correction of biochemical abnormalities and increased fetal monitoring helps in preventing any adverse fetal outcomes.

Synonyms

Obstetric cholestasis, prurigo gravidarum.

Etiology

It is complex[18] but may be due to the increased levels of bile salts in the blood due to the effect of maternal estrogens on hepatocytes.

Clinical Presentation

This usually starts in the late second or third trimester. The patient presents with intense pruritus which begins on the palms and soles and then may become generalized. There are *no primary skin lesions* but excoriation marks and prurigo-like lesions.[18] Itching is often worse at night leading to insomnia. Ten percent of patients only develop jaundice[19] usually after the onset of pruritus.

Laboratory Findings

Liver function tests are deranged and the serum bile acids are raised. Liver ultrasound is normal.

Prognosis

Pruritus resolves soon after delivery. However, recurrence is seen in subsequent pregnancies. Fetal risks include premature birth, fetal distress and fetal loss. Maternal hemorrhage may result due to impaired vitamin K absorption.

Differential Diagnosis

Atopic eruption of pregnancy (AEP), polymorphic eruption of pregnancy (PEP). Refer to **Flow chart 49.1**.

Treatment

Emollients, topical corticosteroids and oral antihistamines are ineffective in allaying the itching. Ursodeoxycholic acid (UDCA) is the only treatment which reduces the maternal pruritus and reduces the fetal risk. It is given in the dose of 15 mg/kg body weight/day. It is safe during the third trimester of pregnancy although it is not FDA approved. Prompt diagnosis and close surveillance and weekly monitoring is recommended to prevent any maternal and fetal complications.

First-line
- Topical emollients
- Oral antihistaminics
- Oral UDCA

Second-line
- Cholestyramine

Salient Points

- No primary skin lesions are seen
- There is severe pruritus which begins from palms and soles and then becomes generalized
- Increased levels of serum bile acids
- May be associated with adverse maternal and fetal outcomes like postpartum hemorrhage, stillbirths.

PEMPHIGOID GESTATIONIS

This is a rare autoimmune vesiculobullous pruritic disorder with a prevalence ranging from 1 in 7000 to 1 in 50,000 pregnancies.

Synonym

Herpes gestationis.

Etiology

It is an autoimmune disorder. Antibodies are produced against the BP (bullous pemphigoid) antigen in the skin BMZ (basement membrane zone). The cause of antibody production is not known. It is more likely to occur in older patients and those with a history of pemphigoid gestationis in the previous pregnancies.

Clinical Presentation

Pemphigoid gestationis[20] presents abruptly with intense pruritus followed by urticarial papules and plaques involving the periumbilical area which can become polycyclic or targetoid and develop bullous lesions within these areas. The lesions can gradually become generalized but usually spare the face and the mucosal surfaces. Some patients may not develop bullous lesions and the lesions can be confused with urticaria or PEP or erythema multiforme.

Laboratory Findings

Skin biopsy with direct immunofluorescence evaluation confirms the diagnosis.

Prognosis

The course is variable as it may undergo remission during pregnancy and relapse after delivery. Rarely, it can progress to bullous pemphigoid. It often recurs in subsequent pregnancies and is more severe. Some neonates may develop a transient rash due to the maternal antibodies. Small for gestation age weight at birth and preterm deliveries are reported. The chances of adverse outcomes are more if the condition develops early in the pregnancy. Mother is at an increased risk of developing autoimmune disorders like Grave's disease.

Differential Diagnosis

Urticaria, drug eruption, erythema multiforme, PEP (in prebullous stage) and other autoimmune vesiculobullous disorders such as linear IgA disease, dermatitis herpetiformis and pemphigus vulgaris.

Treatment

In mild cases, topical steroids, systemic antihistamines and cool compresses provide relief. In severe cases with generalized bullous lesions, systemic corticosteroids (prednisolone) in the dose of 0.5–1 mg/kg/day is used and then tapered as the lesions subside.[21] Azathioprine may be used in patients who do not respond to systemic steroids. Patients are advised to avoid oral contraceptives after delivery to prevent any relapses.

First-line
- Topical emollients
- Topical steroids
- Oral antihistaminics

Second-line
- Systemic steroids

Third-line
- Azathioprine

Salient Points

- Rare autoimmune disorder
- It may start as urticarial lesions followed by bullous lesions on the body. Face and mucosa are spared
- Fetal risks include fetal growth retardation and premature delivery.

IMPETIGO HERPETIFORMIS

This is an acute pustular eruption in pregnancy without any family history or previous history of psoriasis.

Synonym

Generalized pustular psoriasis of pregnancy.

Etiology

It is attributed to high estrogens and progesterone levels.[21,22]

Clinical Presentation

The eruption usually starts in the third trimester. It manifests as tiny pustular lesions on erythematous patches in the flexural regions which tend to spread to the trunk and extremities. The pustules are sterile and the lesions can become confluent-forming lakes of pus. The lesions can become secondarily infected. The lesions are usually non-pruritic but may be accompanied by fever, chills, malaise and arthralgia. The patients may develop hypocalcemia and signs of hypoparathyroidism like tetany. Fetal monitoring for placental insufficiency should be done at regular intervals for placental insufficiency.

Laboratory Findings

Histopathological examination is suggestive of pustular psoriasis. Peripheral blood picture shows leukocytosis with neutrophilia, raised ESR and hypocalcemia, hypo-albuminemia, and electrolyte imbalance.

Table 49.6: Drug safety				
Sr. No.	Drug category	FDA category	Drug category	FDA category
	Systemic		Topical	
1.	Antibiotics			
	Azithromycin	B	Mupirocin	B
	Cephalosporins	B	Silver sulphadiazine	B
	Penicillin	B	Clindamycin	B
	Metronidazole	B	Erythromycin	B
	Fluoroquinolones	C	Metronidazole	B
	Tetracyclines	D	Benzoyl peroxide	C
2.	Antifungal			
	Terbinafine	B	Clotrimazole	B
	Fluconazole	C	Miconazole	B
	Iatraconazole	C	Terbinafine	B
	Ketoconazole	C	Ciclopirox olamine	B
	Griesofulvin	C	Oxiconazole	C
			Ketoconazole	C
3.	Antiparasitic			
	Ivermectin	C	Permethrin	B
			Lindane	C
			Crotamiton	C
4.	Steroids			
	Prednisone	C	Steroids	C
	Prednisolone	C		
	Methyl prednisolone	C		
5.	Antiviral			
	Acyclovir	B		
	Famcyclovir	B		
	Valacyclovir	B		
6.	Antihistaminics			
	Chlorphenaramine	B		
	Diphenhydramine	B		
	Cetirizine	B		
	Loratadine	B		
	Fexofenadine	C		
	Hydroxyzine	C		
7.	Category X drugs			
	Systemic retinoids (isotretinoin, acitretin)			
	Methotrexate			
	Thallidomide			
	Finasteride			
8.	Miscellaneous			
	Cyclosporine	C		
	Azathioprine	D		
	Dapsone	C		

Prognosis

Maternal risk of sepsis and complications is more if the condition develops early in pregnancy and the lesions are widespread or become secondarily infected. Fetal risks are those of low birth weight babies, intrauterine growth retardation and stillbirth.

Differential Diagnosis

Pustular drug eruption, pemphigoid gestationis, subcorneal pustular dermatitis and other infectious causes of pustular eruptions.

Treatment

Prompt treatment is imperative. The treatment involves correction of electrolyte imbalance and protein loss. Systemic corticosteroids are the first line of treatment. Prednisolone is used in the dose of up to 60–80 mg/day. Cyclosporine is the second drug of choice where steroids are contraindicated.[21] Broad spectrum antibiotics may be added to prevent secondary infection.

First-line
- Emollients
- Topical steroids

Second-line
- Narrow band UVB therapy

Third-line
- Systemic steroids
- cyclosporine

Salient Points

- Pustular lesions develop in the flexures which may later spread to the other areas
- Sterile pustular lesions which can become secondarily infected
- There may or may not be a previous history of psoriasis
- Fetal risks include low birth weight baby, intrauterine growth retardation while maternal risks include hypocalcemia and sepsis.

DERMATOLOGICAL DRUG SAFETY IN PREGNANCY

Treatment of dermatological conditions in pregnancy may have an effect on the mother and or fetus. Therefore, it is important to know the drug safety of commonly used drugs in pregnancy.[23] As described earlier, steroids are commonly used to treat most of the pregnancy-specific dermatosis. Therefore, certain safety guidelines are important to follow to prevent any morbidity because of adverse effects of the drugs. Halogenated corticosteroids should be used when required. Prednisolone is the steroid of choice as it is enzymatically inactivated in the placenta (unlike dexamethasone and betamethasone). The steroids should be used only for short term to avoid risk of cleft lip and cleft palate in the child or adrenal insufficiency in the newborn. Topical steroids are however, safer to use. These agents, if used, should be of low to mid potency and for limited period of time. FDA has a five-lettered pregnancy labeling system outlined in **Table 49.3**.

Commonly used systemic and topical drugs used during pregnancy and their safety according to the US FDA prescribing categories are highlighted in the **Table 49.6**.

REFERENCES

1. Yip, Mc Cluskey J, Sinclair R. Immunological aspects of pregnancy. Actadermatol venereal. 1975;55:11-3.
2. Muzzafar F, Hussein I, Haroon TS. Physiological skin changes associated with pregnancy. Int. J. Dermatol. 1998;37:29-31.
3. Pecoraro V, Barman JM, Astore I. The normal trichogram of pregnant women. In: Montagna W, Dobson RL (Eds). Advances in biology of skin, vol. IX. Hair Growth. Oxford: Pergamon; 1996. pp. 203-20.
4. Ingber A. Endocrine and immunologic alterations during pregnancy. In: Ingber A (Ed). Obstetric dermatology: A practical guide. Berlin, Germany: Springer-Verlag; 2009. pp. 1-5.
5. Hurley HL, Shelly WB. The human apocrine gland in health and disease. Springfield: Thomas; 1960. pp. 65-6.
6. Sobel JD. Use of antifungal drugs in pregnancy: a focus on safety. Drug Saf. 2000;23:7-85.
7. ACOG Practice Bulletin. Clinical management guidelines for obstetrician-gynaecologists. No. 82, June 2007. Management of herpes in pregnancy. Obstet Gynaecol. 2007;109:189-1498.
8. Lyde CB. Pregnancy in patients with Hansen's disease. Arch Dermatol. 1999;133:623-27.
9. Centre for disease control and prevention. Sexually transmitted diseases guidelines. Morb Mort Wkly Rep. 2010:59.
10. Winton GB. Skin diseases aggravated by pregnancy. J Am Acad Dermatol. 1989;20:1-13.
11. Ambros-Rudolph CM. Dermatoses of pregnancy. J Dtsch Dermatolaes. 2006;9:748-61.
12. Krompouzos G, Cohen LM. Dermatoses of pregnancy. J Am Acad Dermatol. 2003;6:236-40.
13. Winton GB. Skin diseases aggravated by pregnancy. J Am Acad Dermatol. 1989;20:1-13.
14. Ingber A. Atopic eruption of pregnancy. J Eur Acad Dermtol Venereol. 2010;24:974.
15. Kroumpouzos G, Cohen LM. Pruritic folliculitis of pregnancy . J Am Acad Dermatol. 2000;43:132-4.
16. Ambros-Rudolph CM, Black MM, Vaughan Jones S. The papular and pruritic dermatoses of pregnancy. In: Black MM, Ambros-Rudolph C, Edwards L, et al (Eds). Obstetritic and gynaecologic dermatology, 3rd edn. London, England: Mobsy Elsevier; 2008. pp. 73-7.
17. Smith A. Burkhart CG. Pruritus in pregnancy. Cutis. 1984;34: 86-8.
18. Cicek D, Kandi B, Demir B, et al. Intrahepatic cholestasis occurring with prurigo of pregnancy. Skin med. 2007;6:298-301.
19. Haemmerli UP. Jaundice during pregnancy. Acta Med Scand. 1996;179 (Suppl).
20. Shornick JK, Bangert JL, Freeman RG, et al. Herpes gestationis: clinical and histologic features of twenty eight cases. J Am. Acad Dermatol. 1983;8:21-224.
21. Tauscher A, Fleischer Jr AB, Phelps KC, et al. Psoriasis and pregnancy. J Cutan Med Surg. 2002;6:561-70.
22. Winzer M, Woff HH. Impetigo Herpetiformis. Hautarzt. 1998;39:110-13.
23. Briggs GG, Freeman RK, Yaffe, SJ (Eds). Drugs in pregnancy and lactation, 7th edn. Lippincot William & Wilkins, Philadelphia; 2005.

Chapter 50

Pregnancy and Oral Health

Shivani Dwivedi, Pushpa Pandey, Richa Baharani

INTRODUCTION

A woman's health is essential to the good health of her baby. The storm of hormones which is induced during pregnancy causes changes in the mother's body and are also associated with oral mucosal changes, most of which are reversible clinically. The oral changes which are commonly seen during pregnancy include gingivitis, pyogenic granuloma, mobility, erosion and salivary changes. Among the oral tissues, gingiva is the one that is most commonly affected.

New evidence supports an association between the periodontal status and complications during pregnancy and vice versa, hormonal changes in pregnancy affecting the oral status. Some countries have developed policies and practice guidelines recommend oral care and the control of inflammation of the periodontal tissues through pregnancy. Dental care has been proven to not only be safe and effective during pregnancy, but also necessary to promote sound oral health. Healthcare providers should recognize the importance of good oral health and ascertain the need for dental care during pregnancy and early childhood is met. This chapter will review the bidirectional relationship of pregnancy and periodontal or oral status.

ORAL CONDITIONS EFFECTING PREGNANCY

In recent years, periodontal diseases have been associated with a number of systemic diseases such as rheumatoid arthritis, cardiovascular disease, diabetes mellitus, chronic respiratory diseases and adverse pregnancy outcomes. It has been reported that maternal periodontal disease may be an independent contributor to abnormal pregnancy outcomes including preterm low birth weight (PLBW), miscarriage, risk for pre-eclampsia, mortality, and growth restriction. Dental problems such as caries, erosion, loose tooth, ill-fitting crowns, bridges, and dentures (prostheses) may have special significance during pregnancy especially labor. Increase in tooth decay during pregnancy may be due to change in diet and oral hygiene which results repeated acid attacks on tooth enamel. Nausea and vomiting in pregnancy may cause extensive erosion. A large number of studies have reported positive association between periodontal disease and adverse pregnancy outcomes[1-3] However, studies reporting no significant association,[4,5] constitute a small proportion of the total available evidence collected to date.

There are a number of risk factors associated with adverse pregnancy outcomes including low socioeconomic status, the mother's age, race, multiple births, smoking, drug and alcohol abuse and systemic maternal infection, however, these risk factors are absent in about one-fourth of PLBW cases, leading to continued search for other causes.[6] It has been shown that genitourinary tract infections and bacterial vaginosis, caused by aerobic and anaerobic bacteria, are associated with many adverse pregnancy outcomes including PLBW.[7]

BIOLOGICAL HYPOTHESES LINKING PRETERM BIRTH AND PERIODONTAL DISEASES

It is important to understand the underlying biologic mechanisms for the relationship between periodontal disease and adverse pregnancy outcome in order to provide a rationale for therapeutic interventions **(Flow chart 50.1)**. Considering epidemiological evidence, biological theories have been proposed to link preterm birth and periodontal diseases.[8]

Mainly, three hypotheses have been developed:
1. Bacterial spreading,
2. Inflammatory products dissemination,
3. Role of fetomaternal immune response against oral pathogens.

Bacterial Spreading

The current paradigm indicates that majority of intrauterine infections originate in the lower genital tract. Despite this statement, number of studies report intrauterine infections caused by species not found in urogenital tract.[9]

The bacterial spreading theory is based on the possible dissemination of oral bacteria including periodontal pathogens through blood circulation to the amniotic fluid

Flow chart 50.1: Mechanism linking periodontal infection and preterm labor

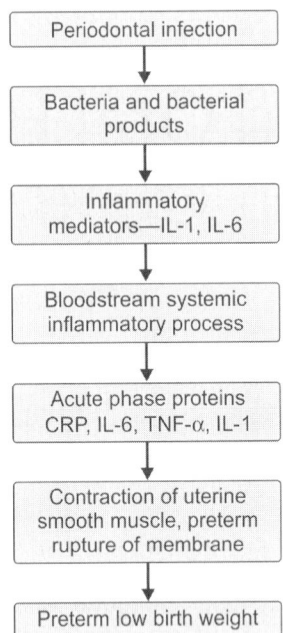

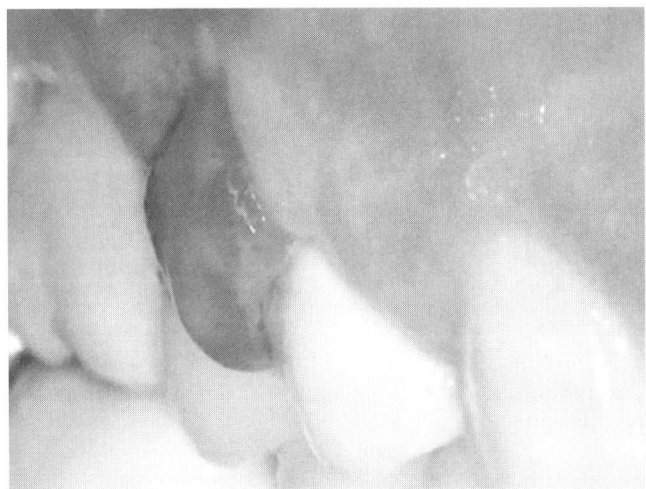

Fig. 50.1: Pyogenic granuloma *(For color version, see Plate 4)*

and leading to chorioamniotic infections.[10] The frequent gingival inflammation of women presenting periodontal diseases, facilitates bacteremia process.[9] Many analyses of amniotic fluid or placenta have been performed and shown the evidence of the presence of different oral pathogens such as *Bergeyella, Eikenella*,[9] *Fusobacterium nucleatum*, or *Porphyromonas gingivalis*.[11-13]

Inside uterus, these pathogens could provoke an inflammatory response. The increase of inflammatory cytokines or metalloproteases synthesis and the neutrophil activation could induce preterm birth process.[9] *In vivo* studies show that the invasiveness of uterine tissues largely depends on the type of bacteria. For example, *Porphyromonas gingivalis* could infect syncytiotrophoblasts, chorionic trophoblasts, decidual cells, and amniotic epithelial cells,[13] and promotes inflammatory process trough toll-like receptor 4.[14]

Hematogenous Dissemination of Inflammatory Products (Fig. 50.1)

The pathogenesis of periodontal diseases is mediated by the inflammatory response to bacteria in the dental biofilm. There is evidence that specific microbes are associated with the progressive forms of the disease; however, the presence of these microorganisms in individuals with no evidence of disease progression suggests that the disease is the net effect of the immune response and the inflammatory processes, not the mere presence of the bacteria. In the various immune mechanisms in the process of gingival inflammation, polymorphonuclear leukocytes (PMNs) are the primary effector cells and appear to play a major role. When stimulated by bacterial pathogens, host cells release proinflammatory cytokines as a part of the immune response. These cytokines recruit PMNs to the site of infection, releasing a variety of biologically active products, such as chemokines, proteolytic enzymes, cytokines, and reactive oxygen species (ROS) and thus indirectly contribute to increase of gingival inflammation, indicating depressed function of neutrophils can be damaging to gingiva.[15,16]

The data about the alteration in chemotaxis, cytokines, enzymes, and antioxidant secreted from PMNs, human gingival fibroblasts (GFs), or periodontal ligament cells (PDLCs) in response to the inflammatory stimuli during pregnancy are reviewed in this chapter.

Chemotaxis

In vitro studies found that progesterone significantly enhanced the chemotaxis of PMNs, while estradiol and progesterone did not alter chemotaxis of monocytes at any concentration tested.[17]

Similarly, when production of chemokines from PDLCs in response to lipopolysaccharide (LPS) was investigated, a differentially regulated chemokine expression in human PDL cells was found at a physiological concentration of the endogenous estrogen (100 nm 17β-estradiol, which was the same concentration of E2 observed in plasma during pregnancy).

Cytokines

When human monocytes, gingival fibroblast, periodontal ligament cells were subjected to bacteria and their products, various cytokines are release. Such release of cytokines was found to be altered in pregnant patients. Due to different concentration of ovarian hormones and different experimental protocol, the results were inconsistent and invariable. Matrix metalloproteinases (MMPs) are involved in periodontal destruction, and it was found that progesterone may control and reduce local production of MMPs by cultured human GFs in response to interleukin-1.[18] Acute inflammation is responsible for a substantial fraction of preterm birth.[19] In 1998, offenbacher et al.[7] suggested that the cytokines produced by local inflammation in periodontal tissues affected by periodontitis have systemic effects after diffusion of such cytokines through blood flow.

During pregnancy, progesterone increases vascular permeability which permits the infection to pass from the gingival tissues to the rest of the body. Numerous reviews indicate that the intra-amniotic levels of prostaglandins especially prostaglandin E-2 (PGE2) and tumor necrosis factor (TNF-α) rise steadily throughout pregnancy until a critical threshold is reached to induce labor, cervical dilation, and delivery. These molecules are also produced within the diseased periodontium which can escape into the general circulation together with other lipopolysaccharides, peptidoglycan fragments, and hydrolytic enzymes.[20,21] This can lead to translocation of periodontal pathogens to the fetoplacental unit precipitating preterm labor.[22]

Fetomaternal Immune Response

The immune and genetic characteristics of fetus and pregnant women are one of the potential mechanisms linking periodontal diseases to preterm birth. Numerous studies have analyzed fetal and maternal antibodies directed against oral pathogens during pregnancy. The presence of IgM is associated to an increased risk of preterm birth. This immune response against oral pathogens could be associated with an inflammatory response, and the synergy between the two mechanisms significantly increases the risk.[23]

The genetic predisposition is also important. Polymorphisms of genes coding for proinflammatory cytokines such as TNF-α, IL-1 or IL-6 are associated to a hyperinflammatory response. The consecutive overexpression of these cytokines increases the risk of preterm birth.[24-26]

Pregnancy Effecting Oral Conditions

It is well known that hormonal changes during pregnancy are associated with oral mucosal changes most of which are reversible clinically. Periodontium is a unique structure composed of two fibrous (gingival and periodontal ligament) and two mineralized (cementum and alveolar bone) tissues. For the reason that pregnancy probably has an effect only on the gingiva and has no permanent effects on periodontal attachment, meantime, the effect of female sex hormones on periodontal ligament and tooth supporting alveolar bone has rarely been investigated; the effects, mainly focuses on the impact of progesterone and estrogen on two fibrous tissues (gingival and periodontal ligament). The changes seen during pregnancy are mainly attributed to the hormonal changes seen in pregnancy. Majority of these alterations revert back to normal postpartum, but specific factors do aggravate a few conditions. The levels of oral microflora, plaque, and local irritants determine the severity and the duration of these conditions.

Mechanism for the Possible Effect of Pregnancy on Periodontium

Estrogen and progesterone are the principle female sex hormones produced and play an important role in the physiological changes seen in women from puberty. Elevated levels of these hormones have a significant influence on the major organ systems, including the periodontium[27,28]

Estrogen, Progesterone, and their Receptors

Receptors for these hormones are found in the gingiva.[29,30] These hormones increase vascular permeability and the flow rate of gingival crevicular fluid. They may also alter the immune system.[31] Estrogen receptors have also been found in periosteal fibroblasts as well as in periodontal ligament fibroblasts.[32] Thus, they directly affect the periodontal tissues. Also it was found in mitochondria of human PDLCs, demonstrating that estrogen, probably via ER-β, influences mitochondrial function and energy metabolism in human PDLCs.[33] Estrogen firstly decreases collagen production and keratinization of gingival epithelium and secondly induces proliferation of fibroblasts and decreases the collagen and no collagen proteins, blocks the turnover of the gingival tissue, thereby reducing the capacity of gingival tissue to repair. The result is an increase in the permeability of the epithelial barrier and an increased response to plaque bacteria.[34]

Alterations in Subgingival Microbiota

Periodontium acts as a reservoir of subgingival bacteria. Changes in the subgingival microbiota have been proposed as a potential mechanism for exacerbated gingival inflammation during pregnancy.

Progesterone or estrogens acted as substitutes for the naphthoquinone requirement of the pathogens and thus acted as a growth factor for the bacteria, supporting the marked increase in proportions.[28]

A positive correlation was found between an increase in estradiol and progesterone and an overgrowth of *P. intermedia*.[35-38] Similarly positive correlation was also observed between an overgrowth of *Porphyromonas gingivalis, Tannerella forsythia*[34] and *Campylobacter rectus*[40] and an increase in estradiol concentrations.

The subgingival microflora was found to be increased in second trimester of pregnancy, maintained during the second quarter and reduced during the third trimester to postpartum.[35,36,39,40]

Changes in Host Immunoinflammatory Response

During pregnancy, some degrees of immunosuppression occur, to minimize the risk of fetal rejection. Progesterone and glucocorticoids share important anti-inflammatory and immunosuppressive properties. Increases in progesterone and prostaglandins modulate the immune system during pregnancy. Both hormones have potent antiproliferative effects in mitogen activation and cytotoxic T-cell generation. These hormones also regulate T-cell cytokine profile, decrease CD4/CD8 ratio, and reduces the number of blood lymphocytes. A high dose of progesterone induces production of IL-4, which is anti-inflammatory. Progesterone also upregulates HLA Class I type G gene expression, which is the NK inhibitory ligand,[41] suppresses the proliferation of CD4+ lymphocytes[42] and induces apoptosis in activated CD8+ lymphocytes.[43] Progesterone also downregulates IL-6 production, rendering the gingiva less efficient at resisting the inflammatory challenges produced by bacteria.[18]

A decrease in neutrophil chemotaxis has been observed during pregnancy, which may be due to the effects of sex hormones.[17] These changes in the immune system may explain the susceptibility to infection during pregnancy and can support the clinical observation of complications in pregnant women with periodontitis.

Gingival Conditions

An exaggerated gingival response to dental biofilm among pregnant women has been extensively reported in previous literature suggesting that hormonal changes can have varied manifestations in periodontal tissues.

Following are the oral changes observed:

Gingivitis

The normal healthy gingiva is characterized by its pink color and its firm consistency. Interdentally, the healthy gingival tissues are firm, do not bleed on gentle probing and fill the space below the contact areas between the teeth. Healthy gingiva often exhibits a stippled appearance, and there is a knife-edge margin between the soft tissue and the tooth. Gingivitis is defined as an inflammation of the gingiva. It is characterized by redness and edema of gingival tissue, bleeding on provocation, changes in contour and presence of calculus or plaque with no radiographic evidence of crestal bone loss.

The gingival changes seen during pregnancy were reported as early as 1877. The pregnancy exacerbates the pre-existing gingivitis and this is first noticeable during the 2nd month of pregnancy and peaks in the 8th month. A definite decrease in gingivitis is generally seen in the last month, and immediately postpartum the gingival tissues return to the earlier state similar to the 2nd month of pregnancy.[44] It seemed that good oral hygiene in pregnancy was able to partially neutralize hormonal effect.

Periodontitis

The clinical feature that distinguishes periodontitis from gingivitis is the presence of clinically detectable attachment loss. The amount of periodontal destruction is commensurate with oral hygiene or plaque levels, local predisposing factors and systemic risk factors including smoking, stress, diabetes, HIV and inherent host defense capabilities of the patient. Periodontitis is characterized clinically by apical migration of epithelium along the root surface or clinical attachment loss, deepened pockets, and crestal bone loss. Researches had shown pregnant women with higher Gingival Index and probing pocket depth (PPD), with same plaque index when compared to nonpregnant women. The clinical parameters (PPD and GI) increased in parallel with the increase in the stage of pregnancy, which reached the maximum at the eighth month.[45]

Clinical parameter such as clinical attachment level (CAL), when was observed it was found that, the increased inflammation was detected in the gingival region rather than in other periodontal sites, indicating that pregnancy only has reversible effect on the gingiva without inducing periodontal attachment loss.

Pyogenic Granuloma

Pyogenic granuloma (PG) is also well known as 'Pregnancy Tumor' or 'Granuloma Gravidarum' as it develops in up to 5% of pregnancies. PG is a kind of inflammatory hyperplasia that arises in response to various stimuli such as low-grade local irritation, traumatic injury or hormonal factor. It predominantly occurs in the second decade of life of young females, possibly because of the vascular effects of female hormones. Oral PG is most commonly found in gingiva (75%), followed by lips, tongue, and buccal mucosa as next most common sites. Clinically, lesion manifest as small, red, erythematous papules on a pedunculated or sometimes sessile base, which is usually hemorrhagic and compressible[46-48] **(Fig. 50.1)**. Young PGs are highly vascular and redder in color, whereas older lesions are pink in color due to more collagen content. Generally, it appears in the 2nd–3rd month of pregnancy. During first month of pregnancy, it serves as a base for development of hyperplastic mass, cumulative action of hormonal stimuli and plaque-induced inflammation results in such granulomas. Molecular mechanism behind development and regression of PG during pregnancy has been studied. The profound endocrine upheaval in pregnancy changes the structure and function of the blood and lymph microvasculature of the skin and mucosa. Estrogen leads to granulation tissue formation by stimulating production of various growth factors such as, nerve growth factor (NGF) in macrophages, granulocyte-macrophage-colony stimulating factor (GM-CSF) in keratinocytes and basic fibroblast growth factor (bFGF) and transforming growth factor-beta 1 (TGF-β1) in fibroblasts. Similarly, vascular endothelial growth factor (VEGF) production in macrophages are enhanced by estrogen, which is related to the development of PG during pregnancy.[49] Excisional surgery is the main line of treatment for PG, but removals of causative irritants such as plaque, calculus, foreign material, source of trauma are equally important.

Other Changes Associated with Pregnancy

It include chloasma, facial telangiectasia, sialorrhea, tooth surface loss usually related to vomiting (hyperemesis gravidarum), increase mobility of teeth, changes in severity of oral apathies. Severe bleeding which may or may not be associated with disseminated intravascular coagulation may occur.

Effects of Periodontal Therapy on Pregnancy Outcomes

Randomized controlled clinical trials testing the effects of periodontal therapy on the adverse outcomes of pregnancy have shown that nonsurgical periodontal therapy (scaling and root planning) can reduce the risk of preterm births in mothers who are affected by periodontitis.[50-55] Periodontal intervention resulted in a significantly decreased incidence for preterm delivery. Therefore pregnant women who were periodontally healthy and treated for periodontitis showed less incidence of preterm and low birth weight (PTLBW) deliveries, whereas pregnant women with periodontitis who were not treated showed higher incidence of PTLBW deliveries. Pregnancy without periodontal treatment was associated with significant increases in probing depths, plaque scores, GCF IL-1β, and GCF IL-6 levels. Periodontal treatment was safe, improved clinical status (attachment level, probing depth, plaque, gingivitis, and bleeding on probing scores) and prevented periodontal disease progression. Microbiologically and immunologically significant decrease in periodontal pathogen load was found, and a decrease in both serum IL-6sr, and GCF IL-1β.

Evidence supported the potential benefits of periodontal treatment on pregnancy outcomes 3.8-fold reduction in the rate of preterm delivery, serum markers of IL-6 response.[56]

However, some research has yielded negative results. For example, contradictory studies which state periodontal therapy is not related to the outcome of pregnancy are also available. These studies have reported that periodontal therapy in pregnant women improved only the periodontal condition, however, not incidences of PTLBW deliveries.[57,58] In most of the studies performed, periodontal treatment was provided during the second trimester of pregnancy, ultimately leading to PTLBW deliveries due to a delay in diagnosis. Periodontal treatment, if administered before pregnancy, may produce more beneficial results.[59] Furthermore, the appropriate time for providing periodontal treatment should be researched and the results applied to pregnant women so as to ensure a successful and safe delivery.

Pregnant Women as Dental Patients

Appropriate and timely dental care can lead to improved pregnancy outcomes as well as greater comfort for the woman. The treatment of periodontitis, as well as the use of local anesthetics, amalgams, and X-ray scans, do not pose an increased risk to the developing fetus and is, in fact, important in contributing to maintaining optimal health for mother and baby. Dental care has been proven to not only be safe and effective during pregnancy, but also necessary to promote sound oral health. It is imperative that dental treatment be coordinated among obstetric and oral healthcare providers. Oral healthcare needs should be a part of the training of medical students, nurses, and healthcare workers so as to enable them to identify the main dental manifestations of pregnancy. They should also be able to advise pregnant women on how to maintain good dental health. During pregnancy, careful oral hygiene, removal of dental plaque and use of correct brushing techniques are important to avoid occurrence and recurrence of various oral pathologies such as pyogenic granuloma. This will aid in bridging the gap between the obstetricians and the dental clinicians to provide an effective healthcare to the pregnant women and prevent the associated complications.

Emergency dental procedures can be performed during any trimester when a delay in necessary treatment could result in significant risk to the mother and an indirect risk to the fetus. Special precautions may need to be taken during these instances. The second trimester is the safest time to perform routine dental care, and should include dental procedures aimed towards elimination of problems that can arise in due course of pregnancy **(Table 50.1)**.

Prenatal Oral Health Counseling

The objective of prenatal counselling is to educate parents about their own oral health and to create behaviors that will ensure oral health of their unborn child. Mutans streptococci

Table 50.1: Dental treatment consideration in pregnant patient			
	First trimester	*Second trimester*	*Third trimester*
Type of dental treatment	Controlling plaque	Controlling plaque	Controlling plaque
	Teeth cleaning by dental professional	Teeth cleaning by dental professional	Teeth cleaning by dental professional
	Oral hygiene prophylactic instructions	Oral hygiene prophylactic instructions	Oral hygiene prophylactic instructions
	Only emergency or urgent treatments	Regular routine dental treatments	Regular routine dental treatments with short treatment time (first half)

are detected in all the children with early childhood dental caries[60] and research clearly indicates that this organism transmits from mother to child.[61]

Therefore reducing maternal microflora lowers levels of dental caries in their children. Uses of chlorhexidine varnish and xylitol consumption should be encouraged in pregnant women, after delivery. It was found that, habitual xylitol consumption by mothers was associated with a statistically significant reduction of the probability of mother-child transmission of MS assessed at two years of age. The effect was superior to that obtained with either chlorhexidine or fluoride varnish treatments performed as single applications at six-month intervals.[62] Similarly, lower levels of MS as well as delayed colonization in newly born for up to 4 months were found with pregnant women who underwent proper dietary counseling, oral hygiene instructions and professional prophylaxis.[63]

CONCLUSION

Proper assessment, intervention, and patient educations about dental problems during pregnancy can help to enhance pregnancy outcomes and decrease infant dental caries. Knowledge of these conditions are important so as to minimize the effects or complications until childbirth when these conditions regress. Therefore role of obstetricians and gynecologists is vital in encouraging their patients for a regular oral check ups.

REFERENCES

1. Dortbudak O, Eberhardt R, Ulm M, Persson GR. Periodontitis: a marker of risk in pregnancy for preterm birth. J Clin Periodontol. 2005;32(1):45-52.
2. Siqueira FM, Cota LO, Costa JE, Haddad JP, Lana AM, Costa FO. Intrauterine growth restriction, low birth weight, and preterm birth: adverse pregnancy outcomes and their association with maternal periodontitis. J Periodontol. 2007;78:2266-76.
3. Pitiphat W, Joshipura KJ, Gillman MW, Williams PL, Douglass CW, Rich-Edwards JW. Maternal periodontitis and adverse pregnancy outcomes. Community Dent Oral Epidemiol. 2008;36(1):3-11.
4. Mitchell-Lewis D, Engebretson SP, Chen J, Lamster IB, Papapanou PN. Periodontal infections and pre-term birth: early findings from a cohort of young minority women in New York. Eur J Oral Sci. 2001;109(1):34-9.
5. Noack B, Klingenberg J, Weigelt J, Hoffmann T. Periodontal status and preterm low birth weight: a case control study. J Periodontal Res. 2005;40:339-45.
6. Scannapieco FA. Systemic effects of periodontal diseases. Dent Clin North Am. 2005;49:533-50.
7. Offenbacher S, Jared HL, O'Reilly PG, et al. Potential pathogenic mechanisms of periodontitis associated pregnancy complications. Ann Periodontol. 1998;3(1):233-50.
8. Pretorius C, Jagatt A, Lamont RF. The relationship between periodontal disease, bacterial vaginosis, and preterm birth. J Perinat Med. 2007;35(2):93-9.
9. Fardini Y, Chung P, Dumm R, Joshi N, Han YW. Transmission of diverse oral bacteria to murine placenta: evidence for the oral microbiome as a potential source of intrauterine infection Infect Immun. 2010;78(4):1789-96.
10. Seymour GJ, Ford PJ, Cullinan MP, Leishman S, Yamazaki K. Relationship between periodontal infections and systemic disease. Clin Microbiol Infect. 2007;13(4):3-10.
11. Goncalves LF, Chaiworapongsa T, Romero R. Intrauterine infection and prematurity. Ment Retard Dev Disabil Res Rev. 2002;8(1):3-13.
12. Barak S, Oettinger-Barak O, Machtei EE, Sprecher H, Ohel G Evidence of periopathogenic microorganisms in placentas of women with preeclampsia J Periodontol. 2007;78(4):670-6.
13. Kotz J, Chegini N, Shiverick KT, Lamont RJ. Localization of P. gingivalis in preterm delivery placenta. J Dent Res. 2009;88(6):575-8.
14. Arce R. M, Barros SP, Wacker B, Peters B, Moss K, Offenbacher S. Increased TLR4 expression in murine placentas after oral infection with periodontal pathogens. Placenta. 2009;30(2):156-62.
15. Lamont RJ, Jenkinson HF. Life below the gumline: pathogenic mechanisms of Porphyromonas gingivalis. Microbiol Mol Biol Rev. 1998;62(4):1244-63.
16. Sculley DV, Langley-Evans SC. Salivary antioxidants and periodontal disease status. P Nutr Soc. 2002;61(1):137-43.
17. Miyagi M, Aoyama H, Morishita M, Iwamoto Y. Effects of sex hormones on chemotaxis of human peripheral polymorphonuclear leukocytes and monocytes. J Periodontol. 1992;63(1):28-32.
18. Lapp CA, Lohse JE, Lewis JB, et al. The effects of progesterone on matrix metalloproteinases in cultured human gingival fibroblasts. J Periodontol. 2003;74(3):277-88.
19. Han YW, Fardini Y, Chen C, et al. Term stillbirth caused by oral *Fusobacterium nucleatum*. Obstet and Gynecol. 2010;115(2):442-5.

20. Page RC. The role of inflammatory mediators in the pathogenesis of periodontal disease. J Periodontal Res. 1991; 26(3 Pt 2):230-42.
21. Dasanayake AP, Russell S, Boyd D, Madianos PN, Forster T, Hill E. Preterm low birth weight and periodontal disease among African Americans. Dent Clin North Am. 2003;47(1):115-25, x-xi.
22. Fernando Oliveira Costa, Alcione Maria Soares Dutra Oliveira, Luís Otávio Miranda Cota (2013). Interrelation between periodontal disease and preterm birth, preterm birth. Dr Offer Erez (Ed.), InTech. DOI:10.5772/54977.
23. Boggess KA, Moss K, Madianos P, Murtha AP, Beck J, Offenbacher S. Fetal immune response to oral pathogens and risk of preterm birth. Am J Obstet Gynecol. 2005;193(3):1121-6.
24. Dashash M, Nugent J, Baker P, Tansinda D, Blinkhorn F. Interleukin-6-174 genotype, periodontal disease and adverse pregnancy outcomes: a pilot study. J Clin Immunol. 2008;28(3):237-43.
25. Genc MR, Onderdonk A. Endogenous bacterial flora in pregnant women and the influence of maternal genetic variation. BJOG. 2011;118(2):154-63.
26. Harper M, Zheng SL, Thom E, et al. Cytokine gene polymorphisms and length of gestation. Obstet Gynecol. 2011;117(1):125-30.
27. Amar S Chung KM. Influence of Hormonal variation on the periodontium in women. Periodontol 2000. 1994;6:79-87.
28. Mariotti A. Sex steroid hormones and cell dynamics in the periodontium. Crit Rev Oral Biol Med. 1994;5:27-53.
29. Vittek J, Hemandez MR, Wenk EJ, Rappaport SC, Southern AL. Specific estrogen receptors in human gingiva. J Clin Endocrinol Metab. 1982;54:608-12.
30. Kawahara K, Shimazu A. Expression and intracellular localization of progesterone receptors in cultured human gingival fibroblasts. J Periodontal Res. 2003;38:242-6.
31. Mealey BL, Moritz AJ. Hormonal influences: effects of diabetes mellitus and endogenous female sex steroid hormones on the periodontium. Periodontol 2000. 2003;32:59-8
32. Nanba H, Nomura Y, Kinoshita M, Shimizu H, Ono K, Goto H, et al. Periodontal tissues and sex hormones. Effects of sex hormones on metabolism of fibroblasts derived from periodontal ligament. Nihon Shishubyo Gakkai Kaishi. 1989;31:166-75.
33. Jönsson D, Nilsson J, Odenlund M, et al. Demonstration of mitochondrial oestrogen receptor-β and oestrogen-induced attenuation of cytochrome C oxidase subunit I expression in human periodontal ligament cells. Arch Oral Biol. 2007;52(7):669-76.
34. Markou E, Eleana B, Lazaros T, Antonios K. The influence of sex steroid hormones on gingiva of women. Open Dent J. 2009;5 (3):114-9.
35. Kornman KS, Loesche WJ. The subgingival microbial flora during pregnancy. J Periodontal Res. 1980;15(2):111-22.
36. Muramatsu Y, Takaesu Y. Oral health status related to subgingival bacterial flora and sex hormones in saliva during pregnancy. Bull Tokyo Dent Coll. 1994;35(3):139-51.
37. Gursoy M, Pajukanta R, Sorsa T, Könönen E. Clinical changes in periodontium during pregnancy and post-partum. J Clin Periodontol. 2008;35(7):576-83.
38. Carrillo-de-Albornoz A, Figuero E, Herrera D, Bascones-Martínez A. Gingival changes during pregnancy: II. Influence of hormonal variations on the subgingival biofilm. J Clin Periodontol. 2010;37(3):230-40.
39. Adriaens LM, Alessandri R, Spörri S, Lang NP, Persson GR. Does pregnancy have an impact on the subgingival microbiota? J Periodontol. 2009;80(1):72-81.
40. Yokoyama M, Hinode D, Yoshioka M, et al. Relationship between *Campylobacter rectus* and periodontal status during pregnancy. Oral Microbiol Immunol. 2008;23(1):55-9.
41. Yie SM, Xiao R, Librach CL. Progesterone regulates HLA G though a novel progesterone response element. Hum Reprod. 2006;21:2538-54.
42. Bainbridge DRJ, Ellis SA, Sargent IL. HLA-G suppresses proliferation of CD4+ T Lymphocytes. J Reprod Immunol. 2000;48:17-26.
43. Ebersole JL, Steffen MJ, Holt SC, Kesavalu L, Chu L, Cappelli D. Systemic inflammatory responses in progressing periodontitis during pregnancy in a baboon model. Clin Exp Immunol. 2010;162:550-9.
44. Loe H, Silness J. Periodontal disease in pregnancy. I. Prevalence and severity. Acta Odontol Scand. 1963;21:533-51.
45. Taani DQ, Habashneh R, Hammad MM, Batieha A. The periodontal status of pregnant women and its relationship with sociodemographic and clinical variables. J Oral Rehab. 2003;30(4):440-5.
46. Eversole LR. Clinical outline of oral pathology: diagnosis and treatment, 3rd edn. BC Decker, Hamilton; 2002. pp. 113-4.
47. Neville BW, Damm DD, Allen CM, Bouquot JE. Oral and maxillofacial pathology, 2nd edn. WB Saunders, Philadelphia; 2002. pp. 437-95.
48. Regezi JA, Sciubba JJ, Jordan RCK. Oral pathology: clinical pathologic considerations, 4th edn. WB Saunders, Philadelphia; 2004. pp. 115-6.
49. Kanda N, Watanabe S. Regulatory roles of sex hormones in cutaneous biology and immunology. J Dermatol Sci. 2005: 38:1-7.
50. López NJ, Da Silva I, Ipinza J, Gutiérrez J. Periodontal therapy reduces the rate of preterm low birth weight in women with pregnancy associated gingivitis. J Periodontol. 2005;76(11 Suppl):2144-53.
51. Michalowicz BS, Hodges JS, DiAngelis AJ, Lupo VR, Novak MJ, Ferguson JE, et al. Treatment of periodontal disease and the risk of preterm birth. N Engl J Med. 2006;355(18):1885-94.
52. Tarannum F, Faizuddin M. Effect of periodontal therapy on pregnancy outcome in women affected by periodontitis. J Periodontol. 2007;78(11):2095-103.
53. Sadatmansouri S, Sedighpoor N, Aghaloo M. Effects of periodontal treatment phase I on birth term and birth weight. J Indian Soc Pedod Prev Dent. 2006;24(1):23-6.

54. Gazolla CM, Ribeiro A, Moysés MR, Oliveira LA, Pereira LJ, Sallum AW. Evaluation of the incidence of preterm low birth weight in patients undergoing periodontal therapy. J Periodontol. 2007;78(5):842-8.
55. Lopez R. Periodontal treatment in pregnant women improves periodontal disease but does not alter rates of preterm birth. Evid Based Dent. 2007;8(2):38-40.
56. Offenbacher S, Lin D, Strauss R. Effects of periodontal therapy during pregnancy on periodontal status, biologic parameters, and pregnancy outcomes. J Periodontol. 2006;77 (12):2011-24.
57. Goldenberg RL, Culhane JF. Preterm birth and periodontal disease. N Engl J Med. 2006;355(18):1925-7.
58. Mealey BL. Periodontal medicine: Impact of periodontal infection on systemic health. In Carranza's Clinical periodontology, 10th edn. St. Louis, Missouri; 2006. pp. 312-29.
59. Newman HN. Focal infection. J Dent Res. 1996;75(12):1912-9.
60. Caufield PW. Dental caries: A transmissible and infectious disease revisited: a position paper. Pediatr Dent. 1997;19: 491-8.
61. Caufield PW, Cutter GR, Dasanayake AP. Initial acquisition of mutans streptococci by infants: evidence for a discrete window of infectivity. J Dent Res. 1993;72:37-45.
62. Söderling E, Isokangas P, Pienihäkkinen K, Tenovuo J. Influence of maternal xylitol consumption on acquisition of mutans streptococci by infants. J Dent Res. 2000;79(3):882-7.
63. Brambilla E, Felloni A, Gagiliani M, Malerba A, GarciaGodoy F, Strohmerger L. Caries prevention during pregnancy: results of a 30 month study. J Am Dent Assoc. 1998;129:871-7.

Chapter

51

Epilepsy in Pregnancy

Deepti Gupta

INTRODUCTION

Epilepsy is a neurological condition characterized by predisposition to generate seizures and its associated neurobiological, cognitive, psychological and social consequences. Epilepsy is defined as 2 or more unprovoked seizures without any immediate identifiable cause.[1] Estimated incidence ranges from 0.5% to 2%. In India, incidence is estimated to be about 1% in general population with incidence in rural population being more than that of urban.[2]

It is estimated that almost 50% of WWE (women with epilepsy) in India are in the reproductive age group. This figure is important because not only is epilepsy a concern during pregnancy, but it affects girls and women before conception also. Menstrual abnormalities, hirsutism and polycystic ovaries have been associated with valproate and carbamazepine.[2] Epilepsy can also alter hypothalamo-pituitary-ovarian axis and lead to changes in reproductive hormone levels, thus contributing to infertility.

Convulsive disorders are second most common and most serious neurological condition in pregnant women. Epileptic seizures can be:
- Generalized (tonic-clonic or grand mal)
- Complex partial (loss of awareness or staring with mild motor movements)
- Focal motor or sensory (Jacksonian with no loss of awareness)
- Absence or Petit mal
- Myoclonic jerks
- Auras of déjà vu/fear or abnormal odor.

While encountering a patient with epilepsy in pregnancy, it is important to remember that 95% have a history of epilepsy or have been taking anticonvulsant medication.

ETIOPATHOGENESIS

Most cases are idiopathic wherein no identifiable cause is found. About 30% of these have an associated family history of epilepsy. Epilepsy in pregnancy is called secondary when there is an underlying pathology like:[3]

- Previous brain surgery
- Intracranial mass lesions (meningiomas, arteriovenous malformations, AVM enlarge during pregnancy. If first seizure occurs during pregnancy, AVM should be considered)
- Eclampsia
- Cerebral vein thrombosis
- Stroke
- Subarachnoid hemorrhage
- Drug and alcohol withdrawal
- Infections.

INVESTIGATIONS

Detailed neurologic workup with thorough history
- Blood pressure, urinalysis, platelet count, clotting screen, blood film
- Blood glucose, serum calcium, serum sodium, serum urea, serum creatinine, liver function tests
- CT scan with shielding or MRI
- EEG.

DIFFERENTIAL DIAGNOSIS

- Other forms of loss of consciousness like syncopal episodes/hysteric attacks/hyperventilation. These conditions usually do not have postictal confusional state; neither is there loss of bladder/bowel control or tongue biting.[4]
- Noncentral nervous system causes like hypoxia/hypoglycemia/hypocalcemia/hyponatremia.
- Rarely seizures may also result from withdrawal of certain drugs/medications, exposure to toxic substances, including heavy metal toxicity.

PRECONCEPTION COUNSELING

This is extremely important on women known to have seizure disorders planning to conceive. Adequate seizure control before onset of pregnancy, good neurological evaluation, achieving seizure-free period of 2 years, planned conception, and folic acid supplementation for at least 3 months should be done.[4] Avoiding polytherapy and valproate is important. Risk of recurrence of seizure is about 25% by 1 year after drug withdrawal and 40% by 2 years. Risk of recurrence is more in women with known structural lesion/abnormal EEG.

PREGNANCY AND DISEASE PROGRESSION

- Onset of epilepsy not increased during pregnancy
- 95% of patients with seizure in pregnancy have history of epilepsy or on anticonvulsant
- If adequately controlled, deterioration unlikely during pregnancy
- If history of frequent uncontrolled seizures, then expect same pattern during pregnancy, especially first trimester
- Breakthrough seizures likely in third trimester due to poor sleep.

Congenital Anomalies

Risk of anomalies in infants exposed to AED is 2 folds of general population. However, this risk is not increased in women with history of seizure disorder who are not taking any antiepileptic medication. Major malformations include orofacial clefts, neural tube defects, congenital heart disease. Minor malformations include craniofacial anomalies, short neck, and hypoplastic fingernails. Fetal hydantoin syndrome affects 3–5% of exposed offspring and includes mental retardation, small for gestational age, craniofacial anomalies and limb defects. A mild form of phenytoin associated syndrome may be present in as many as 8–15% babies but is obvious only on careful observation for first 3 years.

MANAGEMENT OF PREGNANCY AND DELIVERY[3,4]

Seizures can cause maternal and fetal injury, spontaneous abortion, preterm delivery, fetal bradycardia. Per se epilepsy in pregnancy not an indication for planned cesarean section. Mode of delivery should be determined by other factors.

Antenatal Management

- All women on antiepileptic drug (AED) should be given folic acid 5 mg/day for 12 weeks prior to conception.
- Ideally target should be monotherapy of AED as multiple AED increases teratogenic risk. Most effective drug in lowest necessary dose should be given.
- Valproate should be avoided and, if at all, it has to be given, it should be given in 3–4 divided doses or sustained release preparation so as to decrease peak serum levels and decrease teratogenic risk.
- Decreased protein binding, increased plasma volume, alteration in absorption/excretion of drugs, high hepatic metabolism (lamotrigine, phenytoin, phenobarbital, carbamazepine), noncompliance, morning sickness all contribute to low levels of antiepileptic drugs in serum in pregnancy.
- Blood level measurements should be used to monitor and maintain therapeutic range. Blood level testing should be done at least once in each trimester and before delivery. Always check serum-free drug levels.
- Stress on importance of good and adequate sleep as breakthrough seizures can precipitate from lack of sleep, especially towards third trimester.
- For refractory seizures, increase dose of one drug to maximum before adding another because treatment with 2 or more AED doubles the risk of major malformation.
- *Status epilepticus*: Lorazepam 2 mg IV followed by 2 mg IV every minute to 0.1 mg/kg first-line treatment. Phenytoin 20 mg/kg slow IV if seizures still persist. Last resort is general anesthesia. Cerebral edema is very common in these cases and may be reduced with dexamethasone, mannitol and hyperventilation.
- According to North American AED pregnancy registry, major malformation 10.7% with valproic acid, especially at daily dose >1000 mg. Phenobarbital has malformation rate of 6.5%; others like carbamazepine, phenytoin and lamotrigine have 3%. It is important to note that treatment with 2 antiseizure drugs roughly doubles the risk of congenital malformation.

Intrapartum Management

- About 1–2% women have seizure during labor and another 1–2% in 24 hours after delivery. Hence, intrapartum and postpartum, women should never be left unattended.
- Ensure good hydration, oxygenation and electrolyte balance during labor as hypoxia/hypoglycemia/hyponatremia/hypocalcemia may all trigger seizure.
- Start vitamin K 10 mg/d from week 36 onwards and give vitamin K to infant after delivery.

Postpartum Management

Mothers should be counseled regarding infant safety and breastfeeding. If the breastfed infant is too sedated, it could be a result of antiepileptic medication. The pediatrician should be consulted and breastfeeding may be stopped with top-feed supplements. Mothers with frequent seizures should avoid tub bath and prefer sponge bath preferably with use of strap to secure the baby **(Table 51.1)**.[5]

Contraception: Women taking hepatic enzyme-inducing drugs like phenytoin, primidone, carbamazepine, phenobarbitone will require higher dose contraceptive pills. Injectable depot contraceptives and intrauterine LNG-releasing devices are not affected by these drugs hence may be used in same dose.

Table 51.1: Various antiepileptic drugs (AED) and their doses

Drug	Starting dose	Maintenance dose	Dosing schedule	Monitoring
Phenobarbital	3 mg/kg	3–6 mg/kg	QD-BID	CBC, LFT, serum levels
Phenytoin	4 mg/kg	4–8 mg/kg	QD-TID	CBC, LFT, serum levels
Valproic acid	15 mg/kg	15–45 mg/kg	TID-QID	CBC, LFT
Carbamazepine	10 mg/kg	10–35 mg/kg	TID	CBC, LFT
Ethosuximide	15 mg/kg	15–40 mg/kg	QD-BID	CBC, LFT
Gabapentine	10 mg/kg	25–50 mg/kg	TID	Weight
Lamotrigine	0.15–0.5 mg/kg	5–15 mg/kg	BID	CBC, LFT
Levetiracetam	10 mg/kg	40–100 mg/kg	BID	Behavior
Oxcarbazepine	8–10 mg/kg	30–46 mg/kg	BID	Hyponatremia
Topiramate	1–3 mg/kg	5–9 mg/kg	BID	Weight

KEY MESSAGES

- All women on AED should get preconception counseling and folic acid supplementation.
- Lowest possible dose of AED should be given, monitored with serum levels during pregnancy, monotherapy always better than polytherapy
- Emphasize on medication compliance, avoid seizure triggers.
- Potential risk of injury to mother and infant, hence team work very important, never leave woman alone.

REFERENCES

1. William's Textbook of Obstetrics, 22nd edition, 1231-3.
2. Subbareddy SN, Sinha S, Satishchandra P. Epilepsy: Indian Perspective. Ann Indian Acad Neurol. 2014;17(Suppl 10): S3-S11. Doi: 10.4103/0972-2327.128643.
3. Piercy CN. Handbook of Obstetric Medicine. CRC press, 5th edition; 163-71.
4. Decherney AH, Nathan L, Goodwin T M, Laufer N. Current diagnosis and treatment obstetrics and gynecology. McGraw Hills 10th edition, 399-401.
5. Page B Pennell. Using Current Evidence in Selecting Antiepileptic Drugs for Use during Pregnancy. Epilepsy Curr. 2005;5(2):45-51.

SECTION 10: COMPLICATIONS DURING DELIVERY

Chapter 52

Rupture Uterus

Tripti Nagaria

Rupture uterus is one of the most dreaded complications in obstetrics responsible for a very high maternal and perinatal morbidity and mortality. It indirectly indicates the standard of obstetric care the population is receiving.

It is defined as disruption of the uterine muscle extending to and involving the uterine serosa or disruption of the uterine muscle with extension to the bladder or broad ligament while uterine dehiscence is defined as disruption of the uterine muscle with intact uterine serosa.[1]

Meta-analysis of pooled data from 20 studies in the peer-reviewed medical literature published from 1976–2009 indicated an overall incidence of pregnancy-related uterine rupture of 1 per 1,536 pregnancies (0.07%).[2] According to WHO systematic review on maternal morbidity and mortality, for unselected pregnant women, the prevalence of uterine rupture reported was considerably lower for population-based (median 0.053, range 0.016–0.30%) than for facility-based studies (median 0.31, range 0.012–2.9%). It is difficult to be sure of the extent to which women with previous cesarean section contributed to these numbers, and the proportion with previous cesarean section may have varied considerably between populations studied.[3] There is a vast difference in the incidence of rupture uterus amongst the developed and developing countries of the world. The prevalence tended to be lower for countries defined by the United Nations as developed, 0.012–0.059%[3-7] than the less or least developed countries where the reported incidence ranged to the extent of 0.5–1.6%.[8-10] With the improvement in the maternal healthcare services in the developed countries the incidence of rupture uterus with unscarred uterus is extremely low 0.0045–0.007%,[6,11,12] though in the less developed countries, it ranged from 0.012 to 0.045%[13] but there is an increase in the incidence to 22–74/10,000[1,14-16] deliveries following a previous cesarean section, if vaginal birth is attempted. Incidence of rupture uterus varies from 0.23/1000 to 7/1000 deliveries in India accounting for 5–10% of all maternal deaths.[17-19]

CLASSIFICATION OF RUPTURE UTERUS

According to type:
- Complete—involving all the layers of uterus including the serosa
- Incomplete—serosa not involved
  - *According to timing of occurrence in relation to pegnancy*:
    - During pregnancy
    - During labor without dystocia
    - During labor following obstructed labor or difficult delivery
  - *According to mode of occurrence*:
    - Spontaneous
      - Unscarred uterus
      - Scarred uterus
    - Traumatic
    - Iatrogenic
  - *According to site of rupture*:
    - Fundal
    - Upper uterine segment (UUS)
    - Lower uterine segment (LUS)
    - *Wall of uterus*:
      - Anterior
      - Posterior
      - Lateral.

Rupture of Uterus During Pregnancy

Almost all the cases belonging to this group are previously scarred uterus. However, certain conditions making the myometrium thin or weak can result in spontaneous rupture at any time during pregnancy. Accidental trauma resulting in rupture is a rare cause for uterus to rupture.

Etiology

The causes of rupture uterus during pregnancy are as shown in **Table 52.1**.

Table 52.1: Causes of rupture uterus during pregnancy

Spontaneous	Scar rupture	Iatrogenic/trauma
Thinning of myometrium: • Prior D and C • MRP • Perforation of uterus • Sacculation of uterus *Congenital malformation:* • Pregnancy in • Bicornuate uterus • Unicornuate uterus • Rudimentary horn *Defective connective tissue:* • Marfan syndrome • Ehlers-Danlos syndrome • Corticosteroid long-term therapy • Cocaine use • Couvelaire uterus • Placenta previa	*Previous scarred uterus:* • Classical cesarean section (CS) • Lower segment cesarean section (LSCS) • Hysterotomy • Rupture uterus repair • Uterine corrective surgery • Myomectomy scar • Deep cornual resection of interstitial fallopian tube in ectopic pregnancy	• Forcible external version • Fall • Accident • Blow over abdomen

Table 52.2: Sign and symptoms in cases of rupture during pregnancy

Spontaneous complete	Incomplete	Silent dehiscence
Symptoms: • Sudden severe abdominal pain • Feeling of something has given way *Signs:* • Collapse • Signs and symptoms of internal hemorrhage—fall of BP, tachycardia and increasing pallor • No vaginal bleeding as the os is closed • Fetal parts superficially palpable • Absence of fetal heart sound • Uterus is contracted and felt as a separate suprapubic mass	*Symptoms:* • Persistent abdominal pain • Pain/tenderness at the site of uterine scar *Signs:* • Tachycardia • Fetal bradycardia may be initial sign of scar dehiscence • Loss of fetal heart sound • Condition may closely resemble abruption placenta • Fetus partly or fully retained in the uterus and the diagnosis is often missed	Gradual dehiscence of scar with slight bleeding into the peritoneal cavity followed by infection. *May present with* • Fever • Abdominal pain • Loss of fetal movements • Abdominal distension* • Tenderness over the site of scar is sign of impending rupture • Can result into secondary abdominal pregnancy with herniation of the fetal sac through the scar and getting vascular supply from the surrounding structures. • Uterus retracts, as it does so no more bleeding into the peritoneal cavity and absence of any symptoms

*According to the features may be confused with intestinal obstruction with peritonitis.

Clinical Features

Depends upon the duration of pregnancy and whether occult or overt. If occur in early pregnancy, sign and symptoms are like ruptured ectopic pregnancy. In midtrimester, it presents with features of acute abdomen. Clinical features are as shown in **Table 52.2**.

Rupture During Labor

- Spontaneous
- Iatrogenic
- Traumatic

Causes of rupture uterus during labor are as shown in **Table 52.3**.

Table 52.3: Causes of rupture uterus during labor

Spontaneous		Scar rupture	Iatrogenic/trauma
Obstructive causes		*Previous scarred uterus*	• Forcible version IPV
Bony obstruction:	*Fetal causes*	• Classical CS	• Forceps application vaccum application
• Congenital anomalies of bony pelvis	• Malpresentations	• LSCS	• Destructive operation
• Fracture pelvis	• Malposition	• Hysterotomy	• Breech extraction through incompletely dilated cervix
• Osteophytes	• Macrosomia	• Rupture uterus repair	• Injudicious use of oxytocics
• Bony tumours	• Hydrocephalus	• Uterine corrective surgery	
	• Fetal ascites	• Myomectomy scar	
Soft tissue obstruction:	• Fetal tumors		
• Cervical dystocia	• Locked twins		
• Fibroid in LUS, broad ligament	• Conjoint twins		
• Impacted ovarian tumor			
• Nongravid horn of uterus			
• Cerclage stitch, if not removed			
• Vaginal septa			
Nonobstructive causes			
• Grand multiparity			
• Pendulous abdomen			
• Dextrorotation of uterus			

Use of misoprostol in uncontrolled dosages for labour induction was identified as the cause in several cases. There have been reports of uterine rupture, when misoprostol was used in dosages above 25 µg vaginally.

The causes of rupture uterus during labor are considerably different in different parts of the world. Spontaneous rupture still account for significant number of rupture uterus in the underdeveloped or developing countries. Reports from Nigeria, Ghana, Ethiopia and Bangladesh indicated that about 75% of cases of uterine rupture were associated with unscarred uterus.[20] In contrast in the developed countries, rupture uterus is most often encountered, while attempting vaginal birth after cesarean section, prevalence being in the region of 1% as against <1/10,000 for women without previous cesarean section.[3] Results from the Belgian Obstetric Surveillance System reported a 81.1% of all the ruptures occured in cases who had at least one previous cesarean section.[5] According to one study the risk experienced is 50 times higher, if the mother had a cesarean section.[21] A number of other variants also increase the risk of rupture uterus in present pregnancy, if trial of labor is attempted after previous cesarean section or uterine surgery as shown in the **Table 52.4**.

Clinical presentation in different types of rupture uterus is as shown in **Table 52.5**.

Rupture at the site of a previous uterine scar may occur with few warning signs because the scar is relatively avascular.

Site of Rupture

Complete uterine rupture can occur involving LUS with or without extension upwards involving UUS.

About 70% are on the anterior wall, sometimes posterior wall is involved, if nipped against sacral promontory. Extension to the cervix vagina and bladder occurs in 3–10% of cases. Rupture often involves the lateral wall, particularly left lateral, because of the dextrorotation of the uterus.[31]

Direction of Rupture

- Often oblique
- Longitudinal often involving the lateral wall
- Transverse may encircle the uterus dividing into two
- Rarely transverse in the upper part or fundus only
- Lateral often involve the uterine vessels, broad ligament may extend anteriorly in the uterovesical space, posteriorly retroperitoneally upto the kidneys and may tear through into the peritoneal cavity
- Traumatic rupture often extend upto the fornices, cervix and lateral wall of the uterus

MANAGEMENT OF RUPTURE UTERUS

Rupture uterus is an obstetric emergency where the most crucial steps in the management that can reduce the maternal

Table 52.4: Risk of rupture uterus in women with previous uterine surgeries attempting vaginal delivery

Variants	Risk of rupture uterus	Reference
One previous CS	0.68%,[21] .2–1.5[22]	RCOG guidelines[21], SOGC[22]
Previous section with low transverse incision	0.5–0.9%[24]	ACOG guidelines (practice Bulletin—115)[24]
CS with inverted T or J incision	1.9%[1] 4–9[24]	Londan[1] ACOG 2004[24]
CS with low vertical incision	2%[1] 1–7[24] 1–1.6[23]	Londan[1] ACOG[24] SOGC[23]
CS with high vertical incision involving UUS	2–9%[25, 26]	Guise JM, Hashima J, Osterweil P.[25] Turner MJ. Uterine rupture.[26]
Previous rupture uterus	41.7%[27]	AU Usta IM, Hamdi MA, Musa AA, Nassar AH[27]
Two or more cesarean section	92/10,000[22]	RCOG guidelines[22]
Previous myomectomy	0.75%[28] 0.93% (0.45–1.92%) 0.47% for trial of labor after myomectomy[29]	J Claeys, I Hellendoorn,[28] Zita Gambacorti-Passerini[29]
Induction of labor	7.7% without PG[30] 24.5% with PG[30]	Lydon-Rochelle,[30]

Table 52.5: Clinical presentation in rupture during labor

Complete rupture	Incomplete rupture	Scar dehiscence
Symptoms • Severe abdominal pain followed by sudden cesation of pain • Usually persistent abdominal discomfort • Shoulder tip pain • Vaginal bleeding may be scanty/profuse • Loss of fetal movement *Signs* • Features suggestive of shock • Tender abdomen • Abdominal distension/free fluid • Loss of uterine contour • Cessation of uterine contractions • Superficially palpable fetal parts • Loss of fetal heart sounds • Recession of presenting parts on per vaginal examination • Loose hanging cervix • Bleeding • Hot dry vagina in cases obstructed labor • Hematuria	*If the rupture is extraperitoneal*: • Pronounced localized fullness and tenderness • Suprapubic pain • Bladder tenesmus • Blood stained urine found in catheter sample • Progressive increase in pain in lower abdomen • Increasing severity of collapse.	• Prolonged fetal bradycardia is the first sign in >70% • 8% presented with pain • 3% with bleeding • Typical feeling of something giving way • If there is an atypical pattern of pain, or pain previously controlled by analgesia (epidural or otherwise) which becomes more severe • Shoulder tip pain may indicate peritoneal irritation • Suprapubic pain may reflect local, including bladder, irritation • Hematuria

and fetal catastrophe are establishing an early diagnosis and shortest diagnosis to definitive surgical intervention interval. As a rule, the time available for successful intervention after frank uterine rupture and before the onset of major fetal morbidity is only 10–37 minutes.[32-36] Therefore, once the diagnosis of uterine rupture is considered, all available resources must quickly and effectively be mobilized for successful stabilization of the mother and the delivery of the fetus. Institution of timely surgical treatment results in favorable outcomes for both the newborn and the mother.

- Inform consultant on call to attend
- Summon help
- IV access (use 2 size 14–16 G) and cross match 4–6 units of blood
- Stop syntocinon infusion if in use
- Volume replacement
- Airway + oxygenation
- Left lateral position
- Catheterise and monitor urine output
- Once stabilised, evaluate fetal condition
- Patient and relatives must be made aware preoperatively of the possibility of a hysterectomy and this should be reflected in the consent form.
- Correct any blood loss
- Arrange blood and blood product as required

Delivery of the Fetus

If general condition of the patient is stable and is fit for surgery, or is poor, then with blood transfusion and ongoing resuscitative measures immediate laparotomy and delivery the fetus should be done. Even if the fetus is partially extruded as an attempt to deliver the baby vaginally will increases the tear or rupture. If there is no choice left but to deliver the case as in remote area exploration of the uterus for extent of rent after the delivery should be done, give oxytocin to let the uterus contract and refer the case the case to tertiary centre for further management.

Surgical Management of Uterus

- Repair of rupture uterus
- Hysterectomy—subtotal/total

After the fetus is successfully delivered, the type of surgical treatment for the mother whether uterine repair or hysterectomy should depend on the following factors:

- Type of uterine rupture
- Extent of uterine rupture
- Degree of haemorrhage
- General condition of the mother
- Mother's desire for future childbearing

Table 52.6: Management of rupture uterus: Indications for repair of rupture uterus/ hysterectomy

Repair of rupture uterus	Hysterectomy
• If patient is stable	• Patient is in shock
• Minimal risk of infection	• Intractable uterine bleeding
• Edges of rupture site are clean cut	• Multiple site rupture
• No extension to upper uterine segment, broad ligament, or cervix or para colpos	• Extension to upper segment, broad ligament, cervix and vagina
• Low transverse uterine rupture	• Edges ragged and necrotic
• Easily controllable uterine hemorrhage	• Uterus not salvageable
• No clinical or laboratory evidence of an evolving coagulopathy	• Sepsis
• Family not completed	• Family completed

Indications of repair or hysterectomy are as shown in **Table 52.6**.

CAUTIONS WHILE DOING REPAIR

In most of the cases, repair of the rupture uterus can be done. While repairing following precautions should be taken to avoid complications to occur.

- While freshening the edge, too much time should not be wasted in it.
- Separate the bladder thoroughly before repair
- For deep tear extending into the pelvis, start repairing from upper end place, traction suture at the upper end to draw the lower edge out of the deeper part of broad ligament, then start working from below upwards.
- Great care must be taken to avoid including the ureter while suturing
- Vaginal tears can also be repaired from vaginal route, if needed
- Vac drain may be left in place
- Antibiotic therapy

In case of broad ligamentary/incomplete rupture, there is formation of paracervical hematoma and broad ligamentary hematoma reaching as high as upto the round ligament.[13] After delivery of fetus, hysterectomy may be difficult and hazardous, if cellular tissue is disrupted extensively.

- Retraction of the torn vessels is major problem. To control bleeding pack, press the bleeding points.
- Press the aorta
- Ligation of anterior division of internal iliac artery.
- Restore the lost blood volume.

Hysterectomy

Some of the cases may require emergency hysterectomy, such as if uterus is irreparable with extensive tears, torrential hemorrhage, hemodynamically instable patient, etc.

Advantages

- Safe
- Prevent consequences of next pregnancy
- Removes source of infection
- Provides smooth convalescence

- Subtotal hysterectomy is faster and easier than total especially when the case is unstable.
- However, removal of cervix and suture of vaginal vault reduces the risk of continued bleeding from this area.

RUPTURE UTERUS IF DETECTED AFTER DELIVERY

Many are detected after extraction of the fetus while exploring the uterus when a rent may be detected. These are often incomplete, occurring in between the broad ligament. Small incomplete rent may be managed conservatively. However, if a large rent detected or persistent hemorrhage exploratory laparotomy and appropriate management should be done.

Complications

Maternal outcome

Maternal death as a consequence of rupture uterus varies in different parts of the world. In less and least developed countries, maternal mortality due to rupture uterus ranged from 1% to 14.7% as against only 0–1% in the developed countries.[3,5,7,9,10,19,37] In India, reported maternal mortality ranged from 0–9.3%.[8,17,18] In the Second Report on Confidential Enquiries into Maternal Deaths in South Africa (1999–2001), ruptured uterus caused 6.2% of deaths due to direct causes and 3.7% of all deaths (1.9% due to rupture of an unscarred uterus and 1.8% due to rupture of a scarred uterus).[3] Mokgokong and Marivate noted that the maternal mortality rate associated with uterine rupture largely depends on whether the diagnosis is established before or after delivery; these rates were 4.5% and 10.4%, respectively.[38]

Other complications are:
- Shock
- Postoperative infection
- Bladder and ureter injuries, fistula formation
- Amniotic fluid embolus
- Massive obstetric hemorrhage and disseminated intravascular coagulation (DIC)
- Pituitary failure

Fetal Outcomes

Perinatal outcome depends upon time elapsed between the diagnosis of uterine rupture to the definitive management, i.e. the delivery of the fetus. A high perinatal death 74–92%[3,9,10,17,19] is still associated with rupture uterus as generally only 10–37 minutes are available before clinically significant fetal morbidity and mortality becomes available.[39-43]

Perinatal morbidities associated are:
- Hypoxia or anoxia
- Acidosis (umbilical artery cord pH <7)
- Depressed Apgar scores (Five-minute Apgar score <7)
- Admission to neonatal intensive care unit.

Prevention

Risk of rupture uterus varies depending upon various factors associated with the current pregnancy and the risk out of the previous pregnancy management. The risk in women with unscarred uterus is extremely low as against with scarred uterus. The most direct prevention strategy for minimizing the risk of pregnancy-related uterine rupture is to minimize the number of patients who are at highest risk.

- Counsel for tubectomy along with classical cesarean section or rupture uterus repair (except in low parity cases of scar dehiscence)
- If tubectomy was not done in such cases, then careful monitoring of the cases during subsequent pregnancy and do elective LSCS
- Careful monitoring of cases during subsequent pregnancy and labor with previous history of perforation during D and C, CuT insertion or myomectomy, hysterotomy, previous history of MRP, uterine malformation corrective surgeries
- Avoid multiparity
- Use of partogram in labor
- Judicious use of oxytocics during pregnancy
- Careful selection of cases for LSCS, particularly in primi gravida from rural area who may not be followed up during next pregnancy and come for institutional delivery
- Careful monitoring of previous LSCS delivered case, if trial of labor is being given according to the guidelines for VBAC
- Early detection of the signs and symptoms of scar dehiscence and prompt management
- Elective cesarean section in cases with previous documented classical cesarean section, rupture uterus repair, etc.

FUTURE PREGNANCY

If tubectomy is not done during repair of the ruptured uterus:
- If LSCS scar dehiscence, the patient will behave like a case of previous LSCS scar and managed accordingly with elective LSCS at 38–39 weeks

- If rupture had involved the upper uterine segment extensively or a dehiscence of the classical scar the patient should be counseled against pregnancy as chances of rupture are very high.

CONCLUSION

Rupture uterus is a preventable cause of maternal and perinatal morbidity and mortality. As the outcome is largely dependent on early diagnosis and timely definitive management, while managing the high-risk pregnancies a high level of suspicion regarding the potential diagnosis of rupture uterus and a quick definitive management is of paramount importance.

REFERENCES

1. Landon MB, Hauth JC, Leveno KJ, Spong CY, Leindecker S, Varner MW, et al. Maternal and perinatal outcomes associated with a trial of labor after prior cesarean delivery. N Engl J Med. 2004;351:2581-9.
2. Kurdoglu Z, Kurdoglu M. The risk of uterine rupture in labour induction of women with previous caesarean delivery. Crescent Journal of Medical and Biological Sciences. 2016;3:8-13.
3. WHO systematic review of maternal mortality and morbidity: the prevalence of uterine rupture. BJOG. 2005;112:1221-8.
4. Fitzpatrick KE, Kurinczuk JJ, Alfirevic Z, et al. Uterine rupture by intended mode of delivery in UK: a national case control study. PLos Med. 2012;9;e1001184.
5. Vandenberghe G, MD Blarere, V Van leeuw, K Roelens, Y Englert, M Hanssens, H verstraelen. Nationwide population-based study of uterine rupuature in Belgium: results from the Belgian Obstetric Surveillance System. BMJ Open. 2016;6:e010415.
6. Z Wart JJ, Richters JM, Ory F, et al. Uterine rupture in the Netherland: a nationwide population-based cohort study. BJOG. 2009;116:1069-78.
7. Colmon LB, Petersen KB, Jalobson M, et al. The Nordic Obstetric surveillance Study: a study of complete uterine rupture, abnormally invasive placenta, peripartum hysterectomy and severe blood loss at delivery. Acta Obstet Gynaecol. 2015;94:734-44.
8. Kadowa I. Ruptured uterus in rural Uganda: prevalence, predisposing factors and outcomes. Singapore Med J. 2010; 51:35-8.
9. Akaba GO, Onafowokan O, Offiong RA, Omonua K, Ekele BA. Uterine rupture: trends and fetomaternal outcome in a teaching hospital. Niger J Med. 2013;22:304-8.
10. Qazi Q, Akhtar Z, Khan K, Khan AH. Women Health: uterus rupture, its complications and management in teaching hospital, Bannu. Pakistan. Maedica. 2012;7:49-53.
11. Miller DA, Goodwin TM, Gherman RB, Paul RH. Intrapartum rupture of the unscarred uterus. Obstet Gynecol. 1997;89: 671-73.
12. Al-Zirqi I, Stray Pedersen B, Forsen L, et al. Uterine rupture trends over 40 years. BJOG. 2016;123:780.
13. Gibbons KJ, weber T, Holmgren CM, et al. Maternal and fetal morbidity associated with uterine rupture of the unscarred uterus. Am J Obstet Gynecol. 2015;21:382.
14. Chauhan SP, Martin JN Jr, Henrichs CE, Morrison JC, Magann EF. Maternal and perinatal complications with rupture uterus in 142,075 patients who attempted vaginal birth after caesarean delivery: a review of the literature. Am J Obstet Gynecol. 2003; 189:408-17.
15. Wen SW, Rusen ID, Walker M, et al. Comparison of maternal morbidity and mortality between trial of labour and elective caesarean section among women with previous caesarean delivery. Am J Obstet Gynecol. 2004;19:1263-9.
16. Mozurkewich EL, Hutton EK. Elective repeat cesarean delivery versus trial of labor: a meta-analysis of the literature from 1989 to 1999. Am J Obstet Gynecol. 2000;183(5):1187-97.
17. Sunitha K, Indira I, Suguna P. Clinical study of rupture uterus: assessment of maternal and fetal outcome. IOSR Journal of Dental and Medical Sciences. 2015;14:39-45.
18. Rajaram P, Agrawal A, Swain S. Determinants of maternal mortality: a hospital based study from South India. Indian J Matern Child Health. 1995;6(1):7-10.
19. Partha Saradh, Reddy G, Pateel A. A Study of Rupture Uterus Maternal and Foetal Outcome. IOSR Journal of Dental and Medical Sciences. 2016;15:26-9.
20. Hofmeyr GJ. Obstructed labor: using better technologies to reduce mortality. Int J Gynecol Obstet. 2004;85:62-72.
21. Esraa Hamed. Rupture of uterus in pregnancy and labour in Al-yarmouk Teaching Hospital Iraqui. J Comm Med. 2010; 23(2).
22. Royal College of Obstetrician and Gynaecologists Green top Guideline No. 2007;15.
23. SOGC clinical practice guidelines. Guidelines for vaginal birth after previous caesarean birth. Number 155 (Replaces Guideline Number 147), February; 2005.
24. ACOG Practice bulletin no. 115: Vaginal birth after previous caesarean delivery. Obstet Gynecol. 2010;116:450-63.
25. Guise JM Hashima J, Osterweil P. Evidence-based vaginal birth after caesarean section. Best Prac Clin Obstet Gynecol. 2005;19:117-30.
26. Turner MJ. Uterine rupture. Best Prac Clin Obstet Gynecol. 2002;16:69-79.
27. Usta IM, Hamdi MA, Musa AA, Nassar AH. Pregnancy outcome in patients with previous uterine rupture. Acta Obstet Gynecol Scand. 2007;86(2):172.
28. Claeys JJ, Hellendoorn I, Hamerlynck T, Bosteels J, Weyers S. The risk of uterine rupture after myomectomy: a systematic review of literature and meta-analysis. Gynecol Surg. 2014;11(3): 197-206.
29. Zita Gambocorti-Passerini, Alexis C Gimovsky, Anna Locatelli, Vincenzo Berghela. Trial of labour after myomectomy and uterine rupture: a systematic review. Acte Obstetrica Et Gynecologica Scandinavica. 2016;95:724-34.
30. Lydon-Rochelle, Victoria L. Holt, Thomas R Easterling, Diane P Martin. Risk of uterine rupture during labor among women with a prior cesarean delivery. N Engl J Med. 2001;345:3-8.
31. Deepti Goswami, Sangeeta Bhasin, Swaraj Batra. Obstetric and gynaecological emergencies. Jaypee Brothers Medical Publishers; 2012.

32. Blanchette H, Blanchette M, McCabe J, Vincent S. Is vaginal birth after cesarean safe? Experience at a community hospital. Am J Obstet Gynecol. 2001;184(7):1478-84.
33. Leung AS, Leung EK, Paul RH. Uterine rupture after previous cesarean delivery: maternal and fetal consequences. Am J Obstet Gynecol. 1993;169(4):945-50.
34. Menihan CA. Uterine rupture in women attempting a vaginal birth following prior cesarean birth. J Perinatol. 1998;18:440-3.
35. Yap OW, Kim ES, Laros RK Jr. Maternal and neonatal outcomes after uterine rupture in labor. Am J Obstet Gynecol. 2001;184:1576-81.
36. Bujold E, Gauthier RJ. Neonatal morbidity associated with uterine rupture: what are the risk factors? Am J Obstet Gynecol. 2002;186:311-4.
37. Nahum G. Uterine rupture; 2012.
38. Mokgokong ET, Marivate M. Treatment of the ruptured uterus. S Afr Med J. 1976;50(41):1621-4.
39. Blanchette H, Blanchette M, McCabe J, Vincent S. Is vaginal birth after cesarean safe? Experience at a community hospital. Am J Obstet Gynecol. 2001;184(7):1478-84.
40. Bujold E, Mehta SH, Bujold C, Gauthier RJ. Interdelivery interval and uterine rupture. Am J Obstet Gynecol. 2002;187(5):1199-202.
41. Leung AS, Leung EK, Paul RH. Uterine rupture after previous cesarean delivery: maternal and fetal consequences. Am J Obstet Gynecol. 1993;169(4):945-50.
42. Menihan CA. Uterine rupture in women attempting a vaginal birth following prior cesarean birth. J Perinatol. 1998;18:440-3.
43. Yap OW, Kim ES, Laros RK Jr. Maternal and neonatal outcomes after uterine rupture in labor. Am J Obstet Gynecol. 2001;184(7):1576-81.

Chapter 53

Medical Management of Postpartum Hemorrhage

Madhuri Alwani

INTRODUCTION

Maternal mortality globally is estimated at 529,000 deaths per year, a ratio of 400 maternal deaths per 100,000 live births. Postpartum hemorrhage (PPH) is most common cause of maternal mortality and accounts for one quarter of all maternal deaths worldwide.[1] And its incidence in developed world is increasing.[2] In developing countries, PPH accounts for one third of all maternal death.[3] About 14 million cases of PPH occur each year with a case fatality rate of 1%.[4] According to the recent confidential enquiry into maternal and child health (CEMACH) report, obstetrics hemorrhage occurs in around 3.7 per 1000 births with uterine atony being the most common cause.[5] Worldwide, PPH continues to contribute to significant maternal morbidity and mortality mainly due to 'too little being done too late'.[6] Severe obstetric morbidity may be a more sensitive measure of pregnancy outcome than mortality alone and Waterston et al.[7] have shown that of obstetrics complications, the disease specific morbidity per 1000 deliveries is highest for hemorrhage.

DEFINITION

There is no single, satisfactory definition of PPH. Quantitative definition is arbitrary and is related to the amount of blood loss in excess of 500 mL following birth of the baby (WHO). It may be useful for statistical purpose. As the effect of the blood loss is important rather than the amount of blood lost, the clinical definition which is more practical states "any amount of bleeding from or into the genital tract following birth of the baby up to the end of the puerperium, which adversely affects the general condition of the patient evidence by rise in the pulse rate and falling blood pressure is called postpartum hemorrhage." The average blood loss following vaginal delivery, cesarean delivery and cesarean hysterectomy is 500 mL, 1000 mL and 1500 mL, respectively. Depending upon the amount of blood loss, PPH can be (1) Minor (<1L); (2) Major (>1L) or Severe (>2L).

Incidence is about 4 to 6% of all deliveries.

PPH is classified as primary and secondary. Primary PPH occurs within the first 24 hours following birth of the baby and in secondary PPH hemorrhage occurs beyond 24 hours and within puerperium.

ETIOLOGY AND RISK FACTORS ASSOCIATED WITH PPH

The most common cause of postpartum hemorrhage is uterine atony due to the failure of myometrium to contract and retract after the delivery of the fetus to stop bleeding from the raw placental site. Common risk factors for PPH are mentioned in **Table 53.1**. However, PPH can occur even in women without identifiable risk factors. Numerically, more women without risk factors have atonic PPH compared to those with risk factors. They are related to an over distended uterus due to multiple pregnancy, polyhydramnios or fetal macrosomia.

Table 53.1: Risk factors of PPH[20]

- Placenta previa
- Abruptio placentae
- Multiple pregnancy
- Pre-eclampsia/hypertension
- Asian ethnicity
- Previous PPH
- Obesity (BMI >35)
- Anemia (Hb <9.0 g)
- Induced labor
- Emergency/elective cesarean section
- Mediolateral episiotomy
- Operative vaginal delivery
- Big baby weight >4 kg
- Prolonged labor >12 hrs
- Age > 40
- Pyrexia in labor

Abbreviations: PPH, postpartum hemorrhage; BMI, body mass index

Table 53.2: The 'four Ts': causes of postpartum hemorrhage[21]

Four 'T's cause	Approximate incidence (%)
• Tone-atonic uterus	80
• Trauma—lacerations, hematoma, inversion, rupture	10–15
• Tissue-retained tissue	3–5
• Thrombin-coagulopathies	1–2

PPH is commonly due to abnormalities of one or a combination of four basic processes, referred to in the 4Ts pneumonic **(Table 53.2)**.

MANAGEMENT

Preventon

A large number of risk factors for PPH have been identified but most cases of PPH have no identifiable risk factor. For those women known to have risk factors for PPH appropriate management should be instigated in both the antenatal and intrapartum periods to minimize this risk. Importantly, this should include discussion with the woman and her family about the most appropriate place for delivery. Women with significant risk factors for PPH should deliver in a unit with rapid access to blood and blood products and have antenatal correction of anemia.

The prediction of PPH using antenatal risk assessment is poor. Only 40% of women who develop PPH have an identifiable risk factor.[8] Management of PPH invariably involves addressing the causes of bleeding, commonly known as 'the four Ts'. A fifth 'T' has been added to emphasize the important role of theater and surgery in managing all causes of PPH. The International Confederation of Midwives (ICM) and the International Federation of Gynaecology and Obstetrics (FIGO) have launched a worldwide initiation to promote to active management of third stage of labor for all women.[9]

The intrinsic contribution of each component of the 'active management of the third stage of labor' was examined in light of new available evidence, and relevant recommendations were made. The usual components include administration of uterotonic agents, controlled cord traction and uterine massage after delivery of the placenta. This approach reduces the risks of PPH, postpartum anemia, blood transfusion requirements, prolonged third stage of labor and use of therapeutic drugs for PPH.[10]

Injectable oxytocin has been recommended for routine use in the active management of third stage of labor. It is a synthetic nonpeptide that is routinely administered for prevention and treatment of PPH. Oxytocin is a first line agent because it is effective 2–3 min after injection and, as it has minimal secondary effects, it can be used in all women. If oxytocin is not available, other uterotonics can be used, such as ergometrine maleate 500 μg IM or ergometrine with oxytocin 5 IU/mL or misoprostal.

Misoprostal, a prostaglandin E1 analog, is more stable than oxytocin and has been administered by oral, sublingual and rectal routes.[11] However, there are concerns that misuse of misoprostal can lead to significant maternal morbidity. The main side effects are nausea, vomiting and diarrhea. Shivering and elevated body temperature has also been reported with the use of misoprostal in third stage of labor. Rectal misoprostal causes less pyrexia and shivering than oral misoprostal.

TREATMENT (FLOW CHART 53.1)

A systematic and stepwise management of PPH can be achieved with the use of the mnemonic "HAEMOSTASIS" following each step in rapid succession **(Table 53.3)**. The pneumonic is conveniently divided into two parts—medical and surgical.

H: Ask for Help

Massive PPH should be managed appropriately with a multidisciplinary input. Senior obstetricians and anesthetists, midwives and theater staffs, hematologists and blood bank and the intensive care unit should be alerted.

A: Assess (Vital Parameters, Blood Loss) and Resuscitate

Early recognition, prompt resuscitation and rapid restoration of the circulating blood volume are the key components of the initial management of PPH. General resuscitation measures include assessment of hemodynamic status by monitoring patient's vital signs—level of consciousness, blood pressure, pulse and oxygen saturation. Two large bore cannulae should be inserted and blood samples taken for full blood count, group and save or cross-match (depending on the severity of hemorrhage), coagulation screen and renal and liver profile.

Fluid resuscitation in PPH is often overly conservative because of underestimation of volume and rapidity of blood loss. It is important to remember that symptoms of hypovolemia are often delayed due to compensatory mechanisms. Moreover, concerns that fluid overload may lead to pulmonary edema, or failure may be misleading. A loss of 1 liter of blood requires replacement with 4 to 5 liters of crystalloid (0.9% normal saline or lactated ringer's solution) or colloids until cross-matched blood is available, as most of the infused fluid shifts from the intravascular to the interstitial space.[12]

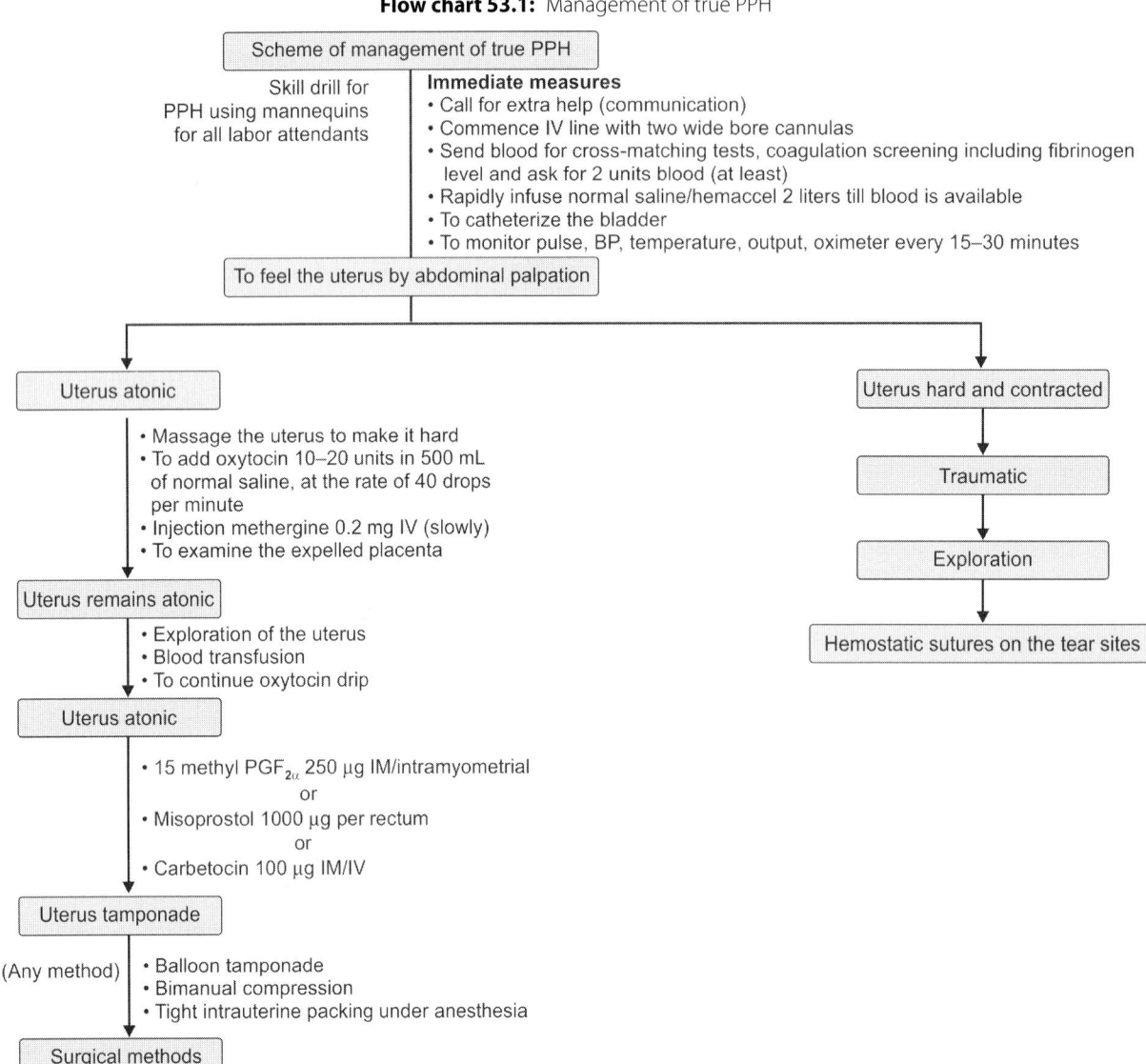

Flow chart 53.1: Management of true PPH

Table 53.3: HAEMOSTASIS mnemonics
General medical management
H Ask for help
A Assess (vital parameters, blood loss) and resuscitate
E Establish etiology, "4T's"-tone, tissue, trauma, thrombin
M Massage the uterus
O Oxytocin infusion, prostaglandins (intravenous, rectal, intramuscular, intramyometrial)
Specific surgical management
S Shift to operation theater
T Tissue and trauma to be excluded and proceed to tamponade balloon, uterine packing
A Apply compression sutures
S Systematic pelvic devascularization
I Interventional radiology
S Subtotal or total abdominal hysterectomy

Golden First Hour and the Rule of 30

Severe hemorrhage can lead to cardiovascular failure as more time elapses between the onset of severe shock and resuscitation, the chances of survival decrease because metabolic acidosis sets in. "The golden hour" is the time at which resuscitation must be commenced to ensure the best chance of survival. The probability of survival decreases sharply after the first hour, if the patient is not affectively resuscitated.

For the general acute management of PPH, 'A rule of 30' has been proposed. If the patients systolic blood pressure (SBP) falls by 30 mm of Hg, heart rate (HR) rises by 30 bpm, respiratory rate (RR) increases to more than 30 breaths per minute and hemoglobin (Hb) or hematocrit (Hct) drop by 30% and or urinary output is less than 30 mL/hour, then the patient is most likely to have lost at least 30% of blood volume and is in moderate shock leading to severe shock.[13]

E: Establish Etiology, Ecbolics and Ensure Availability of Blood

- Establish etiology—'4Ts', tone, tissue, trauma and thrombin
- Ecbolics (syntometrine, ergometrine, bolus syntocinon)
- Ensure availability of blood and blood products.

A systematic assessment for identifying the cause of bleeding should be made using mnemonic "4Ts". Thorough assessment of the uterine size and tone should be followed by vigorous uterine massage and administration of therapeutic uterotonic agents if the uterus is atonic. If bleeding persists despite well-contracted uterus, examination under anesthesia should be performed to look for extended tears in the cervix or high in the vaginal vault, as these may extend into the uterus or the broad ligament or they may cause retroperitoneal hematomas. Pressure or packing over the tears may be useful to achieve hemostasis and prevent of formation of hematomas. If retained tissue or trauma is excluded and bleeding continues despite a well-contracted uterus, a defect in the coagulation is unlikely cause.

A uterine atony is the most common cause, medical management usually consists of oxytocin 10 units by slow intravenous injection, ergometrine 0.5 mg by slow intravenous injection, methergine 0.2 mg intramuscularly, oxytocin infusion, 15-methyl PGF-2α intramuscularly or intramyometrially, dinoprostone vaginally or rectally, or misoprost.

Blood and blood product transfusion should be commenced, if bleeding is continuing, if the estimated blood loss is over 30% of the blood volume, or if the patient is hemodynamically unstable despite aggressive resuscitation. Group-specific or group O Rh-negative blood should be transfused until cross-matched blood becomes available. 1 liter of fresh-frozen plasma should be administered (15 mL/kg) with every 6 units of blood transfused. Cryoprecipitate which provides a more concentrated form of fibrinogen and other clotting. Factors (VIII, XIII, von Willebrand factor), may be required if there is DIC, or if the fibrinogen level is less than 10 g/L.

M: Massage the Uterus

Uterine massage, either manually (hand on the fundus) or bimanually (vaginal hand in the anterior fornix; abdominal hand on the posterior aspect of the fundus) is a simple and a very effective firstline measure and reduces bleeding even if the uterus remains atonic, allowing resuscitation to take effect with a reduced blood loss. If uterine atony continues after oxytocics are given, then bimanual compression is undertaken.

O: Oxytocin Infusion, Prostaglandins (Table 53.4)

Oxytocin can be administered as a slow IV bolus (10 units) or as an infusion (40 units in 500 mL of 0.9% normal saline, infused at the rate of 125 mL/hr) in order to maintain uterine contraction. Although there are no absolute contraindications, an antidiuretic effect with volume overload may develop with high cumulative doses. If the uterus remains atonic after initial oxytocin therapy, syntometrine or ergometrine should be repeated.

Carboprost is a prostaglandin F2 analog, which is administered intramuscularly or intramyometrially. This is 80–90% effective in stopping PPH in cases that are refractory to oxytocin and ergometrine. It is contraindicated in asthma as it has bronchoconstrictor properties.

Misoprostol is a synthetic prostaglandin E1 analog, which has been used in the management of PPH. A recent Cochrane review concluded that there is insufficient evidence to show

Table 53.4: Commonly used oxytocics in the management of PPH[22-24]

Drug	Dose	Route	Dose frequency	Side effects	Contraindications
Oxytocin	10–40 units in 1 L of crystalloid solution	*First line:* IV *Second line:* IM (10 units)	Continuous IV	• Nausea • Water intoxication	Not as IV bolus, otherwise none
Methergine	0.2 mg	*First line:* IM/IV *Second line:* PO	Every 2–4 hours	• Nausea • Vomiting • Hypertension	• Hypertension • Pre-eclampsia
15 methyl PGF$_{2\alpha}$	0.25 mg	*First line* IM: *Second line:* Intrauterine	Every 15–90 min (8 doses maximum)	• Nausea • Vomiting • Diarrhea • Chills	• Bronchial asthma • Active cardiac, renal or hepatic disease
Misoprostol (PGE$_1$)	600–1000 µg	*First line:* PR *Second line:* PO	Single dose	• Fever • Tachycardia	None

that addition of misoprotol is superior to the combination of oxytocin and ergometrine alone for the treatment of primary PPH.[14] The peak serum concentration of oxytocin is much shorter than oral misoprostol which reaches its serum peak concentration at 20 minutes, a combination of these two agents could provide a sustained uterotonic effect.

Carbetocin functions as an agonist at peripheral oxytocin receptors, particularly in the myometrium, with lesser affinity for myoepithelial cells. During pregnancy, the synthesis of oxytocin receptors in the uterus greatly increase, reaching a peak during labor and delivery. The dose of this drug is 100 µg IM/IV.

Recombinant Activated Factor VII

A number of case reports of empirical 'off-label' use of rFVIIa show that it may be an alternative hemostatic agent when the standard treatment is ineffective. Recombinant activated factor VII (rFvIIa, NovoSeven; Novo nordisk A/S, Bagsvaerd, Denmark) was originally used in treating hemorrhage in patients with hemophilia with inhibitors, acquired hemophilia or other inherited bleeding disorders. In recent years, it has been used in nonhemophiliac hemorrhage, including life-threatening obstetric hemorrhage. A number of case reports of empirical "offlabel" use of rFVIIa show that it may be an alternative hemostatic agent when the standard treatment is ineffective. The Scottish Confidential Audit of Severe Maternal Morbidity recommends that if conservative measures fail to control hemorrhage, surgical hematosis should be commenced 'sooner rather than later'. In addition, recommendations have been made that all hospitals with delivery units should aim to provide an emergency interventional radiology service as these have the potential to save lives of patients with catastrophic PPH.[15,16]

To improve the preparedness and efficiency of treatment in PPH, a low cost, portable, comprehensive obstetrics emergency box **(Table 53.5)**, PPH drug box **(Table 53.6)**, PPH Trauma inspection tray and balloon tamponade tray are kept separately **(Figs 53.1 and 53.2)**.

PPH Trauma Inspection pack **(Fig. 53.3)**:
- 4 sponge holders
- 2 large Sim's speculum
- 4 inch ribbon gauze—a large ball approx 3 meters
- Long needle holder
- Toothed forceps
- Straight scissors.

Condom tamponade:
- Single use condom
- IV set
- Silk thread.

Table 53.5: List of contents of the obstetrics emergency box[25]

Contents	Numbers
IV Cannula	Gray #1
	Green #1
Blood Sample Bottles	Pink #1
	Blue #1
	Red #1
Syringes	20 mL #2
	10 mL #4
	5 mL #2
	2 mL #6
Plaster to fix the cannula	1
Foley's catheter size 16	1
Urobag	1
Distilled water 10 mL	1
Infusion set	1
Blood set	1
Sterile gloves size 6½	1 pair
Cotton swabs	
Pair of scissors	1
Ringer lactate	1 Unit
3 way	1
Oxygen mask	1
Airway (Medium)	1

Table 53.6: PPH drug kit[22-24]

Oxytocin	10 amp
Ergometrine	2 amp
PGF$_{2\alpha}$ 250 µg	4 amp
Misoprostol 600 µg	2 tab

Tamponade with Balloon or Uterine Packing

Uterine Packing

This has long been considered safe, quick and effective for controlling PPH.[15] The use of uterine packing in the management of PPH fell in to disfavor after 1950s following concerns that it: (i) was a potentially traumatic and time-consuming procedure; (ii) might conceal on-going hemorrhage; (iii) might predispose to the development

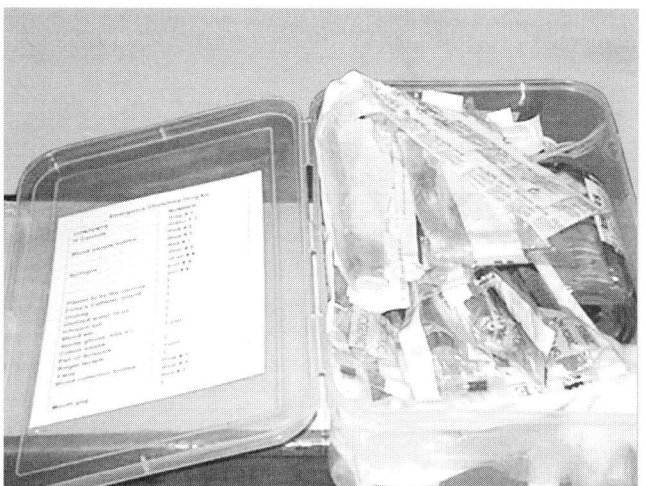

Fig. 53.1: Emergency obstetric drug box

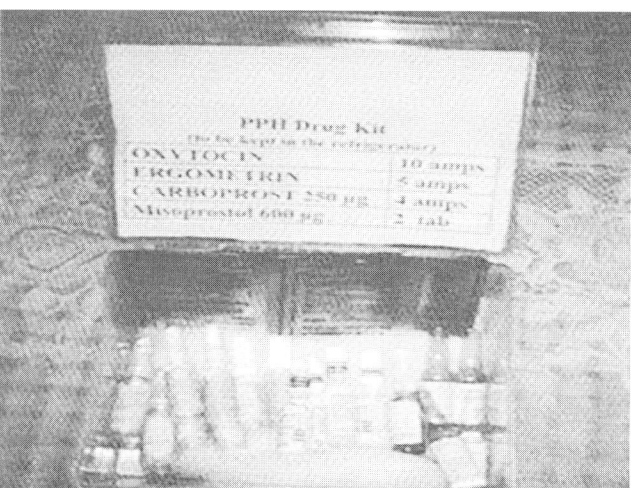

Fig. 53.2: Postpartum hemorrhage drug box

of infection; and (iv) represented a 'nonphysiological approach'.[16] More recently, it has been concluded that uterine packing is a safe, quick and effective procedure for controlling PPH.

Intrauterine Tamponade

Using different types of balloon has been suggested as an effective, easy and minimal invasive method to control uterine bleeding temporarily. Multiple types of balloons are available, including Bakri balloon, BT-cath balloon tamponade catheter, Foley's catheters, Rusch balloon, condom catheters and Sengstaken-Blakemore tube. The Bakri postpartum balloon and BT-cath balloon tamponade catheters are specifically designed for postpartum intrauterine tamponade. More recently, success has been reported with the use of 'Shivkar pack'. In this method, a collapsed condom is introduced into the atonic uterine cavity. The end of an intravenous infusion set connected to a saline infusion bottle is introduced into the condom and the free end of the condom tied firmly around the infusion tubing about 3–4 inches distal to its end. By raising the saline bottle to a height of about 2 feet the saline is permitted to run into the condom and distend the same. The ballooned condom adapts itself very well to the uterine cavity and exerts uniform lateral pressure all around thereby obliterating the bleeding sinuses; heavy bleeding comes promptly under control. Intrauterine balloon pressure is maintained for about 2 hours; thereafter the distended condom is progressively deflated and finally removed. This method has been found to be very effective in emergency situations when very little help is available—it has often spared the patient the need for surgery and helped retain the uterus. It must be emphasized that this method has a special place in rural obstetric practice as the materials

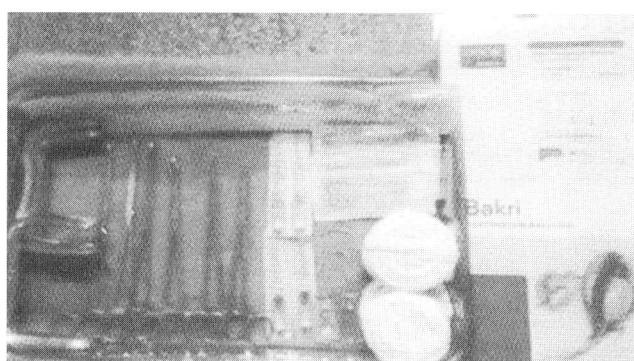

Fig. 53.3: PPH trauma inspection pack

used are easily available. The method helps to buy time whilst arrangements are being made to transfer the patient to a hospital. In desperate situation, further delay and persistence with conservative measures seen unwarranted, a surgical option has to be exercised.

WHAT IS NEW IN THE MANAGEMENT OF POSTPARTUM HEMORRHAGE?

Transfusion Strategies

Fluid replacement is the initial resuscitating step of PPH to normalize blood volume and current recommendation is to infuse crystalloids and colloids. However, this significantly worsens existing coagulopathy and enhances fibrinolysis.[17] A ratio of FFP:platelets:RBC 1:1:1 was associated with a significant reduction in mortality. (40% versus 60%) as compared to the traditional one unit of FFP, one unit of platelets for every four unit of blood transfused (1:1:4 ratio).

Massive Transfusion Protocols (Flow chart 53.2)

The morbidity and mortality associated with massive PPH is often accompanied by a triad of hypothermia, acidosis and coagulopathy. This has led to development of pre-defined protocol driven early transfusion of RBC, platelets, FFP and crystalloid solutions which may allow significant improvement in outcomes. *Massive transfusion is defined*, in adults, as replacement of >1 *blood* volume in 24 hours or >50% of *blood* volume in 4 hours (adult *blood* volume is approximately 70 mL/kg).

Tranexamic Acid

Although, the role of tranexamic acid (TXA) in surgical and trauma patients has been extensively studied, its role in obstetric hemorrhage is still under evaluation. A recent French study reported that the use of TXA was associated with a lower median blood loss, increased likelihood of stopping bleeding within 30 minutes and less chance of progressing to severe PPH in women undergoing vaginal delivery when compared with controls.[18] The role of TXA in postpartum hemorrhage is currently evaluated by multicentre RCT.[19]

CONCLUSION

PPH is a leading cause of maternal morbidity and mortality. Although identification of risk factors antenatally and during labor may be useful in the prevention and management of PPH, severe life-threatening hemorrhage is often unpredictable.

Prompt resuscitation of the patient with restoration of circulating blood volume and identification of the cause of bleeding should be performed by multidisciplinary approach. Rapid succession of treatment measures in a stepwise, systematic management of PPH can be facilitated using the algorithm 'HAEMOSTASIS' and assessment tools such as the 'rule of thirty'. Protocols for the prevention and management of PPH should be in place in every maternity unit. Training in

Flow chart 53.2: Massive transfusion protocol (MTP) template

```
The information below, developed by consensus, broadly covers areas that should be included
in a local MTP, this template can be used to develop an MTP to meet the needs of the local
institution's patient population and resources
           ↓
Senior clinician determines that patient meets criteria for
MTP activation
           ↓
Baseline
Full blood count, coagulation screen (PT, INR, APTT, fibrinogen),
biochemistry, arterial blood gases
           ↓
Notify transfusion laboratory (insert contact no.) to:
Activate MTP
```

Laboratory staff
- Notify hematologist/tranfusion specialist
- Prepare and issue blood components as requested
- Anticipate repeat testing and blood component requirements
- Minimize test turnaround times
- Consider staff resources

Hematologist/transfusion specialist
- Liaise regularly with laboratory and clinical team
- Assist in interpretation of results, and advise on blood component support

Senior clinician
- *Request:*
  - 4 units RBC
  - 4 units FFP
- *Consider:*
  - 1 adult therapeutic dose platelets
  - Tranexamic acid in trauma patients
- *Include:*
  - Cryoprecipitate, if fibrinogen < 1g/L

Bleeding controlled?
Yes / No
→ Notify transfusion laboratory to: Cease MTP

Optimize
- Oxygenation
- Cardiac output
- Tissue perfusion
- Metabolic state

Monitor (every 30–60 mins)
- Full blood count
- Coagulation screen
- Ionized calcium
- Arterial blood gases

Aim
- Temperature >35°C
- pH > 7.2
- Base excess <–6
- Lactate <4 mmol/L
- Ca^{2+} > 1.1 mmol/L
- Platelets >50 × 10^9/L
- PT/APTT <1.5 × normal
- INR ≤ 1.5
- Fibrinogen > 1.0 g/L

the management of this common obstetric emergency should include regular 'fire drills' involving all the members of staff. The use of tranexamic acid may help improve outcomes.

REFERENCES

1. World Health Organisation. The World Health Report 2005. Make every mother and child count. Geneva: WHO; 2005.
2. Lalonde A, Herschdorfer K. Postpartum hemorrhage today:ICM/FIGO initiative 2004-2006. Int J Gynecol Obstet. 2006;243-53.
3. Khan KS, Wjoydyla D, Say L, Gulmezoglu AM, Van Look PF. WHO analysis of causes of maternal death: a systematic review. Lancet. 2006:1066-74.
4. Department of Reproductive Health and Research, World Health Organisation. Maternal mortality in 2000: estimates developed by WHO, UNICEF and UNFPA. Geneva: WHO; 2004.
5. Saving mothers lives: reviewing maternal deaths to make motherhood safer; 2006-2008. The eighth report of the confidential enquires into maternal deaths in the United Kingdom. BJOG. 2011;118;1-203.
6. Why mother die? Triennial report 2000-02. confidential enquiries into maternal and child death. UK; 2004.
7. Waterstone M, Bewley S, Wolfe C. Indicators and predictors of severe obstetric morbidity: case-control study. BMJ 200;322:1089-93, discussion 1093-1094. ACOG Practice Bulletin: Clinical Management Guidelines for Obstetricians and Gynaecologists Number 76, October 2006: postpartum haemorrhage. Obstet Gynecol. 2006;108:1039-47.
8. Sherman SJ, Greenspoon JS, Nelson JM, Paul RH. Denitrifying the obstetric patient at high risk of multiple unit blood transfusions. J Report Med. 1992;37:649-52.
9. Lalonde A, Daviss BA Acosta A, Herschderfer K. Postpartum haemorrhage today; ICM/FIGO initiative 2004-2006. Int J Gynaecol Obstet. 2006;94:243-53.
10. Prendiville WJ, Ebourne D, Mcdonald S. Active versus expectant management in the third stage of labour. Cochrane Database Syst Rev. 2000(3):CD000007.
11. Hofmeyr GJ, Walraven G, Gulmezgolu AM, Maholwana B, Alfirevic Z, Villar J. Misoprostol to treat postpartum haemorrhage: a systematic review. Br J Obstet Gynaecol. 2005; 112:547-53.
12. Ramanathan G, Arulkumaran S. Postpartum haemorrhage. J Obstet Gynacol Can. 2006;28:967- 73.
13. Chandrahan E, Arulkumaran S. Massive postpartum haemorrhage and management of coagulopathy. Obstet Gynaecol Reprod Med. 2007;17:119-22.
14. Mousa HA, Alfirevic Z. Treatment for primary postpartum haemorrhage. Cochrane database Syst Rev. 2007(1):CD003249.
15. Royal College of Obstetricians and Gynaecologists. The Role of Emergency and Elective Interventional Radiology in Postpartum Haemorrhage. Good Practice Guidelines. London: RCOG; 2007.
16. Investigations into 10 maternal deaths at, or following delivery at, Northwick Park Hospital, North West London Hospitals NHS Trust, between April 2002 and April 2005. London: Healthcare Commission; 2006.
17. Chandraharan E, Rao S. The Triple—P procedure as a conservative surgical alternative to peripartum hysterectomy for placenta percreta: International Journal of Genecology and Obstetrics. 2012;117(2):191-4.
18. Huissoud C, Carrabin N, Audibert F, et al. Bedside assessment of fibrinogen level in postpartum haemorrhage by thromboelastometry. BJOG. 2009;116(8):1097-102.
19. Gungorduk K, Yildirim G, Asicioglu O, et al. Efficacy of intravenous tranexamic acid in reducing blood loss after elective cesarean section: a prospective, randomized double blind, placebo-controlled study. Am J Perinatal. 2011;28 (3):233-40.
20. Lill Trine Nyfløt, Irene Sandven, Babill Stray-Pedersen, Silje Pettersen, Iqbal Al-Zirqi, Margit Rosenberg, et al. Risk factors for severe postpartum hemorrhage: a case-control study. BMC Pregnancy Childbirth. 2017;17:17.
21. Evensen A, Anderson JM, Fontaine P. Postpartum hemorrhage: prevention and treatment. Am FAM Physician. 2017;95(7):442-9.
22. Varatharajan L, Chandraharan E, Sutton J, Lowe V, Arulkumaran S. Outcome of the management of massive postpartum hemorrhage using the algorithm "HEMOSTASIS". Int J Gynaecol Obstet. 2011;113(2):152-4. doi: 10.1016/j.ijgo.2010.11.021. Epub 2011 Mar 10.
23. Toppozada M. The use of prostaglandins in postpartum haemorrhage. J Egypt Soc Obstet Gynecol. 1991;17(1):9-18..
24. Mirteimouri M, Tara F, Teimouri B, Sakhavar N, Vaezi A. Efficacy of rectal misoprostol for prevention of postpartum hemorrhage. Iran J Pharm Res. 2013 Spring; 12(2):469-74.
25. Bajwa SK, Bajwa SJS. Delivering obstetrical critical care in developing nations. Int J Crit Illn Inj Sci. 2012;2(1):32-9.

Chapter 54

Balloon Tamponade in Postpartum Hemorrhage

Nalini Mishra, Devanshi Mishra Vyas, Kanchan Gulbani, Mamta Sai

INTRODUCTION

Though the Millennium Development Goals came to end in 2015, many resource-poor countries have fallen short of achieving the same.[1,2] The new Sustainable Development Goals set the objectives of reducing global maternal mortality ratio to less than 70 per 100,000 live births by the year 2030.[3] This needs urgent strategies to reduce the deaths due to postpartum hemorrhage (PPH) which is the major contributor to maternal mortality (accounting for up to 35% cases) in the developing countries.[4]

There is evidence of substandard care in most of deaths due to PPH mainly at the level of primary care in resource-poor settings due to lack of facility for surgery or blood transfusions. If the first-line medical measures are not effective in arresting the ongoing hemorrhage, women with severe PPH are often referred to a higher center in a critical state and many of them succumb on the way. These deaths are largely preventable.[5]

As per the WHO and FIGO, the use of intrauterine balloon tamponade (UBT) is recommended for the treatment of PPH due to uterine atony (which is the cause for nearly 80% cases of PPH) if women do not respond to uterotonics or if uterotonics are not available.[6,7] The balloon tamponade is reported to be successful in 80–100% cases.[8] It is an emergency management where the surgical management is not available and even if available; most of the times is not needed after the balloon placement. It may be a lifesaving intervention in the woman who would otherwise have died during the course of transfer to a higher facility. Advantages of this method include avoidance of laparotomy as well as easy and rapid insertion. It can even be performed by relatively inexperienced personnel. The removal is easy and success rate is at par with surgical interventions which carry significant morbidity and necessitate operation theater facilities along with trained medical team.

TAMPONADE TEST

A 'positive test' (control of PPH following inflation of the balloon) indicates that laparotomy is not required.

A 'negative test' (continued PPH following inflation of the balloon) is an indication to proceed to laparotomy.

History: Historically, uterine packing with roller gauze was reported as early as 1856 to treat refractory uterine atony. This method fell out of favor due to the risk of uterine injury due to blind insertion, infection and concealed hemorrhage associated with it.

Later on, a group of silicone Foley catheters (eight to be precise), each filled with 35–75 mL of N-saline were tried for uterine tamponade but the problem was that when applied individually (without an overbag), they did not readily conform to uterine anatomy; and therefore, the potential for effective site-specific tamponade could not be achieved. On the other hand if they were applied jointly in a plastic covering or overbag, this did not allow for proper drainage with a fear of concealed uterine hemorrhage. In general, the application of multiple Foleys was cumbersome.

Balloon tamponade: In modern obstetrics, uterine tamponade is achieved by balloon catheters to avoid these complications. Various devices are used for uterine tamponade.

TYPES OF BALLOON TAMPONADE

Uterine-specific balloon tamponade devices such as Bakri balloon®, BT-Cath® and EBB®. All these balloons have a drainage channel and insufflation system. Bakri balloon is the most studied and used device. It has a capacity of 500 mL and is made of silicon. The drainage channel allows direct measurement of blood drainage from the uterine cavity but the major disadvantage is the cost (around 250$, i.e. 13000–15000 Rupees) and, therefore, it is not feasible in developing countries with low resources.

Non-uterine specific balloon tamponade devices such as the Sengstaken-Blakemore tube, Rusch balloon, Foley's catheter and the condom catheter balloon. Out of these, the first two are not commonly found in a basic obstetric setup. The capacity of the bulb of common largest size Foleys catheter (24 Fr) is not more than 150 mL. Condom balloon has a definite edge over others in that the condoms are widely available in health facilities in low resource settings and are relatively cheap. Additionally, the Foley's catheter, intravenous infusion sets are common in every labor ward. A simple Condom Balloon uterine Tamponade (CBT) device which is assembled on the spot using these basic minimum resources is, therefore, the most feasible second-line intervention for management of PPH in these settings.[9]

VARIETIES OF CONDOM BALLOON TAMPONADE PREPARED ON THE SPOT

Conventional CBT

It is prepared in the following way: Arrange the following items on a sterile towel laid on a side trolley.
- A catheter
- A condom
- Sterile No. 0 or 1 suture
- A bottle of warmed saline
- Intravenous infusion set released from the pack.

Take the catheter out of the packing and unfold the condom over the end of the catheter to about two thirds of its length (in case it is Foley's). Hand tie it to the catheter firmly, using several rounds of sterile suture at a point about 2 cm distal to the open end of the condom. Have an assistant connect the infusion set to the bottle of warmed normal saline suspended 4–6 feet above the patient. Connect the other end to the catheter, run saline into the condom to make sure the system is water tight by holding the catheter tip upwards, afterwards, empty the balloon of the saline and wash the condom with either warm saline or 5% povidone iodine.

Insertion of balloon: Place the woman either in the dorsal or lithotomy position and expose the cervix by using one or two Sim's speculae. Grasp the anterior lip of the cervix with a sponge holder. Now insert the entire condom catheter system into the uterus. One can keep the condom catheter between the index and middle fingers and introduce it like exploring the uterus (or doing a pelvic examination).

Insufflation: Reconnect the catheter to a giving set and start filling the condom with warmed saline until the balloon conforms to the shape of uterus and the uterine fundus become firmly palpable or bleeding is controlled (whatever is earlier). Keep watching the cervix for the balloon to start bulging out of it and stop filling it any further than 500 mL is instilled. The cessation of bleeding from the uterine cavity may be noticed. If the bleeding stops, pack the vagina with a vaginal pack (two-inch ribbon gauze pack or a gauze towel) around the catheter in a circumferential manner. The other end of the catheter is folded and a tight tie placed on it or else a clamp may be applied to prevent backflow.

During CS: The balloon is placed in a transabdominal manner (retrograde) after placing the CBT in the uterine cavity through the uterine incision, the catheter shaft is traversed through the cervical canal into the vagina where it is pulled out by an assistant. The balloon is inflated after closing the uterine incision but before closing the abdominal wall which is done after the control of bleeding is achieved.

Inconsistencies of conventional CBT: There are some inherent problems associated with the conventional CBT particularly when prepared by inexperienced health professionals. These are mostly related to thread or suture material used to tie the condom to catheter. It is time consuming and may lead to a very tight knot which occludes the lumen and hinders inflation of balloon or it may be a loose knot causing leakage of saline and thereby defeating the whole purpose. Sometimes, the string cuts through the condom material with consequent leakage of the distending fluid and thereby forfeiting the whole purpose. Another problem is that after placement and inflation of conventional CBT, the distal end needs to be occluded. The usual practice is to do so with string or knotting the catheter on itself. Sometimes, a clamp is used but is inconvenient to the woman and is often not recovered after transfer. Lastly, since there is no drainage port in conventional CBT, the direct measurement of ongoing intrauterine bleeding cannot be done and one has to rely on indirect measures like regularly checking the vulval pad for estimating the amount of bleeding which has dribbled down from the uterine cavity. The diagnosis of ongoing hemorrhage may be delayed as well as inaccurate by this indirect method.

All these inconsistencies can cause reluctance to use the method. To overcome these hassles and to further reduce the cost of this lifesaving intervention, two innovative CBTs are being used successfully and are as follows.

Innovative Condom Balloons

Easy Balloon

This is an endeavor to make the assembly of CBT very fast and consistent. It begins by rolling the condom over the Foley's catheter of any available size (usually 16 or 18 Fr). Care is taken to ensure placement of catheter tip into the blind tip of condom. Now two rings of 1 millimeter width are cut from the drainage port of Foley's catheter **(Fig. 54.1)**. First of these rings is used to tie the condom to the catheter by encircling twice over it just in the manner of tying a ponytail with a rubber band. Another ring is used to occlude the distal end of balloon catheter after the placement and insufflation of the device in the uterus **(Fig. 54.2)**. The bulb inflation port of the Foley's catheter may be excised optionally to facilitate placement of ring. Occlusion of distal end of catheter with this ring is quick to perform, allows further inflation if needed as well as very easy deflation.

Method of use: The device is to be dipped in antiseptic solution for at least 3 minutes. The anterior lip of cervix is caught

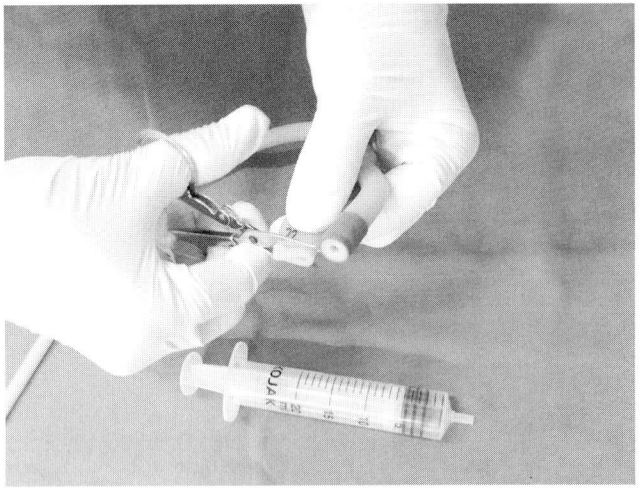

Fig. 54.1: Foley's catheter

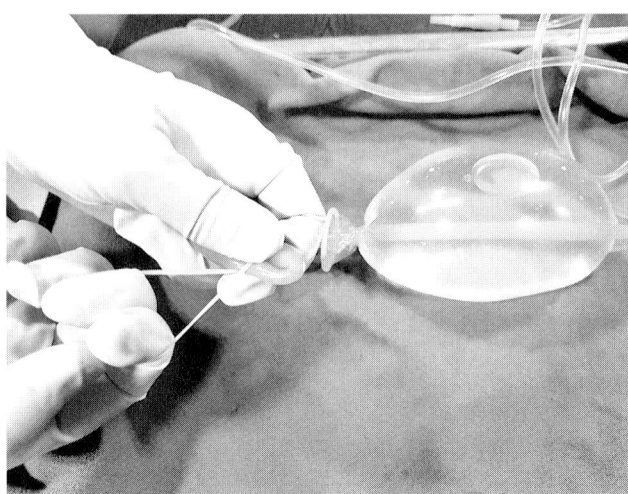

Fig. 54.2: Easy balloon

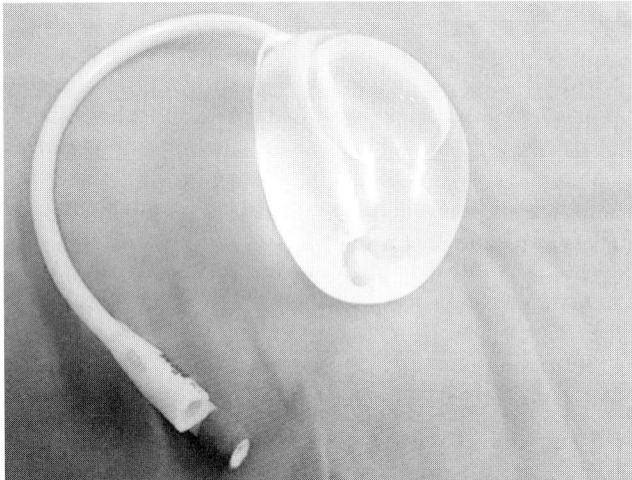

Fig. 54.3: CG balloon

with the help of sponge-holding forceps and the device is introduced in the uterine cavity by holding it between two fingers till the rim of condom comes at external cervical os. The device is then inflated with saline by connecting the catheter to a drip set till the bleeding stops or an amount of 500 mL is reached. After hemostasis, vagina is packed and the distal end is occluded with the second ring by wounding around it twice or thrice.

Easy balloon can also be used successfully in cases of cesarean sections with closed cervix having PPH which is not responding to oxytocic agents. In these situations, after placing the Easy Balloon in the uterine cavity through the uterine incision, the bulb inflation port may be excised to reduce the dimensions of the distal end of catheter to facilitate the retrograde passage of catheter through the narrow cervical canal. Rest of the process is similar to conventional CBT.

This simple, consistent, easiest to assemble and easy to deflate CBT is named Easy Balloon. This device can be assembled and used by trained frontline workers at peripheral health facilities to reduce blood loss during transfer and thereby lowering maternal mortality.

This device is particularly useful when a fast assembly and faster insufflations is required

CG Balloon

This innovative CBT has a drainage port for direct assessment of ongoing blood loss. It requires a Foley catheter (minimum 20–22 Fr and preferably 24 Fr) in addition to a condom, scissors, two 20 mL syringes, and saline. It is prepared manually in following steps:

Cut two rings of approximately 1–2 mm in width from the distal end of the drainage tube of the catheter in a manner similar to Easy Balloon. About 5 mL of air is now introduced into the bulb of the catheter followed by excision of bulb completely, the condom is then unfolded over one third of the proximal end of the catheter and the condom is secured over the catheter at both ends keeping 1–2 cm away from each end. This is done by encircling these rings twice over the condom in the same manner as tying a ponytail. The assembly of the device is completed by excising together, the tip of the Foley catheter and condom. This creates the drainage hole at the top in a manner similar to that of uterine-specific devices. **(Fig. 54.3)**.

Method of use: The device should be dipped in antiseptic solution and inserted into the uterine cavity in a manner similar to Easy Balloon. The balloon here is filled with saline (maximum 500 mL) through the bulb-inflation port of the catheter using syringes in an alternating repetitive manner until the bleeding is controlled. The rim of the CG Balloon

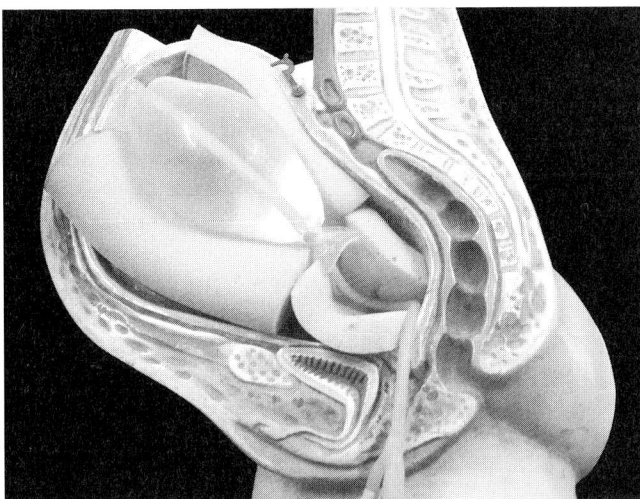

Fig. 54.4: Balloon in uterus

should be at the level of cervical os **(Fig. 54.4)**. Once the hemorrhage is arrested, the vagina is packed with gauze and bleeding is assessed at the outflow port, which is connected to a collecting bag.

Post-placement care of condom balloon tamponade (all varieties): In all CBTs, after vaginal packing, mark the level of the fundus as well as the lateral margins of the uterus on the abdomen with a marker pen. Start oxytocin 10 units in 500 mL @40 drops per minute. Monitor vital signs and uterine height closely. Start antibiotic prophylaxis.

Deflation: If there is no vaginal bleeding, no change in the height of the uterus and vital signs are stable, plan to remove the catheter at a convenient time 6–24 hours later. Generally it is removed after 12–24 hours. In conventional CBT the tie/knot or clamp is released and in case of Easy Balloon, the deflation is done by simply pulling the two arms of the folded distal end of the catheter in opposite directions which allows the saline to come out. In case of CG Balloon, the saline is withdrawn with the help of a syringe. Do not remove the pack at this stage. Observe for recurrence of bleeding for next 30 minutes. Remove the vaginal pack now without removing the condom catheter. If there is no further bleeding for another 30 minutes, release the total volume of instilled saline and remove the condom catheter gently.

CONTRAINDICATIONS TO USE OF CBT

- Allergy to latex
- Chorioamnionitis
- Cancer Cx
- Arterial bleeding requiring exploration and ligation or angiographic embolization
- Cases indicating hysterectomy

- Where uterine rupture is suspected
- Malformation of uterus
- Retained products of conception.

Theoretical complications like perforation, necrosis and rupture of the uterus are largely based on the use of balloons in other organ systems such as the esophagus and also reported for the Sengstaken–Blakemore tube in the esophagus.

To date, there have only been one such report of uterine rupture complicating sequential curettage and Bakri balloon tamponade to control secondary PPH. Woman with two previous cesarean sections underwent dilation and evacuation procedure under GA and bled, managed by medical management and tamponade. Later a uterine defect at the site of the cesarean section scar was detected. The opinion was that most likely it was a dehiscence rather than an iatrogenic injury that occurred at the time of uterine evacuation.[10]

So far, there is no other report of perforation of the balloon devices through the uterus following placement.

Extended Use

- Placenta previa, morbidly adherent placenta in placenta accreta, conservative method, i.e. Affronti sutures combined with external (B-lynch suture) and internal (ut. balloon) uterine compression can be considered an Option in the management of selected cases.
- PPH secondary to vaginal lacerations, an important observation concluded that after a vaginal delivery vaginal tissues can be edematous, friable and very difficult to suture. Vaginal balloon tamponade can be a solution in difficult cases of intractable vaginal hemorrhage or occult vaginal bleeding causing vaginal hematoma. A self-retaining vaginal balloon tamponade device can be a safe and effective solution. Vaginal balloon tamponade is well tolerated by the patients.[11]
- In the prevention of recurrent uterine inversion
- In the absence of blood resources and facilitating the transfer of patients to tertiary centers
- In DIC secondary to excessive blood loss.

(Although not indicated for the use in the presence of DIC, however, in such a situation the use of the balloon may reduce the loss of blood to facilitate resuscitation and correct the coagulopathy before a more definitive procedure such as laparotomy is performed).

Discussion: When medical management fails, contraindicated or not available further management measures are divided into two interventions—Operative and nonoperative. The first category includes arterial embolization, uterine compression sutures, uterine artery ligation, and, ultimately hysterectomy. All these measures are highly invasive, require extensive resources, require expertise and are associated with significant morbidity and, above all, may not be available at all levels of healthcare facilities. In sharp contrast, the nonoperative option of uterine balloon tamponade is available, effective, requires minimum resources and expertise, preserves fertility and is minimally invasive with minimum morbidity.

In a systemic review, the cumulative outcomes showed success rates of 90.7% (95% confidence interval [CI], 85.7–94.0%) for arterial embolization, 84.0% (95% CI, 77.5–88.8%) for balloon tamponade, 91.7% (95% CI, 84.9–95.5%) for uterine compression sutures, and 84.6% (81.2–87.5%) for iliac artery ligation or uterine devascularization.[12] It concluded that there is no evidence to suggest that any one method is better for the management of severe postpartum hemorrhage. As balloon tamponade is the least invasive and most rapid approach, it would be logical to use this as the first step in the management.

If the patient is undergoing cesarean section and bimanual compression of the uterus successfully arrests the bleeding, then compression sutures may be of value. Particularly the modification of original B-Lynch suture technique is quite easy which is a great advantage, and fertility is also preserved. The obvious disadvantages are the need for laparotomy in case the woman has delivered vaginally. Complications include pyometra, partial ischemic necrosis of the uterus, uterine cavity synechiae and uterine necrosis.

Pelvic devascularization also requires laparotomy, arterial ligation are technically challenging procedures carrying well-documented risks. They can be time-consuming, require substantial surgical expertise. Complications are post-ischemic lower motor neuron damage; obstruction of right common iliac artery wound dehiscence and broad ligament hematomas.

Radiological management of PPH namely arterial embolization is not available in most facilities, very expensive, and requires a hemodynamically stable patient and there are some reported complications of the procedure like uterus and bladder necrosis after uterine artery embolization.

Mechanism of action of balloon tamponade: The precise mechanism of action for UBT is still unclear. However, the following explanations are offered for the haemostatic effect.
- The placenta is a low-pressure system, so when the placenta is the source of hemorrhage, the direct pressure of the balloon, even well below systemic pressure, will halt the bleeding.
- When the hemorrhage is instead from an arterial source in the endometrium, it is possible that the balloon's exerted pressure exceeds the arterial pressure and thus promotes clot formation.
- Exerts hydrostatic pressure on the capillaries and veins in the uterus.[13] Acts like a hemostatic cushion by exerting "inward-to-outward pressure" that is greater than the systemic arterial pressure to prevent continual bleeding.
- It may be due to the hydrostatic pressure effect of the balloon on the uterine arteries.
- There is some evidence of stimulation of uterine contractions by the balloon.[14]

Merits of innovative balloons: The inconsistencies of conventional CBT are overcome by the two innovative balloons. Both the innovative balloon devices, i. e. Easy balloon and CG balloon have replaced thread used in conventional CBT with rings. These rings are made out of the catheter material itself which is presterilized and are always optimally tight. The CG balloon successfully provides a drainage port and facilitates rapid identification of failed cases. In general, it works as efficiently as commercially available uterine-specific devices but at 100 times less the cost.[15,16]

Another important factor is that of cost. If a catgut or silk or vicryl is used for tying, it raises the cost of device three to four times, i.e. the total cost comes to around Rs 300–400 (100 for catheter + 200 or 300 for the cost of suture material). If one can save this amount in every CBT, the country can save a huge sum over the years which can be utilized for betterment of health facilities. If to cut the cost, thread is used, the sterilization of the thread has to be ensured which is difficult in emergency situation like PPH.

CONCLUSION

The balloon tamponade device is a quick, affordable, reliable and, above all, an available device which can be assembled at the point of use using basic things. This device can go a long way in reducing maternal mortality particularly when the technique is made easier (as in case of Easy Balloon) and far superior (as in case of CG balloon which is as good as a commercially available and popular uterine-specific device costing around $250). The CBT is prepared only in Rs 100 (almost 1.5 $) and is three to four times cheaper than the conventional CBT.

Overall the condom balloon tamponade devices avoid death and avert surgery effectively. These very effective, consistent and satisfying devices can go a long way to bring down the maternal mortality rate in low-resource settings as well as reducing the cost of this life-saving intervention.

Note: The video of making of CG balloon can be accessed through the link for video provided in www.ijgo.org/article/S0020-7292(16)00043-6 DOI: http://dx.doi.org/10.1016/j.ijgo.2015.10.014.

REFERENCES

1. UN. Official List of MDG Indicators. United Nations. 2008. Available at http://mdgs.un.org.
2. WHO. Trends in maternal mortality: 1990 to 2015: Estimates by WHO, UNICEF, UNFPA, World Bank Group and the United

Nations Population Division. World Health Organization; 2015.
3. UN. Sustainable Development Goals: 17 Goals to Transform our World. United Nations; 2015.
4. Countdown to 2015: maternal, newborn and child survival. [Internet]. WHO and UNICEF; 2012. http://www.countdown 2015 mnch.org/documents/2012Report/2012-Complete.pdf. Last accessed. 2012;1.
5. Trends in maternal mortality: 1990 to 2010. WHO, UNICEF, UNFPA and The World Bank estimates. Geneva: WHO; 2012. http://whqlibdoc.who.int/publications/2012/9789241503631_eng.
6. World Health Organization (WHO). WHO recommendations for the prevention and treatment of postpartum haemorrhage. Geneva: World Health Organization (WHO); 2012.
7. FIGO. FIGO guidelines: prevention and treatment of postpartum hemorrhage in low-resource settings. Int J Gynaecol Obstet. 2012;117:108-18.
8. Georgiou C. A review of current practice in using Balloon Tamponade Technology in the management of postpartum haemorrhage. Hypertens Res Pregnancy. 2014;2:1-10.
9. Tindell K, Garfinkel R, Abu-Haydar E, et al. Uterine balloon tamponade for the treatment of postpartum haemorrhage in resource-poor settings: a systematic review. BJOG. 2013;120 (1):5-14.
10. Ajayi OA, Sant M, Ikhena S, Bako A. Uterine rupture complicating sequential curettage and Bakri balloon tamponade to control secondary PPH. BMJ Case Rep. 2013; 2013 Feb 6. doi: 10.1136/bcr-2012-007709.
11. Giuseppe Ghirardini, et al. Egypt Gynecol Obstet Invest. 2012;74:320-3.
12. Stergios K Doumouchtsis, Aris T Papageorghiou, Chiara Vernier, Sabaratnam Arulkumaram. Management of postpartum hemorrhage by uterine balloon tamponade: Prospective evaluation of effectiveness. Acta Obstetricia et Gynecologica Scandinavica. 2008;87(8):849-55.
13. Georgiou C. Balloon tamponade in the management of postpartum haemorrhage: a review. BJOG. 2009;116:748-57.
14. Yorifuji T, Tanaka T, Makino S, Koshiishi T, Sugimura M, Takeda S. Balloon tamponade in atonic bleeding induces uterine contraction: attempt to quantify uterine stiffness using acoustic radiation force impulse elastography before and after balloon tamponade. Acta Obstet Gynecol Scand. 2011;90:1171-2.
15. Mishra N, Shrivastava C, Agrawal S, Gulabani K. The CG balloon is an innovative condom balloon tamponade for the management of postpartum hemorrhage in low-resource settings. International Journal of Gynecology and Obstetrics (2016). http://dx.doi.org/10.1016/j.ijgo.2015.10.014.
16. Nalini Mishra, Sumi Agrawal, Kanchan Gulabani, Chandrashekhar Shrivastava, et al. Use of an Innovative Condom Balloon Tamponade in Postpartum Haemorrhage: A Report. The Journal of Obstetrics and Gynecology of India (January–February. 2016;66(1):63-7.

Surgical Management of Postpartum Hemorrhage: A Review

Chapter 55

Kavita N Singh, Shweta Sirsikar

INTRODUCTION

Postpartum hemorrhage (PPH) is still a major cause of maternal mortality and morbidity.[1] It is an obstetric emergency which every obstetrician has to face often unexpectedly. Fortunately, techniques for dealing with it have improved so that mortality from this cause continues to decline. Most common cause of PPH is atonic followed by traumatic PPH.

"4 T's" mnemonic to remember causes of PPH
Tone, Tissue, Trauma, and Thrombosis

Although risk factors for PPH are known, it is not possible at times to successfully prevent it. Rapid recognition and diagnosis of PPH is essential for successful management. The determining factor as to which method is to be used usually will depend upon the experience of the surgeon. This article is a review of the surgical approach in management of PPH.

Surgical approach includes:
- Uterine compression sutures
  - B-lynch suture (Brace suture)
  - Hayman suture } Modified B-lynch suture
  - Cho square suture
- Uterine and ovarian artery ligation (stepwise devascularization)
- Internal iliac (hypogastric) ligation
- Hysterectomy
- Logothetopulos pack
- Arterial embolization.

UTERINE COMPRESSION SUTURES

B-Lynch Suture (Brace Suture) (Figs 55.1A to D)

B-Lynch suture, also known as the 'Brace Suture', was described by Christopher B-Lynch in 1997, on account of five cases,[2] where compression of the uterus was achieved following cesarean section using this technique. It can stop PPH without the need for pelvic surgery and potentially preserving fertility. Absorbable suture can be left *in situ* and would typically not lead to problems with future pregnancies.

Technique of B-Lynch Suture (Use Vicryl No. 1 or Chromic catgut No. 2).
- Suture in left lower edge of the uterine incision
- Suture at left upper edge of the uterine incision
- Suture passed above the fundus
- Suture at the posterior wall of the uterus
- Suture back through the posterior wall into the uterine cavity
- Suture through right of uterine cavity to posterior wall
- Suture at the right posterior wall of the uterus
- Suture at the right anterior wall of the uterus
- Suture at the right upper edge of the incision into the uterine cavity
- Suture at the right lower edge of the incision through uterine cavity.

Modified B-Lynch Suture

Dr Richard Hayman and Professor Arulkumaran in Derby modified this procedure of B-Lynch suture independently. Here there is no need to open the uterine cavity and the suture on straight needle is used to transfix uterus from front to back first above reflect of bladder and tied at fundus of uterus.

The Hayman Uterine Compression Suture: Clinical Points (Fig. 55.2A)[3]

- Lower uterine segment or uterine cavity not opened
- Uterine cavity not explored under direct vision
- Probably quicker to apply
- No feedback data on fertility outcome
- Morbidity feedback data limited
- Unequal tension leads to segmented ischemia secondary to slippage of suture—'shouldering' with venous obstruction.

Cho Multiple Square Sutures (Fig. 55.2B)

The Cho multiple square sutures: Clinical points[4]
- Multiple full-thickness square sutures applied, probably time-consuming, if many square sutures required

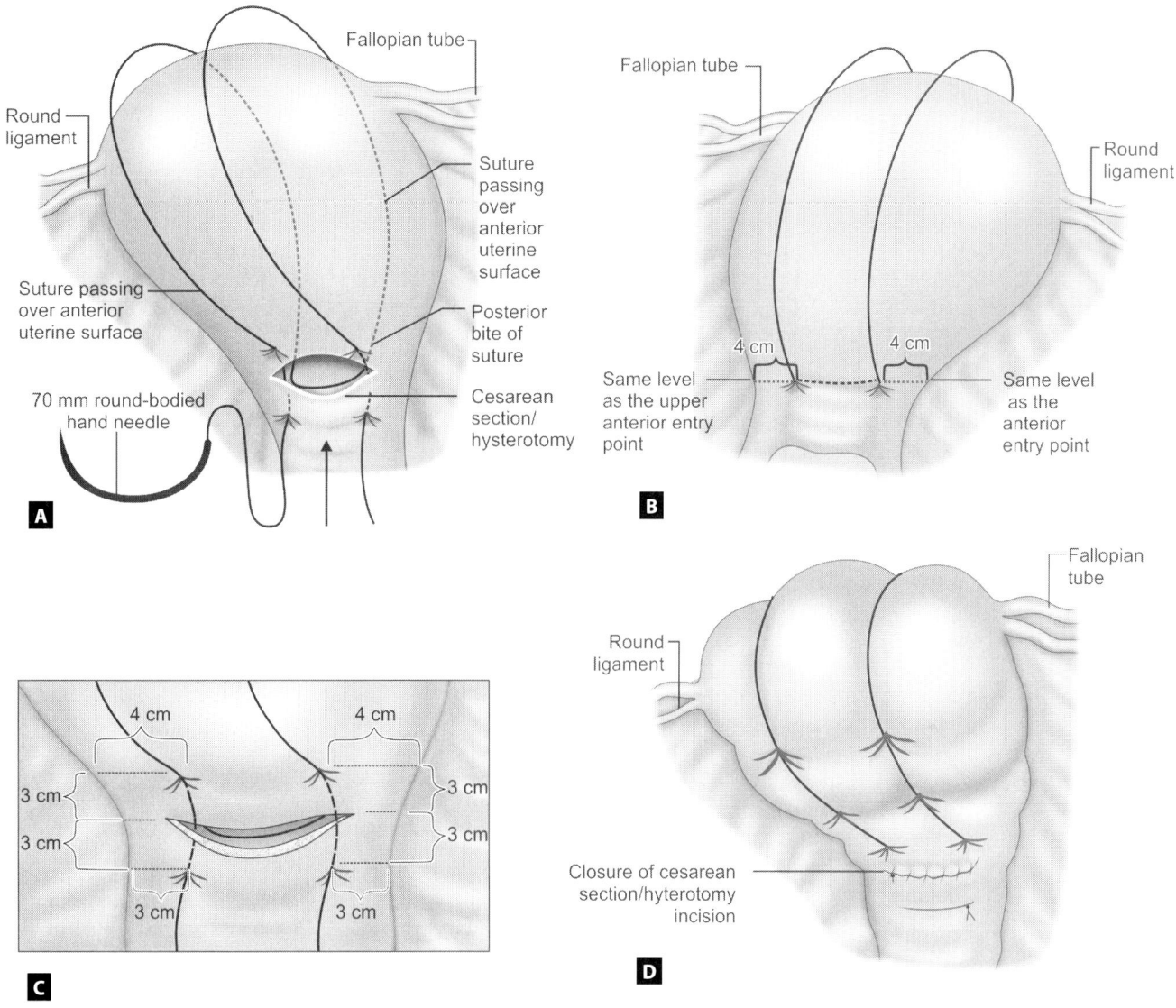

Figs 55.1A to D: Summary of the application of the B-Lynch procedure

- Uterine cavity drainage restriction—pyometra risk
- No feedback data on fertility outcome
- Morbidity feedback data limited
- Rhythmic contraction not facilitated and involution impeded
- The production of multiple uterine synechiae.

UTERINE AND OVARIAN ARTERY LIGATION (STEPWISE DEVASCULARIZATION OF THE UTERUS)

A novel technique which is effective and safe for management of uncontrolled PPH with preservation of the uterus. This technique entails five successive steps, so if bleeding is not controlled by one step, the next step is taken until bleeding stops. Stepwise devascularization **(Fig. 55.3)** of the uterus in the management of PPH has been described in a report from Egypt.[5] The steps are:

1. Unilateral uterine artery ligation
2. Bilateral uterine artery ligation (at the upper part of the lower uterine segment)
3. Low uterine vessel ligation after mobilization of the bladder
4. Unilateral ovarian vessel ligation
5. Bilateral ovarian vessel ligation.
   – Myometrium is included in the ligatures in steps 1 to 3.

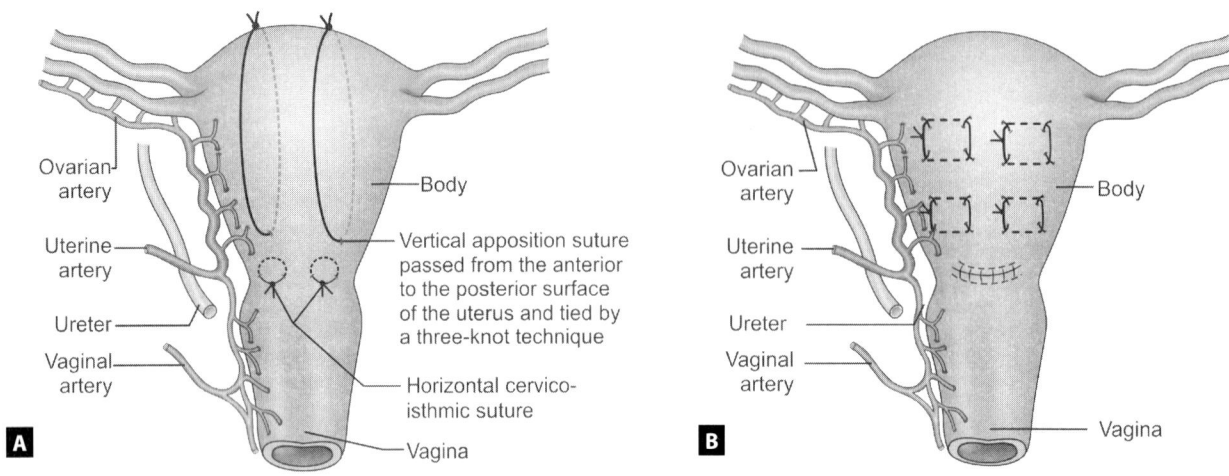

Figs 55.2A and B: Modified B-Lynch suture

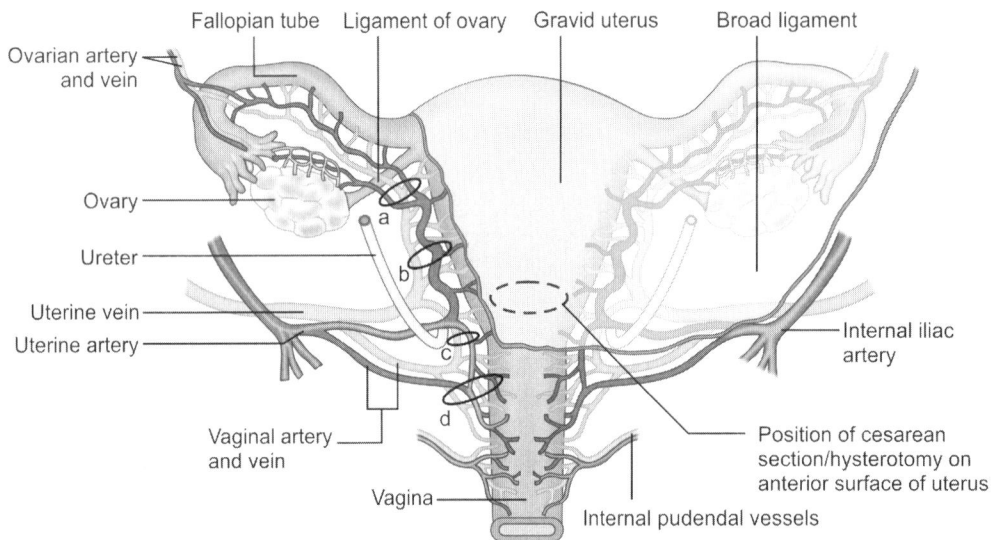

Fig. 55.3: Stepwise devascularization of uterus—ligation sites

UTERINE ARTERY LIGATION[6]

If use of a simple compression suture is unsuccessful, then ligation of the uterine arteries can be tried next and is often effective. The objective of ligation of uterine arteries is to decrease blood flow to the uterus as about 90% of the uterine blood supply in pregnancy comes from these vessels. After passing over the ureter, the uterine artery divides at the level of the internal cervical os into a main ascending and a smaller cervicovaginal branch. After ligation of the uterine arteries, if bleeding is not controlled, then the next step is to ligate the ovarian arteries.

OVARIAN ARTERY LIGATION

Ovarian artery arises directly from the aorta and ultimately anastomoses with the uterine artery in the region of the uterine aspect of utero-ovarian ligament. Identify the ovarian artery just below the fallopian tube where it enters the meso-ovarian. A suture should be placed carefully around the ovarian artery through an avascular window in the meso-ovarian taking care not to involve the fallopian tube in the suture. If not possible to identify the ovarian artery, then tie off the whole infundibular ligament.

VAGINAL UTERINE ARTERY LIGATION

Vaginal uterine artery ligation as an approach for PPH management has been suggested by many obstetricians. It is a simple effective and minimal invasive technique for treating intractable PPH. Indeed, one suspects that uterine artery ligation is sometimes performed inadvertently when a lower segment incision extends during a difficult delivery (for example, of a large baby) and extensive suturing into the broad ligament is necessary to control the resultant bleeding. There appear to be no consequences for future pregnancies of such ligation, presumably because a collateral circulation develops from other vessels (particularly the ovarian arteries) to compensate.

INTERNAL ILIAC (HYPOGASTRIC) ARTERY LIGATION AND AORTIC COMPRESSION

There has long been controversy about when ligation of the internal iliac artery should be attempted.[7] It is a difficult maneuver because of the proximity of the internal iliac vein, which can be torn during mobilization of the artery and is difficult to repair, and the external iliac artery, which if ligated in error results in an ischemic leg. A practical point is that when the artery is mobilized using an artery clamp, this should be done laterally to medially, so that the tip of the clamp points away from, rather than into, the internal iliac vein. In the hands of experts who perform the procedure regularly, the results can be good.[8] It should probably not be undertaken by the obstetrician who performs it, for example, only once every 5 years, but instead the assistance of a gynecological oncologist or vascular surgeon should be sought. If there is a delay in obtaining assistance from such an expert, direct compression of the aorta against the spinal column can reduce bleeding by ~40% and this can be lifesaving in some cases. Complete occlusion of the aorta by clamping below the renal arteries is even more effective and flow to the legs can be completely stopped for 4 hours or more without irreversible damage. However, analogous to the problem with ligating the internal iliac artery, damage to the vena cava can be catastrophic and so such clamping should only be applied by an experienced vascular surgeon.

HYSTERECTOMY

In women wishing to retain their fertility, cesarean hysterectomy is the procedure of last resort; but, as has been repeatedly emphasized in the Confidential Enquiries into Maternal and Child Health (CEMCH), it should not be left until the woman is *in extremis*, but instead should be carried out promptly if the previously described procedures prove to be ineffective and there are signs of impending cardiovascular decompensation. Anesthetists will be the people most in touch with the woman's condition, and if they declare that the pulse rate is continuing to rise and the blood pressure to fall despite conservative measures, hysterectomy becomes inevitable. The precise timing of this intervention must, of course, always remain a matter of clinical judgment.

It is often a good idea to do subtotal hysterectomy first. This is often sufficient to arrest the bleeding, if the main cause is an atonic corpus, because the two major pedicles clamped, cut and tied include both the ovarian and the uterine arteries. Even if there is continuing bleeding, removing the body of the uterus improves access to and visibility of the pelvic floor. It allows identification of the cervix, and therefore reduces the chance of taking a pedicle too low and including the ureter. Once the bleeding is controlled, any temptation to remove more tissue, for example, the cervix, should be resisted, as this may simply restart the bleeding.

LOGOTHETOPULOS PACK

If bleeding continues following hysterectomy, it becomes mandatory to include surgeons with additional experience of dealing with major hemorrhage, such as a gynecological oncologist or vascular surgeon. In the meantime, pelvic tamponade with a Logothetopulos pack[9] will usually staunch the flow. The principle is straightforward. A flexible plastic bag larger than the pelvic cavity is filled with gauze swabs or anything similar to hand. The neck is firmly tied to a length of tubing, which is passed from the pelvis out through the vagina, and then attached to a liter bag of fluid which is allowed to hang freely over the end of the bed. This applies a steady tamponade which molds itself to the pelvic cavity and will stop all but the most major arterial bleeding.

ARTERIAL EMBOLIZATION

This is a relatively new technique, which requires the help of a trained interventional radiologist and a good fluoroscopy setup.

Procedure: The catherization is carried out usually through the femorals with both sides being occluded through a single puncture. The catheters—several types available, are ideally small smooth hydrophilic ones, enough to not produce vascular spasm. Initially, an arteriogram is taken to visualize the arterial arcade. The catheter is introduced to the uterine artery and the vessel identified and occluded. However, if in the arteriogram extravasation of blood is seen from another branch, then selective angiography must be done and the vessel identified and occluded. Bleeding from tears in the lower cervix and vagina can be treated effectively by occluding the vaginal artery.

SPECIAL SITUATIONS

Uterine Inversion

This is a rare cause of PPH with neurogenic shock, but it is important to recognize it promptly as the situation will not be resolved until the inversion is corrected. If the woman has had adequate analgesia, prompt manual correction of the inversion is feasible and will be effective in many cases. If the placenta is still adherent to the uterus, it should be left *in situ* until the uterus has been replaced. If there is a delay while the woman is resuscitated and anesthesia provided, then hydrostatic replacement (the O'Sullivan technique) may be necessary. Several liters of warmed Hartmann's solution instilled into the vagina is usually enough to stretch the cervix and generate enough pressure to push the uterus back into a normal position. Traditionally, the lower vagina was plugged with the Accoucheur's hand, but a better seal can be obtained using a silicone-vacuum extractor (ventouse1).[10]

Placenta Previa and Accreta

With the considerable rise in the rate of cesarean section in recent years, the incidence of placenta previa and placenta accreta has risen substantially. The risk of placenta previa in a first pregnancy is only about 1 in 400, but it rises to 1 in 160 after one cesarean section, 1 in 60 after 2, 1 in 30 after 3 and 1 in 10 after 4.[11]

Practical aspects of preparation and care in the operating theater when placenta accreta is suspected. The average blood loss in cases of placenta accrete is 3–5 liter,[12] so proper prior liaison with the hematologist to ensure an appropriate supply of cross-matched blood is essential.

The most appropriate abdominal incision is a midline, which gives the best access in case of heavy bleeding. Ensure that uterine incision should be away from the placenta, so as to allow delivery of the baby before there is any attempt at removing the placenta. It is useful to give oxytocics (such as an intravenous infusion of oxytocin and 1000 µg of misoprostol rectally) once the baby is safely delivered and then wait to see, if the placenta separates. If it does, and there is good uterine retraction with minimal bleeding, then once the placenta is extruded by uterine contraction the uterus can be closed. If the placenta does not separate spontaneously within 10 minutes, do not make any attempt to separate it provided, there is no bleeding, but instead close the uterus and wait for the placenta to discharge spontaneously in the puerperium. If, however, there is substantial bleeding, then proceed straight to hysterectomy without making it worse by trying to remove the placenta piecemeal.

CONCLUSION

For most of the last century, the management of major PPH relied upon the use of oxytocic agents, followed by hysterectomy, if these failed. However, the last 10 years has witnessed the introduction of many useful additional surgical procedures, in particular uterine compression sutures. These are now widely used and are effective in ~90% of cases. However, reports of both short- and long-term complications are now appearing, and it is important not to reduce the perfusion of the uterus so much that it becomes devitalized. Uterine artery ligation can be carried out safely by an obstetrician. Hysterectomy still has an important place. If bleeding continues after the uterus has been removed, the Logothetopulos pack can be used to stabilize the situation and arterial embolisation can be life-saving. With the increasing incidence of cesarean section, the possibility of placenta accrete should always be considered in the next pregnancy and ultrasound/magnetic resonance imaging are important. Anticipation and careful preparation of the operating theater, facilities, blood products and trained experienced obstetricians remains the key to successful management.

REFERENCES

1. Joseph KS, Rouleau J, Kramer MS, Young DC, Liston RM, Baskett TF. Investigation of an increase in postpartum haemorrhage in Canada. BJOG. 2007;114:751-9. doi:10.1111/j.1471-0528.2007.01316.
2. Lynch C, Coker A, Lawal AH, Abu J, Cowen MJ. The B-Lynch surgical technique for the control of massive postpartum haemorrhage: an alternative to hysterectomy? Five cases reported. Br J Obstet Gynaecol. 1997;104:372-5.
3. Hayman RG, Arulkumaran S, Steer PJ. Uterine compression sutures: surgical management of postpartum hemorrhage. Obstet Gynecol. 2002;99:502-6. doi:10.1016/S0029-7844(01)01643.
4. Cho JH, Jun HS, Lee CN. Hemostatic suturing technique for uterine bleeding during cesarean delivery. Obstet Gynecol. 2000;96:129-31.doi:10.1016/S0029-7844(00)00852-8.
5. Cho JY, Kim SJ, Cha KY, Kay CW, Kim MI, Cha KS. Interrupted circular suture: Bleeding control during caesarean delivery in placenta previa accrete. Obstet Gynaecol. 1996;56:151-3.
6. O'Leary JA. Uterine artery ligation in the control of postcesarean hemorrhage. J Reprod Med. 1995;40:189-93.
7. Chew S, Biswas A. Caesarean and postpartum hysterectomy. Singapore Med J. 1998;39:9-13.
8. Joshi VM, Otiv SR, Majumder R, Nikam YA, Shrivastava M. Internal iliac artery ligation for arresting postpartum haemorrhage. BJOG 2007;114:356-61. doi:10.1111/j.1471-0528.2006.01235.
9. Robie GF, Morgan MA, Payne GG, Jr., Wasemiller-Smith L. Logothetopulos pack for the management of uncontrollable postpartum hemorrhage. Am J Perinatol. 1990;4:327-8. doi:10.1055/s-2007-999514
10. Ogueh O, Ayida G. Acute uterine inversion: a new technique of hydrostatic replacement. Br J Obstet Gynaecol. 1997;104:951-2.
11. Clark SL, Koonings PP, Phelan JP. Placenta previa/accreta and prior cesarean section. Obstet Gynecol. 1985;66:890-92.
12. Clark SL, Yeh SY, Phelan JP, Bruce S, Paul RH. Emergency hysterectomy for obstetric hemorrhage. Obstet Gynecol. 1984;64:376-80.

SECTION 11: MISCELLANEOUS

Chapter 56

Intrauterine Fetal Death
(Its Impact on Maternal Morbidity and Mortality and Preventive Strategies)

Rujuta Fuke

INTRODUCTION

Intrauterine fetal demise (IUFD) is defined as a death of fetus in uterus after 20 weeks of gestation which results in delivery of a stillborn baby.[1] Before 20 weeks of gestation, IUFD has distinct etiology and termed as abortions.

Approximately 1 out of every 160 deliveries in India ends in stillbirth, a devastating experience for women and their families, yet its causes remain poorly understood. Though most stillbirths are avoidable, surprisingly the issue is overlooked and neglected in developing countries like India.

Most of the stillbirths are associated with the high-risk pregnancy and its complications, thus adding to increased maternal morbidity and mortality. In an effort to help prevent stillbirths by improving the understanding of its risk factors and causes, health policy makers are trying to get to the root cause of this problem but stillbirth, one of the most common negative pregnancy outcomes remains an unanswered question because of the lack of proper diagnosis and apathetic attitude towards autopsy.

EPIDEMIOLOGY

The problem of stillbirths is global but more so in developing countries such as India. Approximately, 3.2 million stillbirths occur annually in low and middle income countries. There were over 2.6 million stillbirths globally in 2009, and 98% occurred in low and middle income countries. In 2009, 76.2% of stillbirths occurred in South Asia and sub-Saharan Africa. A study to be published in *The Lancet* medical journal has found that an average of 2.6 million stillbirths occurred every year between 1995 and 2009, 23.2% of which were from India.[2] This means an average of 1,680 babies were born dead every day in the country in that time.

RECENT NOMENCLATURE[3]

Fetal Death

The International Classification of Diseases, Revision 10 (ICD 10) defines a fetal death as 'death prior to the complete expulsion or extraction from its mother of a product of conception, irrespective of the duration of pregnancy; the death is indicated by the fact that after such separation the fetus does not breathe or show any other evidence of life, such as beating of the heart, pulsation of the umbilical cord, or definite movement of voluntary muscles' without specification of the duration of pregnancy.

Early Fetal Deaths

According to the ICD10, an early fetal death is death of a fetus weighing at least 500 g (or, if birth weight is unavailable, after 22 completed weeks gestation, or with a crown heel length of 25 centimeters or more).

Late Fetal Deaths (Stillbirths)

A late fetal death is defined as a fetal death weighing at least 1000 g (or a gestational age of 28 completed weeks or a crown heel length of 35 centimeters or more). The ICD10 recommends this definition for the purposes of international comparison.

RISK FACTORS

Hypertension and diabetes, both risk factors for IUFD, are two of the most common medical conditions that occur along with pregnancy.[4] Research indicates that women who have diabetes prior to pregnancy have a two- to five-fold increased risk of stillbirth. Obesity is associated with an increased risk of both miscarriage and stillbirth. The risk of stillbirth is 8 per 1,000 births among obese pregnant women with a body mass index (BMI) between 30 and 39.9 and is even higher among pregnant women with a BMI greater than 40 (11 per 1,000). Obesity remains an independent risk factor for stillbirth even after controlling for smoking, gestational diabetes, and pre-eclampsia.[5]

Multiple gestations also are related to higher stillbirth rates. A pregnancy with two or more fetuses has a stillborn rate four times higher than a singleton pregnancy. Advanced maternal age (older than 35) is yet another risk factor for stillbirth, even after taking into account other risk factors such as hypertension, diabetes, placenta previa, and multiple gestations. Older women having their first pregnancy appear to be at greater risk than older women who have given birth previously.[6]

CAUSES

The factors leading to IUFD are classified into: maternal (5–10%), fetal (25–40%) and placental (20–35%) and Idiopathic (25–35%). A significant portion of stillbirths remains unexplained despite a thorough evaluation, according to ACOG.[7] The lack of uniform protocols for evaluating and classifying stillbirths in India, coupled with unwillingness on part of parents for fetal autopsy, has hindered the study of specific causes. In most cases, fetal death certificates are filled out before a full investigation has been completed, and amended death certificates are rarely filed when additional information from the stillbirth evaluation surfaces.

Fetal growth restriction (FGR), when a fetus does not grow in size appropriately, is one known cause of stillbirth and is associated with certain genetic defects, fetal infections, maternal smoking, hypertension, autoimmune disease, obesity, and diabetes.[8] Placental abruption, a condition in which the placenta separates away prematurely from the uterine wall, is another common cause of stillbirth. Cocaine and other illegal drug use, smoking, hypertension, and preeclampsia all significantly contribute to placental abruption.[9]

Chromosomal and genetic abnormalities can be found in approximately 8 to 13% of stillborn fetuses. The most common identifiable abnormalities found among stillborns include Down syndrome, Turner syndrome, Edward's syndrome, and Patau syndrome.[10] Infections such as parvovirus, cytomegalovirus, syphilis, and *Listeria monocytogenes* are all causally associated with stillbirth.[11-13]

Thrombophilias and other lupus anticoagulants are possibly one of the causes of IUFD as evidenced by intravascular thrombosis in placental vessels.[14]

Although umbilical cord problems and abnormalities are frequently blamed for stillbirths, ACOG's guidelines state that other causes should be excluded before making this diagnosis because cord abnormalities are found in nearly one-third of all normal live births. A stillbirth attributed to a cord problem should have evidence of obstruction or circulatory compromise.

The causes are summarized in **(Table 56.1)**.

DIAGNOSIS

Symptoms: Lack of fetal movements previously perceived by the patient.

Signs

- Progressive decrease in the fundal height of the uterus
- Decrease in the tone of the uterus; uterus feels flaccid with easy palpation of fetal parts
- Fetal movements are not perceived during palpation
- On auscultation, fetal heart sounds are not appreciated
- There are no tracings on cardiotocography.

Investigations

- *Ultrasonography*: Real-time ultrasonography is the confirmatory for the diagnosis of IUFD. It shows lack of fetal movements and cardiac standstill. Spalding's sign in the form of collapsed cranial bones are evident. It usually occurs 7 days after IUFD. Robert's sign with gas in the heart and great vessels is also seen. It appears as early as 12 hours after IUFD. It also shows associated conditions responsible for IUFD, such as oligohydramnios, retroplacental clot, cord around neck of the fetus, fetal edema, fetal ascites, structural abnormalities of the fetus, etc.

Table 56.1: Causes of IUFD[15]

Maternal	Fetal	Placental	Iatrogenic	Idiopathic
Hypertensive disorders of pregnancy)	Chromosomal abnormalities	Placental insufficiency	Inadvertent use of oxytocics	Cause remains unknown
Diabetes in pregnancy	Congenital anomalies	Antepartum hemorrhage	External cephalic version	
Maternal infections	Intrauterine growth restriction of fetus	Cord accidents	Amniocentesis	
Hyperpyrexia	Intrauterine infections	Twin transfusion syndrome	Drugs	
Autoimmune conditions	Rh-incompatibility			
Thrombophilias	Nonimmune hydrops			
Abnormal labor				
Post-term pregnancy				

- Spalding's sign is also seen on straight X-ray abdomen. Hyperflexion of the spine, crowding of the ribs are some of the other signs seen.
- *Blood*: Blood coagulation studies, blood fibrinogen levels and partial thromboplastin time should be determined periodically when the fetus is retained for more than 2 weeks.

COMPLICATIONS OF IUFD

- *Psychological trauma*: This is to be addressed in a very sympathetic way.
- *Infections*: As long as the membranes are intact, infection is unlikely but as soon as membranes rupture, the dead nonviable cells favor growth of *Clostridium welchii*, gas-forming bacteria with dreadful complications. Patients can land up in septicemia and septicemic shock.
- Blood coagulation disorders are less common and occurs if the fetus is retained for more than 4 weeks in the uterus. There occurs silent disseminated intravascular coagulopathy due to gradual absorption of thromboplastin liberated from the dead placenta and decidua in the maternal circulation.

Management[16,17]

Prevention

As there is a small possibility of recurrence in the next pregnancy mostly because of diabetes, fetal anomalies, chromosomal defects, hypertensive disorders, thrombophilias, hereditary disorders, following measures are advised to prevent stillbirths.
- Prenatal and pre-conceptional counseling to prevent occurrence in future pregnancy
- Prenatal diagnosis by amniocentesis in suspected genetic disorders
- Supplementation of periconceptional and prenatal folic acid
- Identification and management of at risk women during antenatal period.

Psychological counseling in case of IUFD: Many strategies have been described for discussing bad news. Late IUFD poses particular difficulties as it is often sudden and unexpected. A crucial component is to determine the emotional feelings and needs of the mother and her companions. This empathetic approach seeks to identify and understand women's thoughts and wishes but without trying to shape them. Women with an IUFD and their partners value acceptance and recognition of their emotions highly. If the woman is unaccompanied, an immediate offer should be made to call her partner, relatives or friends. Discussions should aim to support maternal/parental choice. Parents should be offered written information to supplement discussions.

Management of IUFD: Treatment of the underlying cause of the IUFD is undertaken like control of blood pressure and deranged blood glucose levels, antepartum hemorrhage, treatment of infections, correction of endocrine abnormality, etc.

Expectant management: The patients with IUFD tend to undergo spontaneous labor within 2 weeks in 80% of the cases, and hence expectant management can be carried out. Psychological counseling plays an important part in expectant management as patient and relatives are likely to be very upset. In that case the idea of carrying a dead fetus is usually not welcomed by the patient and relatives. In this management, serum fibrinogen levels are to be monitored twice weekly to identify the early signs of DIC.

Active interference: Now-a-days with availability of early and definite diagnosis and better pharmacotherapy, active management of IUFD pregnancy is preferred.

The indications are:
- If patient shows signs of infection in case of prolonged rupture of the membranes
- If the dead fetus is retained for prolonged duration
- In case of early signs of coagulation failure
- Psychological upset of the patient which happens to be the most common indication.

Mode of delivery: Delivery of the dead fetus is the main aim. Except few indications, cesarean section is avoided. The principle during labor is to keep the membranes intact as far as possible to prevent infection, and secondly to facilitate easy dilatation of the cervix and progress of labor. Intrapartum management includes strict watch on progress of labor and maternal general condition. Signs suggestive of obstruction, abnormal presentation, change in the contour of the uterus, non-progress of labor, maternal exhaustion, dehydration, impending eclampsia, bleeding per vaginum, etc. are to be looked for and managed accordingly. After delivery retained placenta and postpartum hemorrhage are known complications and needs active management.

Following are the methods of induction:
- *Misoprostol (PGE1)*: Tablet misoprostol is safe and now the treatment of choice for induction of labor. The dose is usually 25 to 50 µg repeated every 4 hourly. Vaginal route is preferred than the oral route. It is safe, effective and cheap.
- *Misoprostol and mifepristone combination*: It has now become the treatment of choice for IUFD management. Mifepristone tablet in the dose of 200 mg followed by misoprostol tablets (25 µg 4 hourly) in the usual dose is

found to be very effective. Tab Mifepristone alone can be given 600 mg orally daily for 2 days.
- *Prostaglandins*: Vaginal administration of PGE2 gel is equally effective, especially in conditions of unfavorable cervix. It needs to be supplemented by oxytocin infusion after 6–8 hours.
- *Oxytocin infusion* is the most popular method in case of favorable cervix. To begin with 5–10 units are started in 500 mL of Ringer's solution to be augmented accordingly.

A word of caution, repeated attempts to induce the labor by oxytocics points towards, ectopic or abdominal pregnancy and should be kept in mind.

Role of Cesarean Section

Role of cesarean section is restricted to very few conditions, such as abnormal presentation, obstructed labor, impending scar rupture, placenta previa, previous 2 cesarean section, etc.

Postpartum Care

Lactation suppression: Lactation suppression by cabergoline, if not contraindicated, is required after delivery or alternatively pyridoxine tablets can be given for lactation suppression.

Sympathetic attitude by staff, treating physicians and relatives.

Psychological counseling by counselers as these patients are prone for postpartum depression.

Recovery in postpartum ward is to be avoided.

RECOMMENDED EVALUATION OF A STILLBORN[18]

After a stillbirth, sensitivity to the family's emotional state is important. Parents should be given the opportunity to hold their baby and perform cultural or religious activities. The issue of performing an autopsy is especially sensitive, but clinicians should emphasize that the results may be valuable in planning future pregnancies. Less invasive evaluation methods such as photographs, X-rays, ultrasound, magnetic resonance imaging, and samples of skin or blood of the stillborn may help identify a cause for parents, who object to a full autopsy.

Parents want answers when they have a stillbirth, so clinicians should not be afraid to request an autopsy. Without a thorough evaluation, it will be difficult to counsel women on their risk of having another stillbirth.

A general examination of the stillborn fetus should be performed promptly after delivery for gross structural abnormalities, pallor, macrosomia, growth restriction. Examination of the placenta and the umbilical cord is an essential component of stillbirth evaluation for any abnormality, such as large edematous placenta, small placenta, retroplacental or intraplacental hemorrhage, calcifications and necrosis, cord entanglement, single umbilical artery, etc. American College of Obstetricians and Gynecologists (ACOG) recommends that genetic testing be performed in all stillbirths after parental permission is obtained. Samples from the viable skin tissue and blood is to be obtained, if possible for cytogenetic studies to determine aneuploidy and single gene disorders. Placenta should be sent for histopathological examination to determine the underlying cause.

A thorough maternal history also should be taken, including obstetric history, exposure to medications and viruses, and family history. Maternal testing for such things as blood group and Rh-typing, Kleihauer-Betke test, Glycosylated hemoglobin, blood glucose, lupus anticoagulant, anticardiolipin antibodies, antinuclear antibodies, thrombophilia study, thyroid function tests, serum prolactin level, venereal disease research laboratory (VDRL), and antibodies to human parvovirus, Toxoplasmosis, Other (Syphilis, Varicella-Zoster, Parvovirus B19), Rubella, Cytomegalovirus (CMV), and Herps (TORCH) group of infections as well certain genetic conditions may provide information that could affect future pregnancies.

COUNSELING AND PREVENTION

Counseling women on their risk of having another stillbirth may be quantifiable when specific risk factors are identified. In low-risk women with an unexplained stillbirth, the risk of recurrence after 20 weeks' gestation is estimated at 7.8 to 10.5 per 1,000 births with most of the risk occurring before 37 weeks' gestation. After 37 weeks, the risk of recurrence drops to 1.8 per 1,000. Women with a history of live birth complicated by FGR, however, have a much higher stillbirth rate of 21.8 per 1,000. Diabetes, hypertension, and a history of placental abruption also carry higher rates of recurrent fetal loss.

Although, there is no sure-fire method to prevent stillbirths, losing weight, quitting smoking, and abstaining from drugs and alcohol are all lifestyle modifications that women can make before becoming pregnant. Women with diabetes should get their glucose levels under tight control before becoming pregnant and throughout pregnancy. Preconception and prenatal care can also help identify and screen women for other risk factors that may increase stillbirth risk.

In terms of preventing stillbirth, women should try to optimize their health prior to pregnancy. This includes getting enough folic acid before they become pregnant and getting both preconception and prenatal care. We also need to educate women that delaying their first birth until after age 40 is associated with an increased risk of adverse outcomes, including an increased risk of stillbirth. We could help in dealing with the cause of IUFD and stillbirths by encouraging physicians to request, and families to agree to, an autopsy so that we can gain a better understanding of the causes of stillbirth and thereby decreasing perinatal mortality as well as maternal morbidity and mortality.

KEY POINTS

- Diagnosis of intrauterine fetal demise (IUFD) is disheartening to the patient resulting in psychological setback.
- There are many risk factors for IUFD such as increasing maternal age, obesity, smoking and some of the medical conditions.
- Out of the high-risk factors, some are modifiable, and hence prevention is possible in these cases.
- However, some factors such as inherited thrombophilias and congenital malformations are nonmodifiable. Here the role of preconceptional counseling and quality antenatal care with assessment of fetal wellbeing plays an utmost important role.
- In case of IUFD, pregnancy can be terminated either by surgical or medical methods depending on the obstetric indications.
- In that case to find out the cause of stillbirth, physician should request on performing autopsy of the stillborn.
- Strong emotional support and psychological consultation should be offered to the couple with IUFD.

REFERENCES

1. Joseph KS, Kinniburgh B, Hutcheon JA, et al. Rationalizing definitions and procedures for optimizing clinical care and public health in fetal death and stillbirth. Obstet Gynecol. 2015; 125:784.
2. Roy MP. Mitigating the stillbirth challenge in India. Lancet. 2016;387(10032):1995. doi: 10.1016/S0140-6736(16)30460-3. PubMed PMID: 27203766.
3. Allanson ER, Tunçalp Ö, Gardosi J, Pattinson RC, Francis A, Vogel JP, Erwich J, Flenady VJ, Frøen JF, Neilson J, Quach A, Chou D, Mathai M, Say L, Gülmezoglu AM. Optimising the International Classification of Diseases to identify the maternal condition in the case of perinatal death. BJOG. 2016. doi:10.1111/1471-0528.14246. [Epub ahead of print] PubMed PMID: 27527550.
4. DiMario S, Say L, Lincetto O. Risk factors for stillbirth in developing countries: a systematic review of the literature. Sex Transm Dis. 2007;34:S11.
5. Nohr EA, Bech BH, Davies MJ, et al. Prepregnancy obesity and fetal death: a study within the Danish National Birth Cohort. Obstet Gynecol. 2005;106(2):250-9.
6. Raymond EG, Cnattingius S, Kiely JL. Effects of maternal age, parity, and smoking on the risk of stillbirth. Br J Obstet Gynaecol. 1994;101:301.
7. ACOG Practice Bulletin No. 102: management of stillbirth. Obstet Gynecol. 2009;113:748.
8. Frøen JF, Gardosi JO, Thurmann A, et al. Restricted fetal growth in sudden intrauterine unexplained death. Acta Obstet Gynecol Scand. 2004;83:801.
9. Getahun D, Ananth CV, Kinzler WL. Risk factors for antepartum and intrapartum stillbirth: a population-based study. Am J Obstet Gynecol. 2007;196:499.
10. Stillbirth Collaborative Research Network Writing Group. Causes of death among stillbirths. JAMA. 2011;306:2459.
11. Goldenberg RL, McClure EM, Saleem S, Reddy UM. Infection-related stillbirths. Lancet. 2010;375:1482.
12. Iwasenko JM, Howard J, Arbuckle S, et al. Human cytomegalovirus infection is detected frequently in stillbirths and is associated with fetal thrombotic vasculopathy. J Infect Dis. 2011;203:1526.
13. Williams EJ, Embleton ND, Clark JE, et al. Viral infections: contributions to late fetal death, stillbirth, and infant death. J Pediatr. 2013;163:424.
14. Many A, Elad R, Yaron Y, et al. Third-trimester unexplained intrauterine fetal death is associated with inherited thrombophilia. Obstet Gynecol. 2002;99(5 Pt 1):684-7.
15. Eller AG, Branch DW, Byrne JL. Stillbirth at term. Obstet Gynecol. 2006;108:442.
16. Weeks JW, Asrat T, Morgan MA, et al. Antepartum surveillance for a history of stillbirth: when to begin? Am J Obstet Gynecol. 1995;172:486.
17. Silver RM. Fetal death. Obstet Gynecol. 2007;109(1):153-67.
18. Silver RM, Varner MW, Reddy U, et al. Work-up of stillbirth: a review of the evidence. Am J Obstet Gynecol. 2007;196(5): 433-44.

Chapter 57
Cerebrovascular Accidents in Pregnancy

Jignesh Shah

INTRODUCTION

Stroke, the sudden onset of brain dysfunction from a vascular cause, is one of the most common causes of long-term disability. Although rare during childbearing years, stroke is even more devastating when it occurs in a young woman trying to start a family. Pregnancy and the postpartum period are associated with an increased risk of ischemic stroke and intracerebral hemorrhage, although the incidence estimates have varied. There are several causes of stroke that are in fact unique to pregnancy and the postpartum period, such as pre-eclampsia and eclampsia, amniotic fluid embolus, postpartum angiopathy and postpartum cardiomyopathy. Data regarding these individual entities are scant. Most concerning is the lack of data regarding both prevention and acute management of pregnancy-related stroke. The purpose of this article is to summarize existing data regarding incidence, risk factors and potential etiologies, as well as treatment strategies for stroke in pregnancy **(Fig. 57.1)**.

Recent studies suggest that the risk of cerebral infarction is increased during the puerperium but not during pregnancy itself. Most of the known causes of ischemic stroke in the young have been reported during pregnancy. In most of these conditions, it is uncertain whether pregnancy is coincidental or plays a role in the occurrence of stroke. Eclampsia is the main pregnancy-specific cause, which may be associated with focal neurological deficits of sudden onset, consistent with a clinical diagnosis of stroke. However, the precise pathogenesis of these stroke-like focal deficits remains poorly understood. The two other pregnancy-specific conditions (choriocarcinoma and amniotic fluid embolism) are rarely responsible for focal cerebral ischemia. In a significant number of patients, the cause of the stroke remains undetermined, despite an extensive etiological investigation. Whether a hypercoagulable state and vessel wall changes associated with pregnancy may play a role in the occurrence of these otherwise unexplained ischemic strokes remains unknown. The occurrence of cerebral venous thrombosis is clearly linked to the puerperal state, suggesting a direct role of the latter. However, cerebral venous thrombosis during pregnancy or the puerperium has been related to various etiologies, stressing the need for an etiological study, particularly when the thrombosis occurs during pregnancy. Pregnancy may increase the risk of subarachnoid hemorrhage, The most common cause is rupture of an arterial aneurysm. Although this is a controversial issue, the increased tendency of an aneurysm to bleed with advancing gestational age suggests that hemodynamic, hormonal or other physiological changes of pregnancy may play a role in aneurysmal rupture. The classic notion that rupture of an arterial aneurysm occurs more frequently during labor has not been confirmed. Most authors agree that surgical management after subarachnoid hemorrhage in pregnancy should be the same as that in the non-pregnant state. Data specifically devoted to intraparenchymal hemorrhage in pregnancy are scarce. Pregnancy and in particular the puerperium seem to be associated with an increased risk of intracerebral hemorrhage. The most common causes are eclampsia and ruptured vascular malformations. Whether pregnancy increases the risk of rupture of an arteriovenous malformation is controversial.

POSSIBILITY AND RISK FACTORS

Approximately 10% of strokes occur before delivery period, 40% occur proximate to intrapartum, and 50% occur puerperium and after discharge.[1-4]

During complete pregnancy and the postpartum period are allied with a noticeable rise in the relative risk and a small increase in the absolute risk of ischemic stroke and intracerebral hemorrhage, with the highest risk during the puerperium.[2,5-9]

Some data are contradictory for the occurrence of aneurysmal subarachnoid hemorrhage during pregnancy, delivery, and the postpartum period. Some clinical studies have reported an amplified risk,[10,11] while others determined that aneurysmal rupture is not very common.[12]

The danger of hemorrhage from a cerebral arteriovenous malformation is debated, and no definitive data exist.[13,14]

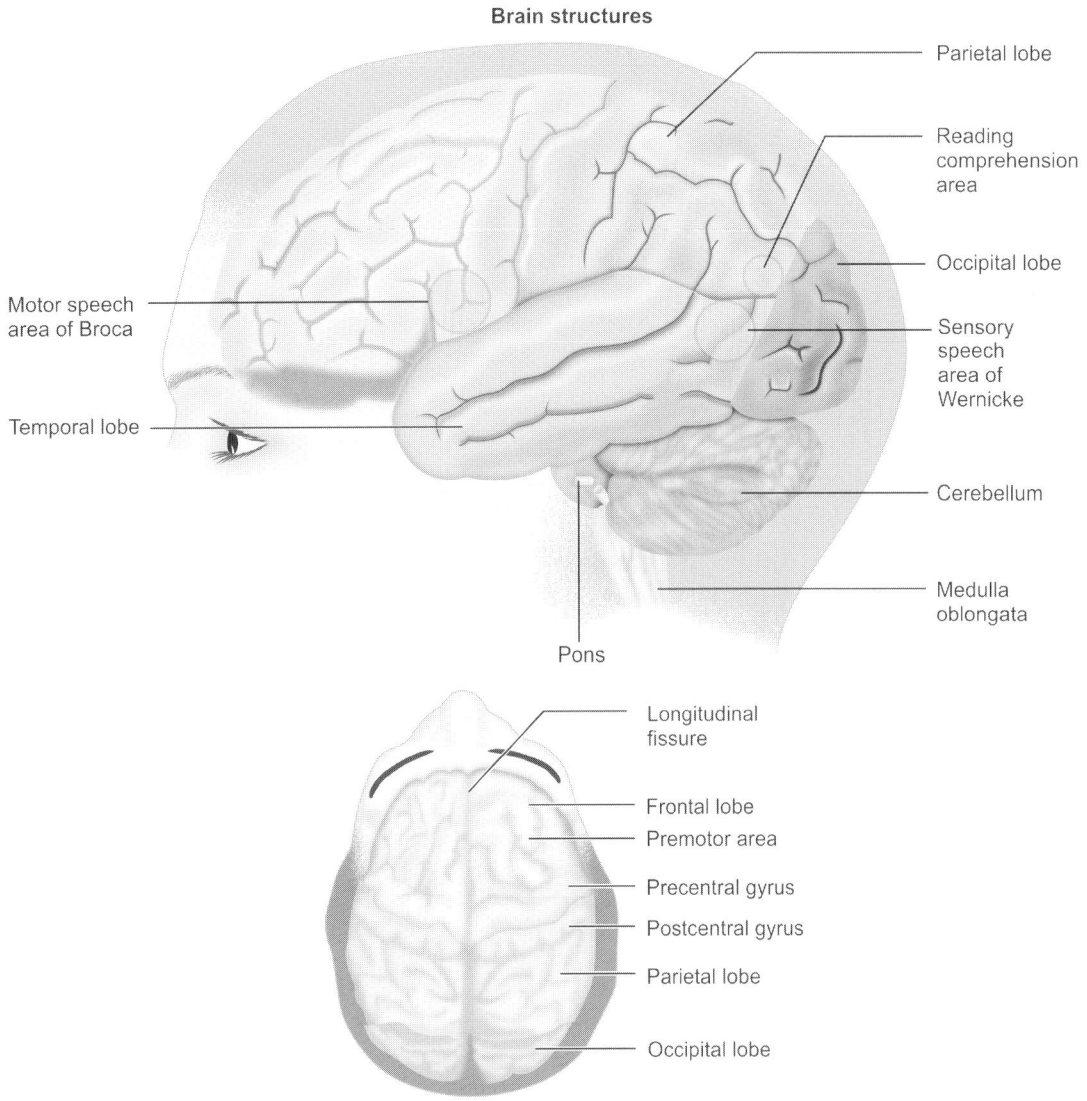

Fig. 57.1: The brain

Major Causative Factors

- Risk factors for stroke related to pregnancy include cesarean delivery, pregnancy-induced hypertension[8]
- Postpartum infection[2]
- Possibly multiple gestation,[15] although the latter has not been evaluated as an independent risk factor.

Amniotic fluid embolism is a significant cause of pregnancy-related morbidity and mortality, but is thought to be a very rare etiology of focal cerebral ischemia in pregnancy.[16,17]

The risk of stroke in women with pre-eclampsia/eclampsia is discussed in detail separately.

Clinical characteristics of PFO stroke in pregnancy refer **Table 57.1**.

ETIOLOGY (TABLE 57.2)

All types of stroke can be seen in perinatal period:[18]
- *Hemorrhagic stroke from aneurysms:*[5,6,19,20]
  - Arteriovenous malformations
  - Pre-eclampsia/eclampsia
- Ischemic stroke
  - Cerebral venous sinus thrombosis
  - Pre-eclampsia/eclampsia
  - Cardioembolism related to valvular heart disease.[21-24]
- *Cerebral venous thrombosis:* Cerebral venous thrombosis (CVT) is rare, but occurs more commonly in association with pregnancy.[25-28] It presents most often in the third trimester of pregnancy and the puerperium.[29,30]

Table 57.1: Clinical characteristics of PFO stroke in pregnancy

	PFO (n = 24)	Non-PFO (n = 46)	P values
Mean delivery ages (years)	29.87 (15–39)	32.91 (24–40)	NS
Race			
• African American	1 (4.17%)	6 (13.04%)	0.240
• White	23 (95.83%)	39 (84.78%)	0.168
• Asian	0 (0%)	1 (2.17%)	0.169
HTN	2 (8.33%)	13 (28.26%)	0.054
Hyperlipidemia	1 (4.17%)	3 (6.52%)	0.687
Gestational diabetes	2 (8.33%)	5 (10.87%)	0.737
Obesity	0 (0%)	5 (10.87%)	0.094
Pre-eclampsia	3 (12.5%)	8 (17.39%)	0.594
May-Thurner syndrome	5 (20.83%)	0 (0%)	0.001
Migraine with aura	13 (54.17%)	10 (21.74%)	0.006
Hypercoagulability	20 (83.33%)	18 (39.13%)	0.0004
Smoke	7 (29.17%)	12 (26.(%)	0.783
Illicit drug using	2 (8.33%)	2 (4.35%)	0.495
EtoH	1 (4.17%)	2 (4.35%)	0.972

Table 57.2: Relative risk of stroke in pregnancy and post-partum versus non-pregnant

	Third trimester	Peripartum	Postpartum
Ischemic stroke	2.2	33.8	8.3
Intracerebral hemorrhage	0.3	95.0	11.7
Subarachnoid hemorrhage	0.8	46.9	1.8

Other rare causes are:
- Hypercoagulable state
- Antiphospholipid syndrome
- Prothrombin gene mutation
- Deficiency of antithrombin, protein C, or protein S Although these abnormalities typically cause venous thrombosis, we suggest a laboratory evaluation for an inherited or acquired thrombophilia for a woman presenting with a nonhemorrhagic ischemic neurologic event during pregnancy.

Other: Cervical manipulation **(Table 57.3)**.

DIAGNOSTIC WORK-UP

Types of strokes:
- Transient ischemic attacks
- Ischemic
- Hemorrhagic.

Symptoms of a Cerebrovascular Accidents

Depends upon the area of the brain affected. Usually, a sudden development of one or more of the following: Weakness/Paralysis of an arm, leg, side of face, or any part of the body, visual changes/disturbances, slurred speech or difficulty in understanding speech, difficulty in reading or writing, swallowing, difficulty in reading or drooling, vertigo, loss of balance or coordination, personality changes, mood changes (depression), drowsiness, lethargy, loss of consciousness, uncontrollable eye movements or eye drooping and memory loss **(Table 57.4)**.

Transient Ischemic Attacks (TIA)

- Temporary neurologic deficits caused by impaired cerebral blood flow
- Considered a warning sign
- Characterized by focal neurological deficits, typically lasting minutes to hours in duration.
- When symptoms present more than 24 hours but then disappear, the patient is said to have reversible ischemic neurologic deficits.

Clinical Manifestations of Transient Ischemic Attacks

- Dizziness
- Momentary confusion
- Difficulty with speech
- Visual disturbances
- Weakness of paralysis on one side of the body
- Ptosis
- Tinnitus.

Diagnosis of TIA

- Health history.
- Clinical presentation.
  The diagnostic evaluation and treatment of stroke in pregnant women is similar to that in nonpregnant individuals.[16]
- Noncontrast head CT
- MRI is safe during pregnancy
- Avoid in pregnancy iodine and gadolinium-based contrast

Table 57.3: Probability of stroke or serious adverse events following cervical manipulation		
Source	Method	Risk per manipulation
Dvorak	Survey of 203 members of Swiss Society of Manual Medicine (all non-chiropractors)	1 serious complication/400,000
Patijn	Review of computerized registration system In Holland	1 complication/518,000
Haldeman	Extensive literature review to formulate practice guidelines	1–2 strokes/1 million
Jaskoviak	Clinical files of National College	0 complication/5 million 15-year period
Henderson/Cassidy	Canadian Memorial Chiropractic College Clinic	0 complication/5 million 9-year period
Hurwitz	Randomised cervical study literature review	0.64 serious complications/1 milllon; 0.27 deaths/1 milllon
Carey	Claim review: Canada's largest malpractice insurance company	1 CVA/3 million; 0 deaths 5-year period
NCMIC	Claim review: Principal chiropractic malpractice insurance company within US	1 CVA/2 million 3-year period
Haldeman	Claim review: Canada's largest malpractice insurance company	0.17 CVA/1 million 10-year period
Thiel	UK survey of 28,807 treatment consultations	No adverse events

Table 57.4: Difference between right and left hemisphere injuries	
Right side brain damage changes	Left sided brain damage changes
Left-sided paralysis	Right-sided paralysis
Decreased attention span and focus	Loss of speech
Memory loss	Inability to understand words
Spatial relationships	Inability to understand written words
Orientation	Scientific function and reasoning
Ability to recognize faces	

Other Tests[31,32]

- Electrocardiogram
- Complete blood count
- Peripheral blood smear
- Urine

Management

Treatment of TIA
- Aimed at cause.
- Hypertension management.
- Decrease platelet aggregation.
  - Ticlid (Ticlopidine)
  - Plavix (Clopidogrel)
  - Aspirin.
- Coumadin (Evarparin)
- For carotid stenosis > 70% endarterectomy.

Ischemic Strokes (Fig. 57.2)

- Thrombotic or embolic.
- Obstruction in blood flow from a clot, atherosclerotic plague or the combination of the two.
- Account for 80% of strokes.
- Thrombotic—atherosclerotic plaques
- Embolic—atrial fibrillation, valvular stenosis; MI

Hemorrhagic Strokes (Fig. 57.3)

- Account for 20% of strokes.
- Rupture of blood vessel with bleeding into brain tissue.
- Intracerebral-associated with trauma, hypertension, aneurysms.
- Subarachnoid hemorrhage, subdural hemorrhage or ventricular hemorrhage.
- Phencyclidine, crack, cocaine, amphetamines and heroin have been associated with hemorrhagic stroke.
- Can be permanent on resolve in time.
- Can vary depending on time and location.

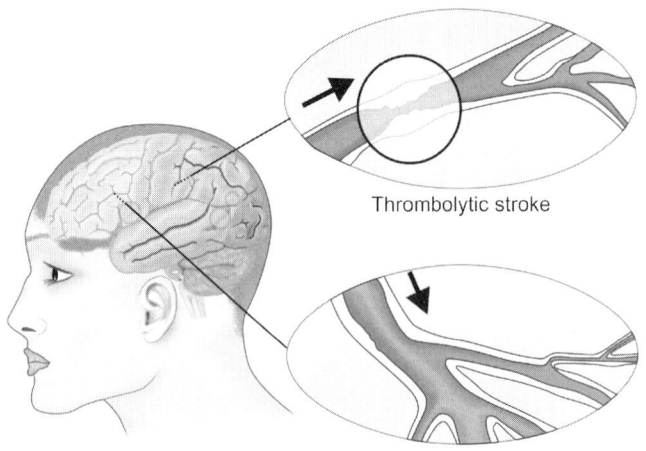

Fig. 57.2: Ischemic strokes

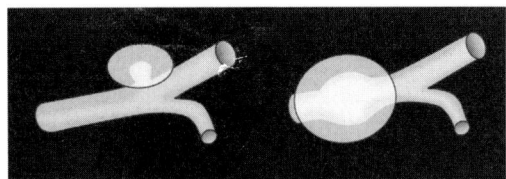

Fig. 57.3: Hemorrhagic strokes: Aneurysms

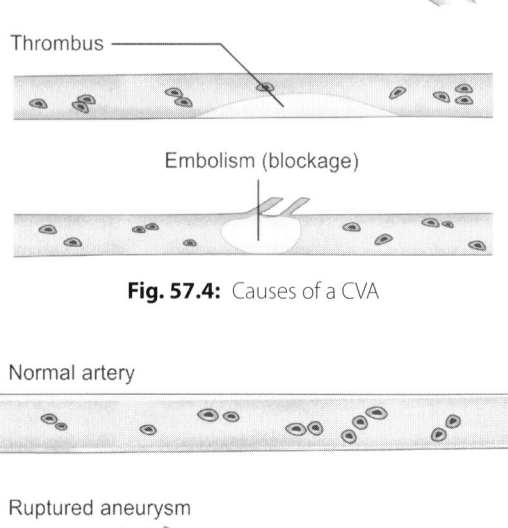

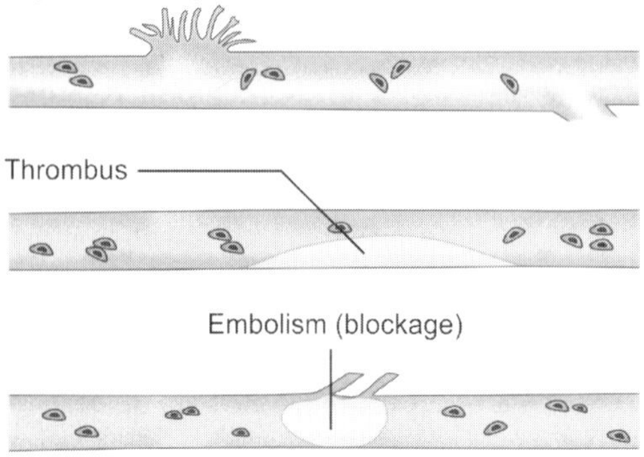

Fig. 57.4: Causes of a CVA

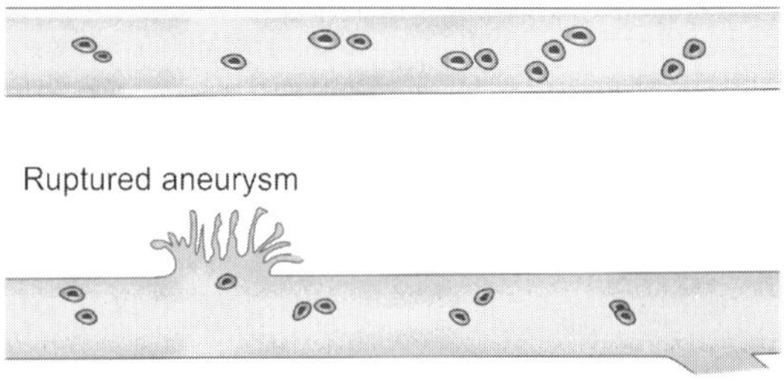

Fig. 57.5: Hemorrhagic strokes: Ruptured aneurysms

SIGNS AND SYMPTOMS OF STROKE

- Aphasia
  - Expressive
  - Recessive
  - Global
- Dysarthria.
- Dysphagia.
- Dyspraxia (Partial loss of the ability to coordinate and perform certain purposeful movements and gestures, in the absence of other motor and sensory impairments such as multiple sclerosis or Parkinson's disease).
  - Hemiplegia.
  - Altered sensation.
  - Unilateral neglect.
  - Homonymous hemianopsia.
  - Emotional liability.
  - Impaired judgment.
  - Incontinence.

CAUSES OF CVA (FIG. 57.4)

- Ruptured aneurysm (**Fig. 57.5**).
- Thrombus.
- Embolism (Blockage).

Modifiable Risk Factors

- Hypertension (greatest risk factor)
- Smoking.
- Coronary artery disease
- Diet.
- Diabetes.
- Some medications.
- Cocaine.
- Alcohol abuse.

Non-modifiable Risk Factors

- Age.
- Sex.
- Family history.
- Bleeding disorders.
- Pregnancy
- Post-pregnancy.

The management of stroke during pregnancy depended on cause of stroke.[33]

Magnesium sulfate is the drug of choice for the prevention of recurrent eclamptic seizures. Platelet transfusion is indicated in HELLP (hemolysis, elevated liver enzymes, and low platelets) syndrome, if there is significant maternal bleeding, or if the platelet count is <20,000 cells/mL.

Treatment of TTP or HUS: For the majority of patients with suspected thrombotic thrombocytopenic purpura (TTP) during pregnancy, urgent plasma exchange therapy is the appropriate treatment.

An exception is a woman with known hereditary TTP or a strong suspicion of hereditary TTP based on hereditary TTP in a sibling. For these individuals, plasma infusion is the appropriate treatment.

For patients with suspected complement-mediated hemolytic uremic syndrome (HUS), which often presents in the postpartum period, the risk for end-stage renal disease is high. It may be reasonable to initiate anti-complement therapy urgently in order to limit preventable renal damage while the diagnosis is being confirmed (or excluded).

Importantly, unlike pre-eclampsia and HELLP syndrome, there is no evidence that delivery alters the course of TTP or HUS. If TTP or HUS is the presumptive diagnosis, delivery should only be performed for obstetric reasons.

Treatment of Postpartum Angiopathy

As with all of the central nervous system vasculopathy syndromes, there is no proof that any therapeutic intervention is effective for postpartum angiopathy. The syndrome is usually self-limiting. Some patients have received glucocorticoids (especially those with findings that suggest possible isolated central nervous system vasculitis), calcium-channel blockers, and/or magnesium.[22] Progressive deterioration is usually a relatively early finding (within the first few weeks) and may be due to increasing brain edema.

The prognosis of postpartum angiopathy was thought to be good, but in one of the largest series (n = 18), a complete recovery was achieved by 9 patients (50%), while a fulminant course followed by death affected four patients (22%).[22] There is no evidence of a high risk of recurrence in future pregnancies,[34] although at least one recurrent case has been reported,[35] or of an increased risk of eclampsia/preeclampsia in future pregnancies.

Acute Ischemic Stroke

The treatment of acute ischemic stroke in pregnancy is mostly guided by the same principles as in the general population. These are discussed separately.

Early aspirin therapy is recommended for patients with acute ischemic stroke who are not receiving alteplase, intravenous heparin, or oral anticoagulants. This recommendation is in accord with current guidelines.[36,37] Aspirin should be given within 48 hours of stroke onset and may also be used in combination with subcutaneous heparin for deep vein thrombosis prophylaxis.

Thrombotic strokes associated with hypercoagulable states are generally treated by anticoagulation (to prevent recurrence) and possibly by acute thrombolysis.

Fibrinolytic (thrombolytic) therapy: Among the fibrinolytic agents, only alteplase (recombinant tissue plasminogen activator) is approved for use in acute stroke. Treatment with intravenous alteplase is beneficial in selected patients with acute ischemic stroke who can be treated within 4.5 hours of symptom onset. Issues related to such therapy are discussed in detail separately.

The efficacy and safety of thrombolytic therapy for acute ischemic stroke in pregnant women are unknown.[38-42]

Given these data, we believe that alteplase can be given in pregnancy after careful discussion of the potential risks and benefit.[43,46-48]

Secondary prevention of ischemic stroke: An antiplatelet agent for secondary prevention is recommended for patients with a history of noncardioembolic stroke or transient ischemic attack (TIA) of atherothrombotic, lacunar (small vessel occlusive type), or cryptogenic type.

Aspirin, clopidogrel, and the combination of aspirin-extended-release dipyridamole are all acceptable options for preventing recurrent noncardioembolic ischemic stroke. An aspirin dose of 60 to 81 mg/day is considered safe in pregnancy.[49-51]

The evaluation and management of the inherited thrombophilias is discussed in greater detail separately.

Cerebral venous sinus thrombosis: The mainstay for the treatment of symptomatic cerebral venous sinus thrombosis, with or without hemorrhagic venous infarction, is anticoagulation therapy with intravenous heparin or subcutaneous low molecular weight heparin. For women with cerebral venous thrombosis during pregnancy, guidelines from the American Heart Association/American Stroke Association conclude that low molecular weight heparin in full anticoagulant doses should be continued throughout pregnancy, and low molecular weight heparin or a vitamin K antagonist with a target INR of 2 to 3 should be continued for at least six weeks postpartum for a total minimum duration of therapy of six months.[52,53] Symptomatic management issues include control of seizures and intracranial hypertension.

Intracranial hemorrhage: Subarachnoid and/or intracerebral hemorrhage during pregnancy or the postpartum period is most often caused by aneurysmal rupture or bleeding from a vascular malformation.[18] Pre-eclampsia/eclampsia/HELLP is another important cause of hemorrhagic strokes during pregnancy.

One retrospective study reported 154 women with intracranial hemorrhage during pregnancy or the puerperium who had an identified vascular lesion.[54] The cause of the hemorrhage was cerebral aneurysm or arteriovenous malformation in 77 and 23%, respectively. Aneurysm rupture during pregnancy occurred most frequently in the third trimester (55%), and less so in the second trimester (31%), first trimester (6%), or postpartum period (8%). Hemodynamic, angiogenic, and endocrine changes associated with pregnancy may affect the growth and rupture of aneurysms in the gravid patient.[55] However, there is conflicting evidence regarding whether the risk of aneurysmal subarachnoid hemorrhage (SAH) is increased with pregnancy and the puerperium.

One old retrospective study found that among 37 pregnant women in good condition after SAH from a verified intracranial aneurysm, recurrent bleeding during the same pregnancy from surgically untreated aneurysms occurred in 13 (35%).[56] The overall incidence of rebleeding after initial SAH in the modern era is uncertain. Limited data from older literature suggest that the maternal case fatality rate of aneurysmal SAH is approximately 50%,[54] which is similar to that of the general population The fetal case fatality rate is approximately 17%.[54]

Intracerebral aneurysms and arteriovenous malformations can be managed by surgical (i.e., clipping) or endovascular (e.g., embolization) treatment of the causative lesion.[57]

In general, ruptured intracranial aneurysms in pregnant women are treated as they would be in patients who are not pregnant. Endovascular coiling is preferred to surgical clipping for appropriately shaped aneurysms. A number of reports have described successful endovascular coiling of intracranial aneurysms associated with term or near-term births.[58-61] However, aneurysms with broad necks, a low neck-to-fundus ratio, distal segment lesions, and a number of giant aneurysms are not amenable to endovascular therapy. Stable, unruptured asymptomatic aneurysms can usually be observed without intervention during pregnancy, whereas symptomatic or enlarging unruptured aneurysms can be treated.[3,62]

Similarly, symptomatic arteriovenous malformations in pregnant women are treated as they would be in patients who are not pregnant. There are a few case reports of successful embolization of hemorrhagic arteriovenous malformations during pregnancy via the endovascular approach, followed by surgical resection of the AVM.[63,64] CT angiography with shielding of the abdomen during pregnancy can be performed prior to the embolization procedure to delineate any pre-nidal or intra-nidal aneurysms that might be the source of the bleed.

As noted above, retrospective data suggest that severe preeclampsia/eclampsia/HELLP is the cause of 14 to 55% of hemorrhagic strokes in pregnancy. In such cases, management goals are to stabilize the mother, prevent recurrent convulsions, treat severe hypertension to reduce or prevent cerebral edema and hemorrhage, and initiate delivery of the fetus.

Delivery: Women who have had the cause of their cerebral hemorrhage treated (e.g., clipping or embolization of a cerebral aneurysm or arteriovenous malformation) may undergo labor and delivery. However, there is considerable controversy regarding management of labor and delivery with ruptured aneurysms or arteriovenous malformations that have not been definitively treated. The two major alternatives are: (1) Prophylactic cesarean delivery, and (2) regional anesthesia with instrumental delivery to eliminate cerebral hemodynamic fluctuations associated with pain and the Valsalva maneuver.

There are no data from large series or randomized trials, but it appears that maternal and fetal mortality rates are the same with both methods. As a result, cesarean delivery should be reserved for the usual obstetrical indications.[54] Aneurysm rupture has occurred during elective cesarean birth; thus it is not completely protective. Therefore, regardless of the mode of delivery, it is important to control hypertension and minimize fluctuations in blood pressure.

Some experts believe that selected patients who are stable after intracranial hemorrhage can be managed supportively until the pregnancy is taken to term.[57] The lesion can then be treated by surgical or endovascular means after delivery. However, emergency surgery is indicated, if there is neurologic deterioration caused by recurrent bleeding.

PREVENTION OF CVA

The risk of initial stroke during the first trimester is not increased compared to the nonpregnant state. The risk of recurrent stroke during the first trimester might also be assumed to be low as compare with late pregnancy or the postpartum period. Aspirin due to low cost and ease of use has been the most popular choice for secondary prevention of ischemic stroke during the first trimester. Although case control studies have suggested a possible association of aspirin use with several rare conditions such as pulmonary hypertension in newborn, gastroschisis, premature closure of the ductus arteriosus, low dose aspirin is considered to be relatively safe and to have generally positive effects on reproductive outcomes. Available evidence suggests that low dose (less than 150 mg/day) aspirin during the second and third trimesters is safe for both mother and fetus.

Various treatment options for prophylaxis in high risk cases (Past history of pregnancy induced hypertension (PIH), eclampsia, chronic hypertention, diabetes, extreme obesity)
- No treatment throught first trimester
- Aspirin 75 mg daily
- Aspirin 325 mg daily
- Clopidogrel 75 mg daily
- Acetyl salicylic acid/Dipyridamole one capsule twice daily
- Subcutaneous low molecular weight heparin
- Subcutaneous unfractionated heparin.

SUMMARY AND RECOMMENDATIONS

- The risks of both cerebral infarction and intracerebral hemorrhage are increased in the six weeks after delivery but not during pregnancy itself.

- Women with transient neurological events appearing during pregnancy should be investigated for inherited thrombophilias. Such a diagnosis may have important implication for both mother and fetus as these patients may be at increased risk for recurrent vascular complications, antithrombotic treatment should be considered.
- It is recommended a complete neurologic work-up on the patient before the pregnancy in high-risk cases
- Pregnancy induced hypertension should be closely monitored and controlled.
- Chronic hypertension carries the highest risk for CVA
- Low dose aspirin (less than 150 mg/day) during the second and third trimesters is safe for both mother and fetus when used for prophylaxis.
- Death registration should include cause of death in eclampsia, which would be due to CVA (60% cases). But because of lack of documentation and post mortem, cases in our country go unnoticed.
- There is no need to advise against pregnancy in women with an increased risk of subarachnoid hemorrhage and no evidence to advise against vaginal delivery in such women as the risk of SAH is not increased during pregnancy.
- Stroke is more common in pregnant women, especially in the puerperium.
- Pre-eclampsia/eclampsia is one of the most common
- causes of both ischemic infarction and hemorrhagic stroke in pregnancy. Other causes are listed in the **Table 57.1**.
- The diagnostic evaluation and treatment of stroke in pregnant women is similar to that in nonpregnant individuals. A head CT scan is usually the first imaging modality obtained because it is both informative and readily available. However, brain MRI is more sensitive than CT for the detection of small infarcts and for visualization of very early infarction when diffusion-weighted imaging is employed.
- The management of stroke during pregnancy is guided by the stroke etiology and subtype.
- With pre-eclampsia/eclampsia/HELLP, the goals are to stabilize the mother, prevent recurrent convulsions, treat severe hypertension to reduce or prevent cerebral edema and hemorrhage, and initiate prompt delivery.
- Early aspirin therapy is recommended for patients with acute ischemic stroke who are not receiving alteplase or anticoagulants.
- An antiplatelet agent for secondary prevention is recommended for patients with a history of noncardioembolic stroke or transient ischemic attack (TIA) of atherothrombotic, lacunar (small vessel occlusive type), or cryptogenic type.
- The treatment of symptomatic cerebral venous sinus thrombosis, with or without hemorrhagic venous infarction, is anticoagulation therapy.
- Subarachnoid and/or intracerebral hemorrhage due to aneurysmal rupture or bleeding from a vascular malformation can be managed by surgical (i.e., clipping) or endovascular (e.g., embolization) treatment of the causative lesion.
- The risk of recurrent stroke in future pregnancy is probably low, but data are sparse.

REFERENCES

1. Petitti DB, Sidney S, Quesenberry CP Jr, Bernstein A. Incidence of stroke and myocardial infarction in women of reproductive age. Stroke. 1997;28:280.
2. James AH, Bushnell CD, Jamison MG, Myers ER. Incidence and risk factors for stroke in pregnancy and the puerperium. Obstet Gynecol. 2005;106:509.
3. Davie CA, O'Brien P. Stroke and pregnancy. J Neurol Neurosurg Psychiatry. 2008;79:240.
4. Scott CA, Bewley S, Rudd A, et al. Incidence, risk factors, management, and outcomes of stroke in pregnancy. Obstet Gynecol. 2012;120:318.
5. Kittner SJ, Stern BJ, Feeser BR, et al. Pregnancy and the risk of stroke. N Engl J Med. 1996;335:768.
6. Sharshar T, Lamy C, Mas JL. Incidence and causes of strokes associated with pregnancy and puerperium. A study in public hospitals of Ile de France. Stroke in Pregnancy Study Group. Stroke. 1995;26:930.
7. Bateman BT, Schumacher HC, Bushnell CD, et al. Intracerebral hemorrhage in pregnancy: frequency, risk factors, and outcome. Neurology. 2006;67:424.
8. Lanska DJ, Kryscio RJ. Risk factors for peripartum and postpartum stroke and intracranial venous thrombosis. Stroke. 2000;31:1274.
9. Kamel H, Navi BB, Sriram N, et al. Risk of a thrombotic event after the 6-week postpartum period. N Engl J Med. 2014;370:1307.
10. Fox MW, Harms RW, Davis DH. Selected neurologic complications of pregnancy. Mayo Clin Proc. 1990;65:1595.
11. Salonen Ros H, Lichtenstein P, Bellocco R, et al. Increased risks of circulatory diseases in late pregnancy and puerperium. Epidemiology. 2001;12:456.
12. Tiel Groenestege AT, Rinkel GJ, van der Bom JG, et al. The risk of aneurysmal subarachnoid hemorrhage during pregnancy, delivery, and the puerperium in the Utrecht population: case-crossover study and standardized incidence ratio estimation. Stroke. 2009;40:1148.
13. Brown RD Jr, Flemming KD, Meyer FB, et al. Natural history, evaluation, and management of intracranial vascular malformations. Mayo Clin Proc. 2005;80:269.
14. Horton JC, Chambers WA, Lyons SL, et al. Pregnancy and the risk of hemorrhage from cerebral arteriovenous malformations. Neurosurgery. 1990;27:867.
15. Ros HS, Lichtenstein P, Bellocco R, et al. Pulmonary embolism and stroke in relation to pregnancy: how can high-risk women be identified? Am J Obstet Gynecol. 2002;186:198.
16. Mas JL, Lamy C. Stroke in pregnancy and the puerperium. J Neurol. 1998;245:305.

17. Wabnitz A, Bushnell C. Migraine, cardiovascular disease, and stroke during pregnancy: systematic review of the literature. Cephalalgia. 2015;35:132.
18. Feske SK. Stroke in pregnancy. Semin Neurol. 2007;27:442.
19. Martin JN Jr, Thigpen BD, Moore RC, et al. Stroke and severe preeclampsia and eclampsia: a paradigm shift focusing on systolic blood pressure. Obstet Gynecol. 2005;105:246.
20. Cantu-Brito C, Arauz A, Aburto Y, et al. Cerebrovascular complications during pregnancy and postpartum: clinical and prognosis observations in 240 Hispanic women. Eur J Neurol. 2011;18:819.
21. Singhal AB, Bernstein RA. Postpartum angiopathy and other cerebral vasoconstriction syndromes. Neurocrit Care. 2005;3:91.
22. Fugate JE, Ameriso SF, Ortiz G, et al. Variable presentations of postpartum angiopathy. Stroke. 2012;43:670.
23. Fugate JE, Wijdicks EF, Parisi JE, et al. Fulminant postpartum cerebral vasoconstriction syndrome. Arch Neurol. 2012;69:111.
24. Bakhru A, Atlas RO. A case of postpartum cerebral angiitis and review of the literature. Arch Gynecol Obstet. 2011;283:663.
25. Singhal AB. Postpartum angiopathy with reversible posterior leukoencephalopathy. Arch Neurol. 2004;61:411.
26. Fletcher JJ, Kramer AH, Bleck TP, Solenski NJ. Overlapping features of eclampsia and postpartum angiopathy. Neurocrit Care. 2009;11:199.
27. Jeng JS, Tang SC, Yip PK. Incidence and etiologies of stroke during pregnancy and puerperium as evidenced in Taiwanese women. Cerebrovasc Dis. 2004;18:290.
28. Skidmore FM, Williams LS, Fradkin KD, et al. Presentation, etiology, and outcome of stroke in pregnancy and puerperium. J Stroke Cerebrovasc Dis. 2001;10:1.
29. Witlin AG, Friedman SA, Egerman RS, et al. Cerebrovascular disorders complicating pregnancy—beyond eclampsia. Am J Obstet Gynecol. 1997;176:1139.
30. Liang CC, Chang SD, Lai SL, et al. Stroke complicating pregnancy and the puerperium. Eur J Neurol. 2006;13:1256.
31. Sibai BM, Coppage KH. Diagnosis and management of women with stroke during pregnancy/postpartum. Clin Perinatol. 2004;31:853.
32. Kupferminc MJ, Yair D, Bornstein NM, et al. Transient focal neurological deficits during pregnancy in carriers of inherited thrombophilia. Stroke. 2000;31:892.
33. Treadwell SD, Thanvi B, Robinson TG. Stroke in pregnancy and the puerperium. Postgrad Med J. 2008;84:238.
34. Rémi J, Pfefferkorn T, Fesl G, et al. Uncomplicated pregnancy and delivery after previous severe postpartum cerebral angiopathy. Case Rep Neurol. 2011;3:252.
35. Ursell MR, Marras CL, Farb R, et al. Recurrent intracranial hemorrhage due to postpartum cerebral angiopathy: implications for management. Stroke 1998;29:1995.
36. Lansberg MG, O'Donnell MJ, Khatri P, et al. Antithrombotic and thrombolytic therapy for ischemic stroke: Antithrombotic Therapy and Prevention of Thrombosis, 9th edn. American College of Chest Physicians Evidence-Based Clinical Practice Guidelines. Chest. 2012;141:e601S.
37. Jauch EC, Saver JL, Adams HP Jr, et al. Guidelines for the early management of patients with acute ischemic stroke: a guideline for healthcare professionals from the American Heart Association/American Stroke Association. Stroke. 2013;44:870.
38. Aleu A, Mellado P, Lichy C, et al. Hemorrhagic complications after off-label thrombolysis for ischemic stroke. Stroke. 2007;38:417.
39. Turrentine MA, Braems G, Ramirez MM. Use of thrombolytics for the treatment of thromboembolic disease during pregnancy. Obstet Gynecol Surv. 1995;50:534.
40. Leonhardt G, Gaul C, Nietsch HH, et al. Thrombolytic therapy in pregnancy. J Thromb Thrombolysis. 2006;21:271.
41. Murugappan A, Coplin WM, Al-Sadat AN, et al. Thrombolytic therapy of acute ischemic stroke during pregnancy. Neurology. 2006;66:768.
42. Albers GW, Amarenco P, Easton JD, et al. Antithrombotic and thrombolytic therapy for ischemic stroke: American College of Chest Physicians Evidence-based Clinical Practice Guidelines (8th Edition). Chest. 2008;133:630S.
43. De Keyser J, Gdovinová Z, Uyttenboogaart M, et al. Intravenous alteplase for stroke: beyond the guidelines and in particular clinical situations. Stroke. 2007;38:2612.
44. Broderick JP. Should intravenous thrombolysis be considered the first option in pregnant women? Stroke. 2013;44:866.
45. Demchuk AM. Yes, intravenous thrombolysis should be administered in pregnancy when other clinical and imaging factors are favorable. Stroke. 2013;44:864.
46. Activase® (Alteplase). Full prescribing information. www.gene.com/download/pdf/activase_prescribing.pdf (Accessed on February 02, 2016).
47. Selim MH, Molina CA. The use of tissue plasminogen-activator in pregnancy: a taboo treatment or a time to think out of the box. Stroke. 2013;44:868.
48. Demaerschalk BM, Kleindorfer DO, Adeoye OM, et al. Scientific Rationale for the Inclusion and Exclusion Criteria for Intravenous Alteplase in Acute Ischemic Stroke: A Statement for Healthcare Professionals From the American Heart Association/American Stroke Association. Stroke. 2016;47:581.
49. Sibai BM, Caritis SN, Thom E, et al. Prevention of preeclampsia with low-dose aspirin in healthy, nulliparous pregnant women. The National Institute of Child Health and Human Development Network of Maternal-Fetal Medicine Units. N Engl J Med. 1993;329:1213.
50. Duley L, Henderson-Smart D, Knight M, King J. Antiplatelet drugs for prevention of pre-eclampsia and its consequences: systematic review. BMJ. 2001;322:329.
51. Kernan WN, Ovbiagele B, Black HR, et al. Guidelines for the prevention of stroke in patients with stroke and transient ischemic attack: a guideline for healthcare professionals from the American Heart Association/American Stroke Association. Stroke. 2014;45:2160.
52. Saposnik G, Barinagarrementeria F, Brown RD Jr, et al. Diagnosis and management of cerebral venous thrombosis: a statement for healthcare professionals from the American Heart Association/American Stroke Association. Stroke. 2011;42:1158.
53. Bushnell C, McCullough LD, Awad IA, et al. Guidelines for the prevention of stroke in women: a statement for healthcare professionals from the American Heart Association/American Stroke Association. Stroke. 2014;45:1545.
54. Dias MS, Sekhar LN. Intracranial hemorrhage from aneurysms and arteriovenous malformations during pregnancy and the puerperium. Neurosurgery. 1990;27:855.
55. Marshman LA, Aspoas AR, Rai MS, Chawda SJ. The implications of ISAT and ISUIA for the management of cerebral aneurysms during pregnancy. Neurosurg Rev. 2007;30:177.
56. Pool JL. Treatment of intracranial aneurysms during pregnancy. JAMA 1965;192:209.

57. Qaiser R, Black P. Neurosurgery in pregnancy. Semin Neurol 2007;27:476.
58. Tarnaris A, Haliasos N, Watkins LD. Endovascular treatment of ruptured intracranial aneurysms during pregnancy: is this the best way forward? Case report and review of the literature. Clin Neurol Neurosurg. 2012;114:703.
59. Pumar JM, Pardo MI, Carreira JM, et al. Endovascular treatment of an acutely ruptured intracranial aneurysm in pregnancy: report of eight cases. Emerg Radiol. 2010;17:205.
60. Meyers PM, Halbach VV, Malek AM, et al. Endovascular treatment of cerebral artery aneurysms during pregnancy: report of three cases. Am J Neuroradiol. 2000;21:1306.
61. Piotin M, de Souza Filho CB, Kothimbakam R, Moret J. Endovascular treatment of acutely ruptured intracranial aneurysms in pregnancy. Am J Obstet Gynecol. 2001;185:1261.
62. Stoodley MA, Macdonald RL, Weir BK. Pregnancy and intracranial aneurysms. Neurosurg Clin N Am. 1998;9:549.
63. Dashti SR, Spalding AC, Yao TL. Multimodality treatment of a ruptured grade IV posterior fossa arteriovenous malformation in a patient pregnant with twins: case report. J Neurointerv Surg. 2012;4:e21.
64. Jermakowicz WJ, Tomycz LD, Ghiassi M, Singer RJ. Use of endovascular embolization to treat a ruptured arteriovenous malformation in a pregnant woman: a case report. J Med Case Rep. 2012;6:113.

Chapter 58

ART Pregnancies: Are they Different?

Asha Baxi, Sonam Baxi

INTRODUCTION

With better availability of assisted reproductive technique and its success more and more infertile couples are being assisted to accomplish their dream of parenthood. Assisted reproductive technique (ART) may affect the outcome of pregnancy which may be related to the infertile condition itself or to the technique used. Though multiple gestation is a high-risk factor, even the singleton pregnancies conceived by *in vitro* fertilization (IVF) are at risk.

There is some evidence that ART affects the perinatal outcome, the mode of delivery and the early childhood up to some extent, but this may or may not be that significant.

RISK OF MULTIFETAL GESTATION

With ART, the incidence of multifetal gestation goes up significantly.[1] Multiple gestation itself is associated with higher maternal and fetal morbidity as well as mortality.[2] The perinatal risk increases disproportionately with number of fetus and monozygosity. IVF is associated with 2 fold increase in monozygosity compared to natural birth.[3] In a meta-analysis of 12 studies, it was concluded that IVF twins are at risk of preterm birth and low birth weight.[4] Monozygotic twins are associated with discordant growth and twin-to-twin transfusion. A practice of single embryo transfer may reduce the incidence of multiple pregnancy.

In high order pregnancies, it is important to counsel the couple about the morbidity associated and should be offered multifetal pregnancy reduction. This will reduce the preterm labor, but it is associated with a nearby 4.7% risk of miscarriage.[5] It is a highly skilled procedure, and should be performed by a clinician with the expertise.

Preterm Birth

Multiple pregnancy itself is the main cause of preterm labor and in IVF twins, it is 23% more as compared to twins conceived naturally. With singleton also, there is nearly two-fold increase in preterm and moderate preterm birth, which include elective preterm birth also.[4] Besides multiple pregnancy, the underlying cause of infertility, placental dysfunction and infection may also initiate preterm labor in these women.

Low Birth Weight and Small for Gestational Age

Apart from multiple gestation being a clear risk factor, singleton IVF pregnancies are also associated with low birth weight.[6] Although the preterm labor is important cause of low birth weight, the relative risk of small for dates is increased by 40–60%, suggesting that factors other than preterm labor are responsible for low birth weight.[7] In the case of vanishing twin or multifetal reduction, even if only a singleton is left, chances of small for gestational age fetus are higher, therefore single embryo transfer may reduce the incidence to some extent.

Congenital Anomalies

This is the issue which worries the couple most. Various studies have reported 30–40% increase in major congenital anomalies. It appears that the increased risk is partly due to underlying infertility and its determinants as the couples who take longer than 12 months to conceive also exhibit tendency to increased anomalies, though to a lesser extent than IVF treated couples.[8] A population wide cohort study from South Australia showed that pregnancy conceived through ART had a significant increased risk of birth defects (adjusted OR 1.28, 1.57, 95% CI, 1.30–1.90) although use of IVF without ICSI did not demonstrate an increased risk (adjusted OR 1.07, 95% 1.90–1.26).[9] Another study showed that birth defects incidence has gone down with time which suggests changes in population and ART techniques.[10] The principle anomalies which have been reported are gastrointestinal, cardiovascular and musculoskeletal defects specifically septal heart defects, cleft lip, esophageal atresia and anorectal atresia.[11,12] Though the risk of major congenital anomalies is in the order of 30–40%, the absolute risk is never the less low since the anomalies *per se* are relatively uncommon.

Vertical Transmission of Genetic Diseases

There is an increased prevalence of structural chromosomal anomalies in infertile couples comprising of a 4.6% prevalence of structural chromosomal abnormalities in oligospermic men and 1.14% autosomal reciprocal-balanced translocation in infertile women (general population 0.16%).[13,14] Microdeletion of the long arm of the Y chromosome (Yq) in particular, the ATF region, can also cause spermatogenic failure. However, some who conceived from oligospermic man with Yq microdeletion will inherit this subfertile phenotype and further expansion or *de novo* deletions may occur resulting in a worse phenotype in the offspring.[15,16]

Epigenetic Alteration

Some evidence suggests link between DNA modification such as methylation and genomic printing. A number of genes regulated by imprinting have been shown to be essential for fetal growth and placental function. In IVF, the superovulation and culture conditions are capable of inducing epigenetic changes. Current evidence links three human imprinting syndrome to IVF: Beckwith–Wiedemann syndrome (BWS), Angelman syndrome (AS) and more recently maternal hypomethylation syndrome.[17]

The overall incidence of these condition is very low, i.e. 1:12000, therefore, routine screening is not recommended. Sometimes some subtler effects due to culture media can profoundly affect the birth weight in humans and animals—the so called large offspring syndrome.[18]

Perinatal Outcomes

Compared to spontaneous conception, IVF and ICSI pregnancies are at high-risk for still birth, neonatal deaths, preterm delivery and NICU admission.

Women undergoing ART are at a high risk of obstetrical complications. They need close surveillance so that timely interventions can avoid the complications. In singleton IVF pregnancies, rates of gestational hypertension (2 folds), gestational diabetes (2 folds), placenta previa (3 to 6 folds) and placental abruption (2 fold) are significantly increased.[19]

Compared with mothers of singletons, mothers of IVF twins are more likely to have gestational hypertension but not gestational diabetes, placenta previa or premature rupture of membranes.[20-22]

They are 2–7 times more likely to require hospitalization, although the morbidity during pregnancy is not higher.[22]

Compared with spontaneous conception, IVF pregnancies have a 2 fold increased rate of induction of labor and cesarean delivery.[23,19] IVF/ICSI twins are more likely to have cesarean delivery.[24]

Women with increased age and pre-existent comorbidity face more complications and they should be assessed and counseled before undergoing ART.

Singleton pregnancies following oocyte donation are more likely to be complicated by pregnancy induced hypertension and gestational diabetes.[25]

MANAGEMENT OF ART PREGNANCIES: PRACTICAL TIPS

A good pre-conceptional counseling and vigilant care can avoid many obstetric complications and lead to a good perinatal outcome.

Whether it is ART, conditions leading to infertility, increasing age or high order pregnancies, these women need to be looked after by dedicated units for such pregnancies.

Calculation of EDD

Exact calculation is easy because a day after oocyte retrieval is the day of fertilization and we can calculate the estimated due date (EDD) accordingly. Beta-hCG levels may give some clue as to if it is going to be a multiple order pregnancy, where very high titers may be seen. Sometimes very low titers may be indicative of failing intrauterine gestation or ectopic pregnancy. Serial titers may be helpful.

- During the first transvaginal USG at 6–7 weeks, it is very important to check for multiple gestation. It is easier to pick at this gestation.
- At 6 weeks, even if it is intrauterine pregnancy, check for heterotopic pregnancy.
- Prenatal testing in the form of double marker, noninvasive prenatal testing (NIPT), quadruple test or amniocentesis is very important and all the patients should be counseled.
- Before taking double marker test, make sure that the patient is not on hCG injection because that will alter the double marker results. If it is ovum donation or embryo donation or surrogacy, make sure that age of the biological woman from eggs has been taken, is properly written on the form, otherwise the result may differ.
- Even if the patient is not ready for prenatal diagnosis because of invasive nature of the diagnostic test such as amniocentesis, NIPT which is almost accurate in 99% cases should be offered.
- A good NT scan between 11–13 weeks can detect many congenital malformations and risk of trisomy 21.
- Check the cervical length, transvaginally especially at 20 weeks or earlier because many of these pregnancies may be high-order pregnancies. But there is no role of prophylactic cerclage for all the patients with multiple pregnancies.

- Target scan should be done at a tertiary center.
- Serial ultrasound and growth scans should be performed from 28 weeks to rule out growth restriction.
- As many of these patients are elderly and have polycystic ovary syndrome (PCOS), they should be screened for gestational diabetes.
- Similarly because of age, multiple pregnancy and multiple medical risk factors, one should be watchful for early onset pre-eclampsia.

Prediction of preterm labor, timely administration of corticosteroids and magnesium sulfate can lead to good perinatal outcome in case of preterm labor. During cesarean section, because of possible tuberculosis, previous surgeries, endometriosis, etc. there may be altered anatomy. So senior obstetrician should perform cesarean section.

There is no need for cesarean delivery for these patients. They can be allowed to go into labor like any other patients. But as they being precious pregnancies, they should be delivered at the centers with good intrapartum monitoring, operation theater (OT) and neonatal intensive care unit (NICU) facilities. There are increased chances of adherent placenta in these cases. So, management of third stage of labor may be difficult.

CONCLUSION

While most of the ART pregnancies are uncomplicated and result in birth of healthy baby, they are associated with slightly higher risk. This risk is in the form of maternal morbidity with increased incidence of pregnancy induced hypertension, gestational diabetes, placenta previa, abruption, preterm labor and so on. There is increased incidence of intervention and cesarean and with multiple pregnancy the risk gets further added.

Similarly, perinatal complications in children conceived through ART are high, and there may be a higher risk of abnormalities.

Pre-IVF work-up, counseling, limiting the number of embryos transferred and using soft protocols of ovulation induction may reduce the incidence of complications. Prenatal karyotype, preimplantation genetic diagnosis (PGD) and preimplantation genetic screening (PGS) are coming up in a big way, and may reduce some genetic problems and improve the outcome. During pregnancy use of biochemical screening for trisomy 21, target scan and fetal echo may detect some of the anomalies.

These women are psychologically also very vulnerable, so they need special care and counseling.

Overall ART with improved technology and various guidelines result in healthy mother with healthy child.

REFERENCES

1. Multiple gestation associated with infertility therapy: an American Society for Reproductive Medicine Practice Committee opinion. Practice Committee of American Society for Reproduction Medicine. Fertile Steril. 2012;97:825-34.
2. Multifetal gestations: twins, triplets, and higher-order multifetal pregnancies. Practice Bulletin No. 144. American Coolege of Obstetricians and Gynecologists and Society for Maternal-Fetal Medicine. Obstet Gynecol. 2014;123:1118-32.
3. Human Fertilisation and Embryology Authority. Latest UK IVF figures–2008. London: HFEA; 2011.
4. McDonald SD, HanZ, Mulla S, Murphy KE, Beyene J, Ohlsson A. Preterm birth and low birth weight among in vitro fertilization singletons: a systematic review and meta-analyses. Eur JL Obstet Gynecol Reprod Biol. 2009;146:138-48.
5. Stone J, Ferrar L, Kamrath J, Getrajdman J, Berkowitz R, Moshier E, et al. Contemporary outcomes with latest 1000 cases of multifetal pregnancy reduction (MPR). Am J Obstet Gynecol. 2008;199:406.el-4.
6. McDonald SD, Han Z, Mulla S, Ohlsson A, Beyene J, Murphy KE. Preterm birth and low birth weight among in vitro fertilization twins: a systematic review and meta-analyses. Eur J Obstet Gynecol Reprod Biol. 2010;148:105-13.
7. De Neubourg D, Gerris J, Mangelschots K, Van Royen E, Vercruyssen M, Steylemans A, et al. The obstetrical and neonatal outcome of babies born after single-embryo transfer in IVF/ICSI compares favourably to spontaneously conceived babies. Hum Peprod. 2006;21:1041-6.
8. Zhu Jl, Basso O, Obel C, Bille C, Olsen J. Infertility, infertility treatment, and congenital malformations: Danish national birth cohort. BMJ. 2006;333:679.
9. Davies MJ, Moore VM, Willson KJ, Van Essen P, Priest K, Scott H, et al. Reproductive technologies and the risk of birth defects. N Engl J Med. 2012;366:1803-13.
10. Hansen M, Kurinczuk JJ, de Klerk N, Burton P, Bower C. Assisted reproductive technology and major birth defects in Western Australia. Obset Gynecol. 2012;120:852-63.
11. Reefhuis J, Honein MA, Schieve LA, Correa A, Hobbs CA, Rasmussen SA. Assisted reproductive technology and major structural birth defects in the United States. Hum Reprod. 2009;24:360-6.
12. El-Chaar D, Yang Q, Gao J, Bottomley J, Leader A, Wen SW, et al. Risk of birth defects increased in pregnancies conceived by assisted human reproduction. Fertil Steril. 2009;92:1557-61.
13. Schreurs A, Leguis E, Meuleman C, Fryns JP, D'Hooghe TM. Increased frequency of chromosomal abnormalities in female partners of couples undergoing in vitro fertilization or intra cytoplasmic sperm injection. Fertil Steril. 2000;74:94-6.
14. Clementini E, Palka C, Iezzi I, Stuppia L, Guanciali_Franchi P, Tiboni GM. Prevalence of chromosomal abnormalities in 2078 infertile couples referred for assisted reproductive techniques. Hum Reprod. 2005;20:437-42.
15. Silber SJ, Alagappan R, Brown LG, Page DC. Y chromosome deletions in azoospermic and severely oligozoospermic men undergoing intracytoplasmic sperm injection after testicular sperm extraction. Hum Reprod. 1998;13:3332-7.

16. Lee SH, Ahn SY, Lee KW, Kwack K, Jun HS, Cha KY. Intracytoplasmic sperm injection may lead to vertical transmission, expansion, and de novo occurrence of Y-chromosome microdeletions in male fetuses. Fertil Steril. 2006;85:1512-5.
17. Amor DJ, Halliday J. A review of known imprinting syndromes and their association with assisted reproduction technologies. Hum Reprod. 2008;23:2826-34.
18. Young LE, Sinclair KD, Wilmut I. Large offspring syndrome in cattle and sheep. Rev Reprod. 1998;3:155-63.
19. Jackson RA, Gibson KA, Wu YW, Croughan MS, Perinatal outcomes in singletons followings in vitro fertilization: a meta-analysis, Obstet Gynecol. 2004;103:551-63.
20. Rowe PJ, Comhaire FH, Hargreave TB, Mahmoud AMA. WHO manual for the standardized investigation, diagnosis and management of the infertile male. Cambridge University Press, Cambridge. 2000.pp.1-102.
21. Zaib-un-Nisa S, Ghazal-Aswad S, Badrinath P. Outcome of twin pregnancies after assisted reproductive techniques—a comparative study. Euro J Obstet Gynecol Reprod Biol. 2003;109:51-4.
22. Pinborg A, Loft A, Rasmussen S, Schmidt L, Langhoff-Roos J, Greisen G, et al. Neonatal outcomes in a Danish national cohort of 3438 IVF/ICSI and 10362 non-IVF/ICSI twins born between 1995 and 2000. Hum Reprod. 2004;19: 435-41.
23. Nassar AH, Usta IM, Rechdan JB, Harb TS, Adra AM, Abu-Musa AA. Pregnancy outcome in spontaneous twins versus who were conceived through in vitro fertilization. Am J Obstet Gynecol. 2003;189:513-8.
24. Glazebrook C, Sheard C, Cox S, Oates M, Ndukwe G. Parenting stress in first-time mothers of twins and triplets conceived after in vitro fertilization. Fertil Steril. 2004;81: 505-11.
25. Sheffer-Mimouni G, Mashiach S, Dor J, Levran D, Seidman DS. Factors influencing the obstetric and perinatal outcome after oocyte donation. Hum Reprod. 2002;17: 2636-40.

Chapter 59

Adnexal Masses in Pregnancy

Veena Paliwal, Sushma Dikhit, Tasabieh Ali

INTRODUCTION

With increasing use of first trimester aneuploidy screening, the incidental discovery of adnexal masses during early gestation is a clinically relevant problem, which requires careful consideration. Overall prevalence in hospital-based series is 0.2–2% of pregnancies, complicated by an adnexal mass and about 1–6% of these are malignant.[1-4]

As ultrasound is more commonly used in first trimester the reported incidence of adnexal masses has increased. Furthermore as gestational age advances the incidence of adnexal masses gradually decreases likely secondary to spontaneous resolution of many of these masses.[5]

Malignant tumors vary in size but 75% of them are larger than 5 cm in diameter and most of them have solid as well as cystic elements on ultrasound evaluation.[6]

Understanding benign nature and uncomplicated course of ovarian masses diagnosed incidentally by ultrasound has led to a more conservative, but careful and vigilant approach to management of ovarian masses in pregnancy. Emergent surgical intervention is associated with increased risk of adverse outcome for both mother and fetus. Optimal management lies in weighing the risk of expectant management verses intervention.

In a population-based hospital registry, ovarian cancer was the fifth most common cancer diagnosed after breast, thyroid, cervical cancer and Hodgkin's lymphoma.[4]

In another similar study, there were 37 ovarian cancers diagnosed among 9375 ovarian masses during pregnancy (cancer rate 0.93%, 0.018 ovarian cancers diagnosed per 1000 deliveries).[1] There were also high proportion of tumors of low malignant potential (LMN) (n = 115) reported separately with majority of early stage and associated with favorable maternal and neonatal outcome. A retrospective review reported that ovarian cancer was the 6th most common cancer in Asian population.[7]

PATIENT PRESENTATION

In olden days before ultrasound most adnexal masses in pregnant women remained unrecognized until cesarean delivery or until they become symptomatic, mostly in the postpartum period. Now many are diagnosed incidentally on routine ultrasound.[7-10]

Adnexal masses that have not been diagnosed antepartum may be identified at cesarean delivery. In a retrospective study of 46,500 term cesarean section for various indications, 151 women (0.3%) had surgery for adnexal masses, which was an incidental finding at surgery in just over half of women (83 of 151:55%).[11]

OTHER CLINICAL PRESENTATIONS

- *Nonspecific symptoms* of ovarian cancer such as abdominal or back pain, constipation, abdominal swelling and urinary symptoms are common during pregnancy and their presence is not very useful in diagnosis.[12]
- *Palpable masses* if found on abdominal or pelvic examination later evaluated by ultrasound.
- *Acute abdomen* adnexal torsion occurs in about 5% of pregnant women with adnexal mass.[13] On study review, adnexal masses between 6–8 cm diameters had a significantly higher rate of torsion (22%) than either smaller or larger masses.[13] About 60% of torsions occurred between 10th and 17th weeks of gestation: only 6% occurred after 20 weeks.

Elevated Tumor Markers

Depending on the timing of women's first ultrasound one of the first indicator of pelvic mass may be elevation in maternal serum analytics obtained as part of the triple screen for Down's syndrome or neural tube defects. When significant alpha-fetoprotein (AFP) elevation is identified, concern for germ cell tumors should arise and to be excluded by ultrasound, if not already performed **(Table 59.1)**.[14]

TYPES OF ADNEXAL MASSES

In review of 7 studies, there were 563 adnexal masses. Simple and complex masses **(Figs 59.1 and 59.2)** were 48% and 53% respectively. Malignancy rate was 1% in simple and 9% in complex masses.

CHAPTER 59: Adnexal Masses in Pregnancy

Table 59.1: Ultrasound appearances of adnexal pathology[41]

Pathology	Ultrasound appearance
Teratoma	Complex mass with solid and cystic areas due to presence of fat, bone, sebaceous material and hair
Endometrioma	Diffuse 'ground-glass' pattern due to presence of old blood ('chocolate') within the cyst
Malignant/borderline ovarian tumor	Complex, multiseptate mass with solid and cystic areas
	Papillary projections or mural nodules
	Ascites may be present
	Appearance may be bilateral in up to 25% of cases
Hydrosalpinx	Tubular-shaped structure with anechoic content and incomplete septum of tubal wall. Always stays the same size during pregnancy
Leiomyoma	Hypoechoic, round, solid masses
	Cystic change may occur, if red degeneration develops

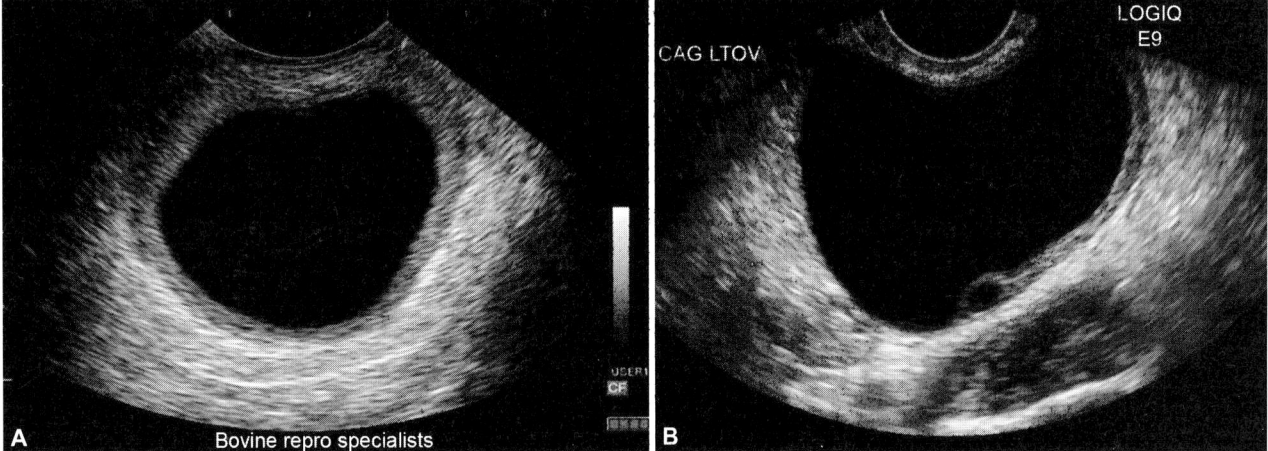

Figs 59.1A and B: Simple ovarian cysts: (A) Corpus luteum cyst; and (B) Large left ovarian cyst—common.
Source: Wikiimage.org.

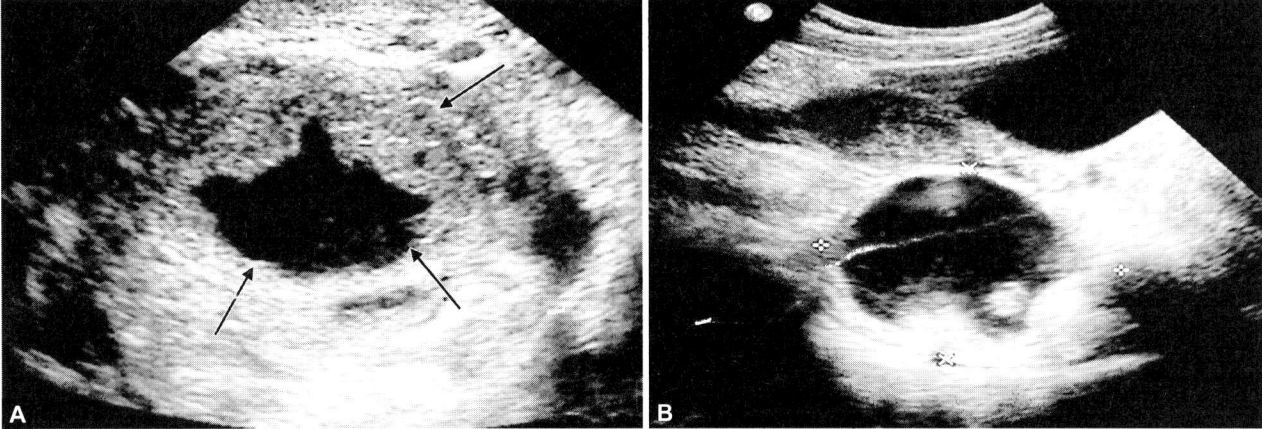

Figs 59.2A and B: Complex cysts: (A) Large hemorrhagic cyst; (B) Dermoid cyst—common.
Source: Wikiimage.org.

Table 59.2: Ultrasound appearances of common ovarian cysts in pregnancy and resolution rate		
Type of mass	Ultrasound appearance	Resolution rate (%)
Simple ovarian cysts (follicular, corpus luteal)	Unilocular, thin-walled, anechoic	90–100, if 5 cm in diameter
Hemorrhagic cysts	Anechoic with echogenic material within cyst	90–100
Hyperstimulated ovaries	Massively enlarged, thin-walled, multilocular cysts. Ascites may be present	>90

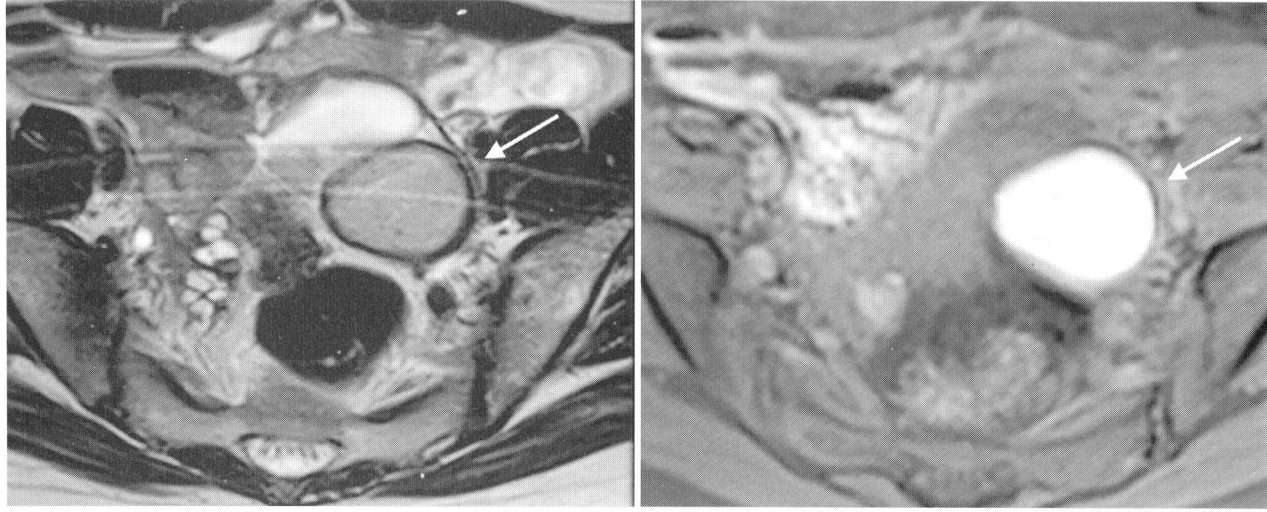

Fig. 59.3: Endometrioma—common.
Source: Wikiimage.org.

Benign Neoplasms

Vast majority of masses detected during routine early obstetric ultrasound are simple cysts and < 5 cm in diameter. Most of them are physiological like functional ovarian cyst, either follicular or corpus luteum cyst. About 70% of them resolve spontaneously by beginning of the second trimester.[15] Persistent masses are 0.07%[16] and majority of them are mature teratomas, other pathologies include endometrioma, para-tubal cyst and cyst adenoma (**Table 59.2**).

Role of CT and MRI

MRI is safe to be used but expensive and needs more time than ultrasound. MRI is particularly good for endometriotic and dermoid cyst.[17,18] MRI has an advantage of better resolution and lack of ionizing radiation as compared to CT scan.[19] Contraindications to use MRI in pregnancy are ferro-magnate aneurysm clips and severe maternal claustrophobia. MRI is particularly useful in characterizing a pedunculated myoma, red degeneration of myoma, endometrioma, decidualized endometrioma and massive ovarian edema and to differentiate from ovarian cancers[20,21] (**Fig. 59.3**).

CT scanning has little place in modern obstetric practice. Fetal ionizing radiation dose of single CT through pelvis is 0.035 gy. As per evidence available fetal radiation exposure of <0.05 gy has not been associated with an increased risk of miscarriage, congenital anomalies, growth restriction or perinatal mortality. There remains concern regarding possible increase in the risk of childhood cancer.[22,23] Use of iodinated contrast agent with CT carries a risk of transient suppression of the fetal thyroid.

Tumor Markers in Ovarian Malignancy with Pregnancy

Tumor markers are routinely done in non-pregnant patient for diagnosis and for prognosis of treatment of ovarian malignancy. During pregnancy, it is not recommended as pregnancy associated pelvic masses are rarely malignant and there is difficult interpretation due to gestational age and other factors. If malignancy is proven, then the appropriate tumor marker can be done in immediate postpartum period.

During pregnancy, however, serum AFP, CA125, CEA, beta-hCG and inhibin levels are involved in biological function associated with fetal development, differentiation and maturation. The levels are normally elevated during pregnancy and vary with gestational age and may be abnormal placentation or fetal abnormalities (Pre-eclampsia, Down's syndrome, open neural tube defects).

Serum CA125

Serum CA125 levels are elevated during pregnancy[24] due to decidual cell production.[25] Some researchers suggested using cut-off level 112 u/mL as upper limit of normal compared to 35 u/mL in non-pregnant.[26] CA125 value in range of 1000–10,000 is likely (not always) related to cancer.

Alpha-Fetoprotein

High maternal serum alpha-fetoprotein (MSAFP) are seen in some types of ovarian germ cell tumors (e.g. endodermal sinus tumor, embryonal carcinoma and mixed tumors), these levels are usually 1000 ng/mL or even up to >10,000 ng/mL[27,28] in pure endodermal sinus (yolk sac) tumors. MSAFP levels are typically <500 ng/mL in pregnancy complicated by open neural tube defects. Multiple of the medians (MoMs) of 2–2.5 are considered abnormal. MSAFP level above 9 MoM should prompt concern for germ cell tumors of either gonadal or non-gonadal origin in the absence of fetal abdominal wall defects or anencephaly.[29]

Lactate Dehydrogenase (LDH)

LDH is raised in ovarian dysgerminoma and is a reliable marker for diagnosis and follow up.[30] LDH is not elevated in normal pregnancy although elevations can occur in PET and (HELLP) [hemolysis, elevated liver (EL) enzymes, low platelet (LP) count] syndrome.

Inhibin

Levels are elevated in early gestation, so not a good marker. There is a twofold rise in Down's syndrome cases.

Human Chorionic Gonadotropins (hCG)

Marker of germ cell tumors (*esp*. Choriocarcinoma) cannot be used as there are high values during pregnancy.

Human Epididymis Protein 4 (HE4)

HE4 is product of WFDC 2 (HE4) gene that is over expressed in ovarian cancer. HE4 biomarkers are unaffected by pregnancy,[31] and therefore may be helpful in evaluation of pelvic masses in pregnancy.

Management in Pregnancy

Most adnexal ovarian cysts noted at first trimester ultrasound are asymptomatic, simple and <5 cm in size. These are functional corpus luteum cysts and approximately 70% resolve spontaneously by early part of second trimester. It is a reasonable option to maintain surveillance with ultrasound in every trimester. In patients who deliver by cesarean section the adnexa should be evaluated.[7] In patients who deliver vaginally repeat imaging should be done 6–8 weeks postpartum.

SURGICAL MANAGEMENT

Patients that have sonographic findings highly suspicious of malignancy or those who develop significant symptoms should undergo surgical resection. This also minimizes the risk of complications such as rupture, adnexal torsion or obstruction of labor and helps in detection of ovarian malignancies.

Timing of Surgery

Optimal time of surgery during pregnancy is after first trimester as:
- Almost all functional cysts will have resolved by this time.
- There are less chances of teratogenicity due to medication as organogenesis is complete.
- Corpus luteum function is replaced by placenta.
- Spontaneous miscarriage due to intrinsic fetal abnormalities is likely to have already been over.

Persistent, simple, unilocular cysts without any solid elements that are larger than 10 cm can be aspirated either vaginally or abdominally under ultrasound guidance using fine needle (20 Gauze).[32]

This is indicated, if cyst is causing pain or obstruction due to location in the pelvis. This is not commonly employed but is a good option in selected women as it is well tolerated without short- or long-term complications. Fluid should be sent for cytological examination. Recurrence rate is 33–50%. This should be done after 14 weeks of pregnancy to avoid disturbance to corpus luteum.

Surgery

Laparoscopy (minimally invasive surgery, MIS) is safe in pregnancy, however, technically difficult in 2nd trimester due to gravid uterus. Whenever possible and expertise is available, this should be favored approach for its well-known advantages. If there is low risk of malignancy, MIS is reasonable and can be done at all stages of pregnancy. In second trimester better is open method (Hasson's technique) for entry.[33]

If malignancy is suspected vertical midline incision should be done. This gives adequate exposure, and minimizes the need for manipulation to access the adnexal mass. After opening of abdomen, peritoneal washings to be collected for staging in case of malignancy. Other adnexa should be carefully inspected and palpated. Ovarian biopsy of contralateral ovary is recommended, if the ovary appears to be involved but routine biopsy is unwarranted. If lesion appears to be benign, it is acceptable to do cystectomy rather than perform a salpingo-oophorectomy. In masses of >10 cm in size, it may not be feasible to perform ovarian cystectomy. If mass is solid, has surface lesions, presence of ascites or has other features of malignancy, then appropriate treatment is ipsilateral salpingo-oophorectomy and tissue is sent for frozen section and pathologist is informed about ongoing pregnancy. Resection of contralateral ovaries should not be performed unless bilateral malignant lesion is confirmed. All suspicious lesions should be biopsied. If frozen section confirms malignancy surgeon should be prepared to do surgical staging procedure and gynecologist should be consulted (**Table 59.3**).

Table 59.3: Staging ovarian, fallopian tube, and peritoneal cancer [TNM and International Federation of Gynecology and Obstetrics (FIGO)]

TNM categories	FIGO stages	Definition
Primary tumor (T)		
TX		Primary tumor cannot be assessed
T0		No evidence of primary tumor
T1	I	Tumor confined to ovaries or fallopian tubes
T1a	IA	Tumor limited to one ovary (capsule intact) or fallopian tube; no tumor on ovarian or fallopian tube surface; no malignant cells in ascites or peritoneal washings
T1b	IB	Tumor limited to both ovaries (capsules intact) or fallopian tubes; no tumor on ovarian or fallopian tube surface; no malignant cells in ascites or peritoneal washings
T1c	IC	Tumor limited to one or both ovaries or fallopian tubes, with any of the following:
	IC1	• Surgical spill
	IC2	• Capsule ruptured before surgery or tumor on ovarian or fallopian tube surface
	IC3	• Malignant cells in the ascites or peritoneal washings
T2	II	Tumor involves one or both ovaries or fallopian tubes with pelvic extension (below pelvic brim) or peritoneal cancer*
T2a	IIA	Extension and/or implants on uterus and/or tube(s) and/or ovaries
T2b	IIB	Extension to other pelvic intraperitoneal tissues
T3	III	Tumor involves one or both ovaries or fallopian tubes, or peritoneal cancer, with cytologically or histologically confirmed spread to the peritoneum outside the pelvis and/or metastasis to the retroperitoneal lymph nodes
T3a	IIIA	Positive retroperitoneal lymph nodes and/or microscopic metastasis beyond pelvis
	IIIA1	Positive retroperitoneal lymph nodes only (cytologically or histologically proven)
	IIIA1 (i)	Metastasis up to 10 mm in greatest dimension
	IIIA1 (ii)	Metastasis more than 10 mm in greatest dimension
	IIIA2	Microscopic extrapelvic (above the pelvic brim) peritoneal involvement, with or without positive retroperitoneal lymph nodes
T3b	IIIB	Macroscopic peritoneal metastasis beyond pelvis up to 2 cm in greatest dimension, with or without positive retroperitoneal lymph nodes
T3c	IIC	Macroscopic peritoneal metastasis beyond pelvis more than 2 cm in greatest dimension (includes extension of tumor to capsule of liver and spleen without parenchymal involvement of either organ), with or without positive retroperitoneal lymph nodes
Regional lymph nodes (N)		
NX		Regional lymph nodes cannot be assessed
N0		No regional lymph node metastasis
N1	III	Regional lymph node metastasis
Distant metastasis (M)		
M0		No distant metastasis
M1	IV	Distant metastasis (excludes peritoneal metastasis)
	IVA	Pleural effusion with positive cytology
	IVB	Parenchymal metastases and metastases to extra-abdominal organs (including inguinal lymph nodes and lymph nodes outside the abdominal cavity)¶
pTNM pathologic classification: The pT, pN, and pM categories correspond to the T, N, and M categories.		

Contd...

Contd...

TNM categories	FIGO stages	Definition	
		Anatomic stage/prognostic groups	
Stage I	T1	N0	M0
Stage IA	T1a	N0	M0
Stage IB	T1b	N0	M0
Stage IC	T1c	N0	M0
Stage II	T2	N0	M0
Stage IIA	T2a	N0	M0
Stage IIB	T2b	N0	M0
Stage IIC	T2c	N0	M0
Stage III	T3	N0 or N1	M0
Stage IIIA	T3a	N0	M0
	≤T3a	N1	
Stage IIIB	T3b	N0 or N1	M0
Stage IIIC	T3c	N0 or N1	M0
Stage IV	Any T	Any N	M1

Note: cTNM is the clinical classification, pTNM is the pathologic classification.
*Dense adhesions with histologically proven tumor cells justify upgrading to stage II.
¶ Transmural bowel infiltration or umbilical deposit are stage IVB.
Source:
1. The American Joint Committee on Cancer, MCC Cancer Staging Manual, 7th edn, New York: Springer, 2010.
2. Prat J. Staging classification for cancer of the ovary, fallopian tube, and peritoneum. Int J Gynaecol Obstet. 2014;124:1.

Each case to be individualized according to pregnancy stage for pros and cons of staging versus potential risk to mother and fetus. Postoperative adjuvant chemotherapy is determined by histologic tumor type. If metastatic ovarian cancer is found, then cytoreduction should be attempted according to individual judgment for expected benefit. If necessary secondary cytoreduction may be undertaken following chemotherapy and successful completion of pregnancy. Survival is poor for all late stage disease. With modern platinum-based adjuvant chemotherapy approximately 70% of patient with advanced disease will respond to chemotherapy even, if they have residual disease remaining after cytoreductive surgery.

For woman with advanced stage ovarian cancer diagnosed before delivery, hysterectomy and secondary cytoreductive surgery are reasonable in postpartum to remove persistent disease. Surgery can be performed following vaginal delivery or in conjunction with cesarean section.

Management of Corpus Luteum

Removal of corpus luteum should be avoided prior to 8 weeks of pregnancy as this is responsible for providing progesterone for maintenance of pregnancy. If it happens progesterone vaginal suppository 50–100 mg is given 8–12 hourly or daily intramuscular injection 50 mg should be given up to 10 weeks as placenta takes over by that time (placental luteal shift), after this supplementation is no longer indicated.[34]

Management of Adnexal Mass at Cesarean Delivery

Any suspicious adnexal mass seen at cesarean section should be resected and sent for frozen section. Complete surgical removal is preferred to aspiration and cytological evaluation, since malignancy can be missed with the latter. If malignancy is present salpingo-oophorectomy to be done and later patient is referred to gynecologist for counseling, staging and possible hysterectomy in 1–2 weeks.

If suspicious adnexal mass is detected antepartum, patient should be counseled and consented properly. Cesarean delivery should be performed by midline incision and gynecologist should be available, if required. After delivery of fetus and placenta and bleeding is controlled, the adnexal mass is resected and sent for frozen section. If there is malignancy full surgical staging can be done.

Chemotherapy

For tumors of low malignant potential (LMP) regardless of stage, chemotherapy is generally not recommended. Epithelial malignancies which are well differentiated and confined to ovary (after comprehensive surgical staging) do not need chemotherapy. For all others, a platinum and taxane-based chemotherapy is standard of care and has been successfully administered in pregnancy.[35,36] Chemotherapy for germ cell tumors, other than for stage 1 dysgerminoma, is typically bleomycin, etoposide, and cisplatin (BEP).[37] Clearly, the use of chemotherapy during ongoing pregnancy carries risk and toxicities not only for mother but also for the fetus. These risks are maximum during first trimester when fetus is undergoing rapid growth and organogenesis.[38] In this situation, women in first trimester may consider pregnancy termination secondary to teratogenic effects of chemotherapy in first trimester. Women with more advanced pregnancies (2nd or 3rd trimester) may consider pregnancy preservation, given the lack of adverse fetal outcomes based on limited clinical data.[39] As pregnancy with ovarian malignancy are rare, cases care should be directed by a multidisciplinary perinatal, neonatal and oncologic team. If chemotherapy is indicated and cannot be postponed, then it is ideal to start chemotherapy in second or early third trimester.

ONCOLOGIC PROGNOSIS

There is no evidence that pregnancy worsens the prognosis of ovarian cancer as compared to non-pregnant patients matched for tumor stage, histology and grade as most of the ovarian cancers are in early stage and of favorable histology. 5-year survival rates for ovarian cancers diagnosed during pregnancy are between 75% and 90%. Presence of ascites at diagnosis implies advanced disease and poor prognosis.[40]

PREGNANCY OUTCOMES

Ovarian neoplasm diagnosed during pregnancy does not seem to have any adverse effects on neonatal outcome such as low birth weight, prematurity neonatal death and neonatal hospital admissions. Decision for termination of pregnancy when diagnosed during first trimester need to be individualized and made by an informed pregnant mother in collaboration with clinician. Early termination does not improve outcome of ovarian cancer, factors which need to be considered are:
- Risk of fetal toxicity or complications from chemotherapy
- Her prognosis and ability to take care of her baby
- Effect of ovarian cancer treatment on future fertility.

CONCLUSION

Number of adnexal masses diagnosed during pregnancy has increased dramatically due to routine use of ultrasound in first and second trimester. The majority resolve spontaneously and those that do not rarely represent malignancy or negatively impact the pregnancy. The conservative or surgical management of pregnant patient with a mass is based on ultrasound features and development of acute symptoms and rate of growth. MRI is safe and useful to evaluate mass where ultrasound is found inconclusive. When surgery is needed, it is best done in second trimester by laparoscopy or laparotomy. If malignancy is diagnosed appropriate staging and debulking should be strongly considered and chemotherapy initiated as appropriate based on cancer histology, stage and grade to have best possible maternal outcome (**Flow chart 59.1**).

SUMMARY AND RECOMMENDATIONS

In hospital-based series, prevalence is 0.2–2% of pregnancies and approximately 1–6% are malignant. Vast majority are benign and asymptomatic, and incidentally found on ultrasound or at cesarean delivery.

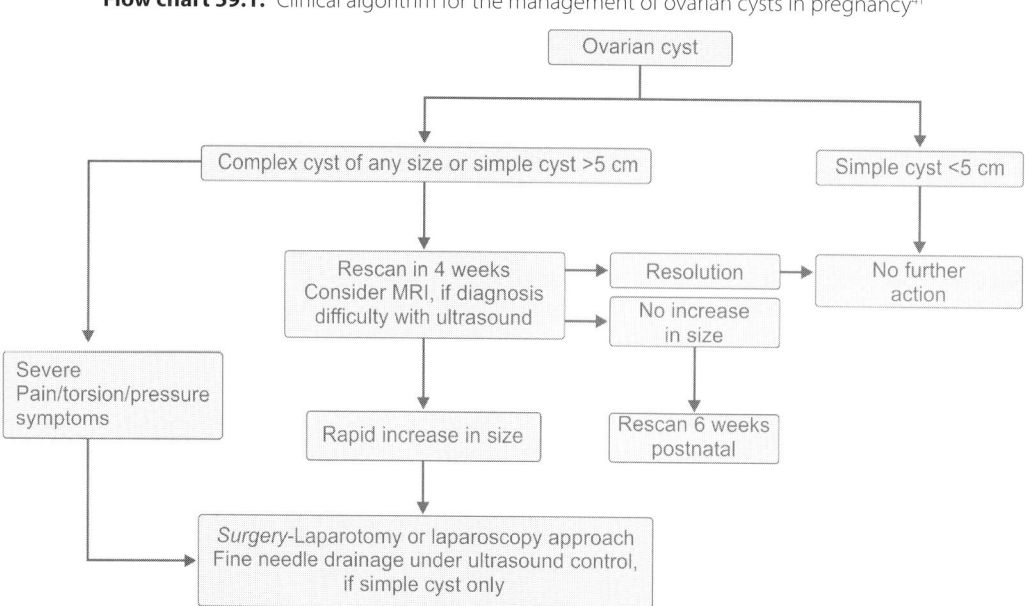

Flow chart 59.1: Clinical algorithm for the management of ovarian cysts in pregnancy[41]

Unexplained elevation of maternal serum analytics (AFP, Inhibin A) obtained in screening for neural-tube defects (NTD) or Down's syndrome can be a sign of ovarian germ cell tumor.

Most adnexal masses are < 5 cm. About 70% of masses detected in first trimester resolve by early second trimester. Majority of persistent masses are dermoids and 10% of them are malignant. About 50% of all ovarian malignancies are epithelial ovarian tumors, and about 30% are germ cell tumors. Definite diagnosis is by histopathology of biopsy.

Pathologist should be expert in diagnosing tumors with ongoing pregnancy and aware of pregnancy of patient.

Surgical treatment is recommended for management of asymptomatic mass after first trimester that are > 10 cm in diameter (grade 2c) or solid or cystic, papillary or septate (grade 2b) as there are more chances of malignancy and also reduces chances of complications of cyst. Expectant management is suggested in corpus luteum cyst, endometrioma and mature teratoma during pregnancy, if diagnosis is reasonably certain based on ultrasound (grade 2c).

Most of the time, preoperative staging work-up with pelvic mass can be limited to ultrasound imaging.

Ovarian cystectomy is treatment of choice for benign cases but if > 10 cm in diameter, it may be difficult. If features suggestive of malignancy, then ipsilateral salpingo-oophorectomy is appropriate and frozen section to be done and all other suspicious lesions should be biopsied.

Adequate surgical staging is important for stage 1 as many of them can be treated with surgery alone. Need for chemotherapy is decided according to tumor characteristics.

Removal of corpus luteum before 8 weeks needs progesterone supplementation.

REFERENCES

1. Leiserowitz GS, Xing G, Cress R, et al. Adnexal masses in pregnancy: how often are they malignant? Gynecol Oncol. 2006;101:315.
2. Webb KE, Sakhel K, Chauhan SP, Abuhamad AZ. Adnexal mass during pregnancy: a review. Am J Perinatol. 2015;32:1010.
3. Schmeler KM, Mayo-Smith WW, Peipert JF, et al. Adnexal masses in pregnancy: surgery compared with observation. Obstet Gynecol. 2005; 105:1098.
4. Smith LH, Dalrymple JL, Leiserowitz GS, et al. Obstetrical deliveries associated with maternal malignancy in California, 1992 through 1997. Am J Obstet Gynecol. 2001;184:1504.
5. Management of adnexal masses during pregnancy. J Obstet Gynaecol Res. 2009.35(3):597-8. PMID: 19527409
6. Sherard GB 3rd, Hodson CA, Williams HJ, Semer DA, Hadi HA, Tait DL. Adnexal masses and pregnancy: a 12-year experience. Am J Obstet Gynecol. 2003;189:358-63.
7. Koonings PP, Platt LD, Wallace R. Incidental adnexal neoplasms at cesarean section. Obstet Gynecol. 1988;72:767-9.
8. Hogston P, Lilford RJ. Ultrasound study of ovarian cysts in pregnancy: prevalence and significance. BJOG. 1986;93: 625-8.
9. Bernhard LM, Klebba PK, Gray DL, Mutch DG. Predictors of persistence of adnexal masses in pregnancy. Obstet Gynecol. 1999;93:585-9.
10. Dgani R, Shoham Z, Atar E, Zosmer A, Lancet M. Ovarian carcinoma during pregnancy: a study of 23 cases in Israel between the years 1960 and 1984. Gynecol Oncol. 1989;33:326-31.
11. Baser E, Erkilinc S, Esin S, et al. Adnexal masses encountered during cesarean delivery. Int J Gynaecol Obstet. 2013;123:124.
12. Goff BA, Mandel LS, Melancon CH, Muntz HG. Frequency of symptoms of ovarian cancer in women presenting to primary care clinics. JAMA. 2004;291:2705.
13. Yen CF, Lin SL, Murk W, et al. Risk analysis of torsion and malignancy for adnexal masses during pregnancy. Fertil Steril. 2009;91:1895.
14. Sarandokou A, Protonotariou E, Rizos D. Tumor markers in biological fluids associated with pregnancy. Crit Rev Clin Lab Sci. 2007;44:151.
15. Giuntoli RL 2nd, Vang RS, Bristow RE. Evaluation and management of adnexal masses during pregnancy. Clin Obstet Gynecol. 2006; 49:492.
16. Platek DN, Henderson CE, Goldberg GL. The management of a persistent adnexal mass in pregnancy. Am J Obstet Gynecol. 1995;173:1236-40.
17. Rieber A, Nussle K, Stohr I, Grab D, Fenchel S, Kreienberg R, et al. Preoperative diagnosis of ovarian tumors with MR imaging: comparison with transvaginal sonography, positron emission tomography, and histologic findings. Am J Roentgenol. 2001;177:123-9.
18. Nishi M, Akamatsu N, Sekiba K. Magnetic resonance imaging of the ovarian cyst: its diagnostic value of endometrial cyst. Med Prog Technol. 1990;16:201-12.
19. Levine D, Barnes PD, Edelman RR. Obstetric MR imaging. Radiology. 1999;211:609-17.
20. Birchard KR, Brown MA, Hyslop WB, et al. MRI of acute abdominal and pelvic pain in pregnant patients. AJR. 2005; 184:452.
21. Telischak NA, Yeh BM, Joe BN, et al. MRI of adnexal masses in pregnancy. AJR. 2008;191:364.
22. ACOG Committee on Obstetric Practice. ACOG Committee Opinion. Number 299, September 2004 (replaces No. 158, September 1995). Guidelines for diagnostic imaging during pregnancy. Obstet Gynecol. 2004;104:647.
23. Harvey EB, Boice JD Jr, Honeyman M, Flannery JT. Prenatal X-ray exposure and childhood cancer in twins. N Engl J Med. 1985;312:541.
24. Bon GG, Kenemans P, Verstraeten AA, Go S, Philipi PA, van Kamp GJ, et al. Maternal serum Ca125 and Ca15-3 antigen levels in normal and pathological pregnancy. Fetal Diagn Ther. 2001;16:166-72.
25. Kobayashi F, Sagawa N, Nakamura K, Nonogaki M, Ban C, Fujii S, et al. Mechanism and clinical significance of elevated CA125 levels in the sera of pregnant women. Am J Obstet Gynecol. 1989;160:563-6.
26. Aslam N, Ong C, Woelfer B, Nicolaides K, Jurkovic D. Serum CA125 at 11–14 weeks of gestation in women with morphologically normal ovaries. BJOG. 2000;107:689-90.
27. Frederiksen MC, Casanova L, Schink JC. An elevated maternal serum alpha-fetoprotein leading to the diagnosis of an immature teratoma. Int J Gynaecol Obstet. 1991;35:343.

28. Nawa A, Obata N, Kikkawa F, et al. Prognostic factors of patients with yolk sac tumors of the ovary. Am J Obstet Gynecol. 2001;184:1182.
29. Elit L, Bocking A, Kenyon C, Natale R. An endodermal sinus tumor diagnosed in pregnancy: case report and review of the literature. Gynecol Oncol.1999;72:123.
30. Buller RE, Darrow V, Manetta A, et al. Conservative surgical management of dysgerminoma concomitant with pregnancy. Obstet Gynecol. 1992;79:887.
31. Gucer F, Kiran G, Canaz E, et al. Serum human epididymis protein 4 can be a useful tumor marker in the differential diagnosis of adnexal masses during pregnancy: a pilot study. Eur J Gynaecol Oncol. 2015;36:406.
32. Caspi B, Ben-Arie A, Appelman Z, Or Y, Hagay Z. Aspiration of simple pelvic cysts during pregnancy. Gynecol Obstet Invest. 2000;49:102-5
33. Al-Fozan H, Tulandi T. Safety and risks of laparoscopy in pregnancy. Curr Opin Obstet Gynecol. 2002;14:375-9.
34. Csapo AI, Pulkkinen MO, Ruttner B, et al. The significance of the human corpus luteum in pregnancy maintenance I. Preliminary studies. Am J Obstet Gynecol. 1972;112:1061.
35. Mendez LE, Mueller A, Salom E, et al. Paclitaxel and carboplatin chemotherapy administered during pregnancy for advanced epithelial ovarian cancer. Obstet Gynecol. 2003;102: 1200-02.
36. Sood AK, Shahin MS, Sorosky JI. Paclitaxel and platinum chemotherapy for ovarian carcinoma during pregnancy. Obstet Gynecol. 2001;83:599-600.
37. Horbelt D, Delmore J, Meisel R, et al. Mixed germ cell malignancy of the ovary concurrent with pregnancy. Obstet Gynecol. 1994;84:662-4.
38. Cardonick E, Iacobucci A. Use of chemotherapy during human pregnancy. Lancet Oncol. 2004;5:283-91.
39. Leiserowitz GS, Managing ovarian masses during pregnancy. Obstet Gynecol Surv. 2006;61(7):463-70. PMID:16787549
40. Zhao XY, Huang HF, Lian LJ, Lang JH. Ovarian cancer in pregnancy: a clinicopathologic analysis of 22 cases and review of the literature. Int J Gynecol Cancer. 2006;16:8. TOG, 2006
41. Robarts, Chris P Spencer/Phil J, Management of adnexal masses in pregnancy, TOG, 2006. UpToDate®, ©2016.

Chapter 60

Medicolegal Aspects of High-risk Pregnancy

Hitesh J Bhatt

INTRODUCTION

After the inclusion of medical services under the ambit of Consumer Protection Act, the awareness among patient about their rights has increased gradually and the rise of social media had added to it. Now doctor is accountable for all his professional conduct towards the patient not only under Medical Council Act but under tort as well as criminal laws. Moreover, the trust in every relation is decreasing and more importance is being given to documentations. Even the sacred Act of marriage needs compulsory registration! So doctors are no excuse and are expected to document everything they do in the best interest of the patient. As a doctor, we have habit of classifying every situation as per medical conditions but the principals of law are not different for different medical conditions. The law remains same for each medical condition and each branch of medicine. Hence, the medicolegal aspect of high-risk pregnancy can be the medicolegal aspect of any medical condition. What is more important is to understand the principal of law and the safe guards.

LEGAL IMPLICATIONS

First of all we must understand a few things as:
- What is negligence?
- What is civil negligence and what is criminal negligence?

What is Negligence?

The negligence is defined as "to do something what a prudent man in similar situation will not do (Act of Commission) and not to do something what a prudent man in similar situation will do (Act of Omission).

So, the conduct of the doctor in question shall be compared with the conduct of similar person, i.e. similarly qualified doctor dealing with similar case under similar circumstances. How such a colleague (Prudent person) would have treated the patient is the main question. This legal test or principal is called Bohlam's test. How to find such a prudent person? This prudent person is a hypothetical situation. So how such a prudent person would have acted is decided by various ways. Court shall consider textbook references, references from the journal and affidavit from a peer authenticating the treatment given by a doctor in question. Here comes the role of situation, court shall also consider that what was the situation at the time of mishap and that situation also becomes a deciding factor for negligence. For example, a case investigated and treatment given at primary health care by a gynecologist for menorrhagia cannot be compared with the similar case handled by similarly qualified gynecologist at tertiary care hospital. The expectation for specific investigations including Pap test, biopsy, blood investigations, CT scan, MRI, laparoscopy, hysteroscopy, etc. whichever is necessary, are expected from a consultant sitting at higher center. Again a treatment given in emergency case cannot be compared with treatment given for planned case. The expectation of preparation to tackle the situation in later case is more than the previous case.

What is Civil Negligence and What is Criminal Negligence?

We also must understand the basic difference between civil and criminal negligence.

Civil negligence, is the breach of a duty to care or failure to fulfill one's duty, or a failure to follow the normal standards of conduct for a reasonable person. The negligent Act must result in some injury or loss or damage to the patient. Then patient claims for such damage in terms of some amount of rupees. The case is between two parties, the patient (plaintiff) and the service provider (the doctor)

Criminal negligence is different because the defendant is accused of intentionally acting in reckless fashion without regard to the safety of others, and as such, the offense falls under criminal codes. It needs high level of negligence, then what is required to prove a civil negligence. The punishment here is fine or imprisonment or both. The case is filed by the State against the accused. There is role of police.

WHAT ARE THE LITIGANT SITUATIONS?

- When treatment is done without consent.
- When some complications have arisen.
- When charges are not communicated properly or charges more for the services and infrastructure.
- Rough behavior of the staff or doctor.

WHAT PREVENTS LITIGATION OR SAVES A DOCTOR IN COURT?

- Proper communication
- Proper documentation.

Communication

Communication includes general communication and consent. It says those who communicate well with patient shall never face the problems. Hiding things from patient or not explaining things for would not of time in busy OPD can put you in trouble. If doctor himself is busy, then he should appoint proper staff or counselors to communicate with the patients but avoiding communication is not the option. Any complication explained before surgery is well accepted by the patient then explaining it after it happens. Way of communication is the reflection of human nature. So if you communicate well, you shall be considered as one with good human nature.

ROLE OF CONSENT

Consent is an important aspect of communication while dealing with patient. After the landmark case of Sameera Kohli versus Dr Prabha Manchanda, where the Apex Court had discussed consent at length, the importance and necessity of consent came into limelight. Taking precedence of this case many other cases were decided where consents were not proper or treatment was done beyond the consent given.

DOCUMENTS

It is said that the things not documented has never happened. We Indians are very poor at documentation. In medical practice, we must have various medical documents including case papers, consents, refer notes, reports, charts, X-rays, forms, etc. Most doctors do not maintain OPD records. We must have copy of every document which our patient has. In court it is said that good documents means good defense, poor documents means poor defense and no documents means no defense. The documents have to be preserved for long time. Various guidelines by various bodies give different time frames as follows:

- Consumer Protection Act—2 years
- Civil Litigations—3 years
- Criminal Laws—No limit
- MTP Act (Section 5.1)—5 years
- PNDT Act (Section 9.6)—2 years
- Income Tax Act—8 years
- FOGSI Guidelines—5 years
- Medical Council Act—3 years
- ART Guidelines—10 years
  We have to destroy documents after public notice.

HIGH-RISK PREGNANCY

This is in particular a safe situation. Though there are more chance of complications, there is a reason for that. If patient is well informed about the risk and something happens to her, they may accept it as an Act of God. While in a normal pregnancy, it is at times difficult to explain to the patient when complication occurs. To avail this benefit, it is advisable to explain the smallest of the risk to the patient. At the same, time the care has to be taken that you do not scare the patient to such an extent that she runs away from you.

Remember in High-risk Pregnancy

- High-risk consent has to be taken
- Take help of colleague in difficult situation
- Have indemnity insurance
- Refer the patient to higher center in time when necessary.

Carry Home Messages

- Most of the medicolegal problems are preventable.
- Communication and documentations are the keys to save you.
- Always keep in touch with current medical practice and update your knowledge regularly.
- In case of medicolegal problem always involve medicolegal expert to guide you.
- Never ignore nor reply to legal notice without consultation with medicolegal consultant.
- Medicolegal problems are part of practice, such as bumps on a road so never get worried for any such problem. Have fearless practice.

Chapter 61

Destination Far Ahead: Strategies to Reduce MMR

Bharti Sahu, Padma Shukla, Ranjana Gupta

INTRODUCTION

Well-known Facts!!!

- More than 287,000 women die annually from complications during pregnancy or childbirth. In sub-Saharan Africa, a woman's maternal mortality risk is 1 in 30, compared to 1 in 3,700 in developed regions.
- Every year, more than 1 million children are left motherless.
- Every day, approximately 800 women die from preventable causes related to pregnancy and childbirth [UNFPA Report 2013].
- Of the 287,000 women who die of pregnancy related complications annually almost all maternal deaths (99%) occur in developing countries[1,2] and 1% in developed countries.
- Every 10 minute one maternal death occurs.
- India alone contributes one quarter of total world maternal demise.[3,4]

Between 1990 and 2010, maternal mortality worldwide dropped by almost 50% but still it is very high. Efforts, mainly through, National Rural Health Mission (NRHM) since 2005 have improved the child and maternal health upto some extent. *Janani Suraksha Yojana* has increased institutional delivery from 0.6 million in 2005 to over 3 million in 2007 and has reached 6 million currently. India is on right path but not much has been achieved in number of measles, mumps, and rubella (MMR) reduction. The MMR is declining slowly, even though the vast majority of deaths are avoidable. Skilled care before, during and after childbirth can save the lives of women and newborn babies. Maternal mortality ratio is a vital index of the effectiveness of prevailing obstetric services and socioeconomic affluence of a country.[5] It also reflects the educational and public health consciousness of a country. Millennium Development Goal targeted to reduce maternal mortality upto or less than 109 per lakh of total live births till 2015 was far away from present level prevailing in India.

The Government of India is committed and struggling to tackle the health and mortality statistics of the rural poor, and of the scheduled caste and tribal peoples, which significantly contribute to the global mortality rates of mothers and children under the age of 5 years.[6]

MATERNAL HEALTH SERVICES

Good quality maternal health services are not universally available and accessible.

- 39% receive no antenatal care.
- ~ 40% of deliveries unattended by skilled provider.
- ~ 60% receive no postpartum care during 1st 6 weeks following delivery.
- 15% unmet need of family planning.
- In the developing countries, only 56% of births in rural areas are attended by the skilled health personnel, compared with 87% in urban area.
- Only half of pregnant women in developing countries receive the recommended minimum of 4 antenatal visits.
- Maternal mortality is higher in women of rural areas and poorer communities.
- Young adolescents face a higher risk of complications and death.

Millennium Development Goal 5 to improve maternal health was to reduce MMR by three-quarters, between 1990 and 2015.

SUSTAINABLE DEVELOPMENTAL GOAL

By 2030, aim is to reduce global MMR to less than 70 per 1,00,000 live births.

- *MMR:*
  - 301 (2001–2003)
  - 254 (2004–2006)
  - 212 (2009–2010)
  - Target—109 by 2015
  - Was expected to reach 135 by 2015 (167 in 2015)
- *Coverage of deliveries by skilled person:*
  - 33% (1992–93)
  - 52% (2007–08)
  - Target universal coverage by 2015
  - Was expected to reach 62% by 2015 (56% in 2015)

BUT WHY ARE WE UNABLE TO SAVE THESE MOTHERS

- Delay in decision to seek care
- Delay in reaching care centers
- Delay in receiving care.

FIRST DELAY (FIG. 61.1)

Delay in deciding to seek care at household level:
- Ignorance and inadequate knowledge about danger signals during pregnancy and labor
- Cultural/traditional practices restricting women from seeking health care
- Gender inequality and acceptance of maternal loss
- Poverty.

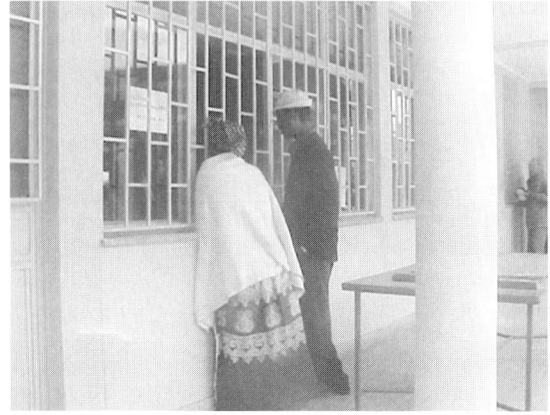

Fig. 61.1: Male involvement is the key

SECOND DELAY (FIG. 61.2)

- Out of reach and inability to access healthcare centers
- Poor roads and communication network
- Supportive environment by community is poor.

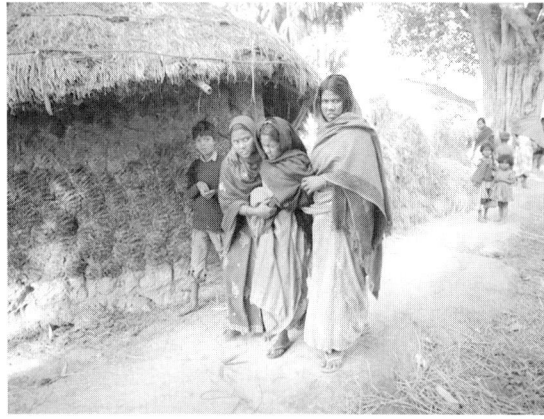

Fig. 61.2: Second delay

THIRD DELAY (FIG. 61.3)

- Time lag between arriving and receiving care at the healthcare center
- Inadequate skilled attendants
- Poorly motivated staff
- Inadequate equipment and supplies
- Weak referral system

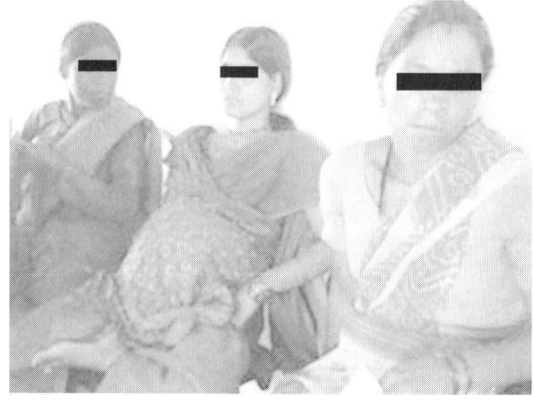

Fig. 61.3: Third delay

CAUSES OF MATERNAL MORTALITY IN INDIA (FIG. 61.4)

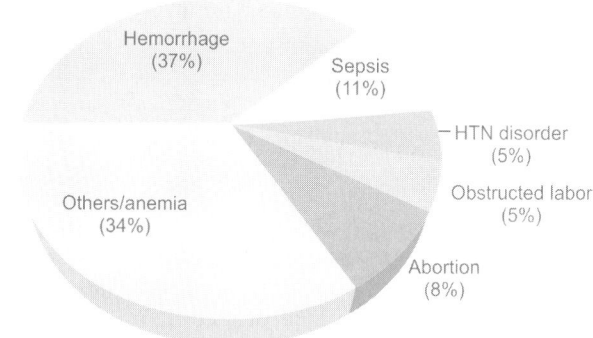

Fig. 61.4: Causes of maternal mortality in India
Source: SRS

CAUSES OF MATERNAL MORTALITY WORLDWIDE (FIG. 61.5)

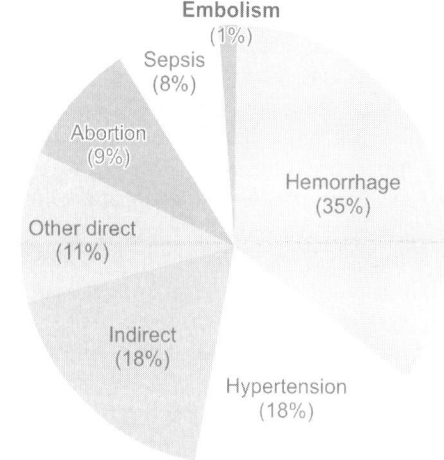

Fig. 61.5: Causes of maternal mortality worldwide
Source: WHO

ROAD BLOCKS!!!

Is it lack of institutional/management capacity?? No, it is lack of commitment.
- Lack of resources.
- Frequent changes in government policies.
- Poor program design.
- Lack of focus on effective strategies—EmOC and skilled birth attendance neglected.
- Lack of monitoring and evaluation.
- Lack of real political and administrative will.
- Inflexibility of schemes
- Lack of specialists and trained staff in rural areas
- Many interventions are not implemented properly, and also there is weak monitoring of implementation—FRUs operationalization, deliveries and EmOC care, maternal deaths.
- Lack of accountability at many levels—50% staff not staying at place of posting.
- Too many activities and programs—no focus on EmOC or delivery care.

What was planned and what happened?

STRATEGIES TO REDUCE MMR (FIG. 61.6)

Over the decades, despite government continuous efforts, the fall in MMR has been slow. Much needs to be done for maternal health care in rural areas. Many studies shows first and second delay are responsible for maximum preventable and treatable deaths .
- Attention should start right from her adolescence, educate and empower girls and women about maternal health issues.
- Our poor village girls are still married early and die young, maternity remaining a preventable cause of these tragic deaths. Discourage early marriage and childbirth.
- Women must have access to skilled care before, during and after they give birth.
- Well trained and more importantly, dedicated health professionals should be providing good antenatal care.
- The quality of the antenatal care is utmost important, as at times the facilities may lack even the most basic resources such as the iron, calcium, the means to measure the blood pressure and hemoglobin. Most of the mothers live in rural areas. Best resources of health facilities in these areas should be made available.
- *Aaganwadi* workers should take due care during antenatal period, they should be trained well to identify high-risk pregnancies, they should sincerely record blood pressure and able to sort out anemics and timely refer high-risk, before it becomes too late.
- Health providers must be trained in emergency obstetric care. Health centers and clinics must have surgical supplies to handle complications.
- Maternal healthcare systems must be strengthened, and communities mobilized and educated to improve deliveries in birth clinics.
- Skilled community-based birth attendants should be trained and posted to increase maternal coverage in remote areas.
- Incentives to peripheral health workers should be given in phases, to motivate them to do their job effectively.
- Contract with private organizations to deliver maternal healthcare services. This will ensure rural areas are covered and will reduce supply shortages, but attention must also be paid to the quality of service provided.
- Educate and empower women and girls about maternal health issues. They compose two-thirds of the world's illiterates and 70% of the world's poorest people. Educated and empowered women can lead healthy lives and can lift their families out of disease.
- Provide transportation services to maternal health centers, which alone can double the utilization of the centers' services.
- Good blood banking and transfusion services will show a positive impact in reducing mortality due to obstetric hemorrhage.
- Empower women's groups so they can deliver political success and tangible health outcomes.
- Launch professional, well-informed advocacy groups to call for action on maternal health.
- Implement streamlined and evidence-based maternal health interventions.
- Implement evidence-based strategies to increase utilization of maternal healthcare services.
- Provision of family planning services, among other factors, can drastically curtail the maternal deaths.
- There should be a good health communication system between health centers, urban slums and tertiary care center.

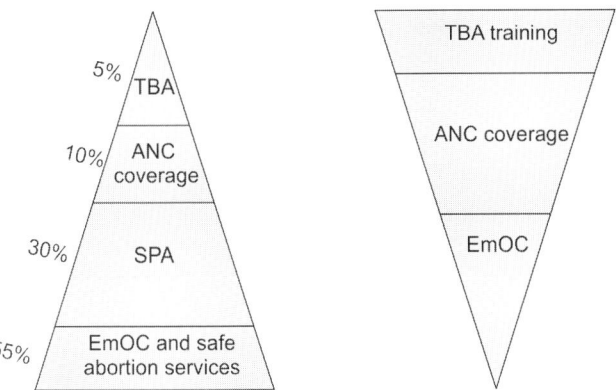

Fig. 61.6: Strategies to reduce maternal mortality rate
Abbreviations: SPA, safe planned abortion; EmOC, emergency obstetric care

- It is necessary even in tertiary centers to channel the working of emergency obstetric care by which 40% MMR can be bought down.
- Evaluate and monitor maternal and child health policies.
- Make sure that the appropriate government ministries are accountable to the public about the performance of investments in maternal health.
- Create strategic alliances between groups representing maternal health, as that will open doors to political and financial support. Currently, maternal health communities have many leaders but no leadership.
- Negligence of societal involvement should also be accountable
- Make child and maternal survival a core national and global health concern.

Death reviews to be attended by all personnel (health and administrative; public and private) involved in the care of pregnant women should be held, and accountability discussed and fixed (presently, there is no such system in place).

Taking appropriate remedial steps for filling lacunaes noted in the management of the cases will be of paramount value in reducing the maternal mortality. If the trend persists, then we may be derailed from the track in achieving the Millennium Development Goal 5 with respect to maternal mortality. Instituting integrated maternal health services with emphasis on primary health care and emergency obstetric care and holistic approach including literacy, nutrition and social and economic empowerment can achieve remarkable improvement, and shed the burden of MMR from India.

By 2030, all countries should reduce MMR by at least two thirds of their 2010 baseline level. The average global is an MMR of less than 70/100 000 live births by 2030.[7] The supplementary national target is that no country should have an MMR greater than 140/100 000 live births (a number twice the global target) by 2030. The ultimate goal of the post-2015 target maternal health strategy is to end all preventable maternal mortality.

IN A NUTSHELL: TO REDUCE MMR

Currently

- Reduce unwanted fertility
- Skilled attendant at delivery
- Emergency obstetrics care.

Reduce Unwanted Fertility

Huge unmet demand for spacing and permanent methods:
- Significant proportion of maternal deaths attributable to unsafe abortions
- Nearly one-third of fertility: Unwanted
- Access to quality contraceptive services will help in reducing unwanted fertility which in turn will reduce numbers of maternal deaths.

Skilled Attendant at Delivery

SBA: An accredited health professional such as midwife, doctor, nurse, who have been educated and trained to proficiency in the skills needed to manage normal pregnancy, child birth and the immediate postnatal period, and the identification, management and referral of complication in women and newborn.
- Proper training for range of skills
- Assess danger signs and recognize onset of complications
- Observe woman, monitor fetus
- Perform essential basic interventions
- Refer mother/baby to higher level of care, if complications arise requiring interventions outside realm of competence.

MYTH

Most Life-threatening Obstetric Complications can be Predicted or Prevented !!!!

Once a woman is pregnant usually most serious obstetric complications cannot be predicted or prevented, but they can be treated.

About 15% do develop obstetric complications. So, all pregnant women need access to emergency obstetric care. Vast majority of deaths (75%) are due to direct obstetric complications. These complications occur even in well-nourished and well-educated women, they cannot usually be predicted or prevented: Some exceptions such as active management of the third stage of labor (AMTSL) for preventing PPH, IP for postpartum infections and provision of safe and early abortion service.

LESSONS AND FUTURE DIRECTIONS

Improve What We Already Have!!
- Systematic process of planning and implementation, with proper monitoring.
- Making FRUs and selected PHCs to provide 24/7 EmOC.
- Increasing skilled birth attendance by ANMs, LHVs, PHC MOs.
- Series of focused and coordinated implementation steps to ensure readiness—training, supplies, efforts to improve quality.
- Addressing policy barriers—delegation and posting and transfers.

KEY TO SUCCESS

Access to:
- Skilled attendance at birth
- Emergency obstetric care

- Family planning
- Prenatal and postnatal care.

Are absolutely essential:

But reduction of MMR to western levels goes beyond health—it requires better nutrition, better hygiene, better education of mothers and better gender equality, in other words, better overall development of people.

What is needed is newer thinking—social health insurance.

India can reduce MMR, but needs societal and political commitment.

Knowing is not enough, we must apply
Willing is not enough, we must do.

REFERENCES

1. Countdown to 2015 for maternal, newborn and child survival: accountability for maternal, newborn and child survival. Geneva: WHO Health Organisation, 2013 (*http//www.countdown2015mnch.org/documents/2013Report/Countdown_2013-Updates_noprofiles.pdf*).
2. Trends in maternal mortality: 1990-2010— estimates developed by WHO, UNICEF, UNFPA and the World Bank. 2012. (*http//www.unfpa.org/public/home/publications/pid/10728*).
3. *www.ibtimes.co.in/every-5-minutes-woman-dies-during-pregnancy-chil. June 13, 2016 - India accounts for one-fourth of maternal deaths worldwide*, the WHO.
4. *www.unfpa.org/.../maternal-deaths-halved-20-years-faster-progress-need. May 16, 2012*. The report "Trends in maternal mortality: 1990 to 2010".
5. Kulkarni Sunanda R, Huligol A. Maternal mortality: 10 years study. J Obstet Gynecol India. 2001;51:73-6. *doi: 10.1159/000052897*. [Cross Ref]
6. World Health Organization and Unicef. Countdown to 2015 Decade Report (2000–2010): Taking Stock of Maternal, Newborn and Child Survival. Geneva: WHO and UNICEF, 2010 [*http//www.childinfo.org/files/countdownReport 2000-2010.pdf*] Accessed 17 August 2011.
7. The EPMM targets and strategies are grounded in a human rights approach to maternal and newborn health, and focus *on eliminating. Who.int/reproductivehealth/topics/maternal_perinatal/epmm/en/FEBRUARY 2015.*

INDEX

Page numbers followed by *b* refer to box, *f* refer to figure, *fc* refer to flow chart, and *t* refer to table

A

Abdomen
    acute 398
    sonography, upper 92
Abdominal circumference 289
Abdominal pain 55
Abdominal palpation 195
ABO incompatibility 66
Aborted pregnancy 87
Abortion 57
    incomplete 105
    services, safe 103
    spontaneous 31
ABPM *See* Ambulatory blood pressure monitoring
Abruptio placentae 5, 57, 82, 83, 178, 190, 204, 360
ACA *See* Anticardiolipin antibody
Accreta 31
ACEI *See* Angiotensin-converting enzyme inhibitors
Acetaminophen 143, 258
Acetylsalicylic acid, low-dose 176
Achondrogenesis 309
Achondroplasia 310
ACI *See* Acute chronic inflammation
Acrochordons 332
Act of
    commission 407
    omission 407
Activin A 3, 171
Acute viral hepatitis 162, 167
    clinical features 167
    management 167
Acyclovir 271, 339
Adam metallopeptidase domain 12 171
Addison's disease 92
Adnexal masses, types of 398
Adnexal ovarian cysts 401
Adnexal pathology, ultrasound of 399*t*
Adolescent childbearing 234
Adolescent girls, childbirth in 236
Adolescent pregnancy and childbirth, factors influencing 234
Advancing maternal age 195
AED *See* Antiepileptic drug
AFP *See* Alpha-fetoprotein
Agenesis of corpus callosum 299
AICD *See* Automated implantable cardioverter defibrillator

Alanine aminotransferase 144
Albendazole 52
Alcohol 235
Alfa-fetoprotein 31
Alloimmune thrombocytopenia 45
Alobar 2
Alpha-fetoprotein 2, 27, 31, 171, 401
    levels of 32
ALT *See* Alanine aminotransferase
AMA *See* Advanced maternal age
Ambulatory blood pressure monitoring 172, 183
Ambulatory peritoneal dialysis, continuous 152
American College of Obstetricians and Gynecologists 171, 180, 289
American Thoracic Society 143
Amikacin 265
Aminophylline 142
Aminotransferase 167
Amiodarone 129
    therapy 138
Amlodipine 137
Amniocentesis 32, 36, 43, 44*f*, 70, 71, 279
    drawbacks of 44
    indications of 43
    risks of 44
    timing of 44
Amnioinfusion 224
    in labor, guidelines for 224
Amnionitis 216
Amnioreduction 230
Amniotic epithelial cells 342
Amniotic fluid
    abnormalities of 311
    embolism 5, 82, 144
    examination of collected 218
    spectrophotometric analysis of 68
    volume 21
Anal atresia 306
Androgen 51
Anemia 45, 151, 235
    caused by
        blood loss 49
        decreased production 49
        increased red cell destruction 49
    causes of 49
    classification of 49
    during pregnancy 49
    laboratory evaluation of 59, 60*fc*
    mild 51

    moderate 52
    of pregnancy physiological 51
    presence of 51
    severe 49, 52
    specific 50
Anemic early second trimester fetus, severely 77
Anencephaly 2, 31, 296, 297*f*
Anesthesia 181, 202
Aneurysms, ruptured 388*f*
Anganwadi workers 8, 411
Angelman syndrome 395
Angiogenic factors 171
Angiogenic functions 173
Angiotensin receptor-blocking 179
Angiotensin-converting enzyme 137
    inhibitors 126
Anisocytosis giant polymorphs 57
Anomalous neonate 314
Anomaly, multiple 243
ANP *See* Atrial natriuretic peptide
Antenatal care 131, 236, 275
    changing trends in 1
    diagnosis 1
    effective 5
    epidemiology 1
    missing dimensions in 7
    physical examination 2
    prognosis 4
    prophylaxis 5
    treatment 3
Antenatal complications 232
Antenatal corticosteroids 180
Antenatal fetal surveillance 18
Antenatal management 350
    of pregnancy 64
Antenatal period 5
Antenatal prophylaxis and protection 67
Antenatal psychological stress 8
Antepartum 119
    classification 20*t*
    complications 239
    infections 240
Antiarrhythmic drugs 138
Antibeta-2 glycoprotein 323
Antibiotic 212
    protocol for management 224*fc*
Antibody to extractable nuclear antigens 318
Anticardiolipin antibodies 87, 323, 328, 382
Anti-*Chlamydia pneumoniae* 135

Anticoagulant 131
   therapy 138
Antiemetics 92
Antiepileptic drug 350
   and doses carbamazepine 351
   ethosuximide 351
   gabapentine 351
   lamotrigine 351
   levetiracetam 351
   low levels of 350
   oxcarbazepine 351
   phenobarbital 351
   phenytoin 351
   topiramate 351
   valproic acid 351
Antiepileptic medication 350
Antigenicity 54
Antihistaminics 339
Antihypertensive medicines 175, 189
   labetolol 189
   nifedipine 189
Antinuclear antibody 317, 382
Antioxidants 175
Antiphosphatidylethanolamine
   antibodies 325
Antiphosphatidylserine antibodies 325
Antiphospholipid 323
Antiphospholipid antibody 87, 328
   activate platelets 324
   and infertility 324
   present 319
   syndrome 87, 88, 131, 323, 328
      diagnosis 324
      differential diagnosis 326
      epidemiology 323
      etiopathogenesis 324
      obstetric implications 324
      primary 31
      recent advances in treatment 328
      treatment 326
Antiphospholipid syndrome 169, 171, 179, 184, 328
Anti-retroviral
   drug 275
   therapy 275
Antithrombin III deficiency 88
Antithrombotic agents 175
Antithyroid
   antibodies, presence of 88
   drug 157, 158
      treatment 158
Antituberculosis drugs 265
Aortic
   compression 377
   dissection 116
   isthmus doppler 292
   regurgitation 125
   stenosis 126, 128, 301
Aortocaval compression 129
Aortopathy 128

Aphasia 388
APLA syndrome 326t
   placental failure in 325f
Aplastic anemia 50
APS *See* Antiphospholipid antibody syndrome
APTT *See* Activated partial thromboplastin time
Arborization test (Ferning) 218
ART *See* Assisted reproductive technique
Arterial embolization 377
   procedure 377
Arteriovenous malformation 249, 349, 390
Asanas 11
Ascites 45
   in hydropic fetus 76f
Ascorbic acid 174
Asphyxiating thoracic dystrophy *See also* Jeune's thoracic dystrophy
Aspirin 174, 176, 260, 389
   low dose 87, 88, 175, 319, 329
   plus heparin, low-dose 175
Assisted reproductive technique 394
   pregnancies 394
      management of 395
   techniques 394
Asthma
   acute severe 142
   exacerbations, treatment of acute severe 142
   fetal risks 141
   in pregnancy, management of 141
   in pregnant women 141
   labor and delivery 142
   management 141
   maternal risks 141
   medications in pregnancy 141
   treatment of 141
Asymptomatic patients 197
Atopic eruption of pregnancy
   clinical presentation 335
   differential diagnosis 336
   etiology 335
   laboratory findings 335
   prognosis 336
   synonyms 335
   treatment 336
Atosiban 213, 214
Atrial fibrillation 131
   presence of 138
Atrial natriuretic peptide 171
Atrial septal defect 125, 300
Atrioventricular block 303
Atrophic gastritis 156
Autoimmune
   disease 179
   hepatitis 162
   thyroiditis 158
Automated implantable cardioverter defibrillator 138

Azathioprine 339
Azithromycin 143, 339

B

Bacterial
   infections 333
   spreading 341
   vaginosis 209, 210, 217
Bacteriuria in pregnancy 2
Bakri balloon 365
Balloon
   easy 369, 370f
   in uterus 371f
   insertion of 369
Balloon tamponade 368, 372
   catheter 365
   in postpartum hemorrhage 368
   types of 368
Barotraumas 187
BCG vaccination 265
Beckwith-Wiedemann syndrome 395
Beclomethasone 142
Bergeyella 342
Beta-blockers 129, 137
   nonselective 138
Betamethasone 79, 180
Betamimetics 56
Beta-thalassemia 25, 33, 53
Bibasilar rales, presence of 119
Bicarbonate 151
Bicornuate uterus 210
Bicuspid aortic valve disease 128
Biochemical miscarriage *See also* Preclinical miscarriage
Biophysical profile 21
Bioprosthetic valves, degeneration of 126
Birth defects, risk factor for 243
Bladder and cloacal exstrophies 305
   diagnosis 305
Bleeding
   in early pregnancy, etiology of 94
   nonobstetrical causes of 100
Blood
   and plasma, components of 83t
   bank 202
   coagulation disorders 381
   components 83
   glucose 382
      levels, rapid normalization of 193
   investigations, normal values of 183t
   loss 361
   pressure 148
      control of 144
      during pregnancy, physiological changes in 178
      measurement of 183
   product transfusion 363
   sample bottles 364
   sugar test 57

transfusion
    in anemia during pregnancy 56*fc*
    in pregnancy, indications of 55
    whole 83
    urea nitrogen 144
Bloom syndrome 33
B-lynch suture 374
    modified 374, 376*f*
    technique of 374
Body edema, generalized 69
Body mass index 179, 238, 360
Body stalk
    anomaly 304
    syndrome 28
Bohlam's test 407
Bolus syntocinon 363
Bone marrow
    iron 52
    transplantation 61
Borrelia 267
Brace suture *See also* B-lynch suture
Bradycardia 302
Bradyzoites 279
Brain 385*f*
Breastfeeding 139, 243, 265
    issues of 320
    management 139
    prognosis 139
    women 16
Bromocriptine 89, 139
    role of 138
BSL *See* Blood surgar test
Budd-Chiari syndrome 162
Budesonide 142
BUN *See* Blood urea nitrogen

C

Cabergoline 89, 138, 139
    use of 138
Caesarean scar pregnancy 248*f*
Calcium 151
    requirements during pregnancy 14
    supplementation 127, 175
Calcium-channel
    antagonists 138
    blockers 137
Campomelic dysplasia 310
Campylobacter rectus 344
Canavan disease 33
Capreomycin 265
CAPS *See* Catastrophic antiphospholipid syndrome
Carbamazepine 349, 350
Carbetocin functions 364
Carbimazole 157
Carboprost 363
Cardiac arrhythmia 45, 128, 302
Cardiac conditions, specific 122
Cardiac defects, major 2

Cardiac disease 123
    in pregnancy, complications of 119
Cardiac events during pregnancy, predictors of 117*t*
Cardiac failure 119
Cardiac function during pregnancy, evaluation of 118
Cardiac lesions, specific 125
Cardiac output 123
Cardiac transplantation 138
Cardiac valve disease 325
Cardiogenic pulmonary edema 143
Cardiomyopathy 129, 130
    dilated 129
Cardiorespiratory involvement 182
Cardiotocography, routine 3
Cardiovascular disease 122, 207
Carvedilol 138
Catastrophic antiphospholipid syndrome 329
Catastrophic hemorrhage 250
Causative factors, major 385
Causative lesion, treatment of 391
CBC *See* Complete blood count
CD4 cells 273
CD4 lymphocytes 273, 344
CD8+ lymphocytes 344
Ceftriazone 143
Cefuroxime axetil 143
Celiac disease 156
Central pontine myelinolysis 92
Central serous chorioretinopathy 193
Cephalocele 296
Cephalosporins 339
Cerebral
    aneurysm 390
    arteriovenous malformation 384
    artery
        Doppler, middle 291, 292*f*
        high middle 187
        middle 71*f*
        peak systolic velocity, middle 71
    edema 127
    ischemia 188
    palsy 9
    vasospasm 187
    vein thrombosis 349
    venous
        sinus thrombosis 389
        thrombosis 385
Cerebroplacental ratio 291
Cerebrospinal fluid, absorption of 297
Cerebrovascular accident 178
    causes of 388
    modifiable risk factors 388
    prevention of 390
    symptoms of 386
Cervical
    cerclage 211
    ectropion 100

    incompetence 86, 217
    insufficiency 97
    length screening 210
    length, short 209
    manipulation 386
    surgery, history of 210
Cervicovaginal branch, smaller 376
Cervix 101
    treatments placed in 104
Cesarean deliveries 232, 248
    management of adnexal mass at 403
Cesarean scar pregnancy 248
    complications 250
    diagnosis of 248, 250
    differential diagnosis 250
    epidemiology 248
    magnetic resonance imaging 249
    management 249
    medical treatment 249
    risk factors 248
    surgical treatment 250
    systemic administration 249
    treatment of 248, 250
Cesarean section 82, 191
    history of 248
    in placenta previa 198
    indications for 320
    previous 195
    rate of 241
    role of 382
Cetirizine 339
CG balloon 370*f*
Chemotaxis 342
Chemotherapeutic agents 79
Chemotherapy 403
    in complicated malaria 255
    in severe malaria 255
Chest pain 55
Chickenpox *See also* Varicella zoster
Chikungunya 283
Childbirth-related complications 234
Childhood and adolescent migraine prevention 129
Chlamydia 235
    trachomatis 211, 217
Chlorhexidine varnish 346
Chloroquine 254-256
    resistant 255
Chlorphenaramine 339
Chlorpromazine 93
Cho multiple square sutures 374
Cho's sutures 198
Cholecystitis 162
Cholelithiasis 162
Chondroectodermal dysplasia 310
Chorioamnionitis
    management of 220*fc*
    signs of 218
Chorioamniotic infections 342
Choriodecidual infection 216

Chorion villus sampling 32
Chorionic tissue, degree of invasion of 201*f*
Chorionic trophoblasts 342
Chorionic villous sampling 36, 42, 62
 indications of 42
Chorionicity 228
Choroid plexus cyst 29
Choroidal dysfunction 192
Chromosomal abnormalities 380
 diagnosis for 27*f*
Chromosomal microarray 32
Chronic inflammation, acute 53
Cisterna magna, enlarged 29
Civil negligence 407
CKD *See* Chronic kidney diseases
Clarithromycin 143
Clinodactyly 29
Clopidogrel 328, 389
Club foot 29, 311*f*
CMA *See* Chromosomal microarray
CMV *See* Cytomegalovirus
Coagulation cascade 82
 normal 81
Coarctation of aorta 128, 301
Cocaine abuse 207
Coformulated tablet of artemether 255
Cohen's transverse incision 198
Coliforms 267
Communication 408
Complement system 87
Complete blood count 52, 57, 144, 183, 329
Condom balloon
 innovative 369
 uterine tamponade 369
Condom balloon tamponade
 contraindications to use of 371
 conventional 369
 inconsistencies of conventional 369
 post-placement care of 371
 varieties of 369
Condom catheters 365
Congenital anomalies 85, 242, 350, 394
Congenital cardiac diseases 116
Congenital diaphragmatic hernia 45, 304, 304*f*
 associated syndromes 304
 diagnosis 304
 management 304
Congenital heart
 block 320, 321
 disease 125, 130
 incidence of 300
Congenital hyperbilirubinemia 162
Congenital hypothyroidism 25
Congenital malformations 25
Congenital rubella syndrome, risk of 268*t*
Congenital toxoplasmosis, clinical signs of 280
Congenital varicella syndrome 271

Conjoined twins (monozygotic) 226, 227*f*
 management of 230
Consent, role of 408
Consumer Protection Act 407
Contingent screening 29
Contraception
 advice of 320
 lack of access to 103
Contraceptive 120
Contraction stress test 20
 interpretation 20
 mechanism of 21*fc*
 method of 21*fc*
Conventional karyotyping 37
Coombs' test 61, 70
Cord clamping, contraindications to delayed 214
Cordocentesis 33, 44, 68, 70
 indications of 45
 risks of 45
Corneal changes 192
Cornerstone 264
Coronary
 artery disease 128
 heart disease 122
Corpus luteum
 cyst 399*f*
  functional 401
  management of 403
  removal of 403
Corticosteroids 92, 206, 327
 administration of 212
 contraindication to 212
 course of 181
 use of 229
Corticotropin-releasing hormone 171
Cortisol and gender steroids 14
Cotrimoxazole 276
 for infants 277*t*
 prophylaxis 276
Coxsackie 267
C-reactive protein 135
Creatinine 144, 149
Criminal negligence 407
Cromolyn 142
Cryoprecipitate 83, 84
CSCR *See* Central serous chorioretinopathy
Cultural constraints 104
Current obstetric status 23
Current pregnancy 18
 fetal 18
 maternal 18
CVD *See* Cardiovascular disease
CVS *See* Chorionic villous sampling
Cyanotic heart disease 124
Cyclizine 92, 93
Cycloserine 265
Cyclosporine 339, 340
Cynocobalamin 51
Cystic fibrosis 33, 36, 143
 management prepregnancy 143

 maternal and fetal risks 143
 pregnancy and labor 143
Cysts, complex 399*f*
Cytogenetic diagnosis, limitations of 33
Cytokines 171, 342
Cytomegalovirus 268, 329, 382
 diagnosis 269
 epidemiology 269
 etiopathogenesis 269
 management 269
 prevention 269
Cytotrophoblastic invasion, stages to 169

D

Dandy-Walker malformation 298, 299*f*
Dapsone 339
De novo appearance 127
Decidual cells 342
Decidual hemorrhage 209
Decidual natural killer cells 200
Decidual veins 200
Deficient endometrium 195
Delayed cord clamping 214
Deliveriy
 decision 189
  and conduct 191
 in women with pre-eclampsia, indications for 150
 interval between 232
 mode of 231, 381
 of dead fetus 381
 of fetus 356
 of women with pre-eclampsia/ eclampsia, timing of 180
 skilled attendant at 412
 timing of 77, 231
Dengue
 case management 262*fc*
 disease 259
 during pregnancy, management of 257
 fever with
  shock on admission 262
  warning sign 262
 patients with warning signs, management for 261*fc*
 treatment in pregnant patient 346*t*
Deoxyuridine suppression test 57
Dermoid cyst 399*f*
Devascularization of uterus, stepwise 375, 376*f*
Dexamethasone 79, 180
Dextran-iron dextran 54
DHA *See* Docosahexaenoic acid
Dhaka regimen 189
Diabetic ketoacidosis 91
Diabetic retinopathy 193
 risk for 193
Dialysis 151, 152
 in pregnancy 150

Diamniotic twins 231
Diaphragmatic hernia 29
Diarrhea 55
Diclofenac sodium 260
Dietary and lifestyle modifications 175
Digoxin 137
Dilation
    low-level 307
    mid-level 306
Dimorphic anemia 50
Diphenhydramine 339
Dipyridamole 174
Disseminated intravascular coagulation 81, 178
    acute 81
    diagnosis 83
    etiology 81
    in pregnancy 81
    management 83
    pathophysiology of 82, 82fc
    prophylaxis 83
    specific treatment 84
    symptoms 83
Dizziness 55
DNA antibody, anti-double-stranded 318
Dobutamine stress test 139
Docosahexaenoic acid 14, 16
Documents 408
Domperidone 92
Doppler velocimetry 22
Down's syndrome 25, 26, 28f, 91, 228
    in multiple gestations 228
Doxycyclin 255
Doxylamine 92
Droperidol 93
Drug safety 339t
Duchenne muscular dystrophy 25, 38
Ductus venosus Doppler 292, 293f
Ductus venous 4
Duodenal atresia 305, 306f
    etiology 305
Dysarthria 388
Dysplastic echogenic kidney, bilateral 308f
Dyspraxia 388

E

Early- and late-onset form 291t
Early pregnancy
    haemorrhage, interpretation of 101
    vomiting in 157
Echocardiographic criteria 135
Echocardiographic evaluation 139
Echogenic bowel 29
Echogenic intracardiac focus 29
Eclampsia 170, 178, 183, 187, 192, 235
    severe 390
Ectopic gestation 99
    clinical features 99

diagnosis 99
differential diagnosis 100
epidemiology 99
etiology 99
risk factors for 99
Ectopic pregnancy 100b, 248
    clinical presentation of 100t
    management of 100
    primary 99
    risk factors 99t
    ultrasound-guided management of 46
EDD *See* Estimated delivery date
Efavirenz 275
Ehlers-Danlos syndrome 353
Eicosapentaenoic acid 14, 16
Eikenella 342
Eisenmenger's syndrome 118, 125, 131, 132
ELISA *See* Enzyme-linked immunosorbent assay
Ellis-Van creveld syndrome 310
Embryonic miscarriage 94
Endocrine factors 89
    in pregnancy losses 88
Endocrine imbalances 91
Endogenous estrogen 342
Endoglin 3
Endometrial polyp 86
Endometrioma 399, 400f
Endomyocardial biopsy 137, 138
Endorphin 11
Endothelial
    adhesion molecules 171
    damage 187
    dysfunction 171
    injury 81
Endothelin 171
    antagonists 125
Energy requirements 13
Enkaphalin 11
Enzyme-linked immunosorbent assay 329
Epidural analgesia, controlled 139
Epigastric pain 182
Epigenetic alteration 395
Epilepsy in pregnancy 349
    differential diagnosis 349
    etiopathogenesis 349
    investigations 349
    preconception counseling 349
Epithelial malignancy 403
Epstein-Barr virus 135
Equivocal hyperstimulation 21
Ergometrine 363, 364
Erythrocyte count 61
Erythrocyte protoporphyrin, evaluation of free 60
Erythromycin 143
Erythropoiesis 51
Esophageal atresia 157, 305
    diagnosis 305
    etiology 305
    management 305

Esophagus 371
Estimated delivery date 27
Estriol 171
Estrogen 343
Ethambutol 265
Ethionamide 265
European Food Safety Authority 14
European Prospective Cohort on Thrombophilia 88
European Registry on Obstetric Antiphospholipid Syndrome 327, 329
European Society of Cardiology 135
Euthyroidism 156
Exomphalos 2
Exomphalos *See also* Omphalocele
Extracellular fluid 147
Extracorporeal membrane oxygenation 138
Extravillous cytotrophoblast 173
Eye
    diseases, pre-existing 193
    in pregnancy 192
    movement, rapid 7

F

Facial clefts 298
Factor V leiden mutation 88
Fallopian tube 402t
Famciclovir 271, 339
Familial dysautonomia 33
Familial inherited disorders 34f
Familial mutation 136
Family planning, advice about 56
Fanconi anemia 33, 50
Fasting blood glucose 319
FEP *See* Free erythrocyte protoporphyrin
Ferric carboxymaltose 54, 55
Ferritin 50, 53
Fertility 238
    treatment 240
Fetal affection, clinical management of previous 73
Fetal and neonatal 130
Fetal anemia
    MCA-PSV suggesting 72f
    severity of 71
    ultrasound, severity of 71
Fetal aneuploidies, screening tests for 2
Fetal arrhythmias, management of 303
Fetal ascites 69
Fetal assessment 180
Fetal blood 70
    group 70
    sampling 36, 73
    transfusion 73
        intraperitoneal transfusion 73
Fetal bradycardia 196
Fetal brain 9

Fetal cardiovascular abnormalities 300
   familial indications 300
      fetal indications 300
      maternal indications 300
Fetal cells 136
   detection of 218
Fetal complications 92, 197, 228, 241
Fetal conditions increasing risk 274
Fetal craniospinal abnormalities 296
Fetal death 31, 170, 379
   early 379
   late 379
Fetal development 8
Fetal disease 33
Fetal distress 242
Fetal DNA, cell-free 174
Fetal dysmorphology 296
Fetal echocardiography 229
Fetal effects 52
Fetal fibronectin 3
Fetal gastrointestinal abnormalities 303
Fetal genitourinary abnormalities 306
Fetal growth restriction 174, 289, 380
   early-onset 290
   examination 289
   late-onset 290
   management of 292, 294
   monitoring 289, 291
   rules of 289
   stage-based classification of 294
Fetal growth, evaluation of 180
Fetal heart 211
Fetal hydantoin syndrome 350
Fetal hydrops 33, 76 *See also* Hydrops fetalis
Fetal lung maturation 45
Fetal maturity, management according to 219*fc*
Fetal membrane, alteration in 210
Fetal microchimerism 129, 136
Fetal miscarriage 94
Fetal movement 19
   counts 20*fc*
      issues relevant for 19
Fetal origins of adult disease 8, 8*fc*
Fetal outcome 18
Fetal physiology and behavior, influence on 8
Fetal pleural effusion 69
   in hydropic fetus 76*f*
Fetal presentation, abnormal lie and 195
Fetal reduction 46
Fetal skeletal abnormalities 309
Fetal surveillance 184
Fetal tachyarrhythmias 129
Fetal therapy 45, 45*t*
   for Rh-immunization 46
   for twin-to-twin transfusion syndrome 45
Fetal transmission with cytomegalovirus, risk of 269*t*

Fetal uropathy 306
   diagnosis 306
   management 307
Fetal well-being, surveillance of 180
Fetofetal transfusion syndrome 45, 232
   signs of 229
   ultrasound for 229
Fetofetal, monitoring for 229
Fetomaternal
   immune response 343
   leak, tests for determination of 68
Fetoplacental dysfunction 241
Fetoplacental unit endocrine dysfunction 171
Fetoscopic laser ablation 230
Fetoscopy 45
Fetotoxicity, severe 127
Fetus
   cell-free DNA of 2
   dead 82
   effect on 57
   from mouth of 11
   investigations of 68
   live 206
   percutaneous procedures in 46
   ultrasound findings in 279
Fetus/infant, previously affected 75*fc*
Fexofenadine 339
Fibrinolytic therapy 389
Fibronectin 171
   measurement 210
FIGLU *See* Formiminoglutamic acid
Filtration fraction 148
Finasteride 339
Fine-needle aspiration cytology 264
First trimester anatomical screening 26
FISH *See* Fluorescence in situ hybridization
Fish oil supplementation 175
Flaviviridae family 282
Flavivirus genus 282
Fluconazole 339
Fluid, microscopy of 218
Fluorescence in situ hybridization 32
Fluoroquinolones 265, 339
Fluticasone 142
FOAD *See* Fetal origins of adult disease
Foley's catheter 184, 188, 364, 365, 368, 369, 370*f*
   port of 369
Folic acid 51, 319
   deficiency 57, 253
   requirements during pregnancy 14
   supplements 14, 57
   tablets 52
Folinic acid 280, 281
Fontan circulation 124
Fontan repair 130
Food, coadministration of 156
Formiminoglutamic acid 57
Fossa cyst, posterior 299*f*

Fox Fordyce's disease (axilla) 333*f*
Fractured limbs 310
Fragile X syndrome 33
Frank pulmonary edema 119
Free erythrocyte protoporphyrin 52, 53, 61
Fresh blood transfusion 262
Fresh-frozen plasma 83
   transfusion 84
Fulminant hepatic failure 167
   clinical feature 167
   management 168
Fungal infections 333
Fusobacterium nucleatum 342

G

Gallbladder, diseases of 162
Garbh sanskar 11
Gardnerella vaginalis 209, 217
Gastritis 156
Gastroesophageal reflux disease 141
Gastrointestinal bleeding 101
Gastroschisis 2, 303
Gastroschisis
   diagnosis 304
   etiology 303
   labor and delivery 304
   management 304
Gaucher disease 33
Gene
   determination 70
   mutations, screening for 33
   polymorphisms 174
Genetic
   abnormalities 380
   diseases, vertical transmission of 395
   disorders 25
      in India, burden of 25*t*
   evaluation 87*fc*
   in prenatal diagnosis, advances in 36
   sonogram 29
   techniques 36
      karyotyping 36
   testing methods, primary 32
Genital tract
   in early pregnancy, bleeding form 101*t*
   infection 210, 217
   inflammations 209
   pathology, lower 100
Genomic hybridization, comparative 32
Genomics and proteomics 174
GERD *See* Gastro-esophageal reflux disease
German measles *See also* Rubella
Gestational age 19, 94, 227
   and chorionicity 227
   small for 3, 28, 289, 293, 394
   specific middle cerebral artery 71*f*
Gestational diabetes 174, 228, 395
   mellitus 238, 239

Gestational hypertension 31, 126, 127, 135, 178, 179, 181, 182
    mild 179
    moderate 179
    severe 180
Gestational hyperthyroidism, management of women with 158
Gestational surrogate 79
Gestational trophoblastic disease 92, 97
    clinical features 98
    diagnosis 98
    epidemiology 97
    etiopathogenesis 97
    histopathological diagnosis 98
    low socioeconomic condition 97
    management 98
    risk factors 97
Gingival
    conditions 344
    fibroblasts 342
    inflammation, process of 342
Gingivitis 344
Glandular changes 332
Glomerular filtration rate 148
Glucocorticoids 320
Glucose-6-phosphate-dehydrogenase 59
Glyceryl trinitrate 213
    dosage 213
    side effects 213
Glycosylated
    dimeric glycoprotein 173
    hemoglobin 382
Gonorrhea 235
Gram-negative bacteria 209
Granulocyte-macrophage-colony stimulating factor 345
Granuloma gravidarum 332*f*
Graves' disease in pregnancy 157, 158
Great vessels, transposition of 301
Griesofulvin 339
Group B *Streptococcus* 217
    prophylaxis 212
Growth retardation 57
GTD *See* Gestational trophoblastic disease

H

H1N1 infection
    clinical manifestation of 257
    in pregnant women prevention 258
    pandemic 258
H1N1 treatment 258
Hair and nail changes 331
Haptoglobin 171
Hashimoto's thyroiditis 156
Hasson's technique 401
Hayman uterine compression suture 374
HBsAg *See* Hepatitis B surface antigen
hCG *See* Human choronic gonadotropin
Headache 55, 182

Health sector pregnancy in adolescents girls, role of 236*fc*
Healthcare
    facilities 372
    professional 237
Heart
    catheterization, right 137
    defects 243
    disease in pregnancy
        effect of 130
        management of 131
    failure 51
    rate, irregular 302
Heinz body anemia 50
Helicobacter pylori 156
HELLP syndrome 187
    classification 190
    criteria for 190
    differential diagnosis 190
    diseases mimicking 190
    etiology 190
    incidence 187
    investigations and treatment 187
    management 187, 190
    maternal mortality 190
    pathophysiology 187
    perinatal mortality 190
    related to
        pregnancy 190
        thrombocytopenia 190
HELLP syndrome *See* Hemolysis, elevated liver enzymes, and low platelets syndrome
Hemagglutinin-1 257
Hematogenous dissemination of inflammatory products 342
Hematuria 150
Hemisphere injuries, right and left 387*t*
Hemodialysis during pregnancy, managing 151*t*
Hemodialysis-induced liver damage 162
Hemodilutional effect 147
Hemodynamic
    monitoring
        continuous 191
        postpartum 132
    stress 129
Hemoglobin 53, 362
    concentration 52
    level 56
Hemoglobinopathy 61
Hemolysis 182
Hemolytic
    anemia 50
    causes 50
    uremic syndrome 389
Hemorrhage 94
    control during surgery, tips for 202
Hemorrhagic cyst, large 399*f*
Hemorrhagic stroke 387, 388*f*
    from aneurysms 385

Hemoglobin, production of 14
Hemolysis 253
Hemophilus influenzae 62
Hemostasis mnemonics 362*t*
Heparin 88, 174
    complications of 327
    efficacy of 131
    unfractionated 87, 119, 131, 327, 329
Heparin-induced thrombocytopenia 132
Hepatic coma 167
Hepatic dysfunction 55
Hepatic enzyme 350
Hepatic failure 167
Hepatic transaminases, elevated 150
Hepatitis
    A 162, 164
        virus 164
    B 162, 164, 272
        chronic 273
        diagnosis 273
        epidemiology 272
        etiopathogenesis 272
        management 273
        prevention 273
        surface antigen 4
    C 162, 164
    chronic 162
    D 162, 164
    E 162, 164
    G 162
Hereditary thrombophilias 88
    treatment of 88
Herpes gestationis 338
Herpes simplex 269, 333
    diagnosis 270
    etiopathogenesis 270
    management 270
Herpes zoster 333
Heterogeneous diseases, group of 97
Hilar moustache 119
HIV 267
HIV/AIDS 273
Hodgkin's lymphoma 398
Holistic health model 10
Holoprosencephaly 2, 298
Home uterine activity monitoring 210
Hormonal and immunomodulatory effects 193
Hormones 51
Host immunoinflammatory response, changes in 344
Howell-Jolly bodies 57
HUAM *See* Home uterine activity monitoring
Human
    chorionic gonadotropin 27, 29, 150, 171, 401
    cytomegalovirus 135
    epididymis protein 4 401

herpes simplex virus 135
malaria 252
papilloma virus 333
placenta 200
development of 200
HUS *See* Hemolytic uremic syndrome
Hydatidiform mole 97
Hydralazine 181
Hydranencephaly 299, 299*f*
Hydrocephalus 297
diagnosis 298
etiology 298
management 298
Hydrocortisone 92
Hydrolytic enzymes 343
Hydronephrosis 45, 306
Hydropic fetus 77*f*, 314
subcutaneous edema in 77*f*
with large placenta 78*f*
Hydrops 29
fetalis 67, 76, 91
ascites 313*f*
scalp edema 313*f*
sonographic features of 69
Hydrosalpinx 399
Hydroxychloroquine 319, 320, 328
of platelet activation 328
role of 328
treatment 328
Hydroxyzine 339
Hyperandrogenism 89
Hyperbilirubinemia, severe 67
Hypercoagulation, tendency of 118
Hyperechogenic bowel 306
Hyperemesis gravidarum 91, 92
complications 92
diagnosis 91
differential diagnosis 91
epidemiology 91
investigations 92
management 92
risk factors 91
treatment 92
Hyperinsulinemia 89
Hyperpyrexia 380
Hyper-reflexia 182
Hyperstimulated ovaries 400
Hypertension 55, 360
antenatally unclassifiable 127
chronic 178, 182, 183
diagnosis of 184
during pregnancy 127
placental origin for 185
pre-existing 127
severity of 182
Hypertensive disease 179
Hypertensive disorder 123, 126, 239
during pregnancy, classification of 178
of pregnancy 51, 169, 178, 182, 239, 380
treatment of 180

Hypertensive encephalopathy 187
Hyperthyroidism 45, 157, 158
during postpartum period, treatment of 158
during pregnancy, treatment of 157
Hypertrophic cardiomyopathy 129
Hypocalcemia 152
Hypoglycemia 255
Hypophosphatasia 310
Hypoplastic left heart syndrome 301
Hypotension 55, 195
Hypothalamopituitary adrenal axis, upregulation of 8
Hypothyroid, treatment of 159
Hypothyroidism 45
cause of 155
develop 154
during postpartum period, treatment of 156
in pregnancy, complications of 155
role of subclinical 88
treatment of 156
Hysterectomy 356, 357, 377
advantages 357
Hysterosalpingogram 89
Hysterosalpingography 86
Hysteroscopic metroplasty 86
Hysteroscopy 86, 248

I

Iatraconazole 339
Iatrogenic causes 101
medications and trauma 101
Ibuprofen 260
Icterus gravidarum 162
IDA *See* Iron deficiency anemia
IDCM *See* Idiopathic dilated cardiomyopathy
Idiopathic dilated cardiomyopathy 137
Iliac artery ligation, internal 377
Iliac balloon catheter, internal 202
Iliac embolization, internal 202
Imferon 54
Immature immune status 274
Immune
abnormal 135
dysregulation 129
modulating therapy 138
Immunoglobulin 139
Immunosuppressive drugs 139
Immunotherapy 142
Imperforate anus 306
Impetigo herpetiformis 338
clinical presentation 338
differential diagnosis 340
etiology 338
laboratory findings 338
prognosis 339
treatment 340
Implantable cardioverter defibrillator 138

Implantation bleeding (physiologic) 100
In utero nutrition 8
In vitro fertilization 33, 248, 394
with preimplantation genetic diagnosis 79
Increta 31
Indomethacin 213
dosage 213
side effects 213
Inevitable delivery during critical phase 263
Infant care 276
Infantile polycystic disease 308
Infants, low-birth-weight 232
Infection 105, 381
Inflammation 135
Inflammatory cytokines 342
Inflammatory pathway 8
Influenza
A 257
and swine flu in pregnancy 257
B 257
C 257
during pregnancy, management of 257
related complications 257
Inhibin 401
A 3, 31, 171
Injectable iron 54*t*
Innovative balloons, merits of 372
Inpatient versus outpatient management 197
Institute for Health and Clinical Excellence 175
Insulin-like growth factor-1 8
Interleukin-6 135
Intermittent presumptive treatment 254
Interstitial fluid compartments 147
Interstitial lung disease 145
Intra-aortic balloon pump 138
Intracerebral
bleeding 191
hemorrhage 386
Intracranial hemorrhage 389
Intrahepatic cholestasis 162
of pregnancy 337
clinical presentation 337
differential diagnosis 337
etiology 337
laboratory findings 337
prognosis 337
treatment 337
risks of 163
Intramuscular administration 54
Intraocular pressure 192
Intrapartum care 181, 281
Intrapartum complications 240
Intrapartum management 350
of twin vaginal delivery 231
Intrauterine
adhesions 86
balloon tamponade 368
death 83, 178, 197

environment 8
fetal death 241, 379, 381
    causes of 380, 380t
    complications of 381
    counseling and prevention 382
    epidemiology 379
    management of 381
    prevention 381
    risk factors 379
fetal demise 379
growth restriction 11, 19, 151, 178, 182, 190
    monitoring for 229
growth retardation 329
infection 9
shunts 46
tamponade 365
Intravascular transfusion 75
Intravenous immunoglobulins 77, 79, 88
Intravenous infusion 369
Intravenous labetalol 181
Invasive fetal tests 32, 70
Iodine
    deficiency 156
    requirements 15
Ipratropium 142
Iron
    balance, negative 51
    binding capacity to 50
    deficiency
        anemia 53, 61t
        erythropoiesis 51
        management of 52
        stages of 51
    gluconate 55
    in pregnancy, daily requirement of 14
    metabolism in pregnancy 50
    requirements during pregnancy 14
    sorbital (jectofer) 54
    sucrose 54
        complex 54
    sulfate 53
Ischemic damage 187
Ischemic stroke 385-387, 388f
    acute 389
    secondary prevention of 389
Isolated hypothyroxinemia 155, 156
Isoxusprine 214
    regimen 214
Isradipine 127
IUGR *See* Intrauterine growth restriction
IVC *See* Inferior vena cava
Ivermectin 339
IVF *See In vitro* fertilization

J

Janani Suraksha Yojana 409
Jaundice 67, 91
    in pregnancy 162

Jejunal and ileal atresia 306
Jeune's thoracic dystrophy 310
Jewish ancestry 33
Joint deformities 311
    rocker bottom feet 311
    talipes 311
Jugular lymphatic obstruction sequence 299

K

Kallikrein *See also* Urinary calcium
Kanamycin 265
Karyotyping
    analysis, common indications for 32
    rapid 33
Kernicterus 67
Ketanserin 174
Ketoconazole 339
Key hole sign-bladder outlet obstruction 307f
Kidney
    abnormalities 308
    disease, chronic 148, 151t
    during pregnancy
        anatomical and physiological changes in 147
        anatomy 147
        physiology 147
    failure 92
    injury, acute 147
Kleihauer-Betke test 382
Korotkoff sound 183

L

Labetalol 127, 179
Labor 240, 276
    abnormal 380
    active management of third stage of 56, 412
    and delivery 132
        during 120
        management of 236
    first stage of 56
    induction of 241
    management 214
        during 56, 138
    precautions during 276
    second stage of 56
    third stage of 56
LAC *See* Lupus anticoagulant
Lacrimal acinar gland, disruption of 192
Lactate dehydrogenase 144, 401
Lamivudine 275
Lamotrigine 350
Landry-Guillain-Barré-Strohl syndrome 327, 329
Langer-Saldino syndrome 309
Laparoscopy 401

Largerhans cells 282
LDH *See* Lactate dehydrogenase
Left heart syndrome 28
Left ventricular assist devices 138
Legal implications 407
Leiomyoma 399
Lentivirinae 273
Leptospirosis 324
Leucovorin 281
Leukocytes, hypersegmentation of 57
Leukotriene antagonists 142
Levofloxacin 143
Levothyroxine 156
    doses of 156
    treatment 156
        effectiveness of 156
LFT *See* Liver function test
Limbs, missing 28
Linezolid 265
Lipopolysaccharide 342, 343
Listeria monocytogenes 267
Litmus paper test 218
Livedo reticularis 325
Liver
    calcification 29
    cirrhosis 162
    damage, drug-induced 162
    disease
        coincidental to pregnancy 162
        in pregnancy 162t
        preceding pregnancy, chronic 162
    disorders caused by pregnancy 162
    enzymes, elevated 182, 193
    function test 57, 92, 162, 163, 184
        abnormal 162
    impairment *See also* Renal impairment
    toxicity 157
    transplantation 162
    tumors 162
Local injection of embryocides 249
Logothetopulos pack 377
Loratadine 339
Low birth weight 274, 394
Lower urinary tract obstruction, percutaneous shunting in 308
Low-molecular-weight heparin 131, 132
Lown-Levine-Ganong syndrome 129
Low-quality evidence 175
Lung infection, acute 144
Lupus anticoagulant 87, 89, 329, 382
Lupus flares, treatment for 320
Lupus pregnancy, treatment of 319
Luteal phase defects 88
Lyme disease 324

M

Macrocytic anemia 50
Macrosomia 174

Macular edema 193
Magnesium
    requirements 15
    sulfate 188, 213, 214
        mechanism of action 188
        side effects 188
        use of 229
Malaria 210
    clinical manifestations of 252
    diagnosis of 253
    during pregnancy 252
        epidemiology 252
        pathophysiology 252
        recurrence of 254
    in pregnancy 252
        clinical diagnosis 253
        energetic 254
        incidence of 252
        management of 254
        management of labor 256
        parasitological diagnosis 253
        prevention of 254
        radical cure 256
        supportive treatment 255
        treatment of 254
    management in pregnancy 255
    on fetus, effects of 253
    on mother, effects of 253
    on pregnant women,
        effects of 253
    pathogenesis of severe 253
Mantoux test 264
Marfan's syndrome 117, 124, 128, 131, 132, 353
Massive parallel sequencing 30, 38
Massive retroplacental clot 82
Massive transfusion protocol 366
    template 366fc
Mast cell stabilizers 142
Maternal age 26
    advanced 94
Maternal and child health 377
Maternal and fetal monitoring 180
Maternal antenatal period 197
Maternal antibody
    screening test, positive 70
    titer determination 70
Maternal assessment 180
    in hypertensive disease of
        pregnancy 182
Maternal cardiac disease on pregnancy,
    effects of 118
Maternal cardiovascular
    mortality, long-term 207
    risk, modified WHO
        classification of 124t
Maternal complications 51, 92, 151, 228
    anemia 228
    hypertension 228
    principles of management 151

Maternal health
    division of Ministry of Health and
        Family Welfare 2
    services 409
Maternal healthcare systems 411
Maternal hypertension, treat 205
Maternal hypomethylation syndrome 395
Maternal infection 267, 380
Maternal intrapartum period 197
Maternal left heart obstruction 125
Maternal medical history/status 23
Maternal microflora lowers levels 346
Maternal morbidity 327, 379
Maternal mortality 243, 328
    causes of 410
    in India, causes of 410, 410f
    rate, strategies to reduce 411f
    worldwide, causes of 410, 410f
Maternal osteoporosis 132
Maternal peripheral blood 136
Maternal placental syndrome 129
Maternal puerperium 197
Maternal relaxation 9
Maternal renal outcome 149
Maternal respiratory system 141
Maternal Rh-immunoglobulin G 66
Maternal risks 312
    fetal risks 312
    investigations 312
    management 312
    of abruption 191
    of premature cardiovascular disease 129
Maternal serum
    alfa-feto-protein 29
    marker analyte, abnormal 31
    screening, abnormal 30, 31
Maternal thyroid disease 156
Maternal weight 3
Matrix metalloproteinase 171, 343
McAfee and Johnson regimen 197
Mean arterial pressure 172
Mean corpuscular hemoglobin 57
    concentration 57
Mean corpuscular volume 49, 57
Measles, mumps, and rubella 409
Mebendazole 52
Mechanical valve 124
    prosthesis 125
Meditation 10, 11f
    dhyan 10
    mantra 10
    pranayama 10
    rajyoga 10
Megacystitis 2
Megaloblastic anemia 56, 57
    causes of 56
    diagnosis of 57
Membranes, prolonged rupture of 267
Memory loss 57, 387
Menadiol sodium phosphate 163

Meningiomas 349
Mental confusion 57
Mental health 7
Mentzer index 61
Metabolic acidosis 152
Metabolic disorders 25
Metabolomics 174
Metalloproteases synthesis 342
Metformin, role of 89
Methergine 363
Methotrexate 249, 339
Methyl prednisolone 339
Methyl tetrahydrofolate reductase
    deficiency 88
Methylprednisolone hydrocortisone 142
Methylxanthines, sustained release 142
Metoclopramide 92, 93
Metoprolol 127, 138
Metronidazole 339
Metroplasty 248
Microalbuminuria 171
Microcytic anemia 50
Microcytic RBCs, etiology 53t
Microtransferrinuria 171
Migraine headache 92
Minimal tissue trauma 191
Ministry of Health and Family Welfare 54
Miscarriage 3, 94
    additional investigations 96
    as gestational age, classification of 94t
    causes of 95t
    clinical classification of 95t
    diagnosis 95
    epidemiology 94
    etiology of second trimester 97
    etiopathogenesis 94
    late 97
    management 96
    medical management 97
    preclinical 94
    risk of 94t
    threatened 100
Misoprostol 132, 361, 363, 364, 381
    and mifepristone combination 381
Missed abortion, sonographic
    criteria of 96b
Mitral regurgitation 125
Mitral stenosis 118, 126
    severe 124
Mitral valve prolapse 124, 128
MMP *See* Matrix metalloproteinase
MMR *See* Measles, mumps, and rubella
Molar pregnancy, preoperative tests in 98b
Molecular genetic diagnosis 33
Molecular weight 54
    heparin, low 87, 327, 329
Monochorionic
    complications, specific 229
    diamniotic placenta 227f
    monoamniotic placenta 227f
    twins 231

Monoclonal antibodies 138
Monosomy X 87
Morphological classification 49
Mucosal changes 332
Multicystic dysplasia 308
Multidrug resistant tuberculosis in
        pregnancy 265
Multifetal
    gestation, risk of 394
    pregnancy 135
Multiorgan failure 328
Multiorgan support systems 138
Multiparous women 172
Multiple gestation 125, 211
    complications with 226
    higher 229
    pregnancy 232
Multiple pregnancy 210, 240, 360, 394
    management of 226
    postpartum care 232
    prevention and management 232
    primary prevention 232
    problems with lactation 232
    screening in 32
    trisomy 21 39
Mural thrombi 138
Muscular dystrophies 36
Musculoskeletal disorders 25
Mycobacterial infections 334
Mycobacterium tuberculosis 264
Mycoplasma pneumoniae 324
Mycoplasma species 209
Myelomeningocele 45
Myocarditis 135
Myoma 210
Myomectomy 248
Myometrium, thinning of 353
Myth 412

N

Nasal bone 4
National Family Health Survey-3 49
National Institute for Health and
        Clinical Excellence 185
National Institute of Child Health and
        Human Development 175
National Rural Health Mission 409
Nausea, severe 157
Neck-cystic hygroma
    abnormality of 299
    diagnosis, abnormality of 299
    management, abnormality of 299
Neisseria gonorrhoeae 211, 217, 218
Neonatal affection, clinical
        management of previous 73
Neonatal care 320
Neonatal complications 130
Neonatal death 232, 242
    causes of 190

Neonatal dengue illness 263
Neonatal events in women with heart
        disease, maternal predictors
        of 125*t*
Neonatal intensive care unit facilities 396
Neonatal lupus syndromes 321
Neonatal outcome 18
Neoplasms, benign 400
Nerve growth factor 345
Neural tube defect 14, 27*fc*, 242, 296
Neuraminidase-1 257
Neuraxial analgesia, administration of 231
Neurobehavioral development 15
Neurokinin B 171
Neutrophil
    activation 342
    hypersegmentation of 57
Nevirapine prophylaxis and dosage 277*t*
New parenteral iron 49
Newer treatment modalities 138
Niacin 15
Niemann-Pick disease 33
Nifedipine 127, 179, 181, 212, 213
Nimes obstetricians and hematologists anti-
        phospholipid syndrome 327, 329
Nitabuch's layer 201
Nitrazine paper test 218
Nitric oxide 125, 178
NOH-APS *See* Nimes obstetricians and
        hematologists antiphospholipid
        syndrome
Noncardioembolic
    ischemic stroke 389
    stroke, history of 391
Noncardiogenic pulmonary edema 144
Noncompliance 350
Noncultured fluid 32
Nonhemophiliac hemorrhage 364
Nonimmune hydrops 313*t*
    fetalis 312
        clinical evaluation 314
        diagnosis 312
        obstetric management 314
        pathophysiology 313
Nonimmune pregnant women 253
Noninvasive prenatal
    screening 29
    testing 2, 38, 70
Non-nutritional anemia 2, 50, 61
    etiology of 59, 60*fc*
    in pregnancy 59
Nonobstetric causes 101*t*
Nonpharmacological management 179
Nonstress test 19, 20*t*, 329
    frequency of testing 19
Non-uterine specific balloon tamponade
        368
Nuchal skin-fold 29
Nuchal translucency 4, 26
    in first trimester 28*f*

    increased 300*f*
    measurement 30
Nucleotide polymorphism
    indications of 30
    technique, single 30
Nulliparity 172
Nutrition 151
Nutritional anemia 50

O

O'Leary stitch 198
O'Sullivan technique 378
Obesity 238
    and pregnancy 238
Obstetric cholestasis 162
    clinical features 162
    effect on pregnancy 163
    etiology 162
    management 163
    prevalence 162
Obstetric complications 130
Obstetric drug box, emergency 365*f*
Obstetric emergency 354
Obstetrical history
    maternal, previous 18
    previous 18
Obstetrics emergency box 364*t*
Obstructed labor in young girls 235
Obstructive sleep apnea 145
Occlusive vascular disorder 193
Ocular adnexal changes 192
OHSS *See* Ovarian hyperstimulation
        syndrome
Oligohydramnios 311
    causes of 311*t*
    development, mechanism of 21*fc*
    etiopathogenesis 311
    fetal risks 311
    investigations 311
    maternal risks 311
Oliguria 195
Omega-3 fatty acids 14
Omphalocele 28, 243, 303
    diagnosis 303
    labor and delivery 303
    management 303
Oncologic prognosis 404
Ondansetron 92, 93
Oocysts 279
Open neural tube defects 296
    anencephaly 296
    cephalocele 296
    labor and delivery 297
    management 297
    spina bifida 296
Optic nerve 57
Oral hygiene prophylactic instructions 346
Oral iron therapy 53
Orthomyxoviridae 257

Oseltamivir 258
Osmolarity 54
Osmotic fragility test 61
Osteogenesis imperfecta 310
Ostium secundum 300
Outflow tract obstruction 301
    management of 301
Ovarian artery ligation 375, 376
Ovarian cancer, nonspecific symptoms of 398
Ovarian cyst
    in pregnancy
        management of 404fc
            ultrasound of common 400t
    large left 399f
    ruptured 100
    simple 399f
Ovarian hyperstimulation syndrome 100
Ovarian malignancy with pregnancy, tumor markers in 400
Ovarian neoplasm 404
Ovarian torsion 100
Overt hypothyroidism 155
Oxygen saturation 184
Oxygenation, maintenance of 187
Oxytocin 361, 363, 364
    infusion 202, 363, 382

P

Packed cells 83
Palpable masses 398
Paracetamol 260
Parasite species 252
Parasitic infections 334
Parasitic placental infection 274
Parathyroid hormone 14
Paravenous leakage 55
Parenteral iron
    dose of 55
    therapy 53
Parenti-Fraccaro syndrome 309
Parkinson's disease 388
Parvovirus B19 135, 267, 285, 382
    clinical presentation 285
    diagnosis 286
    epidemiology 285
    infection 33
    management 286
Parvovirus infection during pregnancy 282
Patent ductus arteriosus 124, 125
Paternal Rh-phenotype and genotype 67
PDA *See* Patent ductus arteriosus
Peak expiratory flow rate 141
Pelvic devascularization 372
Pelvic examination 369
Pemphigoid gestationis 337
    clinical presentation 338
    differential diagnosis 338
    etiology 338
    laboratory findings 338
    prognosis 338
    treatment 338
Penicillin 220, 339
Pentoxifylline 138, 139
Percutaneous umbilical blood sampling 44, 68
    cordocentesis 44f
Perfusion pressure 187
Pericardial effusion 29, 136
Perinatal
    complications 185
    infection 267
    morbidity 328
    mortality 328
Periodontal disease 210
Periodontal infection, mechanism linking 342fc
Periodontal ligament cells 342
Periodontitis 344
Perioral dermatitis 333f
Peripartum cardiomyopathy 119, 123, 129, 135, 139, 143
    clinical features 136
    diagnosis 136
    differential diagnosis 137
    epidemiology 135
    etiology 135
    genetic factors 136
    pathological changes 136
    physical examination 136
    treatment 137
Peripheral blood
    film 52
    smear 49
Peripheral natural killer cells 89
Peripheral vascular resistance 117
Peritoneal cancer 402t
PGD *See* Preimplantation genetic diagnosis
Phenobarbital 350
Phenobarbitone 350
Phenytoin 350
Phosphate 151
Phospholipids, release of 81
Physiological skin changes 331
    during pregnancy 331t
Picornavirus 164
Pigmentary changes 331
Placenta
    dichorionic and diamniotic 226f
    fused dichorionic and diamniotic 226f
    low lying 196
    with retroplacental hemorrhage 204f
Placenta accreta 200, 200f, 378
    diagnosis 201
    high-risk factors 201
    incidence of 201
    management 201
    multidisciplinary approach 202
    operation room plan 202
    risk of 250
Placenta accreta/increta 201
    unsuspected case of 203
Placenta previa 3, 195-197, 360, 371, 378, 395
    anterior 202
    classification 196
    clinical features 195
    complete 196f
    complications of 197
    conduct of expectant management 197
    diagnosis 196
    differential diagnosis 197
    epidemiology 195
    etiopathogenesis 195
    history of 195
    incidence of 195, 201
    management 197
Placental abruption *See also* Abruptio placentae
Placental abruption 170, 204, 208
    classification of 204
    clinical features 204
    etiology 205
    examination 204
    fetal demise 207
    in women, management of 207fc
    initial management 206
    investigations 205
    management 205
    prevention 205
    primary cause of 205
    recurrence 207
Placental biopsy 45, 62
Placental blood smear 253
Placental enlargement 69
Placental growth factor 28, 171, 173
Placental hypoperfusion 179
Placental insufficiency, fetal deterioration in 290f
Placental protein 13 171, 173
Placental separation, degree of 196
Placental trophoblasts, apoptosis of 29
Placenta-related disorders 173
Placentation
    abnormal 170f
    normal 170f
Plasmapheresis 79
Plasmodial infection 252
Plasmodium falciparum 252, 267
    infection 252, 253
    malaria 255
    parasite 254
Plasmodium knowlesi 252
Plasmodium malariae 252
Plasmodium ovale 252
Plasmodium vivax 252, 256
    malaria 255
Platelet 84
    concentrate 83

consumption rate 191
count
    and activation 171
    low 193
Pleural disease 145
Pleural effusion 45
Pneumocystis carinii pneumonia 274
Pneumocystis jiroveci 275
Pneumonia 142, 210
    in pregnancy 142
    management 143
        prepregnancy 143
        maternal and fetal risks 142
        prenatal and postnatal 143
Poikilocytosis 61
Polycystic kidney disease
    adult 309
    autosomal
        dominant 309
        recessive 308
Polycystic ovary syndrome 396
Polydactyly 29
Polyhydramnios 312
    causes of 312*t*
    etiopathogenesis 312
Polymerase chain reaction 279
Polymorphic eruption of pregnancy 336
    clinical presentation 336
    differential diagnosis 337
    etiology 336
    laboratory findings 336
    prognosis 337
    treatment 337
Polymorphonuclear leukocytes 342
Population prevalent genetic diseases, frequency of 33*t*
Porphyromonas gingivalis 342, 344
Post-abortion care 105
Post-delivery 263
Postnatal examination of stillborn 314
Postnatal infection 267
Postnatal management 181
Postpartum 120
    anemia 56
    angiopathy, treatment of 389
    care 236, 382
    complications 243
    depression 235
    hemorrhage 5, 51, 243, 360, 368, 374
        cause of 360, 361*t*
        drug box 365*f*
        drug kit 364*t*
        etiology with 360
        management of 361, 365, 374
        management of true 362*fc*
        medical management of 360
        predictors of 130
        prevention 361
        risk factors of 360, 360*t*
        surgical management of 374
    treatment 361
    type of 204
management 350
mental health issues 232
period 137, 400
prophylaxis 67
thyroiditis 158, 159
women, low-income 56
Potassium requirements 15
Potency
    high 142
    low 142
    medium 142
Preconceptional counseling 116
Predictive test 170
Prednisolone 92, 142, 339
Prednisone 320, 327, 339
Pre-eclampsia 57, 169, 178, 182, 185, 192, 238, 360
    development of 239
    differential diagnosis of 149, 150*t*
    etiopathogenesis of 169
    increased, risk for 172
    prediction and prevention of 169
    prevention of 174
    screening for 3
    severe 390
    signs of severe 127
    superimposed 183
    syndrome, development of 171*t*
    WHO recommendations for prevention of 175
Pre-existing renal disease, differential diagnosis of 149
Pregnancy 234
    acute fatty liver of 163
    adnexal masses in 398
    affecting oral conditions 343
    and breastfeeding 15
    and cardiac disease, registry of 125
    and chronic kidney disease 147
    and delivery, management of 350
    and dengue fever 259
        acute febrile phase 259
        clinical presentation 259
        critical phase 259
        management of 260
        monitor 260
        phase of capillary leak 259
        recovery phase 260
        treatment 260
        warning signs of plasma leak 259
    and disease progression 350
    and oral health 341
    anticipatory malaria in 254
    associated plasma protein-A 3, 28, 173
    asthmatic medications in 142*t*
    carbohydrate requirements during 14
    cardiac diseases in 116
    cardiovascular changes in 122*t*
care of adolescents during 236
careful malaria in 255
causes of
    hypothyroidism in 155
    stress during 8
cerebrovascular accidents in 384
chemoprophylaxis during 254
clinical management of first affected 73
common indices during 148*t*
complications 235, 321
    during 122
    specific risks for 1
consequences of 236
dermatological
    disorders in 331
    drug safety in 340
diabetes in 380
diagnosis of 150
diagnostic interventions in 42
during 151
early 239
effects on 57
elective termination of 230
etiology, acute fatty liver of 164
fat requirements during 13
first trimester of 172, 173
future 357
hemodynamic changes during 117
hemorrhage, early 94
high-risk 408
identification of high-risk 18
in dialysis patients 151
in patient with kidney disease 148
in women, management of 151*t*
induced hypertension 185, 235, 390
investigations, acute fatty liver of 163
loss 85, 86
    anatomic factors implicated in 85
    etiology of recurrent 86*f*
    genetic factors implicated in 86
    immunological factors implicated in 87
    lower frequencies of 232
management in cases of first affected 74*fc*
medicolegal aspects of high-risk 407
morbidity 325
new-onset hypertension in 183
nutrition in 13
of unknown location 101
on periodontium, effect of 343
optimal weight gain in 239*t*
oral
    conditions effecting 341
    iron prophylaxis during 52
outcome of 151*t*, 404
plasma leakage in 259
post-term 380
protein requirements in 13
pustular psoriasis of 338

recurrent jaundice of 162
related complications 238
remember in high-risk 408
renal biopsy during 150
screening methods during 210
specific dermatoses 334, 335t
specific eye diseases 192
stores for 14
stroke in 386t
symptomatology, acute fatty liver of 163
termination of 4, 249
therapeutic indications in 42
treatment, acute fatty liver of 164
triplet 229
ultrasonography-guided
 interventions in 42
with kidney disease management
 protocols 149
with liver diseases 162
with protein A 171
Pregnancy-induced hypertension
 management of 178
 risk of 130
Pregnant mother, harmful effects of
 stress on 8
Pregnant women 16
 as dental patients 345
 interventions for 254
 serologic evaluation of 268t
Preimplantation genetic
 diagnosis 33, 40, 89, 396
 screening 396
Premature rupture of membranes 216,
 217t, 218t
 diagnosis 217
 etiology 216
 incidence 216
 investigation for 218t
 management of 219, 219t, 222fc, 223fc
 pathophysiology 216
 risk factor for 217t
 symptoms of 218t
Prenatal
 aneuploidies, screening for 25
 care 4t
 diagnosis 62
 genetic screening and testing 25
 karyotype 396
 oral health counseling 345
 screening 26
 testing midstream 2
Prepregnancy
 counseling 79, 131
  for women 149
 dilated fundus examination 193
 glycemic control, poor 193
Preterm and low birth weight, incidence
 of 345
Preterm birth 3, 31, 16, 228, 232, 394
 predicting risk of 228

preventing 229
prior 209
process 342
risk of 240
spontaneous 211
subcategories of 209
Preterm delivery 14, 118, 130, 174, 240
 cause 9
 risk of 14, 209
Preterm labor 56, 209, 342fc
 cause of 394
 diagnosis of 209, 211
 interventions 211
 management of 212
 pathophysiology of 209
 prediction of 396
 risk factors 209
 routine investigations for 211
 routine physical examination in 211
 tocolytic therapy in 213t
 treatment 209
Preterm low birth weight 341
Preterm rupture of membranes,
 subtypes of 216
Primaquine 255, 256
Primidone 350
Pritchard regimen 188
 loading dose 188
 maintenance dose 188
Probing pocket depth 344
Procainamide 129
Prochlorperazine 92
Progesterone 343
 dose of 211
 in women with cervical shortening 211
 levels, interpretation of 101
 role of 89
 supplementation 211
Proinflammatory cytokines,
 stimulation of 87
Prolactin 136
Promethazine 92, 93
Prominent pulmonary vasculature 136
Prophylactic iron supplementation 56
Prophylaxis 57, 258
Prostacyclins 125
Prostaglandins 122, 171, 363, 382
 intra-amniotic levels of 343
Prosthetic heart valves 126
Protein
 C deficiency 88
 S deficiency 88
 sources of 13
Proteinuria 150, 185
 measurement of 183, 185
 significant 182
Proteomics 174
Prothrombin G20210A mutation 88
Prothrombin gene mutations 169
Pruritic papular lesions 336f

Pruritus in pregnancy, algorithmic
 approach for 335fc
Pseudomonas aeruginosa 143
Pseudosac and true gestational sac
 features 102t
Psychological trauma 381
Puerperium 51
Pulmonary
 capillary wedge pressure 123
 edema 136, 143, 170, 179, 182, 191
  in pregnancy 144
  in pregnancy, treatment of 144
  with pre-eclampsia 144
 embolism 144
 hypertension 118, 125
 stenosis 124, 301
 vascular resistance 123
Purtscher-like retinopathy 193
Pyelectasis 306
Pyelonephritis, acute 147
Pyogenic granuloma 342f, 344
 on index finger 332f
Pyramid of care 172
Pyrazinamide 265
Pyridoxine 16, 51, 92
Pyrimethamine 254, 281

Q

Quad test 29
Quantitation of anti-D concentration 68
Quinine 255

R

Reactive oxygen species 342
Recurrent ectopic pregnancy 99
Recurrent pregnancy loss 85
 etiology of 85
 evidence-based investigations 85
 managing idiopathic 89
 prevalence and etiology of 85
Red blood cells 49, 253
Renal agenesis 308
 bilateral 308f
Renal anomalies, management of 309
Renal duplication 308
Renal dysfunction 171
Renal function tests 184, 188, 191
Renal hemodynamics 148
Renal hypoplasia 308
Renal impairment 170
Renal plasma flow 148
Residual cervical length 210f
Respiratory diseases
 during pregnancy 141
 in pregnancy 145
Respiratory distress syndrome,
 acute 143, 144

Respiratory physiology during pregnancy, alteration in 141
Restrictive abortion law 103
Reticulocyte count 57
Reticulocyte hemoglobin content 52
Retinal pigment epithelium 192
Retroplacental hematoma 205, 206f
Retroplacental hemorrhage 101
Rh-alloimmunized pregnancy
    alternative treatment modalities 78
    management of 70
    postnatal care 78
RhD antigen determination 70
Rhesus blood type 66
Rhesus disease 33
Rheumatic carditis, acute 119
Rheumatic heart disease 116
Rh-incompatibility during pregnancy 66
    investigations 67
    pathophysiology 66
    prevalence 66
    prevention 67
Rh-negative pregnant 4
Rh-typing 2
Riboflavin 15, 51
Ribonucleic acid 283
    enterovirus 164
Rifampicin 265
Ritodrine 213, 214, 229
Rituximab 328
Rivaroxaban 328
RNA *See* Ribonucleic acid
Robertsonian translocation 30, 87
Rosetting test 68
Rubella 267, 382
    diagnosis 268
    epidemiology 267
    etiopathogenesis 267
    management 268
    prophylaxis 268
Rupture
    direction of 354
    site of 354
Rupture during
    labor 353, 355t
    pregnancy
        sign in cases of 353t
        symptoms in cases of 353t
Rupture of uterus during pregnancy 352
    clinical features 353
    etiology 352
Rupture uterus 352, 358
    classification of 352
    complications 357
    during labor, causes of 353, 354t
    during pregnancy, causes of 352, 353t
    fetal outcomes 357
    management of 354, 356t
    maternal outcome 357
    prevention 357
    repair of 356, 357
    types of 354
Rupture uterus/hysterectomy, indications for repair of 356t
Rusch balloon 365, 368
Russell's viper venom testing, dilute 329

S

SA *See* Sideroblastic anemia
S-adenosyl methionine 163
Salbutamol 142, 213
Salivary estriol 210
Salivation, excessive 91
Salmeterol 142
Salpingitis 100
Sandal gap 29
Scalp edema 77f
Schilling test 57
Second trimester miscarriages *See also* Late miscarriages
Sengstaken-Blakemore tube 365, 368, 371
Septic abortion 97
Serological testing 280
Serum
    antibody titers 68
    B12 level 57
    CA125 401
    electrolytes 92
    ferritin 52
        level 61
    folate level 57
    homocysteine 57
    iron 53
    markers of inflammation, level of 135
    PAPP-A 173
    prolactin level 382
    screen, abnormal 30
    screening
        first trimester 28
        second trimester 29
    transferrin
        receptor 52
        saturation 56
    uric acid 171
    vitamin B12 level 57
Sex chromosome aneuploidy 39
Sexually transmitted diseases 334
Shock
    sign of 195
    symptoms of 195
Short ribbed polydactyly syndrome 310
Siamese twins *See also* Conjoined twins
Sickle cell
    anemia 25, 50
    disease 61, 62
        care during pregnancy 63
        intrapartum 63
        management of patient with 62
        postpartum 63
        preconceptional screening 62
        with pregnancy, complications of 63
    trait, management of patient with 63
Sideroblastic anemia 53
Sildenafil 125
Sim's speculae 369
Sinus bradycardia 302
Skeletal abnormalities, terminology used to 309t
Skin
    conductance latency 8
    disorders in pregnancy, pre-existing 333
    infections
        during pregnancy 333t
        in pregnancy 333
Sleep disturbances 91
Smoking 207, 235
Social health 8
Sodium requirements 15
Soft tissue
    infections 333
    obstruction 354
Soluble endoglin 173
Soluble transferrin receptor 53
Sonohysterosalpingogram 89
Spalding's sign 381
Spider angioma 192
Spina bifida 296
    development of 14
    screening for 3
Spinal muscular atrophy 25
Spiral arteriole, invasion of 200
Spiramycin 280
Spiritual health 9
Spirituality 11
Spirochetal 324
Spontaneous abortion, early 238
Spontaneous miscarriage 97
Sporozoites 279
Stallworthy's sign 196
Staphylococcus 267
    aureus 333
Statins 138, 328
Status asthmaticus 142
Status epilepticus 350
Steroids 79
STFR *See* Soluble transferrin receptor
Stillbirth 3, 241, 379
Stool examination 52
Streptococcus 333
    viridans 119
Streptomycin 265
Striae distensae 332
Striae rubra 332
Stroke
    probability of 387t
    risk factors for 385
    signs of 388
    symptoms of 388
    types of 385

Structural abnormalities, screening for 228
Structural cardiac disease 300
    septal defects 300
    ventricular septal defects 300
Structural chromosomal rearrangements 87
Subarachnoid hemorrhage 349, 386, 390
Subchorionic hemorrhage 95, 101
Subclinical disease 157
Subclinical hypothyroidism 155
Subfertility 238
Subgingival microbiota, alterations in 343
Subgingival microflora 344
Submaximal stress testing 131
Submucous fibroid 86
Substance abuse 235
Subtotal hysterectomy 202
Sudden arrhythmic death syndrome 116
Sudden collapse 51
Sulfadiazine 281, 254
Sulfonamides 280
Sulphadoxine 254
Supraventricular tachycardia 119
    exacerbation of 128
Sweating 195
Swine flu 257
    during pregnancy, management of 257
Symptomatic pregnant women 55
Symptomatic ventricular tachyarrhythmia 138
Syncope 195
Syntometrine 363
Syphilis 235, 324, 382
Systemic hemodynamics 147
Systemic lupus erythematosus 179, 317, 321, 323, 329
    clinical manifestations of 317
    diagnosis 317
    differential diagnosis of 318
    disease flares 320
    in pregnancy 317
    incidence 317
    prepregnancy counseling 318
    serology in 317
Systemic retinoids 339
Systemic steroids 142
Systemic vascular resistance 123, 148
Systolic blood pressure 362

T

Tachyarrhythmia 129
    amiodarone therapy 138
Tachycardia 136, 195, 302
Tachyzoites 279, 280
Tamponade test 368
Tamponade with balloon 364
Tannerella forsythia 344
TB infection, latent 264
T-cell cytokine profile 344
Tea and herbal remedies 104
Teenage girl becoming pregnant 235

Teenage pregnancy 234
    complications 235
    prevention 237
    problems
        during labor and delivery 235
        in antenatal period 235
        in postpartum period 235
Tenofovir 275
Tension 7
Teratoma 45, 399
Terbinafine 339
Terbutaline 142, 213, 214, 229
Tetanus 3
Tetracyclin 255, 339
Tetralogy of Fallot 301
    repaired 124
Thalassemia 33, 50, 61, 61*t*, 63
    diagnosis of 62*fc*
    management of 62*fc*
Thallidomide 339
Thanatophoric dysplasia 309
Theophyline 142
Therapeutic
    amnioinfusion 45
    interventions 53
    procedures in pregnancy, ultrasound-guided 45
    tocolysis 222
Thiamine 15
    supplementation 93
Thrombocytopenia 132, 150, 182, 325
Thromboembolism 240
Thrombolysis, acute 389
Thrombolytic therapy 389
Thrombophilia 184, 380
    study 382
Thromboplastin
    release of 81
    time, activated partial 132, 328
Thromboprophylaxis 93
Thrombosis 132
Thrombotic antiphospholipid syndrome 324
Thyrocalcitonin 14
Thyroglobulin antibodies 158
Thyroid
    diseases, diagnosing 154
    disorders 88
        during pregnancy 154
    dysfunction 155
    function test 92, 382
    peroxidase 154
    peroxidase antibodies 158
    screening 2
Thyroid-stimulating hormone 4, 154
Thyroxine 43, 51, 154
    production of 154
Tissue changes, connective 332
Tocolysis 197, 212
    second-line 212
Tocolysis-associated pulmonary edema 144

Tocolytics
    first-line 212
    use of 229
Total body iron content 50
Total iron-binding capacity 52
Toxic solutions 104
Toxoplasma gondii 278, 280
    infection during pregnancy, prevent primary 280
Toxoplasmosis 267, 382
    during pregnancy 278
    in pregnancy 278
        diagnosis 279
        dose 281
        epidemiology 278
        management 280
        mode of transmission 278
        prevention 280
        preventive measures 280
        routes of transmission 279
Tranexamic acid 366
    role of 366
Transabdominal
    technique 42
    ultrasound 197
Transesophageal electrocardiography 131
Transferrin 171
Transforming growth factor-beta 1 345
Transfusion strategies 365
Transient ischemic attack 386, 389, 391
    clinical manifestations of 386
    diagnosis of 386
    management 387
    tests 387
    treatment of 387
Transient nephromegaly 309
Transmission of varicella, risks of 272*t*
Transplacental hemorrhage, volume of 66
Transvaginal sonography 329
Transvaginal ultrasound, safety of 197
Traumatic postpartum hemorrhage 374
Treponema pallidum 267
Triamcinolone 142
Trichomonas vaginalis 217
Tricuspid regurgitation 300
Triiodothyronine 154
Trimethoprim 276
Triploidies 87
Triploids 91
Trisomy
    16 87
    21 91
    7 87
Trophoblastic invasion 200
Trophoplastic disorder 91
Trophotropisis 195
Troponin-T 137
TSH *See* Thyroid-stimulating hormone
Tubectomy 357
Tuberculin skin test 264

Tuberculosis in pregnancy 264
Tuberculosis in pregnant women
    breastfeeding 265
    diagnosis of 264
    HIV coinfection 265
    treatment 265
Tumor markers, elevated 398
Twin 229
Twin A non-vertex and twin B
        non-vertex 231
Twin A vertex and twin B non-vertex 231
Twin A vertex and twin B vertex 231
Twin pregnancies
    classification of 226
    dichorionic and diamniotic 226
    dizygotic 226
    monochorionic
        and diamniotic 226
        and monoamniotic 226
    monozygotic 226
    principles of management 227
Twin presentation, combinations of 231
Twin, death of single 230
Twin-twin transfusion syndrome 227, 229
    severe 229
Typhoid fever 210
Tyrosine kinase-1 173
Tzanck smear 272

U

Ultrasonography, second trimester 29
Ultrasound 26
    markers 26
Umbilical artery 22
    Doppler 291, 292f
        velocimetry 185
Unconjugated estriol 2, 31
    levels 31
Underlying renal disease 184
Unsafe abortion
    causes of 103
    clinical assessment of 105
    complications 105
    consequences of 103, 104
    heavy bleeding 105
    high-risk group for complications 104
    late complications 105
    magnitude of problem 103
    management 105
    methods of 104
    prevention of 106
    uterine perforation 105
Unwanted fertility, reduce 412
Ureteropelvic junction obstruction 307f
Uric acid 144
Urinary
    calcium 171
    tract
        bleeding 101

infections 210
    obstruction, upper 306
Urine
    analysis 93
    for albumin 188
    protein 144
Urine-routine microscopically 4
Urological preparation 202
Ursodeoxycholic acid 163
Uterine 375
    anomalies, treatment of 86
    artery 3, 372
        Doppler 22, 291, 291f
        Doppler velocimetry 185
        ligation 376
        pulsatility index 5, 173
    compression sutures 374
    contraction 211
    distension 209
    evaluation 86
    instrumentation 210
    inversion 378
    packing 364
    septum 210
Uterine-specific balloon tamponade 368
Uteroplacental circulation 118, 173
Uterus
    massage 363
    surgical management of 356
    through cervix, foreign bodies placed
        into 104
Uveitis 193

V

Vagina and vulva 101
Vagina, treatments placed in 104
Vaginal birth after cesarean section 241
Vaginal bleeding 210
    absence of 205
Vaginal cerclage 211
Vaginal delivery 181, 355t
    operative 241
Vaginal uterine artery ligation 377
Valacyclovir 271, 339
Valproate 349, 350
Valsalva maneuver 390
Valvular heart disease 125
Varicella zoster 267, 271, 382
    diagnosis 272
    epidemiology 271
    etiopathogenesis 271
    immune globulin 272
    immunoglobulin 143
    management 272
    prophylaxis 272
Vasa previa 197
Vascular endothelial growth factor 148, 171,
    173, 200, 345
Vascular prostacyclin 175
Vascular thrombosis 87, 325

Vaso-occlusive disease, increased
    risk of 193
VDRL See Veneral disease research
    laboratory
Vena cava, inferior 123
Veneral disease research laboratory 4
Venous thromboembolism 232
    risk factor for 88
Venovenous hemodialysis, continuous 138
Ventricular ectopic beats 124
Ventricular septal defect 25, 124, 125, 301f
Ventricular tachyarrhythmia 119
Ventriculomegaly 29
Vesicular mole 98b
Vestibular lesions 92
Villus sampling, chronic 27
Viral hepatitis 164, 190
    in pregnancy 164
        clinical features 167
        diagnosis 167
        management 167
        types of 164t
Viral infections 333
    in pregnancy and labor 267
Viral influenza, infections of 257
Viral myocarditis 135
Visual
    disturbances 182
    problems 179
Vital parameters 361
Vital signs 180
Vitamin
    A 16
    B deficiencies 91, 92
    B_{12} 16, 51
        deficiency 16, 56, 57
        deficiency, diagnostic of 57
    B_6 16
    B_6 See Pyridoxine
    C 16, 51
    C See Ascorbic acid
    D
        antithrombotic 174
        levels 15
        requirements 15
    deficiencies 92
    K 163
Vivax malaria, treatment of 255
von Willebrand factor 363

W

Ward technique 198
Warfarin 119, 131, 327
Water requirements during pregnancy 14
Wernicke's encephalopathy 92, 93
Women with cerclage 211
Women with epilepsy 349
Women with heart disease,
    management of 119
Women's immune system 254

Workshop sponsored 196
World Health Organization 103, 238

X

Xanthine 138
Xylitol consumption 346

Y

Y chromosome 395
Yq microdeletion 395

Z

Zafirlukast 142
Zanamivir 258
Zika fever 282
Zika virus
    disease 282
        diagnosis 283
        epidemiology 282
        from mother to child 283
        pathogenesis 282
        precautions and prevention 284
    pregnancy and microcephaly 283
    screening in pregnancy 284
    symptoms of 283
    through mosquito bites 283
    vaccines 285
    virology 282
Zinc 15
    supplements 15
Zuspan IV regimen 188
    loading dose 188
    maintenance dose 188
Zuspan regimen 188